MECHANICAL CIRCULATORY SUPPORT

A COMPANION TO **BRAUNWALD'S HEART DISEASE**

MECHANICAL CIRCULATORY SUPPORT

A COMPANION TO **BRAUNWALD'S HEART DISEASE**

SECOND EDITION

JAMES K. **KIRKLIN**, MD
Professor of Surgery
Division of Cardiothoracic Surgery,
Director
Kirklin Institute for Research in Surgical Outcomes (KIRSO)
Department of Surgery
University of Alabama at Birmingham
Birmingham, Alabama

JOSEPH G. **ROGERS**, MD
Professor of Medicine – Cardiology
Chief Medical Officer
Duke University Health System
Durham, North Carolina

ELSEVIER

Elsevier
1600 John F. Kennedy Blvd.
Ste 1600
Philadelphia, PA 19103-2899

MECHANICAL CIRCULATORY SUPPORT: A COMPANION TO BRAUNWALD'S HEART DISEASE, SECOND EDITION

ISBN: 978-0-323-56699-5

Library of Congress Control Number: 2019943585

Content Strategist: Robin R. Carter
Content Development Specialist: Lisa Barnes
Publishing Services Manager: Deepthi Unni
Project Manager: Beula Christopher
Designer: Renee Duenow
Cover Art: Joe Chovan

Printed in China

Last digit is the print number: 9 8 7 6 5 4 3 2 1

This monograph is dedicated to the physicians, surgeons, and researchers
who have committed their lives to perfecting mechanical solutions to the failing heart;
to the patients so desperately in need of such solutions;
and to our families who provide unconditional love and support
as we carry on this battle.

James K. Kirklin
Joseph G. Rogers

CONTRIBUTORS

Larry A. Allen, MD, MHS
Professor of Medicine
Department of Medicine
Division of Cardiology
University of Colorado School of Medicine
Aurora, Colorado;
Colorado Cardiovascular Outcomes Research (CCOR) Consortium
Denver, Colorado

Francisco A. Arabia, MD, MBA
Director
CSHI Center for Surgical Device Management of Advanced Heart Failure
Department of Cardiothoracic Surgery
Cedars-Sinai Medical Center
Los Angeles, California

Pavan Atluri, MD
Assistant Professor of Surgery
Division of Cardiovascular Surgery
Department of Surgery
University of Pennsylvania
Philadelphia, Pennsylvania

J. Timothy Baldwin, PhD
Program Director and Deputy Chief
Advanced Technologies and Surgery Branch
Division of Cardiovascular Sciences
National Heart, Lung, and Blood Institute
Bethesda, Maryland

Christian A. Bermudez, MD
Associate Professor
Division of Cardiovascular Surgery
Department of Surgery
Hospital of the University of Pennsylvania
Perelman School of Medicine
Philadelphia, Pennsylvania

Emma Birks, MD, PhD, FRCP, MBBS, BSc
Medical Director
Advanced Heart Failure, Transplantation and Mechanical Circulatory Support
Department of Medicine
Division of Cardiovascular Medicine
University of Louisville
Louisville, Kentucky

Robin Bostic, BS
Global Vice President
Health Economics and Reimbursement
Department of Health Economics
Abbott
Windham, New Hampshire

Jennifer Cowger, MD, MS
Medical Director of the Mechanical Circulatory Support Program
Co-Director of the Cardiac Critical Care Unit
Department of Cardiology
Henry Ford Hospital
Detroit, Michigan

Mani A. Daneshmand, MD
Associate Professor
Director
Heart Transplant, Lung Transplant, MCS, and ECMO
Department of Surgery
Emory University
Atlanta, Georgia

Walter Dembitsky, MD
Director
Mechanical Circulatory Support Program
Cardiothoracic and Vascular Surgery
Sharp Memorial Hospital
San Diego, California

Mary Amanda Dew, PhD
Professor of Psychiatry, Psychology, Epidemiology, Biostatistics, Nursing, and Clinical and Translational Science
Director
Quality of Life Research, Artificial Heart Program
University of Pittsburgh School of Medicine and Medical Center
Pittsburgh, Pennsylvania

Stavros G. Drakos, MD, PhD
Heart Failure Program
Division of Cardiology
University of Utah
Salt Lake City, Utah

Yakov L. Elgudin, MD, PhD
Section Chief
Cardiothoracic Surgery
Cleveland VA Medical Center;
Staff Surgeon
Division of Cardiac Surgery
University Hospitals Cleveland Medical Center
Cleveland, Ohio

Daniel J. Goldstein, MD
Professor and Vice Chair
Department of Cardiothoracic Surgery
Montefiore Medical Center
Bronx, New York

Kathleen L. Grady, PhD, RN, MS, FAAN
Professor of Surgery and Medicine
Department of Surgery, Division of Cardiac Surgery
Feinberg School of Medicine
Northwestern University;
Administrative Director
Center for Heart Failure
Bluhm Cardiovascular Institute of Northwestern Memorial Hospital
Chicago, Illinois

Igor D. Gregoric, MD
Chief of Surgical Division
Memorial Hermann Heart and Vascular Institute;
Director
Center of Advanced Heart Failure
The University of Texas Health Science Center-Houston;
Professor
Department of Cardiothoracic and Vascular Surgery
UT Health McGovern Medical School
Houston, Texas

Finn Gustafsson, MD, PhD, DMSci
Professor of Cardiology
University of Copenhagen
Rigshospitalet
Copenhagen, Denmark

J. Thomas Heywood, MD
Director
Advanced Heart Failure and Mechanical Support
Department of Cardiology
Scripps Clinic
La Jolla, California

William L. Holman, MD
Professor of Surgery
Division of Cardiothoracic Surgery
Department of Surgery
University of Alabama at Birmingham
Birmingham, Alabama

Tina Cady Ivovic, BS
Global Senior Director
Field Health Economics and Reimbursement
Department of Health Economics
Abbott
Washington, DC

James K. Kirklin, MD
Professor of Surgery
Division of Cardiothoracic Surgery,
Director
Kirklin Institute for Research in
Surgical Outcomes (KIRSO)
Department of Surgery
University of Alabama at Birmingham
Birmingham, Alabama

Robb D. Kociol, MD, MS, FHFSA
Director of HF Network Integration
Beth Israel Deaconess Medical Center
Boston, MA;
Medical Director, Heart Failure
Beth Israel Deaconess Hospital - Plymouth
Plymouth, MA;
Assistant Professor of Medicine
Harvard Medical School
Boston, MA

Jeff Larose, MSME
Chief Scientific Officer
MCS
Medtronic HeartWare
Miami Lakes, Florida

James W. Long, MD, PhD
Director
Nazih Zuhdi Transplant Institute
INTEGRIS Healthcare
Oklahoma City, Oklahoma

Donald A. Middlebrook, AA, BS
Consultant
Regulatory and Clinical Affairs
MCS Group/HF Division/Abbott
Pleasanton, California

Nader Moazami, MD
Professor of Cardiothoracic Surgery
Department of Cardiothoracic Surgery
New York University
New York City, New York

David Luís Simón Morales, MD
Professor of Surgery and Pediatrics
Clark-Helmsworth Chair of Pediatric Cardiothoracic Surgery,
Director
Congenital Heart Surgery—The Heart Institute
Cincinnati Children's Hospital Medical Center
The University of Cincinnati College of Medicine
Cincinnati, Ohio

Francis D. Pagani, MD, PhD
Otto Gago MD Endowed Professor of Cardiac Surgery
Cardiac Surgery
University of Michigan
Ann Arbor, Michigan

Soon J. Park, MD
Professor of Surgery,
Chief, Division of Cardiac Surgery
University Hospitals Cleveland Medical Center;
Co-Director
UH Harrington Heart and Vascular Institute;
Jay L. Ankeney, MD Chair, Professorship of Surgery
Cleveland, Ohio

Sean Pinney, MD
Director
Advanced Heart Failure and Transplantation Medicine, Cardiology
Mount Sinai Hospital;
Professor of Medicine, Cardiology
Icahn School of Medicine at Mount Sinai
New York City, New York

J. Eduardo Rame, MD, M.Phil, FAHA
Associate Professor of Medicine and Surgery
Health System Director of Mechanical Circulatory Support
University of Pennsylvania
Advanced Heart Failure/Cardiac Transplantation and Mechanical Circulatory Support
Philadelphia, Pennsylvania

Kyle William Riggs, MD
Research Fellow
Department of Cardiothoracic Surgery
Cincinnati Children's Hospital Medical Center
Cincinnati, Ohio

David N. Rosenthal, MD
Professor
Department of Pediatrics
Stanford University
Palo Alto, California

Stuart D. Russell, MD
Regional Director of Heart Failure
Professor of Medicine
Department of Medicine/Division of Cardiology
Duke University School of Medicine
Durham, North Carolina

Erin M. Schumer, MD, MPH
University of Louisville
Louisville, Kentucky

Craig H. Selzman, MD, FACS
Dr. Russell M. Nelson and Dantzel W. Nelson Presidential Endowed Chair,
Professor and Chief
Division of Cardiothoracic Surgery,
Surgical Director
Mechanical Circulatory Support and Heart Transplantation
Division of Cardiothoracic Surgery
University of Utah School of Medicine
Salt Lake City, Utah

Mark S. Slaughter, MD
Professor and Chair
Department of Cardiovascular and Thoracic Surgery
University of Louisville School of Medicine
Louisville, Kentucky

Randall C. Starling, MD, MPH
Professor of Medicine
Cleveland Clinic Lerner College of Medicine, Case Western Reserve University
Kaufman Center for Heart Failure
Cleveland Clinic
Cleveland, Ohio

Lynne Warner Stevenson, MD
Lisa M. Jacobson Professor of Cardiovascular Medicine
Director of Cardiomyopathy
Vanderbilt University Medical Center
Nashville, Tennessee

Garrick C. Stewart, MD, MPH
Associate Physician
Brigham and Women's Hospital;
Instructor
Harvard Medical School;
Associate Physician
Division of Cardiovascular Medicine
Centre for Advanced Heart Disease
Brigham and Women's Hospital
Boston, Massachusetts

Jeffrey Teuteberg, MD
Section Chief of Heart Failure, Cardiac Transplant and Mechanical Circulatory Support
Stanford University School of Medicine
Falk Cardiovascular Research Center
Stanford, California

Daniel Timms, PhD
CTO
Engineering
BiVACOR
Houston, Texas

Nir Uriel, MD, MSc
Director of Heart Failure, Heart Transplant and Mechanical Circulatory Support
Department of Medicine
University of Chicago
Chicago, Illinois

Richard Wampler, MD
Research Associate Professor of Surgery
Oregon Health Sciences University
Portland, Oregon

John T. Watson, PhD
Professor of Bioengineering
Jacobs School of Engineering
University of California, San Diego
San Diego, California

James B. Young, MD
Professor of Medicine and Executive Dean
Lerner College of Medicine of Case Western Reserve University
Cleveland Clinic
Cleveland, Ohio

Those who dreamed of a mechanical pump to permanently replace the functioning heart thought not about subsequent transplantation; no, they envisioned a lifelong mechanical heart pump. But the two are inextricably intertwined. When Alexis Carrel was awarded the Nobel Prize in Physiology or Medicine in 1912 " in recognition of his work on vascular suture and transplantation of blood vessels and organs" at the age of 39, his scientific journey was far from complete. In the 1930's, Carrel and Lindbergh developed a "perfusion pump" resembling an in vitro artificial heart, designed to support organs removed from small animals for several days. Their work has been credited as foundational for the later artificial heart. In humans, the origins of mechanical circulatory support (MCS) rest with Gibbon's development and single successful clinical use of a pump oxygenator to perform open heart surgery in 1953. John Kirklin at the Mayo Clinic followed in 1955 with the world's first successful series of open heart operations using a pump oxygenator, in which four of the first eight patients survived.

As beautifully detailed by Baldwin and Watson in Chapter 1 of this book *(Historical Aspects of Mechanical Circulatory Support)*, an era of excitement about a possible total artificial heart in the 1960s not only consumed a number of leading engineers and physicians (Kolff, Akutsu, DeBakey, Liotta, and Kantrowitz), but also inspired the US Congress to empower the National Heart Advisory Council to target mechanical solutions to heart failure. With an increasing concentration of energy and intellect brought to bear on this challenge, shorter term ventricular assist systems began to outpace the total artificial heart experimental successes. The timeline and challenges of developing these devices between 1963 and 1991 were chronicled in the Institute of Medicine Committee report to "Evaluate the National Heart, Lung, and Blood Institute (NHLBI) Artificial Heart Program" (in which Editor JKK participated as a young surgeon/investigator), which appeared in 1992.

With the formal introduction of cyclosporine immunosuppression into clinical heart transplantation in 1983, a reanimation of the entire field erupted after lying essentially dormant for 25 years. Heart transplantation programs rapidly appeared at many major academic cardiac surgery centers, accompanied by an explosion of transplantation activity and the inevitable donor shortages. As the waiting lists progressively exceeded available donors, patients were dying in large numbers. Researchers and surgeons began to consider a novel use of mechanical devices as "bridge-to-transplant" (BTT) therapy. With reports from Hill and Oyer using the Pierce-Donachy ventricular assist device (VAD) and the Novacor VAD, and Copeland implanting the CardioWest total artificial heart, all as BTT therapy, the field of MCS was awakened in the early 1980's.

But engineers and MCS proponents were frustrated, not satisfied with a limited application of sophisticated MCS systems that simply supported a dying patient through successful heart transplantation and then were discarded. Everything began to change with the REMATCH Trial, initiated in 1998 and completed in 2001. With FDA approval then Centers for Medicare and Medicaid Services (CMS) coverage in 2002-2003, a new world of interest blossomed in MCS therapy. For the first time, selected patients with terminal heart failure not eligible for heart transplantation could be offered life-saving VAD "destination therapy" (DT). While initial DT experiences were evolving with the bulky, flawed, pulsatile XVE, a new generation of continuous flow (CF) devices was under development and entering clinical trials.

With the prospect of thousands of patients being supported long term on these expensive devices, John Watson and his visionary colleagues at the NHLBI sought to pursue the recommendation from the 1992 Institute of Medicine Artificial Heart Program report that "... maintaining a registry of MCS recipients should be considered a routine aspect of this care..." Their initiative generated the birth of INTERMACS in 2006, an NHLBI-funded scientific registry to capture the national experience, facilitate the introduction of new devices, identify risk factors to predict good and bad outcomes with various pumps, quantify ongoing improvements in the field, and inform best practices.

As the field rapidly evolved, whole new areas of specialization and expertise emerged. With the clear superiority of current generation CF devices over prior technology, optimism reigned about ambulatory advanced heart failure patients gaining years and quality of life with these compact, durable devices. Later, in the aftermath of the failed REVIVE-IT trial (in which equipoise for a randomized trial of a CF pump in ambulatory heart failure was violated by a high incidence of pump thrombosis, and no surgical patients were entered), understanding the etiology and possible prevention of adverse events during pump support took center stage as a focus of research.

The first edition of the Braunwald Companion Text on *Mechanical Circulatory Support* was published 7 years ago, and much has evolved since then. In this second edition, existing chapters have been completely updated, some that lack current relevance have been removed, and new chapters of interest have been added. The pathophysiology and risk stratification in advanced heart failure have been updated in Chapters 2 and 3. Candidate selection and decision making has matured over the past 7 years, and this is reflected in Chapter 4. Entirely new chapters on acute (temporary) support and ECMO have been added to address the renewed interest in "bridging" patients in shock to durable devices (Chapters 5 and 6). Given the critical importance of the principles of CF physiology, device hemocompatibility, and the biological response to CF unloading, entirely new chapters (Chapters 7, 8, and 9) have been created. A review of current devices, surgical techniques, and longitudinal patient management has been thoroughly updated in Chapters 10 to 12. Sections on major adverse events and right heart failure have incorporated the most recent information and challenges (Chapters 13 and 14). All relevant clinical trials through 2018 are reviewed in Chapter 15, and health-related quality of life studies are updated in Chapter 16. Entirely new chapters (Chapters 17 and 18) detail the application of CF pumps in pediatric and special populations. The physiology of myocardial recovery during CF pump support and strategies for explant are described in depth in Chapter 19. The newest updates on unique information from registries and the current regulatory landscape provide the content for Chapters 20 and 21. Finally, we paint a prescient picture of future mechanical support in chapter 22.

This comprehensive text is truly a testimony to the phenomenal progress that has accrued with mechanical solutions to the failing heart. Although current devices do not yet rival the expected longevity and quality of life with heart transplantation, the comparative supply is massive and the target population of benefit is huge. After more than 50 years of nearly continuous disruptive innovation, combatants in the field of MCS (with their many associated intellectual peptides) are poised for further scientific and clinical breakthroughs. Yet major challenges remain, and this monograph sets the table for all interested stakeholders, scientists, clinicians, and regulators who embrace the future.

James K. Kirklin
Joseph G. Rogers

CONTENTS

BRAUNWALD'S HEART DISEASE FAMILY OF BOOKS

BRAUNWALD'S HEART DISEASE COMPANIONS

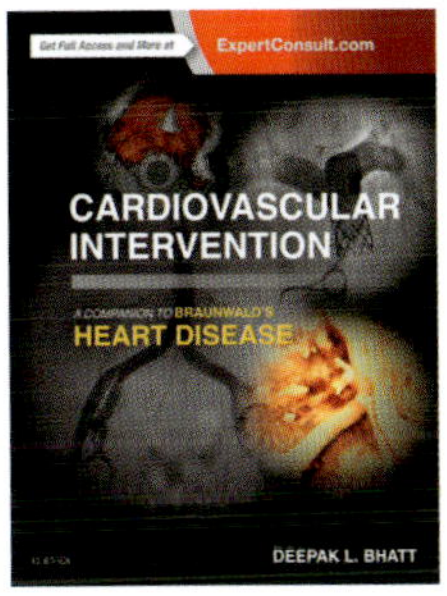

BHATT
Cardiovascular Intervention

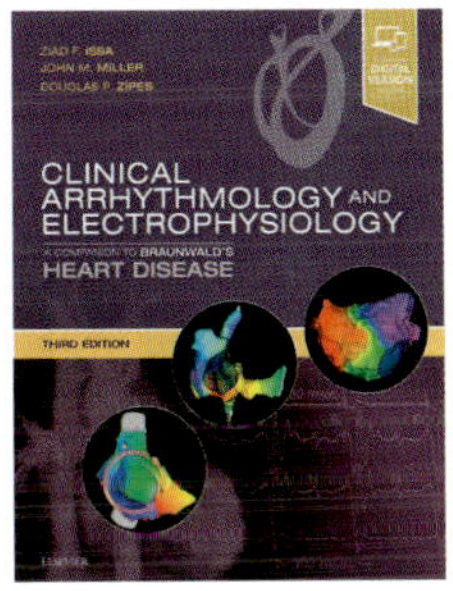

ISSA, MILLER, AND ZIPES
Clinical Arrhythmology and Electrophysiology

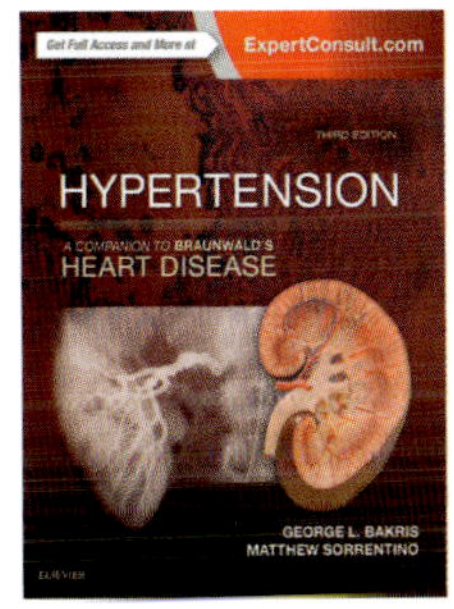

BAKRIS AND SORRENTINO
Hypertension

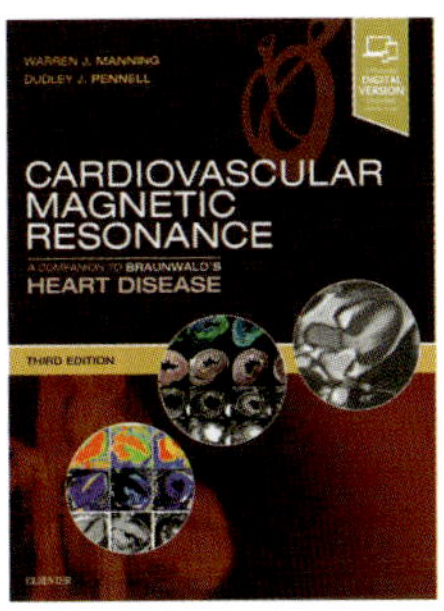

MANNING AND PENNELL
Cardiovascular Magnetic Resonance

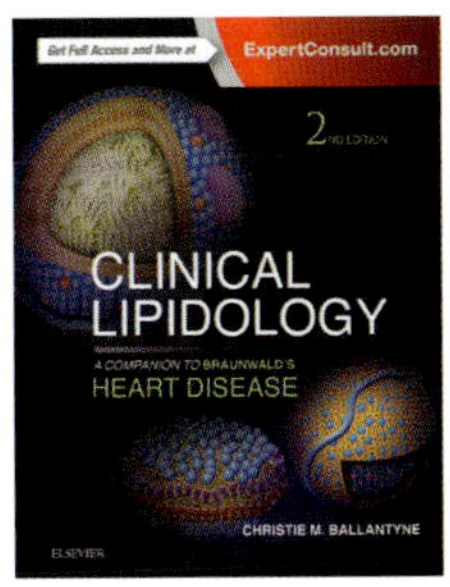

BALLANTYNE
Clinical Lipidology

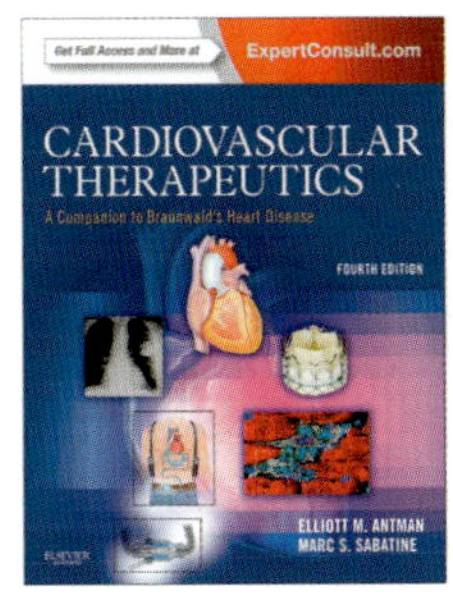

ANTMAN AND SABATINE
Cardiovascular Therapeutics

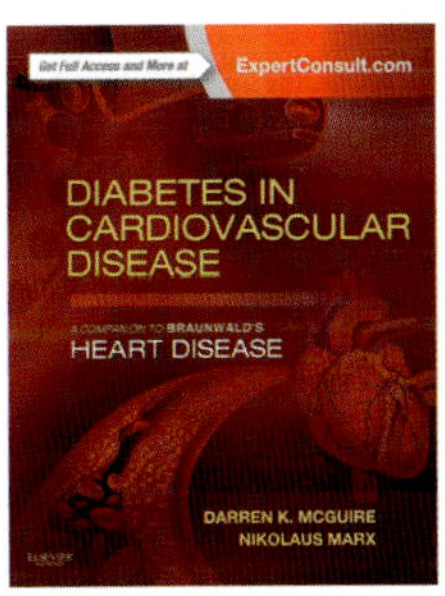

MCGUIRE AND MARX
Diabetes in Cardiovascular Disease

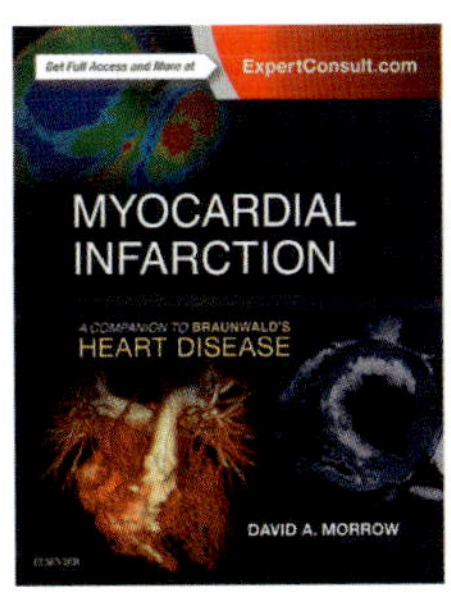

MORROW
Myocardial Infarction

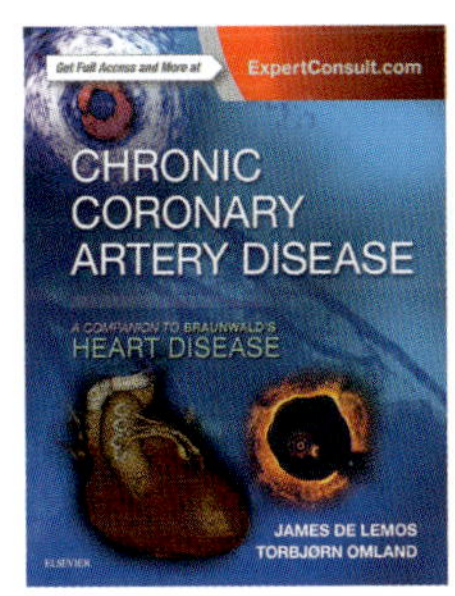

DE LEMOS AND OMLAND
Chronic Coronary Artery Disease

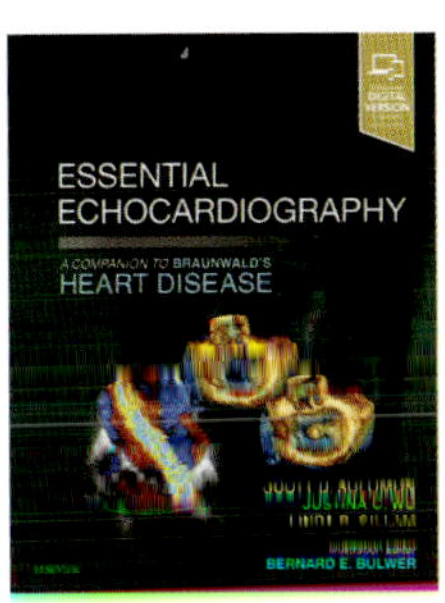

SOLOMON, WU, AND GILLAM
Essential Echocardiography

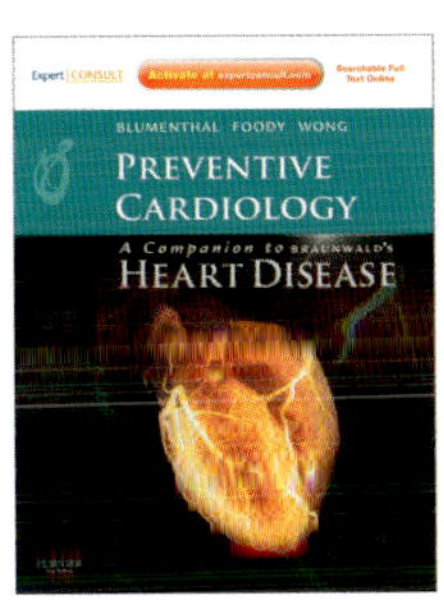

BLUMENTHAL, FOODY, AND WONG
Preventive Cardiology

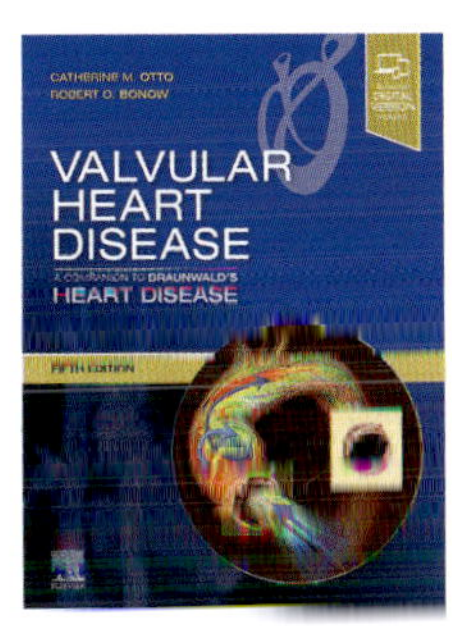

OTTO AND BONOW
Valvular Heart Disease

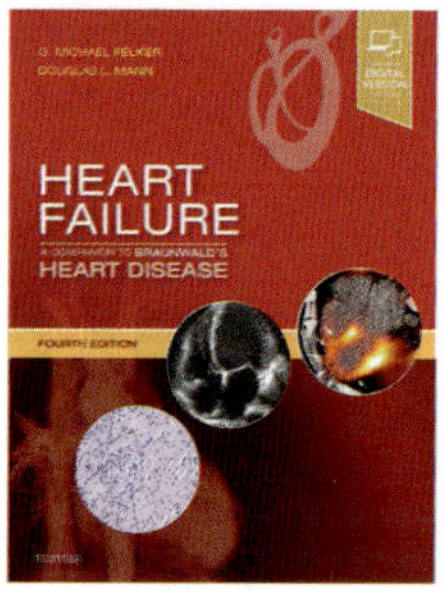

FELKER AND MANN
Heart Failure

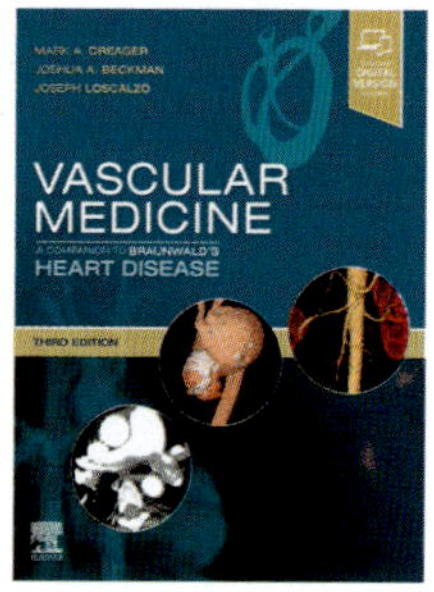

CREAGER
Vascular Medicine

BRAUNWALD'S HEART DISEASE REVIEW AND ASSESSMENT

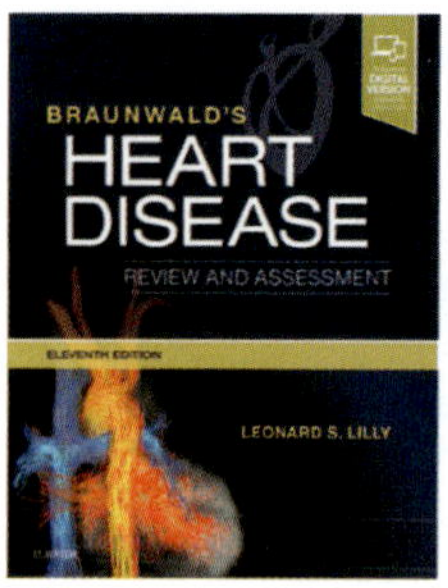

LILLY
Braunwald's Heart Disease Review and Assessment

BRAUNWALD'S HEART DISEASE IMAGING COMPANIONS

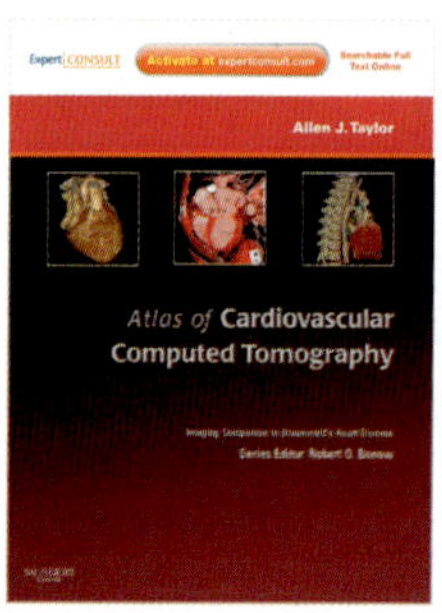

TAYLOR
Atlas of Cardiovascular Computed Tomography

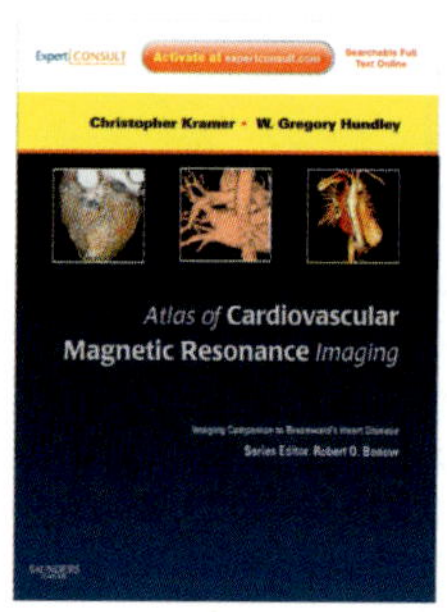

KRAMER AND HUNDLEY
Atlas of Cardiovascular Magnetic Resonance Imaging

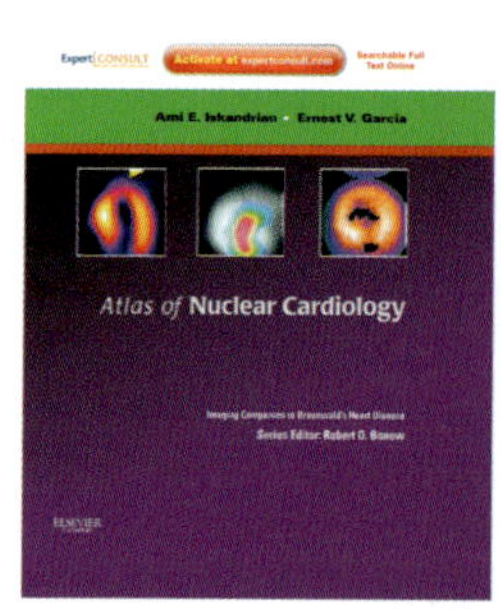

ISKANDRIAN AND GARCIA
Atlas of Nuclear Cardiology

1

Historical Aspects of Mechanical Circulatory Support

J. Timothy Baldwin, John T. Watson

KEY POINTS

Early Mechanical Circulatory Support Devices and Technology Development

Ongoing Technology Developments and Devices

Current State of MCS

EARLY MECHANICAL CIRCULATORY SUPPORT DEVICES AND TECHNOLOGY DEVELOPMENT

Establishing the Concept

In the 1930s, Carrel and Lindbergh[1] developed an in vitro artificial heart-like apparatus for keeping organs alive outside the body. They removed the hearts, kidneys, ovaries, adrenal glands, thyroid glands, and spleens of small animals to watch them develop and function over the course of several days.[2] Acute animal studies in Russia and the United States followed in the 1940s. However, the meaningful origin of the modern era of mechanical circulation support (MCS) can be traced to the development of the heart-lung machine by Gibbon (Table 1.1) and its first successful clinical use in 1953.[3,4] The device was developed for cardiopulmonary bypass so that surgical cardiac procedures that require hours of circulatory support could be performed. The success of the device and the need for prolonged circulatory support for patients who could not be weaned from the heart-lung machine or whose hearts could recover with longer durations of support provided the initial impetus for developing devices that could provide long-term circulatory support. The optimism in the 1950s and 1960s that circulation could be successfully supported for extended periods by an artificial heart spurred its development by pioneers such as Kolff, Akutsu, DeBakey, Liotta, and Kantrowitz.[5] In 1963, DeBakey and Lederberg testified before the US Congress on the need for an artificial heart in very different domains: for patients otherwise healthy except for their failed heart and for isolated travelers on long space journeys.[6] These hearings coincided with the debate about the implications of the Russian Sputnik Program and unbridled national enthusiasm for taking on large technologic challenges such as the program to put the first man on the moon, which had begun just a few years earlier.

In 1964, with special congressional approval, the National Heart Advisory Council established the mission-oriented Artificial Heart Program (AHP) to design and develop devices to assist a failing heart and to rehabilitate heart failure (HF) patients.[7] In the initial planning stages of the program, cardiology and surgery experts recommended that clinical systems be capable of a cardiac output of 10 L/min, be able to maintain normal blood pressure, and be "biocompatible" (a vague physiological term then and now). These and other physiological parameters represented the defined design goals of the first generation of MCS systems.[2] Despite this limited set of design inputs, engineers, biologists, and clinicians created teams and collaborations and used them, when appropriate, as quantifiable engineering design inputs to achieve the physiological goals in the early MCS systems.

Important progress on these early MCS systems resulted from the cooperation and collaboration fostered by the National Heart, Lung, and Blood Institute (NHLBI). In 1977, following a recommendation from the Cardiology Advisory Committee, the NHLBI Devices and Technology Branch (DTB) started the annual Contractors Meeting.[4,8] The primary purpose of the meeting was to provide a public forum for showcasing the progress of the contract research projects. The DTB viewed the meeting as an opportunity for gathering the branch grantees and contractors together to share ideas and network with other teams. After a decade of successful annual meetings sponsored by the NHLBI, the meeting was moved to Louisville, Kentucky, as the "Cardiovascular Science and Technology: Basic and Applied" meeting under the leadership of Jack Norman,[5] then to Washington, DC, with the guidance of Hank Edmunds,[5] and was finally integrated into the Annual Meeting of the American Society of Artificial Internal Organs by then President Bob Eberhart (1993).[7] This progression has preserved the spirit of collaboration of the original Contractors Meeting, which also includes the highly regarded Hastings Lecture dedicated to the memory of Dr. Frank Hastings, the first chief of the NHLBI Artificial Heart Program.

The annual meetings emphasized the importance of developing collaborative venues for the field to share results, both positive and negative, and develop a common language across disciplines with procedural guidelines, which improve the comparability of data between research teams.

During the early period of the program, spanning from 1965 to 1980, progress on implantable, long-term ventricular assist systems outpaced similar work on the more widely publicized total artificial heart (TAH) systems.[9] In fact, short-term ventricular assist systems were being fabricated for use in initial clinical trials in the late 1970s.[10] The Institute of Medicine Committee report to "Evaluate the NHLBI

TABLE 1.1 Mechanical Circulatory Support Milestones

Year	Event
1953	First successful use of heart-lung machine for cardiopulmonary bypass (Gibbon)
1958	First successful use TAH in a dog (Kolff and Akutso)
1963	First successful use of LVAD in human (DeBakey)
1964	Artificial Heart Program established at NIH Six contracts awarded to analyze issues and need for program
1968	First clinical use of intraaortic balloon pump (Kantrowitz)
1969	First artificial heart implant in humans (Cooley)
1977	NHLBI RFPs for blood pumps, energy converters, and energy transmission NHLBI RFA on blood-material interactions
1980	NHLBI RFP for integration of blood pumps designed for 2-year use
1982	Barney Clark received first TAH implant for destination therapy (DeVries)
1984	NHLBI RFP for 2-year reliability studies First use of Pierce-Donachy VAD (Thoratec PVAD) as BTT (Hill) First implant of Novacor VAD First use of electromechanical VAD (Oyer)
1985	First use of CardioWest TAH as BTT (Copeland)
1988	First use of hemopump in humans (Rich Wampler)—first rotary blood pump used (Frazier) NHLBI awards four contracts to develop portable, durable TAHs
1989	Manual of operations for Novacor VAD NHLBI clinical trial completed
1991	First HeartMate VE implant (Frazier)
1994	FDA approval for pneumatic HeartMate VE as BTT
1996	NHLBI IVAS contracts awarded for Jarvik 2000, HeartMate II, CorAide VADS Pilot trial (PREMATCH) for destination therapy begins NHLBI awards two contracts for TAH Clinical Readiness Program (Abiomed, Penn State)
1998	FDA approval for HeartMate XVE as BTT FDA approval for Novacor as BTT REMATCH trial begins First DeBakey VAD implant (Wieselthaler)
1999	First human implant Arrow LionHeart VAD (first use of TETS) (Korfer)
2000	First HeartMate II implant (Lavee) First Jarvik 2000 implant (Frazier)
2001	REMATCH trial completed First implant of the AbioCor TAH (Dowling)
2002	FDA approval of HeartMate XVE as destination therapy
2003	CMS coverage decision for destination therapy
2004	NHLBI pediatric mechanical circulatory support program launched First implant of DuraHeart VAD (Korfer)
2006	First implant of HeartWare HVAD (Wieselthaler) First implant of Levacor VAD (Long) FDA approval of AbioCor TAH (Humanitarian Device Exemption) INTERMACS registry launched (PI: Kirklin)
2007	First implant of Circulite Synergy device (Meyns); advent of miniature VADs Peter Houghton dies after a record 2714 days of VAD support
2008	HeartMate II BTT clinical trial completed
2009	FDA approval of HeartMate II for BTT HeartMate II destination therapy clinical trial completed 850th implant of the CardioWest TAH
2010	FDA approval of HeartMate II for destination therapy
2012	FDA approval of HVAD centrifugal flow pump for bridge-to-transplant therapy
2014	First implant of HM3 (Schmitto)
2017	FDA approval of HVAD for destination therapy FDA approval of HM3 centrifugal flow pump for bridge-to-transplant and bridge-to-recovery therapy

BTT, Bridge-to-transplant; *CMS*, Centers for Medicare and Medicaid Services; *FDA*, Food and Drug Administration; *HM3*, HeartMate; *INTERMACS*, Interagency Registry of Mechanically Assisted Circulatory Support for End-Stage Heart Failure; *IVAS*, Innovative Ventricular Assist System; *LVAD*, left ventricular assist device; *NHLBI*, National Heart, Lung, and Blood Institute; *NIH*, National Institutes of Health; *PI*, principle investigator; *PVAD*, paracorporeal ventricular assist device; *REMATCH*, Randomized Evaluation of Mechanical Assistance for the Treatment of Congestive Heart Failure; *RFA*, request for application; *RFP*, request for proposal; *TAH*, total artificial heart; *TETS*, transcutaneous energy transfer system; *VAD*, ventricular assist device; *VE*, vented electric.

Artificial Heart Program" contains a useful chronology of research and related important events from 1963 to 1991.[11,12]

The first generation (1980) of implantable MCS systems was designed to meet a 2-year operational goal during benchtop reliability testing.[13] Next followed the NHLBI Readiness Program.[14] This program aimed to ensure the functional reliability of the MCS systems that demonstrated the greatest promise. Each awarded contractor placed 12 MCS systems on "Mock Circulations" to assess their function during a simulated cycle of daily life for 2 years without interruption or maintenance. Success was completing the test with no more than one system failure at 2 years.

Clinical Application and Evolution of MCS

These early MSC programs created the engineering design basis for the HeartMate XVE (HM XVE) (Fig. 1.1) that was used in the Randomized Evaluation of Mechanical Assistance for the Treatment of Congestive Heart Failure (REMATCH) trial.[15] In clinical use, the HM XVE and other systems demonstrated that first-generation implantable systems could achieve meaningful physiological objectives for 2 years and improve quality of life. However, many patients suffered serious adverse events such as bleeding, infection, and device malfunction.

Recognizing the initial success of MCS devices by multidisciplinary teams created by the NHLBI programs, in 1994, the NHLBI released the "Innovative Ventricular Assist System" (IVAS) request for proposals to encourage innovation of totally implantable MCS systems that were designed to achieve at least a 5-year functional lifetime with 90% reliability.[16] This program was designed to incorporate the latest advances gained from first-generation MCS systems, the TAH, and in related engineering, clinical, and biology fields.

The IVAS program was crucial to advancing the field of MCS for longer survival and patient quality of life. The program again brought together skilled teams of clinicians, engineers, and biologists working together and collaborating with other teams toward the same defined physiological goals. As a result, the systems with the most promise exceeded the expectations of the program. These included the HeartMate II (HMII) (see Fig. 1.1) and the Jarvik 2000 VAS.[17,18] The HMII, an axial-continuous flow system, became the most clinically successful MCS system. In bench tests, HMII systems met physiological requirements, and some operated indefinitely.

The pivotal clinical trial with the HMII showed significantly improved survival and reduced adverse events for study patients. The unexpected result was underscored in the companion editorial to the release of the multicenter randomized trial. The author compared the REMATCH trial with the HM XVE to the HMII trial using Kaplan-Meier survival graphs.[19] The survival results with HM XVE were exactly the same in 2009 as in 2001, very strongly suggesting that the improved HMII survival was largely due to the engineering design of the systems. This again pointed to the value of the National Institutes of Health/NHLBI initiating the IVAS program.

After the HMII trial, thrombus-related device malfunctions increased without explanation.[20] There was speculation that the dimensionally tight axial-flow channel of the HMII was a contributing factor in thrombus formation. At the same time, magnetically levitated centrifugal-flow systems were on the drawing board. These systems became technically feasible because of advances in permanent magnets. The potential advantage of the centrifugal-flow pump is the dimensionally wider blood flow channels that may reduce the potential for thrombus formation. The importance of design is also seen in the widened internal flow patterns of the HeartMate 3 (HM3), which are likely responsible for the improved rate of "survival free of disabling stroke or reoperation to replace or remove a malfunctioning device" at 2 years compared to the HMII, despite the rates of disabling stroke being similar.[21] The HVAD (Fig. 1.2), also a centrifugal blood pump,

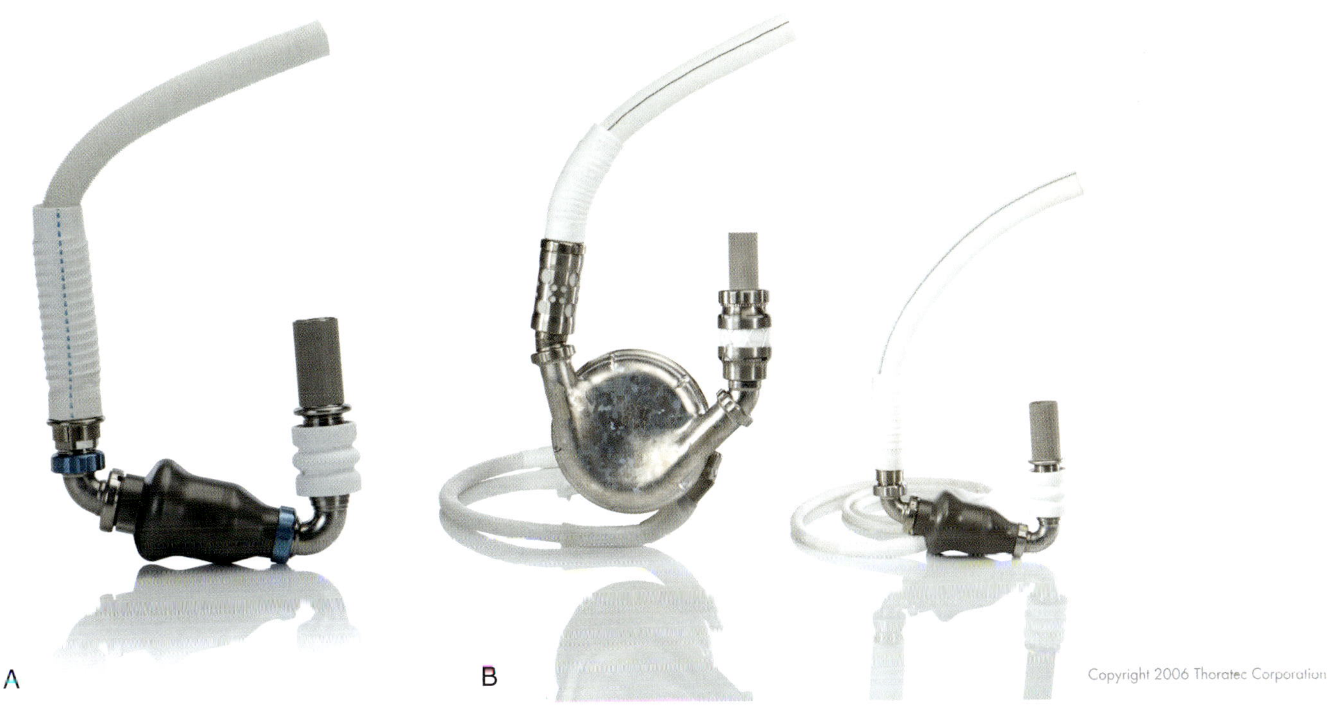

Fig. 1.1 The HeartMate II (A and lower left in B) compared with the HeartMate XVE (B). The HeartMate II was the first rotary ventricular assist device to receive U.S. Food and Drug Administration approval for bridge to transplant and destination therapy. (Courtesy of Abbott.)

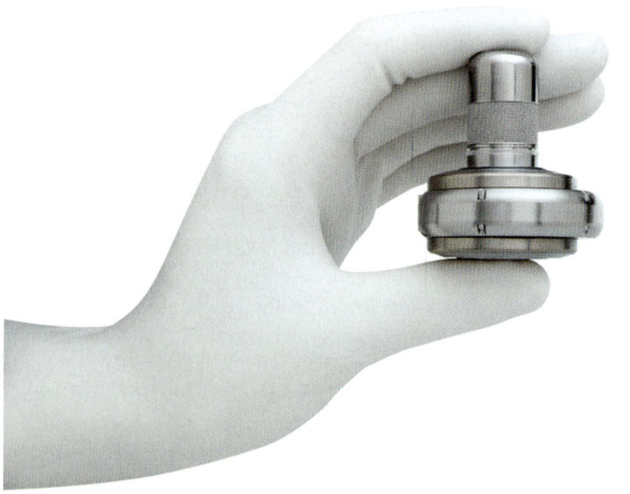

Fig. 1.2 The HeartWare HVAD. (Reproduced with permission of Medtronic, Inc.)

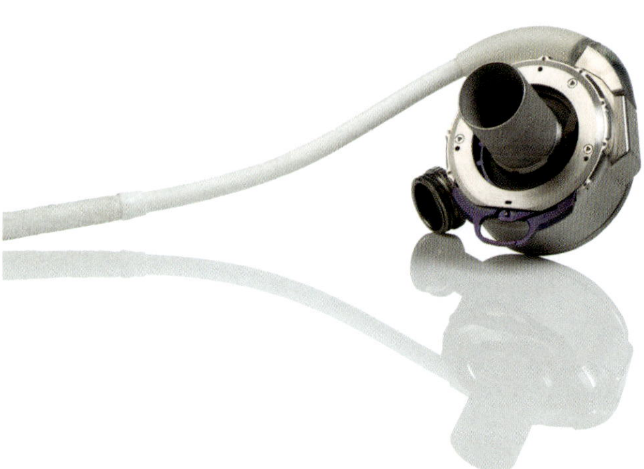

Fig. 1.3 The HeartMate 3, like the HeartWare left ventricular assist device, is a centrifugal pump but, rather than using bearings, has a fully magnetically levitated (Full MagLev) rotor. (Courtesy of Abbot Laboratories, Lake Bluff, IL.)

has different internal flow patterns from the HM3 (Fig. 1.3). In 2017, the Heartware system received Food and Drug Administration (FDA) approval for "Destination" therapy, following prior approval in 2012 as a bridge for cardiac transplantation.[22]

With the growth of MCS in the 1990s and early 2000s and its profound impact on patient outcomes, it was recommended that the NHLBI create a mechanism to assess various MCS technologies as they entered clinical use.[11] To fulfill this vision, the NHLBI elected to develop a registry to collect data to improve patient MCS selection, measure quality of life, meet the FDA regulatory requirements, and inform the Centers for Medicare and Medicaid Services (CMS) regarding reimbursement decisions. This led to a solicitation that resulted in the Interagency Registry of Mechanically Assisted Circulatory Support for End-Stage Heart Failure (INTERMACS).[23]

The NHLBI provided the necessary financial support for the contract to develop and run the registry, which was awarded to the University of Alabama at Birmingham. This substantially reduced triagency administrative factors and allowed the three agencies to join together on the steering committee and address questions relevant to their "agency mission" data collection. INTERMACS exceeded expectations for organizing, collecting, and analyzing clinical data and provided Medical Device Reports for adverse events to the FDA and data for CMS payment decisions.

INTERMACS made an early decision to only curate data generated by patients implanted with FDA-approved durable MCS devices (i.e., devices with the potential for patient discharge).[24] This requirement added additional rigor to the INTERMACS database as the implants were under design controls and thus not subject to random design modifications that may directly influence clinical outcomes. Fourteen device systems met this standard. In recent years, of the 14 systems, 3 adult ventricular assist systems, 1 pediatric device, and 1 TAH system became the primary MCS devices in clinical use, thus providing essentially all the Bridge and Destination therapy data for INTERMACS.

ONGOING TECHNOLOGY DEVELOPMENTS AND DEVICES

The development of new MCS devices has been spurred by innovation, as well as building on the success of earlier concepts. Substantial activity has focused on the development of novel TAHs. To date, the SynCardia TAH (Fig. 1.4), based on the Jarvik-7 TAH developed in the early 1980s, is the only one that has received substantial use, accounting for over 95% of the more than 1700 worldwide TAH implants since the first TAH in 1969.[25] Recent efforts to develop a newer generation of TAH include the CARMAT bioprosthetic TAH,[26] the Cleveland Clinic continuous-flow total artificial heart (CFTAH),[27] and the BiVACOR TAH.[28] The CARMAT TAH, like the SynCardia TAH, is a positive displacement device. However, it utilizes bioprosthetic blood-contacting surfaces, electro-hydraulic pumps to activate the membrane between the two ventricles to product pulsatile flow, and an advanced control system involving implanted sensors to provide flows to meet patient demands. Four patients were implanted with the device in a pilot study, which is anticipated to lead to a pivotal study. The Cleveland Clinic TAH and BiVACOR TAH both involve a single moving part, a rotor with impeller blades on each side, with each side driving the flow in the left and right centrifugal continuous-flow pumps that make up the device. These are considerably smaller than positive displacement TAHs, so small that a pediatric version of the Cleveland Clinical CFTAH is being developed for infants down to 0.3 m^2 body surface area (BSA). The continuous-flow TAHs are both at the stage of animal studies.

Novel, advanced ventricular assist devices (VADs) are being designed and developed to address the outstanding issues with adverse events and special populations. These include a minimally invasive intraaortic balloon pump for long-term support (NuPulseCV, Raleigh, NC) and a valveless VAD that uses magnetically driven pistons to create pulsatile flow, known as the TorVAD (Windmill Technologies, Austin, TX).[29,30] They also include newer generations of continuous-flow VADs such as a miniature implantable pump platform, the Revolution, in which minor modifications of components can be implemented to adjust the pump performance to support the right or left side of the heart (Vadovations, Inc., Oklahoma City, OK).[31,32]

Some of the greatest attention has focused on the development of MSC devices for children, specifically small ones. This was spurred on by the NHLBI Pediatric Circulatory Support Program spanning from 2004 to 2009 and the Pumps for Kids, Infants, and Neonates

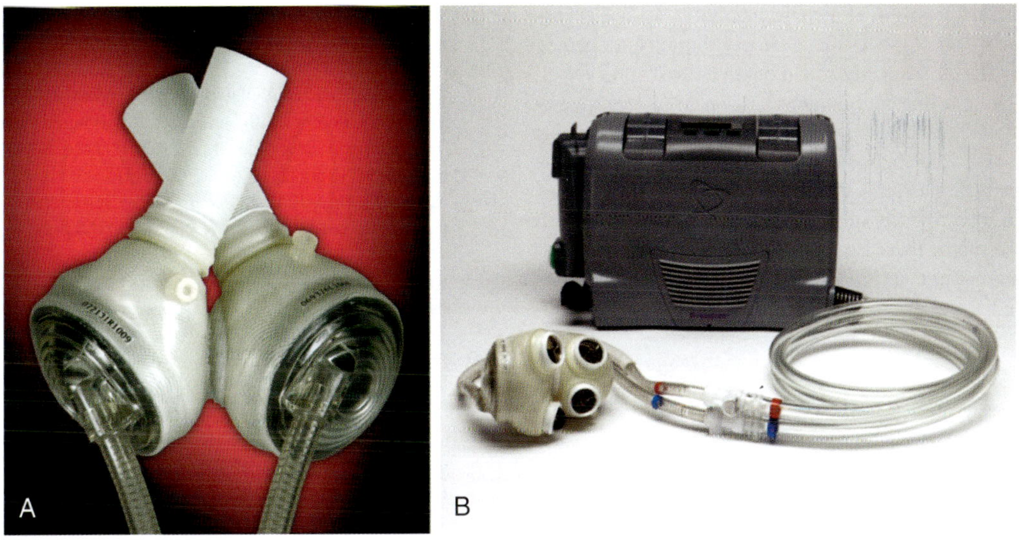

Fig. 1.4 The SynCardia Temporary Total Artificial Heart (A), shown with the wearable driver system (B). (Courtesy of Syncardia Systems, Inc., Tucson, AZ.)

Program, which started in 2010.[31,32] These programs led to the development of various devices for children less than 20 kg with advanced HF because, when the programs began, the only device available for these patients was the Berlin Heart EXCOR, but only through emergency or compassionate use. Since then, the Berlin Heart received FDA approval and currently is the only FDA-approved MCS device for these small children. However, 29% of patients supported by the device experienced strokes in the pivotal trial.[33] Developers hope to lower rates of serious adverse events by incorporating the latest technologies realized in VADs for adults into the new generation of pediatric VADs.

The Jarvik 2015 Ventricular Assist System, which resulted from the NHLBI programs, is poised to begin clinical evaluation.[33] Progress continues on other devices that were developed independently of the NHLBI programs or resulted from them. These include a pediatric rotary flow VAD (Vadovations, Inc., Oklahoma City, OK), the Pediatric TorVAD (Windmill Technologies, Inc., Austin, TX), and the Penn State Pediatric Total Artificial Heart (Penn State University, Hershey and University Park, PA).[34–36]

The development of novel MCS devices like these has been led by a community of multidisciplinary teams. And, like the MCS devices they work on, the MCS community has evolved. Since the days of the DTB Contractors Meetings, the MCS community has continued to grow, collaborate, communicate, and now use other various meetings and organizations to do so such as the Gordon Research Conference on Assisted Circulation,[37] the ITERMACS Registry,[38] the International Society of Heart and Lung Transplantation forum for MCS[39] and the Society of Thoracic Surgeons STS National Database.[40]

CURRENT STATE OF MCS

Over the past five decades, MCS has grown substantially from a small community of researchers working to develop early successful devices to meet modest goals and demonstrate the value of the therapy to one that includes significant numbers of research teams and mature industry leaders in medical devices and has helped thousands of patients with late-stage HF. MCS served as a catalyst for a grassroots coalescing of key disciplines, organizations, and talents dedicated to patient quality of life and the well-being of caretakers. It has attracted clinicians, engineers, and scientists, both senior and recent graduates, who voluntarily committed their careers to MCS research, practice, and patients. Additionally, program coordinators work well beyond their position descriptions to provide 24/7 availability in the management and well-being of MCS patients and caregivers. As a benefit, patients have exceeded expectations in the scope of successful daily and recreational activities.

It is difficult to estimate the worldwide utilization of MCS. Based on increasing accrual rate in the INTERMACS Registry, the annual utilization in the United States may be around 3500 implants. Assuming that MCS use outside of the United States is similar,[41–43] annual worldwide implants may total 6000–7000 units. Of note is that TAH use has grown worldwide, now totaling well over a thousand patients since its first use.[43] With the development of MCS therapy, many patients are living well beyond 5 years, with the longest known patients alive after 15 years. These patients are informing the MCS research community and fellow patients by sharing best practices with their MCS systems through online organizations such as MyLVAD.[44]

An added research benefit of MCS is that while it extends patient survival, it is, in essence, extending the natural history of their physiological condition. With a growing number of patients living 5 years and longer with a device, there is a growing reservoir of opportunities to gain better understanding of the condition of HF itself. For example, the studies of myocardial recovery with device explant may reveal therapeutic strategies that deserve clinical research and trials involving patients without MCS.[45] To this end, the NHLBI held a working group on "Advancing the Science of Myocardial Recovery with Mechanical Circulatory Support" in June 2016.[46] Recommendations from this meeting were made to provide some clear directions to advance the science of cardiac recovery in the setting of mechanical circulatory support, and the hope is that research to address important outstanding questions about myocardial recovery will soon follow.

The interdisciplinary teams of clinicians, engineers, and scientists that began in the early days of the Artificial Heart Program and formed the underpinning of the dynamic MCS field have endured and evolved over the decades. These teams continue working on MCS therapy because patients with MCS devices are still beset by serious adverse events associated with the devices. Progress to address them has been modest because, in part, terms for bleeding, stroke, infection, arrhythmias, and right HF have been incompletely quantified. To take MCS devices to the next level and overcome these issues, comprehensive biology, physics, and engineering parameters that define the device design inputs and goals are needed.

DISCLOSURE

Dr. Baldwin is an employee of the NHLBI, NIH. The comments expressed here are those of the authors and do not reflect official positions of the NHLBI or NIH.

FUNDING

No funding sources were used for this review.

REFERENCES

1. Carrel A, Lindbergh CA. The culture of whole organs. *Science.* 1935;*81*(2112):621–623.
2. Report HEW-NHI. *Cardiac Replacement: Medical, Ethical, Psychological, and Economic Considerations*; 1969.
3. Stoney WS. Evolution of cardiopulmonary bypass. *Circulation.* 2009;119(21):2844–2853.
4. Device and Technology Contractors Meeting Proceedings. Washington, DC, Dec 1997.
5. Annual Meeting Cardiovascular Science and Technology. *Basic and Applied I.* Louisville, KY: Ed. Norman JC; 1989.
6. Annual Meeting Cardiovascular Science and Technology. *Basic and Applied.* Washington, DC: Ed. Edmunds LH; 1991.
7. American Society of Artificial Internal Organs. https://asaio.com/.
8. Frazier OH, Kirklin JK. *Mechanical Circulatory Support (ISHLT Monograph Series).* Elsevier; 2006.
9. DeBakey ME. Development of mechanical heart devices. *Ann Thorac Surg.* 2005;*79*(6):S2228–S2231.
10. Norman JC, Dasco CC, Reul GJ, et al. Partial artificial heart (ALVAD) use with subsequent cardiac and renal allografting in a patient with stone heart syndrome. *Artif Organs.* 1978;2(4):413–420.
11. IOM Committee Report. *The Artificial Heart: Prototypes, Policies and Patients*; 1991.
12. Hogness JR. *Committee to Evaluate the Artificial Heart Program of the National Heart, Lung, and Blood Institute, Division of Health Care Service, Institute of Medicine. The Artificial Heart: prototypes, policies, and patients.* Washington, DC: National Academy Press; 1991.
13. *Request for Proposal RFP NHLBI 80-3, Development of an Implantable Integrated Electrically Powered Left Heart Assist System.* January 1980.
14. *Request for Proposal RFP NHLBI 84-1, Device Readiness Testing of Implantable Ventricular Assist Systems.* October 1983.
15. Rose E, Gelijns A, Moskowitz A, et al. Long-term mechanical left ventricular assistance for end-stage heart failure. *NEJM.* 2001;345(20):1435–1443.
16. *Request for Proposal RFP NHLBI-HV-94-25, Innovative Ventricular Assist System.* August 1994.
17. HeartMate II website: http://heartmateii.com/.
18. Jarvik 2000 website: https://www.jarvikheart.com/products/.
19. Fang JC. Rise of the machines—left ventricular assist devices as permanent therapy for advanced heart failure. *NEJM.* 2009;361:2241–2251.
20. RC1 Starling, Moazami N, Silvestry SC, et al. Unexpected abrupt increase in left ventricular assist device thrombosis. *N Engl J Med.* 2014;370(1):33–40.
21. Mehra MR, Goldstein DJ, Uriel N, et al. MOMENTUM 3 Investigators. Two-year outcomes with a magnetically levitated cardiac pump in heart failure. *N Engl J Med.* Mar 11, 2018. https://doi.org/10.1056/NEJMoa1800866. [Epub ahead of print].
22. Rogers JG, Pagani FD, Tatooles AJ, et al. Intrapericardial left ventricular assist device for advanced heart failure. *N Engl J Med Feb 2.* 2017;375(5):451–460.
23. Kirklin JK, Naftel DC, Stevenson LW, et al. INTERMACS database for durable devices for circulatory support: first annual report. *J Heart Lung Transplant.* 2008;27(10):1065–1072.
24. INTERMACS Device List (Approved and Unapproved): Website http://www.uab.edu/medicine/INTERMACS/INTERMACS-documents.
25. http://www.syncardia.com/2016-press-releases/new-york-times-posts-retro-report-documentary-the-total-artificial-heart-from-1st-implant-to-worlds-most-used-artificial-heart.html (Accessed 2/23/2018).
26. Latrémouille C, Carpentier A, Leprince P, et al. A bioprosthetic total artificial heart for end-stage heart failure: results from a pilot study. *J Heart Lung Transplant.* 2018;37(1):33–37.
27. Fukamachi K, Karimov JH, Sunagawa G, et al. Generating pulsatility by pump speed modulation with continuous-flow total artificial heart in awake calves. *J Artif Organs.* 2017;20(4):381–385.
28. Timms D, Fraser J, Hayne M, Dunning J, McNeil K, Pearcy M. The BiVACOR rotary biventricular assist device: concept and in vitro investigation. *Artif Organs.* 2008;32(10):816–819.
29. Costantini H, Juricek C, Kagan V, et al. Management of a counterpulsation device outside of the intensive care unit. *J Heart Lung Transplant.* 2017;36(4):S356–S357.
30. Letsou GV, Pate TD, Gohean JR, et al. Improved left ventricular unloading and circulatory support with synchronized pulsatile left ventricular assistance compared with continuous-flow left ventricular assistance in an acute porcine left ventricular failure model. *J Thorac Cardiovasc Surg.* 2010;140(5):1181–1188.
31. Wampler R. Heart assist device. *United States Patent US 9.* August 22, 2017;737(651). United States Patent and Trademark Office.
32. Wampler R. Heart assist device. *United States Patent US 9.* December 15, 2015;211(368). United States Patent and Trademark Office.
33. Baldwin JT, Borovetz HS, Duncan BW, et al. The National Heart, Lung, and Blood Institute Pediatric Circulatory Support Program. *Circulation.* 2006;113:147–155.
34. Fraser, C. D., Jr., et al. (2012). Prospective trial of a pediatric ventricular assist device. *N Engl J Med.* 367(6): 532-541.
35. Snyder TA, Coghill P, Azartash-Namin K, Wu J, Stanfield J, Long JW. Design of an implantable blood pump for mechanical circulatory support in pediatric patients. In: *ASME. Frontiers in Biomedical Devices*; 2017. Design of Medical Devices Conference.
36. Gohean JR, Larson ER, Hsi BH, Kurusz M, Smalling RW, Longoria RG. Scaling the low-shear pulsatile TORVAD for pediatric heart failure. *ASAIO J.* 2017;63(2):198–206.
37. Penn State Pediatric TAH (grant reference, but no publications in Pubmedn) n.d.
38. Conferences Gordon Research. https://www.grc.org/find-a-conference/?keywords=assisted+circulation; 2003.
39. Interagency Registry for Mechanical Assisted Circulation Support (INTERMACS). https://www.uab.edu/medicine/INTERMACS/.
40. International Society for Heart and Lung Transplantation (ISHLT). http://www.ishlt.org/.
41. Society of Thoracic Surgery (STS). https://www.sts.org/.
42. Japanese registry for Mechanically Assisted Circulatory Support. *First report, The Journal of Heart and Lung Transplantation.* October 2017;36(10):1087–1096.
43. INTERMACS. *Quarterly Statistical Report Q3.* https://www.uab.edu/medicine/INTERMACS/images/Federal_Quarterly_Report/Federal_Partners_Report_2017_Q3.pdf; 2017.

44. Copeland JG. SynCardia total artificial heart: update and future. *Tex Heart Inst J*. 2013;40(5):587–588.
45. MyLVAD: Living with an LVAD. www.mylvad.com/content/living-lvad.
46. Birks EJ. The promise of recovery. *JACC:HF*. 2016;4(7):577–579.
47. Drakos SG, Pagani FD, Lundberg MS, Baldwin JT. (2017) Advancing the science of myocardial recovery with mechanical circulatory support: a working group of the National, Heart, Lung, and Blood Institute. *JACC Basic Transl Sci*. 2017; 2(3):335–340, *ASAIO J*. 2017 Jul/Aug;63(4): 445–449, *J Card Fail*. 2017 May;23(5):416–421, and *J Thorac Cardiovasc Surg*. 2017 Jul;154(1):165–170.

2

Advanced Heart Failure and Cardiogenic Shock

J. Thomas Heywood, James B. Young

KEY POINTS

- Introduction
- Definition
- Etiology of Cardiogenic Shock
- Hemodynamic Effects of Cardiogenic Shock
- Neurohormonal Response to Cardiogenic Shock
- Inflammatory Pathways
- End Organ Injury
- Conclusion

INTRODUCTION

The term shock first appeared in the English medical literature in a translation by John Clarke of a French treatise on gunshot wounds by Henry LeDran in 1740, *Traité ou Reflexions Tirées de la Pratique sur les Playes d'armes à feu.*[1] In his translation, he used the English "shock" to translate the French word *saisissement*, which at that time might have meant "fright" or "violent emotion."[1] The description only slowly gained acceptance and described more the neurologic reaction, either torpor or agitation, to the trauma of violent injury rather than a physiologic response. The battlefield surgeons of the American Civil War were well acquainted with the condition, "Although the nervous shock accompanies the most serious wounds.... It is recognized by the sufferer becoming cold, faint and pale, with the surface bedewed with a cold sweat; the pulse is small and flickering; there is anxiety, mental depression, with at times incoherence of speech."[2] The measurement of blood pressure, at first invasively and then noninvasively, in the later part of the 19th century added reduced blood pressure to the syndrome.[3,4]

In the late 19th and early 20th centuries, the etiology of shock was thought to be a neurologic reflex or a result of abnormal blood pooling in the mesenteric vessels. World War I led to an intensification of medical interest on the shock syndrome, with insights added from animal models used to scientifically test models for the initiation of shock.

In August 1917, George Crile led the Lakeside Unit from Cleveland into the war. These were the first US Army troops to enter the conflict. A base hospital was established to treat the wounded troops along the German-Allied lines near Rouen, France, and in Belgium's Flanders Field. Several other units from academic medical centers were assembled, including the Harvard Unit, led by Harvey Cushing. Prior to the war, Crile developed an interest in hemorrhagic shock, developing during surgical procedures. He created a number of approaches to blood transfusion after visiting the labs of Alexis Carrel in 1902 and is sometimes credited with the first direct human blood transfusion. A poignant event is described in his autobiography when he was called by his dear friend Harvey Cushing to his outpost, also serving as a forward base hospital in the war. William Osler's only child had been mortally wounded and Crile was called to assist with surgery and to arrange for blood transfusions in a desperate attempt to save his life. Sadly, Revere Osler died despite efforts to ameliorate his shock state, which was multifactorial in nature. Crile's work subsequently led to development of "shock trousers," which were used in the operating room when shock developed.[5] It was also learned during this time that shock from blood loss could be reversed with lactated Ringer's solution.[6]

The current understanding, still incomplete, of cardiogenic shock moved forward in 1927, when Alfred Blalock, prior to the creation of his eponymous shunt with Vivien Thomas and Helen Taussig, began pivotal research on the origins and classification of shock.[7] He was able to show experimentally that it often was not neurologically driven. He also classified its presentation into five clinical syndromes, which form the foundation for approaching shock today, including cardiogenic shock.

1. Shock due to volume loss
2. Neurogenic shock
3. Vasogenic shock, which includes sepsis and anaphylaxis
4. Cardiogenic shock
5. Unclassified conditions

What is described in the following is a current understanding of the pathophysiology of cardiogenic shock. This is by no means to suggest that cardiogenic shock is "understood," a point that is underscored by the persistently high mortality of cardiogenic shock. We are standing on the shoulders of giants, but our vision is still woefully incomplete (Table 2.1).

DEFINITION

Shock is a clinical syndrome, much like heart failure, that is characterized by signs and symptoms recognized by the clinician. These can be horribly apparent, as when cardiac arrest initiates cardiogenic shock with complete absence of vital signs (Fig. 2.1) or so subtle that the patient drifts into shock over the course of weeks or months and even skilled clinicians miss the transition (gradual-onset cardiogenic shock). In general, contemporary definitions of cardiogenic shock are eerily similar to battlefield depictions of severe trauma in the American Civil War, but with the addition of quantitative parameters of reduced urine output and blood pressure. Cardiogenic shock was defined in a

TABLE 2.1 INTERMACS Profiles Inform the Definitions of Cardiogenic Shock

Category	Profile	Shorthand Jargon
INTERMACS Level 1	Critical cardiogenic shock	"Crash and burn"
INTERMACS Level 2	Progressive decline	"Sliding fast on inotropes"
INTERMACS Level 3	Stable/inotrope dependent	"Inpatient/outpatient inotropes"
INTERMACS Level 4	Recurrent severe CHF	"Symptoms on oral Rx at home"
INTERMACS Level 5	Exertion Intolerant	"Housebound and sx with ADL"
INTERMACS Level 6	Exertion limited	"Walking wounded"
INTERMACS Level 7	NYHA Class IIIb	Advanced/not critical CHF

ADL, Activities of daily living; *CHF*, congestive heart failure; *INTERMACS*, Interagency Registry for Mechanically Assisted Circulatory Support; *NYHA*, New York Heart Association; *Rx*, medications; *sx*, symptoms.

Source: Stevenson LW, Pagani FD, Young JB, et al. INTERMACS profiles of advanced heart failure: the current picture. *J Heart Lung Transplant* 2009;28:535–541.

Presentations of Cardiogenic Shock

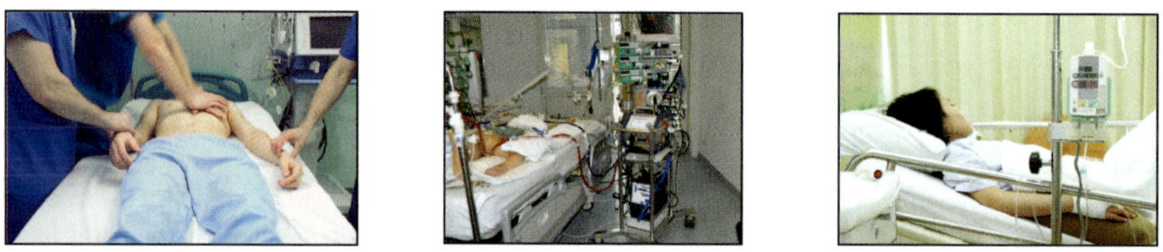

	Catastrophic Shock	Acute Severe Shock	Indolent Progressive Shock
Typical Scenario	Ventricular Fibrillation PEA arrest	Acute Myocardial Infarction Fulminant Myocarditis	Progressive Congestive HF Moving from Stage C to Stage D.
Physiology	Complete cessation of cardiac function.	Severe reduction in CO and BP.	Moderate reduction in CO and BP.
Time Course to Effectively Intervene	<5 minutes to provide adequate CPR or restore cardiac function. <1 hour to restore CO, BP.	Restore CO, BP within 1-6 hours.	Hours to days to improve hemodynamics.
Goals of Therapy	Anoxic brain injury must be avoided.	Avoid SIRS, MOF.	Improve CO, BP and lower filling pressures. Evaluate for TX, LVAD or hospice.

Fig. 2.1 Clinical profiles and outcomes in patients presenting with cardiogenic shock. *BP*, Blood pressure; *CO*, cardiac output; *CPR*, cardiopulmonary resuscitation; *HF*, heart failure; *LVAD*, left ventricular assist device; *MOF*, multiorgan failure; *PEA*, pulseless electrical activity; *SIRS*, systemic inflammatory response; *TX*, cardiac transplant.

recent trial evaluating percutaneous intervention in shock as "a systolic blood pressure of less than 90 mm Hg for longer than 30 minutes or the use of catecholamine therapy to maintain a systolic pressure of at least 90 mm Hg, clinical signs of pulmonary congestion, and signs of impaired organ perfusion with at least one of the following manifestations: altered mental status, cold and clammy skin and limbs, oliguria with a urine output of less than 30 mL per hour, or an arterial lactate level of more than 2.0 mm per liter."[8]

ETIOLOGY OF CARDIOGENIC SHOCK

Acute myocardial infarction is a common, but by no means the only, cause of cardiogenic shock (Box 2.1), and the infarction can result in shock in a number of ways. It can be the result of a catastrophically large infarct or a relatively small infarction in the setting of an ischemic cardiomyopathy. Infarction of the right ventricle with relative sparing of the left ventricle has unique clinical features, including shock. Severe ischemia even in the absence of myocardial injury can reduce cardiac

BOX 2.1 Etiologies of Cardiogenic Shock

- Ischemic
  - Acute myocardial infarction
  - Unstable angina with global ischemia
  - Right ventricular infarction
  - Complications of ischemic heart disease
  - Papillary muscle rupture
  - Acute ventricular septal defect
  - Myocardial rupture
- Valvular
  - Severe aortic stenosis or insufficiency
  - Severe mitral regurgitation or stenosis
  - Severe pulmonic stenosis or regurgitation
  - Severe tricuspid regurgitation or stenosis
- Myocardial disease/unknown
  - Acute myocarditis
  - Giant cell myocarditis
  - Takotsubo stress myocarditis
  - Substance abuse
  - Toxins
  - Chemotherapeutic agents
  - End-stage ischemic or nonischemic cardiomyopathy
- Extracardiac
  - Cardiac tamponade
  - Acute aortic dissection with aortic insufficiency, tamponade, or rupture
  - Large pulmonary embolism
- End-stage congenital heart disease

output substantially with reduced blood pressure. Finally, infarction with tissue necrosis can result in papillary muscle rupture, acute ventricular septal defect, or free wall rupture with severe, often fatal, shock.

In the absence of coronary artery disease, acute myocarditis and especially giant cell myocarditis can result in profound cardiogenic shock such that almost cessation of myocardial contraction can be seen and/or incessant malignant arrhythmias requiring ECMO support. Takotsubo cardiomyopathy can mimic acute myocardial infarction in the emergency room and has a reported incidence of cardiogenic shock of 9%.[9] Long-standing heart failure that has been stable for decades can devolve rapidly or insidiously into end-stage heart failure with hypotension and multiorgan dysfunction. Similarly, chronic valvular abnormalities, when they become severe, can profoundly impair hemodynamics and become life-threatening. Patients with adult congenital heart disease can sink later in life into a shock state with multiorgan failure after years of relatively normal cardiovascular status following early palliative surgery. Large pulmonary emboli can present with syncope and cardiogenic shock from right heart failure, as can end-stage pulmonary arterial hypertension. Finally, long-standing alcohol abuse and illicit drug use with methamphetamines or other sympathomimetic drugs can be responsible for profound cardiac dysfunction.

HEMODYNAMIC EFFECTS OF CARDIOGENIC SHOCK

Reduced Cardiac Output

In general, cardiac output is reduced in cardiogenic shock, although not universally so. Cardiac output is a continuum, so there is not an absolute number below which a patient is in cardiogenic shock. The shock state exists when the output is not sufficient to meet the metabolic needs of the principle organ systems, including the kidneys, liver, central nervous system, and digestive tract. In terms of cardiac output, shock has been defined as a cardiac index less than 1.8 to 2.2 L/min/m^2.[10] That said, not all patients with this reduction in cardiac index are in shock, but it does indicate significant derangement in cardiac function.

Unfortunately, cardiac output requires invasive measurements, and so there are often delays in obtaining this important determinate of shock. Beyond thermodilution estimation of cardiac output, mixed venous saturation can be an important indicator of low output states when corrected for anemia. Mixed venous saturations below 50% or, more frequently, less than 40% are indicative of cardiogenic shock.[11] Echocardiographic determination of the left ventricular outflow time velocity integral can be used to calculate stroke volume and, hence, cardiac output, and extremely low values are associated with poor outcome.[12] Stroke volume can also be estimated by arterial waveform analysis, although this may be less accurate in severe vasodilation or vasoconstriction states.[13]

In some instances of cardiogenic shock, cardiac output may be nearly normal but is associated with profound vasodilation.[14] Vasodilatory shock or systemic inflammatory response, which will be discussed further in the chapter, can develop quickly or during later stages of cardiogenic shock.[15] Calculation of systemic vascular resistance can quickly differentiate between vasodilatory or vasoconstrictive shock versus shock presenting with a normal or increased vascular resistance. These distinctions are vital because the pharmacologic and mechanical support approaches are quite different and initial errors in management can prolong tissue hypoperfusion. Judicious use of vasodilators can result in marked improvement of cardiac output in vasoconstriction, whereas they are absolutely contraindicated in vasodilatory states where vasopressin may be beneficial because of vasopressin depletion.[16,17]

Hypotension

The maintenance of normal blood pressure and primarily to prevent hypotension during changes in posture and abnormal physiologic states (dehydration, hemorrhage) is a critical physiologic function in humans. In common parlance, shock and hypotension are so closely associated that they are often felt to be synonymous. When hypotension is detected by the carotid baroreceptors, this sets off a cascade of neural and hormonal responses that seek to increase cardiac output by increasing heart rate, normalize blood pressure by intense vasoconstriction, and preserve volume by changes in renal handling of salt and water.[18]

The degree and duration of hypotension are critical in both the ongoing pathophysiology of cardiogenic shock and its prognosis. Catastrophic shock associated with cardiac arrest must be corrected or at least ameliorated within minutes to prevent cerebral anoxic injury. Severe hypotension, that is, mean blood pressure <50 mm Hg, may not immediately cause severe brain injury but can result in acute tubular necrosis and liver injury; organ failure at this level may be survivable but complicates and exacerbates shock with poorer outcomes. Milder degrees of hypotension may be present for weeks or even months in chronic heart failure, but frequently lead to more extreme derangement.

Increased Filling Pressures

As cardiogenic shock progresses, filling pressures usually rise. If the genesis of the shock is ischemic, then ischemia itself increases diastolic stiffness by interfering with calcium reuptake in the sarcoplasmic reticulum. When myocardial systolic performance is reduced, then systolic emptying falls and filling pressures rise.[19] An increase in filling pressures may actually be salutary in that they increase cardiac output by the Frank Starling mechanism but, very quickly, the pressures rise to levels that are detrimental.[20] Neurohormonal activation causes increased sodium reabsorption and decreased excretion of free water. Severe prolonged hypotension can result in acute tubular necrosis, so urine output may actually stop, which exacerbates fluid retention. Fluid can shift from the mesenteric bed to the central circulation, further increasing filling pressures.[21] As left atrial pressure rises, fluid moves into the lungs, increasing the work of breathing and reducing gas exchange so that ischemia may be compounded. In primarily right-sided cardiogenic shock, left-sided filling pressures are usually low and may exacerbate systemic hypotension due to inadequate left ventricular preload.

NEUROHORMONAL RESPONSE TO CARDIOGENIC SHOCK

There is a marked activation of the sympathetic nervous system in response to the reduced systemic blood pressure, which is a hallmark of cardiogenic shock. This response is mainly through arterial baroreceptors located in the carotid sinus and the aortic arch.[22,23] Indeed, many of the classic clinical signs of shock are mediated via profound activation of this system, whose key neurotransmitter is norepinephrine. Classical physical signs of shock, such as tachycardia, peripheral vasoconstriction, and cool, clammy skin, are the direct results of norephedrine's effect on the sinus node, vasoconstriction of epithelial arteries near the surface of the skin, and direct effects of the sweat glands. Norepinephrine levels are elevated both in heart failure and in acute myocardial infarction, but the levels are higher and persist longer when cardiogenic shock intervenes.[24] The increases in norepinephrine level are important systemic compensatory mechanisms to both protect blood pressure and increase cardiac output via heart rate increase and myocardial contractility, but this can come at the cost of exacerbating myocardial ischemia and promoting further myocardial cell death via the toxic effect of very high levels of norepinephrine on cardiac myocytes via apoptosis.[25]

Plasma renin levels are also elevated with myocardial infarction and acute decompensated heart failure.[26] These levels are especially elevated when blood pressure is significantly reduced.[27] Elevated renin produces secondary increases in angiotensin II and aldosterone, whose effects include maintenance of blood pressure and sodium retention. Aldosterone levels are elevated in septic shock but have not been reported so in cardiogenic shock, although higher aldosterone levels are associated with worse long-term prognosis following myocardial infarction.[28,29] NT proBNP levels may also increase after myocardial infarction, especially if shock intervenes. Extremely high levels of NT proBNP >12,000 are associated with very poor prognosis in cardiogenic shock, especially when coupled with high interleukin 6 (IL-6) levels.[30] Although angiotensin II levels are elevated in severe heart failure, a recent trial suggests that pharmacologic doses of angiotensin II may improve outcome in vasodilatory shock.[31] In late 2017, this formulation of angiotensin II was approved for clinical use.[32]

Lactic Acidosis

As a consequence of decreased oxygen delivery to tissue due to hypotension and reduced cardiac output, mitochondrial production of adenosine triphosphate (ATP) is impaired and pyruvate levels increase, resulting in increased levels of lactate, a strong acid (Fig. 2.2). A reduction in intracellular and extracellular pH has important physiologic consequences that exacerbate the shock state.[33] Reduced intracellular pH has negative effects on cardiac function by decreasing myofilament sensitivity to Ca^{++} and to adrenergic agonists.[34,35] In addition, it interferes with depolarization by enhancing K^+ egress from the cell, resulting in hyperpolization.[17] Lactic acidosis also causes adrenoreceptor internalization so that sensitivity to norepinephrine is reduced.[36,37] Finally, low intracellular PH stimulates BNIP23, which promotes apoptosis and induces nitric oxide (NO) production, which has detrimental effects.[38]

In smooth muscle cells, hyperpolarization occurs, so these cells critical to the maintenance of blood pressure cannot constrict normally, thus contributing to hypotension. Acidosis also reduces the sensitivity of vascular smooth muscle cells to the vasoconstrictor effects both of NE and angiotensin II.[17] Clearly, in some patients with cardiogenic shock, vasoconstrictive reflexes are still functional. However, as shock is prolonged and/or a vasodilatory state appears, the vascular smooth muscle beds can no longer function normally, and irreversible shock may develop. In patients resuscitated from cardiac arrest out of hospital, presenting lactate levels were highly associated with mortality; 61% of patients survived if the initial lactate levels were <5 mmol/L, whereas only 8% survived if the levels were greater than 10 mmol/L.[39]

Intravascular pH and lactate levels are important indicators of both developing shock and its severity. Lactate is a key biomarker for the detection of early shock, the severity of shock, and its successful management (Box 2.2). High lactate levels correlate strongly with prognosis in cardiogenic shock and shock from other etiologies.[40] Lactate is cleared by both the kidneys and the liver, and as these organs fail, lactate levels remain elevated even when corrective measures have restored blood pressure and cardiac output.[41] Thus, lactate may remain elevated for many hours even though pH has been corrected.

INFLAMMATORY PATHWAYS

In concert with the hemodynamic and neurohormonal abnormalities attendant with cardiogenic shock, an inflammatory response via the cytokine system plays an important role in the progressive circulatory deterioration (Fig. 2.3). IL-6 levels are increased significantly in both cardiogenic and septic shock. The actions of IL-6, which is generated and released by monocytes and T cells, contribute to the inflammatory response by an antiapoptotic effect on T cells. Geppert et al. reported that in patients with cardiogenic shock, IL-6 levels were significantly higher than in other intensive care unit patients without shock and that very high levels of IL-6 were associated with multiorgan failure.[42] IL-6, -7, -8, and -10 levels are also predictive of increased mortality.[43]

Tumor necrosis factor-alpha (TNF-α) is elevated in advanced heart failure and is in part responsible for cardiac cachexia; hence, it is also known as cachexin.[44] Produced by activated macrophages, its release is one component of the acute phase reaction and induces fever and inhibits viral replication. Inhibition of TNF-α has proven successful in some autoimmune conditions but was not successful when applied to heart failure.[45] Peak concentrations of TNF-α were higher in patients with cardiogenic shock compared to patients with acute myocardial infarctions without shock and were higher still in those whose cardiogenic shock and had a vasodilatory component.[46] C-reactive protein, like TNF-α, is also involved in the acute phase reactant produced by hepatic cells and is increased in cardiogenic shock.[47]

While the measurement of most cytokines is not available clinically, procalcitonin is a valuable, routinely used clinical biomarker. It is the precursor of calcitonin, but it has additional biochemical effects that are similar to cytokines.[48] Procalcitonin levels may be elevated in sepsis and may be useful in the early initiation of antibiotics. However, procalcitonin levels may be also elevated in cardiogenic shock without apparent bacterial infection and are indicative of a marked inflammatory response.[46]

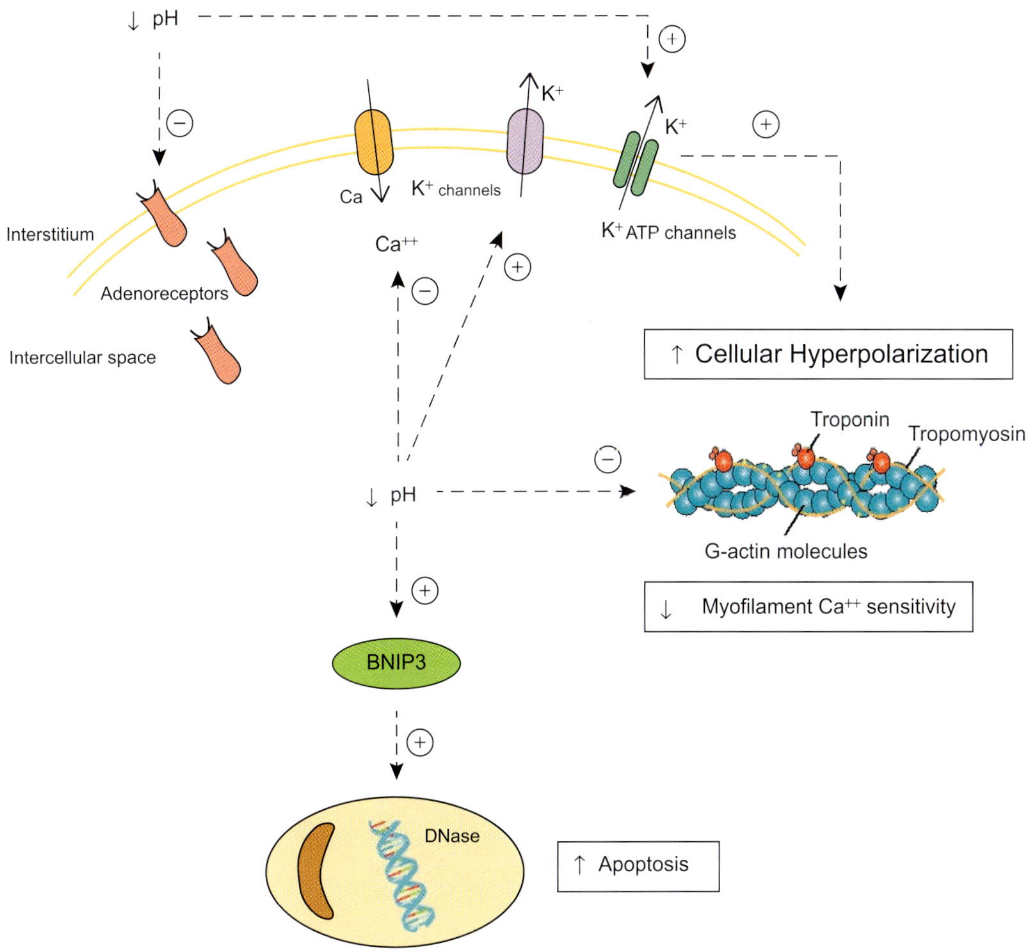

Fig. 2.2 Reduction in pH that occurs with lactic acidosis has a significant, negative impact on cellular function. Lower intracellular pH potentiates K^+ egress from cells, which results in hyperpolarization. In smooth muscle cells this interferes with normal depolarization and contraction, which exacerbates hypotension. Acidosis also is associated with a decrease in adrenergic receptors. Intracellular acidosis interferes with Ca^{++} binding of myocytes which impairs contractility. Acidosis also activates the BNIP3 gene, which is involved in apoptosis. *ATP*, Adenosine triphosphate. (From Antoine Kimmoun, Emmanuel Novy, Thomas Auchet, Nicolas Ducrocq et al, Bruno Lev., Hemodynamic consequences of severe lactic acidosis in shock states: from bench to bedside., Critical Care201721:40. http://creativecommons.org/licenses/by/4.0/.)

BOX 2.2 Generation and Effects of Lactic Acidosis in Cardiogenic Shock

Lactic acidosis—key biomarker in cardiogenic shock

- Elevated lactate levels indicate that oxygen delivery is inadequate to support normal metabolism.
- Indicates transition from aerobic to anaerobic metabolism.
- Higher lactate levels indicate more reliance on anaerobic metabolism with increased acidosis because lactate is a strong acid.
- Survival declines with higher lactate levels and lower pH.
- Organs with high metabolic needs (brain, heart, and kidney) are more dependent on aerobic metabolism and are thus more sensitive to hypoxia.
- Acidosis has multiple detrimental cellular effects, including reduced sensitivity to norepinephrine, impaired contractility, and hyperpolarization of the smooth muscle exacerbating hypotension.
- Reduction in lactate levels with shock treatment is associated with improved prognosis.
- Lactate levels may remain elevated for some time despite reduced production and clearing acidosis because of ongoing kidney and liver disease, which impairs clearance.

Nitric Oxide

NO is an important signaling molecule produced in endothelial cells, neurons, and other mammalian cell lines. The identification of NO and the elegant proof of its pivotal role in biological signaling was recognized by the awarding of the Nobel Prize to Robert Furchgott, Louis Ignarro, and Ferid Murad in 1998.[49,50] It is produced from L-arginine via nitric oxide synthetase (NOS), which is present as several isoforms whose major function in vascular endothelium is to promote vasodilation and inhibit platelet adhesion and aggregation. One isoform of NOS, inducible NOS (iNOS), can be produced in large quantities in sepsis and contribute to hypotension and vasodilatory shock.[51] High levels of NO produced via iNOS in addition can interfere with mitochondrial function and suppress myocardial function.[52,53] The precise mechanism by which iNOS is expressed at high levels is unknown, but IL-6 may play a role.[54]

Inhibitors of NO synthetase exist, and early studies showed beneficial effects in cardiogenic shock.[55,56] A large randomize trial, Tilarginine Acetate Injection in a Randomized International Study in Unstable MI Patients With Cardiogenic Shock (TRIUMPH), was undertaken to evaluate the effects of tilarginine in patients presenting

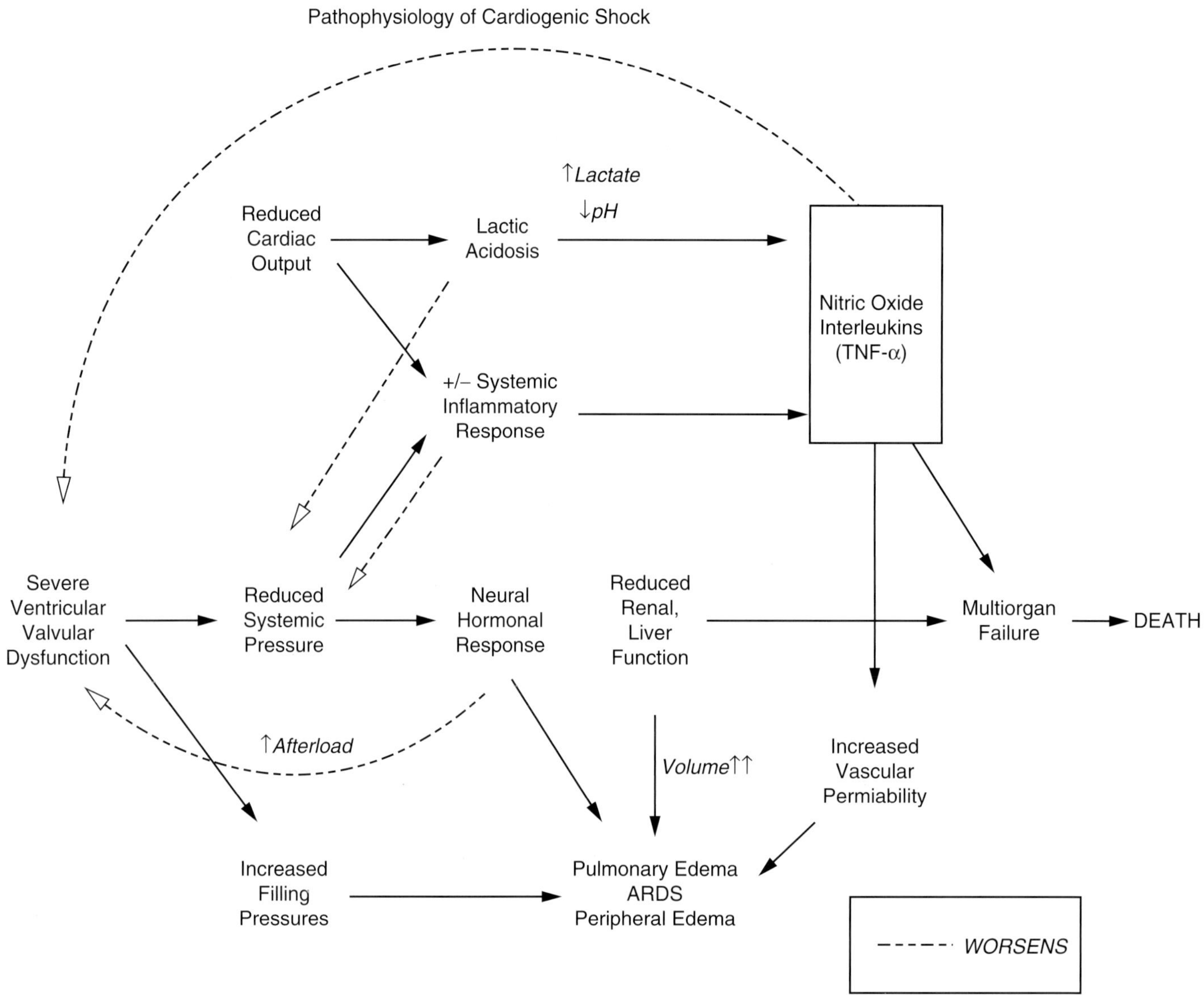

Fig. 2.3 Cardiogenic shock is a complex physiology response to hypotension and/or reduced cardiac output. The primary effect of this is a shift from aerobic to anaerobic metabolism with the elaboration of lactic acid and reduce pH. Neurohormonal and inflammatory pathways are activated by hypotension and acidosis which cause fluid retention and reduce capillary integrity. Impaired oxygen delivery and volume expansion worsen organ function and can result in multiorgan failure. *ARDS*, Acute respiratory distress syndrome; *TNF-α*, tumor necrosis factor-alpha.

with myocardial infarction and cardiogenic shock.[57] Although the agent did increase systolic blood pressure in the treatment group, the study was terminated for futility. Tilarginine is a nonspecific inhibitor of NOS, so all isoforms are affected; therefore, important intracellular isoforms may be inhibited along with the inducible form thought responsible for the high extracellular NO levels.[58]

END ORGAN INJURY

A common criterion included in the clinical definition of shock is reduced urine output. Renal function may be temporarily impaired by the onset of shock or acute tubular necrosis can ensue and renal function may never recover even if the patient survives. Renal dysfunction is common in cardiogenic shock and is a marker for increased mortality. As reported by Koreny et al. in a cohort of patients with cardiogenic shock following myocardial infarction, mortality was 87% in those who developed renal failure in the first 24 hours versus 53% in those who did not.[59] Decreased urine output and worsening renal function are the end result of many factors during the initiation and evolution of shock. Hypotension and reduced cardiac output reduce glomerular filtration pressure, although the preferential shunting of blood to the central organs may forestall this. The effects of hypotension may also be mitigated by increased levels of angiotensin II, which constrict efferent arterioles and thus increase intraglomerular pressure.[60] Conversely, high levels of norepinephrine and sympathetic stimulation cause generalized vasoconstriction, which may further diminish renal blood flow and even lead to renal ischemia. If the systemic vascular resistance is high enough to severely reduce cardiac output careful vasodilation while scrupulously maintaining blood pressure can, in rare instances of early shock, preserve renal function. However, in most cases, blood pressure cannot be supported chemically and mechanical support is required. In any case, preservation of renal function is a critical goal in shock management.

In some cases of cardiogenic shock, a vasodilatory component can occur initially or as shock becomes progressive and unrelenting. Vasodilatory shock makes maintenance of blood pressure extremely difficult as the arteriolar bed becomes resistant to pressors.[17,35] Vasopressin can be useful in some instances of vasodilatory shock because stores of vasopressin are depleted as shock continues.[17] As noted earlier, intravenous angiotensin II may show some benefit in high output shock.[31] Renal failure is almost always seen when vasodilatory shock is present.

Another important component in the setting of worsening renal function is high central venous pressure, which is rarely seen in other forms of shock but is a frequent hemodynamic finding in cardiogenic shock. The increased levels of renin, aldosterone, angiotensin II, and vasopressin all work to increase sodium and free water reabsorption when the kidneys are functioning. When they fail, volume cannot be offloaded except through dialysis and ultrafiltration. The resulting high central venous pressures cause further disruption in renal function by increasing interstitial and abdominal pressures.[61–63] Severe tricuspid regurgitation also significantly impairs renal venous outflow and is associated with a marked reduction in survival in heart failure.[64] Reduction of filling pressures to normal levels via dialysis and continuous renal replacement therapy help to maintain or restore renal function and are important components of shock management.

The liver may also be severely impacted in cardiogenic shock by similar mechanisms as the kidney, that is, passive congestive and ischemic injury.[65] At times, liver failure may be the chief presenting feature of cardiogenic shock; indeed, a cardiac etiology may not be detected initially.[66] Passive congestion of the liver without shock can result in elevation of liver enzymes to several times the normal range and mild elevation of bilirubin. If this elevation persists for years, frank cirrhosis can result. In cardiogenic shock, ischemic hepatic necrosis can be seen. Ordinarily, the liver is resistant to hypoxic injury because hepatocytes are capable of extracting almost all the oxygen from the blood to meet its considerable metabolic needs. When shock persists and necrosis ensues, this presents histologically as centrolobular necrosis of zone 3 hepatocytes without inflammation.[67] Elevations in aspartate aminotransferase (AST) and alanine aminotransferase (ALT) more than 10 times above normal may be seen with much greater increases in bilirubin. Elevations in bilirubin are an independent predictor of mortality in heart failure. Unlike the kidney, where full-blown ATN develops, the liver can recover from the shock state in a matter of days if the shock is reversed quickly enough. If shock persists, liver failure can progress, with reductions in serum albumin and the development of coagulopathies, which increase the risk of mortality.

Respiratory failure due to increased work of breathing and intractable pulmonary edema is a common complication of cardiogenic shock so that mechanical ventilation is extremely common. Elevated filling pressures play an important role, as does breakdown in capillary integrity, which can result in adult respiratory distress syndrome even if filling pressures are controlled by diuretics or renal replacement therapy.[68]

Of all the organs in the body, the central nervous system, because of its extremely high oxygen requirements, is most susceptible to hypotension in cardiogenic shock. Ordinarily, in catastrophic shock with complete cessation of cardiac function, irreversible brain injury can occur unless high-quality cardiopulmonary resuscitation (CPR) is initiated in the first 1 to 2 minutes.

CONCLUSION

Since the introduction of the concept of shock into the medical literature in the 18th century, our understanding of this dreadful and fascinating condition has benefited from the work of physicians on the battlefields, physiologists in the early 20th century, and basic scientists working out complex biochemical effects of neurohormones, cytokines, and apoptosis. As a result of this work, shock can now be diagnosed more quickly and reversed in some cases via well-placed balloons, appropriate pharmaceutical agents, and the rapid application of mechanical pumps. Nonetheless, many more patients are lost to cardiogenic shock than are saved each year. This is a major health care system problem with multiple causes, including inadequate CPR, lack of access to defibrillators, and poor management of shock. On a deeper level, the pathophysiology of shock is still incompletely understood, and thus, the means of reversing its pathophysiologic storm are not yet in our armamentarium.

REFERENCES

1. Millham FH. A brief history of shock. *Surgery*. 2010;148:1026–1037.
2. Chisolm JJ. *A Manual of Military Surgery: For the Use of the Surgeons in the Confederate Army: with an Appendix of the Rules and Regulations of the Medical Department of the Confederate Army (No. 4)*. Norman Publishing; 1861.
3. Mansell-Moulin CW. *On the Pathology of Shock. Dissertation*. London: HG Saunders; 1880.
4. Booth J. A short history of the blood pressure measurement. *Proc Roy Soc Med*. 1977;70:793–799.
5. Crile G. *George Crile: An Autobiography*. 2 Lippincott; 1947.
6. Shires T, Coln D, Carrico J, Lightfoot ST. Fluid therapy in hemorrhagic shock. *Arch Surg*. 1964;88:688–693.
7. Blalock A. Shock and hemorrhage. *Bull NY Acad of Med*. 1936;11: 610–622.
8. Thiele H, Akin I, Sandri M, et al. PCI strategies in patients with acute myocardial infarction and cardiogenic shock. *N Engl J Med*. 2017;377:2419–2432.
9. Templin C, Ghadri J, Diekmann J, et al. Clinical features and outcomes of Takotsubo (stress) cardiomyopathy. *N Engl J Med*. 2015;373:929–938.
10. Holmes DR Jr, Berger PB, Hochman JS, et al. Cardiogenic shock in patients with and without ST-segment elevation. *Circulation*. 1999;100:2067–2073.
11. Muir AL, Kirby BJ, King AJ, et al. Mixed venous oxygen saturation in relation to cardiac output in myocardial infarction. *Br Med J*. 1970;4:276–278.
12. Tan C, Rubenson D, Srivastava A, et al. Left ventricular outflow tract velocity. *Cardiovasc Ultrasound* 2017;15:18–26.
13. Mehta Y, Arora D. Newer methods of cardiac output monitoring. *World J Cardiol*. 2014;6:1022–1029.
14. Kohsaka S, Menon V, Lowe AM, et al. Systemic inflammatory response syndrome after acute myocardial infarction complicated by cardiogenic shock. *Arch Intern Med*. 2005;165:1643–1650.
15. Argenziano M, Chen JM, Choudhri AF, et al. Management of vasodilatory shock after cardiac surgery: identification of predisposing factors and use of a novel pressor agent. *J Thorac Cardiovasc Surg*. 1998;116:973–980.
16. Elkayam U, Janmohamed M, Habib M, et al. Vasodilators in the management of acute heart failure. *Crit Care Med*. 2008;36(1 suppl):S95–S105.
17. Landry DW, Oliver JA. The pathogenesis of vasodilatory shock. *N Engl J Med*. 2001;345:588–594.
18. Creager MA. Baroreceptor reflex function in congestive heart failure. *Am J Cardiol*. 1992;69:10G–16G.

19. Thune JJ, Solomon SD. Left ventricular diastolic function following myocardial infarction. *Curr Heart Fail Rep*. 2006;3:170–174.
20. Sarnoff J. Myocardial contractility as described by ventricular function curves. *Physiol Rev*. 1955;35:107–122.
21. Verbrugge FH, Dupont M. Steels, et al. Abdominal contributions to cardiorenal dysfunction in congestive heart failure. *J Amer Coll Cardiol*. 2013;62:485–495.
22. Leimbach WN Jr, Wallin BG, Victor RG, et al. Direct evidence from intraneural recordings for increased central sympathetic outflow in patients with heart failure. *Ciculation*. 1986;73:913–919.
23. Creager MA, Creager SJ. Arterial baroreflex regulation of blood pressure in patients with congestive heart Failure. *J Am Coll Cardiol*. 1994;23:401–405.
24. Benedict CR, Grahame-Smith DG. Plasma adrenaline and noradrenaline concentrations and dopamine-beta-hydroxylase activity in myocardial infarction with and without cardiogenic shock. *Br Heart J*. 1979;42: 214–220.
25. Mann DL, Kent RL, Parsons B, et al. Adrenergic effects of the biology of the mammalian cardiocyte. *Circulation*. 1992;85:790–804.
26. Vaney C, Waeber B, Turini G, et al. Renin and the complications of acute myocardial infarction. *Chest*. 1984;86:40–43.
27. Dzau VJ, Colucci WS, Hollenberg NK, et al. Relation of the renin-angiotensin-aldosterone system to clinical state in congestive heart failure. *Circulation*. 1981;63:645–651.
28. Moraes RB, Friedman G, Vianna MV, et al. Aldosterone secretion in patient with septic shock: a prospective study. *Arq Bras Endocrinol Metab*. 2013;57:636–641.
29. Palmer BR, Pilbrow AP, Frampton CM, et al. Plasma aldosterone levels during hospitalization are predictive of survival post-myocardial infarction. *Eur Heart J*. 2008;29:2489–2496.
30. Jarai R, Fellner B, Haoula D, et al. Early assessment of outcome in cardiogenic shock: relevance of the plasma N-terminal pro-B-type natriuretic peptide and interleukin-6 levels. *Crit Care Med*. 2009;37:1837–1844.
31. Chawla LS, Busse L, Brasha-Mitchell E, et al. Intravenous angiotensin II for the treatment of high-output shock (ATHOS Trial): a pilot study. *Crit Care* 2014;18:534–543.
32. FDA clears angiotensin II (Giapreza) for septic shock. *Medscape Medical News*; December 21, 2017. Accessed January 22, 2018, https://www.medscape.com/viewarticle/890494.
33. Kimmoun A, Navy E, Auchet T, et al. Hemodynamic consequences of severe lactic acidosis in shock states: from bench to bedside. *Crit Care* 2015;19:175–187.
34. Balnave CD, Vaughan-Jones RD. Effect of intracellular pH on spontaneous Ca^{2+} sparks in rat ventricular myocytes. *J Physiol*. 2000;528:25–37.
35. Huang Y-G, Wong KC, Yip W-H, et al. Cardiovascular responses to graded doses of three catecholamines during lactic and hydrochloric acidosis in dogs. *Br J Anaesth*. 1995;74:583–590.
36. Ives SJ, Andtbacka RHI, Noyes RD, et al. Alpha1-adrenergic responsiveness in human skeletal muscle feed arteries: the impact of reducing extracellular pH. *Exp Physiol*. 2013;98:256–267.
37. Marsh JD, Margolis TI, Donghee K. Mechanism of diminished contractile response to catecholamines during acidosis. *Am J Physiol*. 1988;254:H20–H27.
38. Kusbasiak LA, Hernandez OM, Bishopric NH, et al. Hypoxia and acidosis activate cardiac myocyte death through the BCL-2 family protein BNIP3. *Proc Natl Acad Sci USA*. 2002;99:12825–12830.
39. Cocchi MN, Miller J, Hunziker S, et al. The association of lactate and vasopressor need for mortality prediction in survivors of cardiac arrest. *Minerva Anestesiol*. 2011;77:1063–1071.
40. Lazzeri C, Valente S, Chiostri M, et al. Clinical significance of lactate in acute cardiac patients. *World J Cardiol*. 2015;7:483–489.
41. Attana P, Lazzeri C, Picariello C, et al. Lactate and lactate clearance in acute cardiac care patients. *Eur Heart J Acute Cardiovasc Care*. 2012;1:115–121.
42. Prondzinsky R, Unverzagt S, Lemm H, et al. Interleukin-6, -7, -8 and -10 predict outcome in acute myocardial infarction complicated by cardiogenic shock. *Clin Res Cardiol*. 2012;101:375–384.
43. Levine B, Kalman J, Mayer L, et al. Elevated circulating levels of tumor necrosis factor in severe chronic heart failure. *N Engl J Med*. 1990;323:236–241.
44. Chung ES, Packer M, Lo KH, et al. Randomized, double-blind, placebo-controlled, pilot trial of infliximab, a chimeric monoclonal antibody to tumor necrosis factor-alpha, in patients with moderate to severe heart failure: results of the anti-TNF therapy against congestive heart failure (ATTACH) trial. *Circulation*. 2003;107:3133–3140.
45. Debrunner M, Schuiki E, Minder E, et al. Proinflammatory cytokines in acute myocardial infarction with and without cardiogenic shock. *Clin Res Cardiol*. 2008;97:298–305.
46. Picariello C, Lazzeri C, Chiostri M, et al. Procalcitonin in patients with acute coronary syndromes and cardiogenic shock submitted to percutaneous coronary intervention. *Intern Emerg Med*. 2009;4: 403–408.
47. Meisner M. Update on procalcitonin measurements. *Ann Lab Med*. 2014;34:263–273.
48. Jin M, Khan AI. Procalcitonin: uses in the clinical laboratory and for the diagnosis of sepsis. *Lab Med*. 2010;41:173–177.
49. Furchgott RF, Zawadzki JV. The obligatory role of endothelial cells in the relaxation of arterial smooth muscle by acetylcholine. *Nature*. 1980;288:373–376.
50. Ignarro LJ, Byrns RE, Buga GM, et al. Endothelium-derived relaxing factor from pulmonary artery and vein possesses pharmacologic and chemical properties identical to those of nitric oxide radical. *Circ Res*. 1987;61:866–879.
51. Tsukahara Y, Morisaki T, Kojima A, et al. iNOS expression by activated neutrophils from patients with sepsis. *ANZ J Surg*. 2001;71:15–20.
52. Davidson SM, Duchen MR. Effects of NO on mitochondrial function: pathological relevance. *Cardiovasc Res*. 2006;71:10–21.
53. Tatsumi T, Matoba S, Kawahara A, et al. Cytokine-induced nitric oxide production inhibits mitochondrial energy production and impairs contractile function in rat cardiac myocytes. *J Am Coll Cardiol*. 2000;35:1338–1346.
54. Dawn B, Xuan Y-T, Guo Y, et al. IL-6 places an obligatory role in late precondition via JAK-STAT signaling and upregulation of iNOS and COX-2. *Cardiovasc Res*. 2004;64:61–71.
55. Cotter G, Kaluski E, Milo O, et al. L-NMMA (a nitric oxide synthase inhibitor) is effective in the treatment of cardiogenic shock. *Circulation*. 2000;101:1358–1361.
56. Dzavik V, Cotter G, Reynolds HR, et al. Effect of nitric oxide synthase inhibition on haemodynamics and outcomes of patients with persistent cardiogenic shock complicating acute myocardial infarction: a phase II dose-ranging study. *Eur Heart J*. 2007;28:1109–1116.
57. The TRIUMPH Investigators. Effect of tilarginine acetate in patients with acute myocardial infarction and cardiogenic shock: the TRIUMPH randomized controlled trial. *JAMA*. 2007;297:1657–1666.
58. Ndrepepa G, Schömig A, Kastrati A. Lack of benefit from nitric oxide synthase inhibition in patients with cardiogenic shock: looking for reasons. *JAMA*. 2007;297:1711–1713.
59. Koreny M, Karth GD, Geppert A, et al. Prognosis of patients who develop acute renal failure during the first 24 hours of cardiogenic shock after myocardial infarction. *Am J Med*. 2002;112:115–119.
60. Schoolworth. AC, Sica, DA, Ballermann, BJ, et al. Renal considerations in angiotensin converting enzyme inhibition therapy. *Circulation*. 2001;104:1985–1991.
61. Firth JD, Raine AE, Ledingham JG. Raised venous pressure: a direct cause of renal sodium retention in oedema? *Lancet*. 1988;1(8593):1035–1055.
62. Doty JM, Saggi BH, Sugerman HF, et al. Effect of increased renal venous pressure on renal function. *J Trauma*. 1999;47:1000–1003.

63. Mullens W, Abrahams Z, Francis G, et al. Importance of venous congestion for worsening renal function in advanced decompensated heart failure. *J Amer Coll Cardiol*. 2008;53:589–596.
64. Iida N, Seo Y, Sai S, et al. Clinical implications of intrarenal hemodynamic evaluation by Doppler ultrasonography in heart failure. *JACC Heart Fail*. 2016;8:674–682.
65. Bernal W, Wendon J. Acute liver failure. *N Engl J Med*. 2013;369:2525–2534.
66. Saner FH, Heuer M, Meyer M, et al. When the heart kills the liver: acute liver failure in congestive heart failure. *Eur J Med Res*. 2009;14:541–546.
67. Alvarez AM, Mukherjee D. Liver abnormalities in cardiac diseases and heart failure. *Int J Angiol*. 2011;20:135–142.
68. Siddall E, Khatri Minesh, Radhakrishnan J. Capillary leak syndrome: etiologies, pathophysiology, and management. *Kidney Int*. 2017;92:37–46.

3

Risk Stratification in Advanced Heart Failure

Finn Gustafsson

KEY POINTS

- Introduction
- Acute Versus Chronic Heart Failure
- Heart Failure With Preserved Ejection Fraction
- Sudden Cardiac Death Versus Progressive Heart Failure
- Elderly Versus Transplant Referral Populations
- Renal Dysfunction
- Biomarkers
- Physical Capacity and Mortality Risk in Heart Failure
- Exercise Hemodynamics
- Frailty
- Multivariable Risk Stratification in Heart Failure
- Conclusion

INTRODUCTION

Risk factors or markers for mortality in heart failure (HF) include a long list of clinical parameters, including history, physical examination, laboratory values, hemodynamics, cardiac structure and function, and biomarkers (Table 3.1).[1–3] This chapter reviews predictors of survival in HF and compares acute versus chronic HF, HF with reduced ejection fraction (HFrEF), and preserved ejection fraction (HFpEF), as well as different subpopulations such as transplant candidates and elderly patients.

Although the list of univariable predictors in Table 3.1 is long, there is no perfect prognostic indicator—a variable that, in isolation, would reliably and easily identify a patient's risk. However, some variables are more powerful than others, such as peak oxygen consumption (VO_2), which will be reviewed in detail. Additional key prognostic indicators include the New York Heart Association (NYHA) and Interagency Registry for Mechanically Assisted Circulatory Support (INTERMACS) classifications, severely reduced left ventricular ejection fraction (LVEF), hypotension (systolic blood pressure <90 mm Hg), hyponatremia, elevated B-type natriuretic peptide (BNP or NTproBNP), troponin, and renal dysfunction. However, an ideal biomarker or test—one that has high specificity and sensitivity, is reproducible, has low cost, is generally available, is easily measured, and has been prospectively tested and validated across all demographic groups—does not exist. Hence, prediction of patient prognosis in HF ultimately relies on integration of a careful clinical and laboratory evaluation interpreted in the context of the specific patient. Analysis of the many clinical and laboratory parameters can be performed using statistical models as reviewed at the end of the chapter.

ACUTE VERSUS CHRONIC HEART FAILURE

Most data on risk prognostication are derived from populations with chronic HF. However, populations with chronic and acute HF are obviously intimately connected, and for most patients, the distinction between acute and chronic HF is simply temporal. In fact, approximately two-thirds of patients admitted with HF have an antecedent diagnosis of chronic HF, and likewise, most patients with chronic HF will, at some point in time, have suffered from acute HF.[4]

Acute decompensated HF (ADHF) is a leading cause of hospitalization in the developed world. Although the rate of HF hospitalizations in the United States has decreased from >500 to approximately 400 per 100,000 individuals per year since the early 2000s,[5] more than 900,000 patients are admitted for HF every year.[6] Hospitalization as an event identifies a highly vulnerable period in the HF patient's journey: data from large US registries reveal that mortality is 3%–4% in-hospital, 10%–12% at 30 days, and 30%–40% after 1 year.[7] Rehospitalization rates are high and are generally reported to be 45%–65% within the first year.[7,8]

ADHF encompasses a heterogeneous group of patients whose clinical presentation may identify patients at very high risk. Patients admitted with cardiogenic shock after myocardial infarction have a 30-day mortality that exceeds 40%.[9] The great majority of patients admitted with ADHF are not in cardiogenic shock. In those who are, admission profiles associated with greatest risk include patients with acute myocardial infarction, ischemia as evidenced by electrocardiographic changes or elevated troponin T or I,[3] hypotension (systolic blood pressure <115 mm Hg), renal insufficiency (blood urea nitrogen [BUN] >43 mg/dL and creatinine >2.74 mg/dL), tachycardia, hyponatremia, reduced ejection fraction, increased BNP or NTproBNP, older age, and presence of multiple comorbidities.[10,11] Patients admitted who require vasoactive drugs have a poor prognosis with increased risk of death.[12] The need for inotropic support in the Acute Decompensated Heart Failure National Registry (ADHERE) study corresponded to an in-hospital mortality rate of 12% to 13%, and even higher rates have been reported outside the United States (26% in the Acute Heart Failure Global Survey of Standard Treatment [ALARM-HF] registry).[13]

In contrast, hypertensive patients (systolic blood pressure >160 mm Hg) may appear most acutely ill, but they generally have the best prognosis, with a low 60-day mortality.[14] Similarly, patients presenting with ADHF secondary to medical noncompliance, poorly

TABLE 3.1 Univariable Predictors of Survival in Heart Failure

Demographic parameters	Age, etiology, gender, race
Functional parameters	NYHA class, peak VO_2, % predicted peak VO_2, VE/VCO_2 ratio or slope, anaerobic threshold, circulatory power (peak VO_2 × systolic blood pressure), cardiac power (cardiac output × mean arterial pressure/451), oxygen kinetics (oxygen debt, recovery time), oxygen uptake efficiency slope, exercise oscillatory breathing pattern, chronotropic incompetence (i.e., failure to achieve 85% of age predicted maximum HR or low chronotropic index HR adjusted to maximal exercise test level), HR recovery, 6-minute walk test
Physical signs	↑ HR, ↓ blood pressure, S_3, BMI, mitral regurgitation
Ventricular structure and function	LVEF, ventricular volumes, mitral regurgitation severity, RVEF, tricuspid annular plane systolic excursion
Hemodynamic parameters	RAP, PVR, PCWP, cardiac output, cardiac index, LVSWI, RVSWI, dP/dt, load-corrected PCW
Laboratory values	Sodium, BUN, creatinine, hemoglobin, hypoalbuminemia, ESR, WBC, urine albumin excretion, insulin resistance, cholesterol, INR, bilirubin
Neurohormones	NE, BNP, N terminal-pro BNP, angiotensin II, aldosterone, endothelin, vasopressin, adrenomedullin, IGF-I, testosterone, copeptin, dehydroepiandrosterone, pro-ANP, MR-pro-ANP, galectin-3, tumor necrosis factor, C-reactive protein, interleukin-6, soluble CD 14
Biomarkers	Homocysteine, carbohydrate antigen 125, troponin I, troponin T, cystatin C, neutrophil gelatinase–associated lipocalin, growth differentiation factor 15, ST-2, type 1 collagen telopeptide
Electrocardiogram parameters	↑ QRS duration, ↑ Q-Tc interval, abnormal SAECG, T-wave alternans, ↓ HR variability, atrial fibrillation, ventricular tachycardia
Comorbidities	Diabetes, obesity, renal insufficiency, dementia, sleep apnea, mobility disorders
Medical therapy	Inotropes, inability to tolerate beta blockers or ACEIs
Recent heart failure hospitalization	

ACEIs, Angiotensin-converting enzyme inhibitors; *ANP*, atrial natriuretic peptide; *BMI*, body mass index; *BNP*, brain natriuretic peptide; *BUN*, blood urea nitrogen; *dP/dt*, first derivative of pressure measured over time; *ESR*, erythrocyte sedimentation rate; *HR*, heart rate; *IGF*, insulin-like growth factor type I; *INR*, international normalized ratio; *LVEF*, left ventricular ejection fraction; *LVSWI*, left ventricular stroke work index; *MR-pro-ANP*, mid-regional pro atrial natriuretic peptide; *NE*, norepinephrine; *NYHA*, New York Heart Association; *PCWP*, pulmonary capillary wedge pressure; *PVR*, peripheral vascular resistance; *RAP*, right atrial pressure; *RVEF*, right ventricular ejection fraction; *RVSWI*, right ventricular stroke work index; *SAECG*, signal averaged electrocardiogram; *VE/VCO_2*, minute ventilation to CO_2 production; *VO_2*, oxygen consumption; *WBC*, white blood cell count.

TABLE 3.2 Prognostic Indicators for Acute Decompensated Congestive Heart Failure

Admission Profile Associated With Good Outcome (Low In-Hospital Mortality)	Admission Profile Associated With Poor Outcome
Hypertensive	Elderly
Normal renal function	Blood pressure <100 mm Hg
Serum sodium >136 mEq/L	Creatinine >2.5 mg/dL
Normal troponin	Elevated troponin or ischemic ECG changes
Absence of comorbidity	Pneumonia or significant comorbidity (i.e., dementia, cancer, CVA)
Noncompliance	Good compliance with medications and diet
HFpEF	Markedly elevated BNP

BNP, B-type natriuretic peptide; *CVA*, cerebrovascular accident; *ECG*, electrocardiogram.

controlled hypertension, and normal cardiac troponin I levels also have a good prognosis (Table 3.2).

The INTERMACS classification was recently introduced to capture clinical characteristics of patients with advanced HF, both hospitalized and ambulatory. By defining seven clinically recognizable groups, patients can be categorized with specific focus on potential timing for advanced therapies, especially mechanical circulatory support (Table 3.3).[15] The INTERMACS classification has been shown to correlate with the outcome of patients, even if not managed by mechanical circulatory support. In a study of ambulatory, the 12-month overall survival in non–inotrope-dependent HF patients was 60%, 74%, and 84% in patients in INTERMACS 4, 5, and 6/7, respectively (Fig. 3.1).[16]

Hospitalization as a Prognostic Marker

Hospitalization for HF is an event indicating disease progression, increased mortality, and increased risk of early rehospitalization.[17] Analysis of the health care usage database during the period 2000–2004 in British Columbia, Canada,[18] demonstrated that successive heart failure hospitalizations were associated with incremental mortality. (Fig. 3.2). In ambulatory patients with chronic HF, hospitalization for HF is associated with a marked increase in mortality.[19]

HEART FAILURE WITH PRESERVED EJECTION FRACTION

The clinical profiles of patients with HFpEF versus HFrEF are different, with patients with HFpEF being more frequently female, elderly, hypertensive, and obese, with atrial fibrillation and chronic obstructive pulmonary disease. There is more clinical heterogeneity in HFpEF than in HFrEF. The profile of patients with LVEF in the medium range (LVEF 40%–50%), the so-called HFmrEF, resembles that of HFrEF more than HFpEF, but the prevalence of most clinical characteristics and comorbidities falls in between that of HFpEF and HFrEF.[20]

TABLE 3.3 INTERMACS Classification

INTERMACS Class	Clinical Description
1	Critical cardiogenic shock describes a patient who is "crashing and burning," in which a patient has life-threatening hypotension and rapidly escalating inotropic pressor support, with critical organ hypoperfusion often confirmed by worsening acidosis and lactate levels.
2	Progressive decline describes a patient who has been demonstrated "dependent" on inotropic support but nonetheless shows signs of continuing deterioration in nutrition, renal function, fluid retention, or other major status indicator.
3	Stable but inotrope dependent describes a patient who is clinically stable on mild–moderate doses of intravenous inotropes (or has a temporary circulatory support device) after repeated documentation of failure to wean without symptomatic hypotension, worsening symptoms, or progressive organ dysfunction (usually renal).
4	Resting symptoms describes a patient who is at home on oral therapy but frequently has symptoms of congestion at rest or with activities of daily living (ADL). He or she may have orthopnea, shortness of breath during ADL such as dressing or bathing, gastrointestinal symptoms (abdominal discomfort, nausea, and poor appetite), disabling ascites, or severe lower extremity edema.
5	Exertion intolerant describes a patient who is comfortable at rest but unable to engage in any activity, living predominantly within the house or housebound. This patient has no congestive symptoms but may have chronically elevated volume status, frequently with renal dysfunction, and may be characterized as exercise intolerant.
6	Exertion limited also describes a patient who is comfortable at rest without evidence of fluid overload but who is able to do some mild activity. ADLs are comfortable and minor activities outside the home such as visiting friends or going to a restaurant can be performed, but fatigue results within a few minutes of any meaningful physical exertion.
7	Advanced NYHA Class 3 describes a patient who is clinically stable with a reasonable level of comfortable activity, despite history of previous decompensation that is not recent.

INTERMACS, Interagency Registry for Mechanically Assisted Circulatory Support; *NYHA*, New York Heart Association.

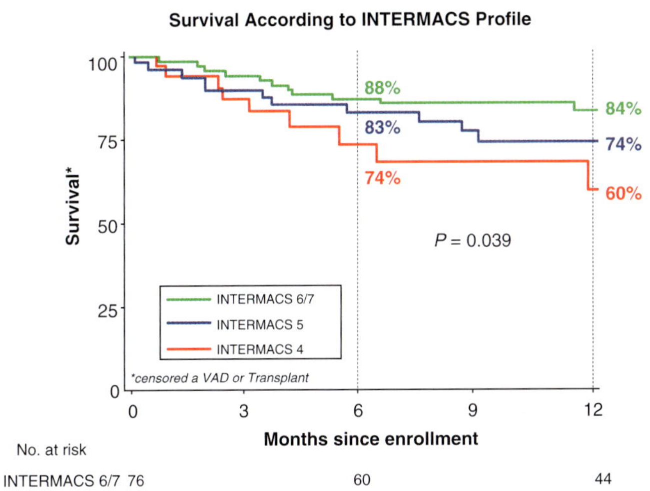

Fig. 3.1 Survival According to INTERMACS Class. Censoring occurred at ventricular assist device *(VAD)* implantation or transplantation. *INTERMACS*, Interagency Registry for Mechanically Assisted Circulatory Support. (From Stewart GC, Kittleson MM, Patel PC, et al. INTERMACS (Interagency Registry for Mechanically Assisted Circulatory Support) profiling identifies ambulatory patients at high risk on medical therapy after hospitalizations for heart failure. *Circ Heart Fail.* 2016;9.)

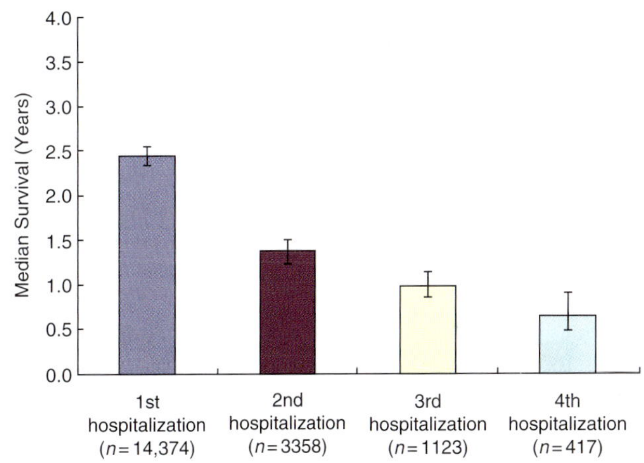

Fig. 3.2 Repeated hospitalizations predict mortality in the community population with heart failure *(HF)*. (From Setoguchi S, Stevenson LW, Schneeweiss S. Repeated hospitalizations predict mortality in the community population with heart failure. *Am Heart J.* 2007;154:260–266.)

The survival rates of patients with HFpEF are mostly reported as better than the survival rates of patients with HFrEF, especially when correcting for the considerable difference in age (Fig. 3.3).[21] The survival of patients with HFmrEF appears to be better than both for patients with HFpEF and HFrEF, underscoring that LVEF is an imperfect tool for risk stratification.[20]

Information about predictors of mortality in HFpEF is less abundant than in HFrEF. As in patients with HFrEF, age, higher NYHA class, higher BNP or NT-proBNP, expired volume-to-carbon dioxide consumption (VE/VCO_2) ratio, pulmonary artery pressures, exercise oscillatory breathing, reduced peak VO_2, renal insufficiency, diabetes, anemia, hyponatremia, dementia, and peripheral arterial disease are associated with reduced survival in HFpEF while male gender and coronary artery disease have not been identified as predictors of reduced survival in this condition.[22,23]

Cardiac amyloidosis, originally thought to be rare, has proven to be a common cause of HFpEF, affecting more than 10% of those with this diagnosis.[24] The later stages of cardiac amyloidosis are characterized by severe restrictive cardiomyopathy, and in some patients, progression to HFrEF is seen. Prognosis in cardiac amyloidosis is worse than in HFpEF associated with other etiologies. In a recent large randomized clinical trial testing tafamidis in patients with

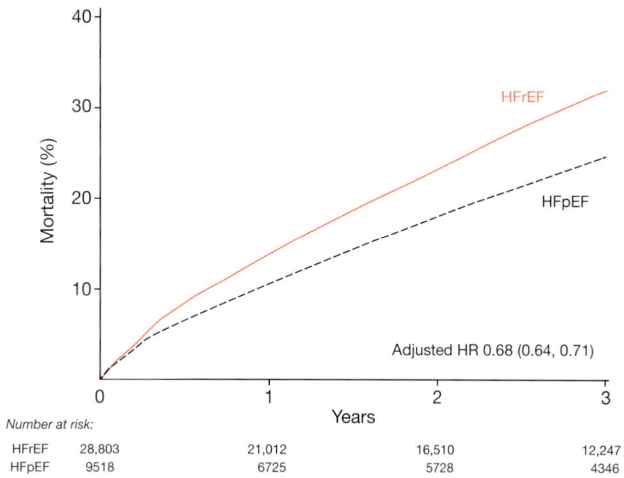

Fig. 3.3 Mortality in patients with heart failure with reduced ejection fraction *(HFrEF)* and patients with heart failure with preserved ejection fraction *(HFpEF)* in the MAGICC registry. *HR,* Hazard ratio. (From MAGGIC. The survival of patients with heart failure with preserved or reduced left ventricular ejection fraction: an individual patient data meta-analysis. *Eur Heart J.* 2012;33:1750–1757.)

transthyretin cardiac amyloidosis (mainly NYHA II–III), 43% of patients in the placebo group had died after 30 months.[25] In patients with the other major form of cardiac amyloid, light chain or primary amyloidosis, mortality is even higher, with reported 2-year mortality rates exceeding 50%.[26] Troponin I or T and especially BNP or NT-proBNP have emerged as potent plasma markers of mortality in cardiac amyloidosis.

SUDDEN CARDIAC DEATH VERSUS PROGRESSIVE HEART FAILURE

Historically, up to 50% of patients with HF have died suddenly, the majority from malignant ventricular arrhythmias. The use of primary and secondary prophylactic defibrillators has changed this picture in populations where defibrillator use is widespread. However, even in populations with low uptake of implantable cardioverter defibrillator (ICD) therapy, the rate of sudden cardiac death (SCD) has declined. In a recent analysis of randomized drugs trials in HF over the last 20 years, the annual rate of SCD decreased from more than 6% to 3%.[27] The proportion of SCD to total mortality, however, was constant at approximately 30%–40% in these trials.

The incidence of SCD is higher in patients with mild HF than in patients with advanced disease, likely because of a higher risk of death from pump failure in the latter population.[28] Data from MERIT-HF (Metoprolol CR/XL Randomised Intervention Trial in Congestive Heart Failure) showed that the distribution of the mode of death changes as HF advances.[29] In patients with NYHA class II chronic HF, 64% of the deaths were classified as sudden death, and 12% were due to progressive HF, whereas in patients with NYHA class IV chronic HF, 33% died suddenly, and 56% died of progressive HF. In particular, beta-blockers and spironolactone have contributed to a reduction in the incidence of both sudden deaths and progressive HF deaths. Parameters that have been identified as prognostic indicators for SCD include the presence of severely reduced LVEF; ischemic etiology; prolonged QRS duration; presence of nonsustained ventricular tachycardia; prior episode of SCD; history of syncope; elevated BNPs; and in patients with an ischemic etiology, abnormal T-wave alternans.[30–32] Elevated ST2, an interleukin-1 receptor family member, which has effects on myocardial fibrosis, has been reported to be predictive of SCD complementary to BNP.[33] In addition, cardiac imaging using gadolinium late enhancement magnetic resonance imaging may identify patterns of myocardial fibrosis associated with a high risk of SCD both in ischemic and nonischemic cardiomyopathy.[34,35]

ELDERLY VERSUS TRANSPLANT REFERRAL POPULATIONS

The incidence of HF rises exponentially with age, and the average age of patients admitted with HF is >75 years in most contemporary epidemiological studies. However, most of the literature describing the prognosis of outpatients has been derived from younger and middle-aged white male patients being evaluated for advanced HF therapies, including clinical trials or cardiac transplantation. The demographic profile of HF in elderly patients is distinct, with a greater percentage of female patients, a higher proportion of HFpEF, and more comorbidities.[36] Recent studies have to some extent addressed this, as seen in studies like Get With the Guidelines (GWTG) study now enrolling >300,000 hospitalized HF patients with a median age of 75 years.[37] However, most studies that include a high proportion of elderly patients fail to provide information about prognostic indicators beyond simple clinical and laboratory values. The use of modalities such as advanced imaging and invasive hemodynamics in elderly individuals and the predictive power of these are still poorly described.

RENAL DYSFUNCTION

Renal dysfunction is extremely common in HF. Among patients hospitalized for decompensated HF, more than 60% have moderate or severely reduced estimated GFR (eGFR) (<60 mL/min) irrespective of cardiac systolic function.[38] Serum creatinine and BUN have been identified in numerous studies as powerful prognostic factors in patients with acute and chronic HF. Hillege and coworkers[39] showed that reduced eGFR was a continuous risk factor and that patients with an eGFR <44 mL/min had twice the long-term mortality of those with normal renal function.

Similarly, development of worsening renal function during hospitalization for HF is associated with poor clinical outcomes. However, recent studies have clearly shown that eGFR cannot be viewed in isolation in HF, since changes induced by angiotensin-converting enzyme inhibitors or mineralocorticoid receptor antagonists (MRAs) are not associated with poor outcomes[40] and since a decrease in eGFR during an admission for HF is detrimental only if accompanied by lack of decongestion.[41] Hence, when using eGFR, creatinine, and BUN to evaluate prognosis in HF, they should be interpreted in a clinical context, incorporating medical therapy as well as the congestive state of the patient.

BIOMARKERS

As discussed earlier, no ideal biomarker has been described yet, but of all the prognostic biomarkers currently identified, BNP comes closest to that ideal parameter. This measurement entails an easily obtainable, rapidly processed, inexpensive blood test that has excellent sensitivity and good specificity for HF. BNP has very significant negative predictive accuracy for the diagnosis of HF.[42] Another valuable biomarker in acute and chronic HF is serum troponin, both in patients with acute coronary syndrome and in patients with nonischemic ADHF.[35]

Natriuretic Peptides

Natriuretic peptides have become a cornerstone in the diagnosis and management of HF. The vast majority of studies have used BNP or

NT-proBNP, but atrial peptides, such as mid-regional pro atrial natriuretic peptide (MR pro-ANP), have also been demonstrated as a reliable biomarker in HF. It is currently a class I recommendation to use natriuretic peptides both for diagnosis and prognostication in HF.[43] A low level of natriuretic peptide effectively rules out HF, whereas elevated levels do not necessarily indicate HF, as peptide specificity is modest, at best, in outpatients or patients presenting with acute dyspnea.[42, 44] Elevated levels of natriuretic peptides are associated with worse outcomes both in patients with mild HF and patients with advanced HF. However, while not necessarily linear,[45] the risk function is continuous. As such, BNP values must be interpreted in a clinical context with the other markers mentioned here. Furthermore, it should be recognized that female gender and low body weight are associated with higher levels of natriuretic peptides irrespective of cardiac function. Also, cardiac (such as atrial fibrillation) and noncardiac conditions (such as renal dysfunction) increase BNP/NT-proBNP and changes should be evaluated in this context. Finally, it should be emphasized that neprilysin inhibitors, such as sacubitril/valsartan, specifically increase BNP, but not proBNP.[46] Consequently, to use natriuretic peptides for monitoring of patients treated with neprilysin inhibitors, NT-proBNP must be applied.

Changes in natriuretic peptides carry even greater prognostic information, and hence, these markers are useful for longitudinal follow up. This finding has led to studies testing the hypothesis that BNP-driven pharmacological strategy would be superior to one guided by clinical judgment. However, so far, outcomes have not been improved convincingly with BNP-guided treatment strategies in HF.[47,48]

Metabolic and Inflammatory Markers

Metabolic markers such as serum cholesterol, uric acid, and hemoglobin have been variably reported to be predictive of outcome in HF patients. An inverse relationship between serum cholesterol and survival has been described in patients with HF, likely reflecting malnutrition and cachexia as poor prognostic factors.[49] Insulin resistance is commonly observed in patients with HF and is associated with worse prognosis.[50] Hyperuricemia is another metabolic abnormality associated with an adverse prognosis.

Elevations in bilirubin and international normalized ratio (INR) are believed to reflect right HF and are important markers of outcome, especially in patients treated with advanced therapies such as left ventricular assist devices (LVADs).

Subclinical inflammation is detectable in many patients with HF. Several biomarkers that have been identified as indicators of poor prognosis may simply reflect the degree of systemic or local inflammation (i.e., C-reactive protein, tumor necrosis factor, and interleukin-6, ST-2).[51]

PHYSICAL CAPACITY AND MORTALITY RISK IN HEART FAILURE

Six-Minute Walk Test

Inability to exercise is the cardinal symptom of chronic HF. Functional capacity is assessed in chronic HF by NYHA criteria, but even if studies show that, indeed, patients with NYHA class II HF have higher exercise capacity than do patients with NYHA class III–IV HF,[52] the assessment of NYHA class remains highly subjective. The 6-minute walk test (i.e., the distance walked over a period of 6 minutes) is less subjective than NYHA functional class but it can be heavily influenced by the motivation of the patient, tester, or both. Additionally, it is important to recognize that the 6-minute walk test is close to a maximal exercise test in some patients with advanced HF, whereas in patients with NYHA class II HF, it is a test of submaximal exercise tolerance. However, the 6-minute walk test has several advantages: it is reproducible, easy to perform, and inexpensive.

Importantly, the 6-minute walk test provides prognostic information as demonstrated by the SOLVD (Study of Left Ventricular Dysfunction) investigators, who showed in a substudy of 898 HF patients in their registry that mortality risk was 3.7 times higher in patients with a 6-minute walk distance less than 350 m compared with patients who walked more than 450 m. Similarly, the risk of HF hospitalization was also higher in patients with reduced walk distance.[53] Subsequent investigators have shown prognostic value of the 6-minute walk test in some cohorts,[54] while others have not.[55]

Maximal Oxygen Uptake and Prognosis in Heart Failure

Determination of peak oxygen uptake during a maximal symptom limited treadmill or bicycle exercise test is the most objective method to assess maximal functional capacity in patients with chronic HF and has been shown to be an excellent indicator of prognosis.

Peak VO_2 can be calculated from the Fick principle: peak VO_2 is the product of peak cardiac output and maximal arteriovenous oxygen difference. Because the maximal arteriovenous difference is similar among most sedentary individuals, peak VO_2 provides an indirect assessment of cardiac output reserve, and this largely underlies the effectiveness of peak VO_2 in risk stratification in HF. Several peripheral factors may also affect peak VO_2, such as the metabolic activity of skeletal muscle mass, endothelial function, and demographics such as age and gender. As HF severity increases, skeletal muscle mass and its metabolic activity both decrease, and endothelial function is progressively impaired, and this may add to the prognostic utility of peak VO_2.

To contribute with valid prognostic information, measurements of peak VO_2 must be accurate and it must be ensured that the value measured is representative of the patient's maximal exercise effort. Patients with comorbidity, such as arthritis, may terminate the test before achieving their peak VO_2. Several methods exist to ensure maximal effort such as a plateau in the VO_2 to power (watt) relationship, greatly elevated plasma lactate (>18 mM), or, most commonly used, an elevated respiratory exchange ratio (RER; the ratio between expired CO_2 and consumed O_2) (Fig. 3.4). An RER >1.05 is generally accepted as a measure of sufficient exercise to validate the peak VO_2 results on a cardiopulmonary exercise test.[56]

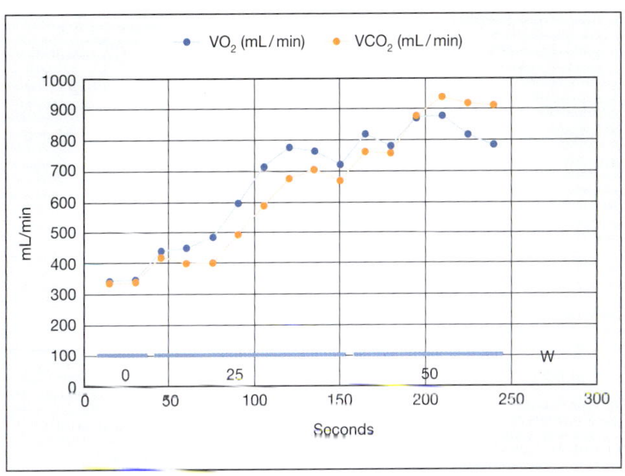

Fig. 3.4 Example of an exercise test with measurement of peak VO_2 dilated cardiomyopathy. *VCO_2*, Carbon dioxide consumption; *VO_2*, oxygen consumption; *RER*, respiratory exchange ratio.

The use of peak VO_2 to determine prognosis in patients with HF was first described by Szlachcic and colleagues.[57] In 27 patients, they reported a 77% 1-year mortality rate for patients with VO_2 less than 10 mL/kg/min and a 21% mortality rate for patients with VO_2 10 to 18 mL/kg/min. In a prospective study of 114 ambulatory patients with chronic HF referred for cardiac transplantation, a VO_2 of less than 14 mL/kg/min was used as a criterion for acceptance for cardiac transplantation.[47] Patients were divided into three groups based on the results of their cardiopulmonary stress tests: patients with a peak VO_2 less than 14 mL/kg/min were accepted as transplant candidates (group 1; $n = 35$); transplant was deferred for patients with a peak VO_2 greater than 14 mL/kg/min (group 2; $n = 52$); and group 3 ($n = 27$) comprised patients with a peak VO_2 less than 14 mL/kg/min who had a significant comorbidity that precluded transplant. Age, LVEF, and resting hemodynamic parameters were similar in all three groups. In patients with VO_2 greater than 14 mL/kg/min, 1-year survival was 94%. Accepted transplant candidates with VO_2 less than 14 mL/kg/min had a 1-year survival of 70%; patients with a significant comorbidity and VO_2 less than 14 mL/kg/min had a 1-year survival of 47%. Patients accepted for transplant had a falsely elevated survival because all transplants were treated as a censored observation. If urgent transplant was counted as death, the 1-year survival decreased to 48%. This approach permitted the identification of candidates whose transplant could be safely deferred.

Analysis of peak VO_2 normalized by a predicted maximum based on age, obesity, and gender has been performed to determine if better prognostication can be achieved using percentage of predicted peak VO_2. Some investigators have suggested the superiority of this approach especially in young patients, whereas others have shown no clear benefit.[58,59]

Use of serial measurements of peak VO_2 has also been shown to effectively identify patients in a low-risk category over time.[60] Conversely, a significant decline usually parallels clinical worsening and a worse prognosis; this is particularly important as the therapy for cardiac diseases continues to evolve and improve. Since the initial report of the value of peak VO_2 in guiding transplant candidate selection in 1991, there have been many advances in the treatment of HF. In particular, the use of beta blockade and ICDs has had a significant impact on long-term survival without significantly improving peak VO_2. Whether VO_2 has retained its predictive power with the advent of beta-blockers and ICDs has been the subject of several reports,[61,62] but in conclusion, peak VO_2 remains a key parameter in the evaluation of candidates for mechanical circulation support cardiac transplantation.

During cardiopulmonary exercise testing, many variables are collected that also provide prognostic information. Ventilatory response to exercise, most frequently measured by the VE/VCO_2 ratio or slope, has been found by several investigators to be even more predictive of outcome than peak VO_2.[63] The abnormal VE/VCO_2 response results from increased ventilation-perfusion mismatching and heightened chemosensitivity and ergoreflex responses. This heightened ventilatory response is present from the onset of exercise, and in contrast to peak VO_2, the VE/VCO_2 relationship does not require a maximal effort. However, there is no consensus on how best to derive this parameter. Both VE/VCO_2 ratios and slopes have been reported (i.e., VE/VCO_2 ratio at anaerobic threshold or at peak exercise and VE/VCO_2 slope from onset of exercise to the anaerobic threshold or throughout the total exercise period). The VE/VCO_2 slope derived throughout exercise testing appears to have the greatest prognostic power. A VE/VCO_2 greater than 34 has been the cut point selected in many studies, but similar to peak VO_2, this parameter is a continuous variable with no absolute cut point. Published studies have shown a VE/VCO_2 ratio greater than 30 conferring increased risk, with the worst prognosis associated with a VE/VCO_2 ratio greater than 40.[64]

VE/VCO_2 correlates more strongly with pulmonary pressures measured during exercise than does peak VO_2. Both peak VO_2 and VE/VCO_2 are frequently found to have independent prognostic power. The combination of VE/VCO_2 and peak VO_2 may provide the strongest determination of risk. A patient with a preserved peak VO_2 and an abnormal VE/VCO_2 remains at greater risk than if the ventilatory response was normal. Similarly, with the converse situation, in which peak VO_2 is severely reduced but VE/VCO_2 is normal, the patient remains at increased risk despite the normal ventilatory response. Patients with severely reduced VO_2 (<10 mL/kg/min) and large VE/VCO_2 (>40) are in the poorest survival group. Peak VO_2 and VE/VCO_2 slope provide independent and complementary data on prognosis and should be used together to assess risk.

Most data on the use of peak VO_2 has been obtained in patients with HFrEF. The cardiopulmonary response of patients with HFpEF is essentially indistinguishable from the response of patients with systolic dysfunction.[65] Recent studies have shown that both peak VO_2 and VE/VCO_2 slope are also independent predictors of mortality in HFpEF and HFmrEF, but more data are required to standardize the use of peak VO_2 for prognostication in HF patients without reduced ejection fraction.[66,67]

EXERCISE HEMODYNAMICS

Invasively measured resting hemodynamics are surprisingly modest indicators of mortality risk in HF. Data from the Evaluation study of congestive heart failure and pulmonary artery catheterization effectiveness (ESCAPE) and other studies have showed that elevated filling pressures (pulmonary capillary wedge [PCW] pressure and/or right atrial pressure) at rest have predictive power, whereas cardiac index does not.[68,69] Small- to moderate-sized studies have investigated the use of hemodynamic parameters obtained during exercise as risk predictors in HF. The prognostic superiority of hemodynamically derived exercise variables over peak VO_2 was first shown by Griffin and associates.[70] In HFpEF, exercise hemodynamic testing is gaining popularity as an important diagnostic tool, and peak PCW pressure corrected for workload has been shown to correlate well with survival.[71]

FRAILTY

Frailty has been recognized as a risk marker in geriatrics for decades and has more recently been introduced in the field of HF, including the subgroup of patients with advanced HF. Frailty is defined as "a biological syndrome that reflects a state of decreased physiological reserve and vulnerability to stressors."[72] Multiple definitions of frailty have been used in cardiovascular medicine, but Fried's phenotype has been used most consistently in HF studies.[73] Fried's criteria include unintended weight loss (>5% or 5 kg within last year), exhaustion (self-reported), inactivity (self-reported, e.g., < 2.5 hours/week), slowness (5-m walk test), and grip strength (measured by a dynamometer). Some studies have suggested that the predictive value of the score is increased if cognitive measures are added.[74] Using most definitions, frailty is present in 30%–60% of patients hospitalized for HF and similarly so in patients referred electively for heart transplantation or LVAD evaluation.[75–77] In the majority of studies, frailty in HF is associated with age and female gender but is independent of ejection fraction, NT-proBNP, and blood pressure.[77]

It was described more than 10 years ago that frailty is associated with HF mortality,[78] but more recently, the predictive power of frailty in patients evaluated for transplantation or MCS has been described. The majority of studies show a significant and independent association between frailty and reduced survival after LVAD implantation.[79,80] However, it should be emphasized that the various components of the frailty complex can be modified by interventions directed against the underlying pathophysiology, such as LVAD therapy in advanced HF. Patients in whom frailty is reversed by advanced HF therapy, such as transplantation or implantation of an LVAD, likely have considerably improved chance of long-term survival. Hence, frailty scores should be used cautiously to exclude patients from destination LVAD therapy or heart transplantation.[81]

MULTIVARIABLE RISK STRATIFICATION IN HEART FAILURE

Risk prediction based on a single variable does not make efficient use of routinely obtained clinical measures of known prognostic significance. Multivariable risk models can incorporate a range of prognostic information, often reflecting different pathophysiologic aspects and phenotypic characteristics of the clinical condition, to improve prognostic accuracy. A large number of models describing outcome in both inpatients and outpatients have been published over the last two decades. Some are purely based on clinical parameters, mostly available at the bedside, whereas others incorporate specific biomarkers beyond plasma sodium and creatinine. Authors of several models provide online calculators for easy determination of 1- or 5-year mortality risk. While these tools have attracted much scientific interest, the role they play in daily management of HF patients is less clear as their use has not been documented to improve patient outcomes. One challenge is that different models may yield very different outcome predictions for the individual patient. Also, the models' distinction between inpatients and outpatients is, to some extent, problematic in practice: if a patient is reviewed the day after a HF hospitalization, would his/her mortality risk suddenly change dramatically compared with 2 days earlier, just before discharge? These factors underscore that the survival models can be used only as supportive tools for decision making, and if used, it is advisable to apply at least two models. They are, however, particularly useful when considering advanced therapies, such as cardiac transplantation or LVADs, as they may inform discussions with patients and relatives, as well as other stakeholders in the therapeutic process, for instance, payers. Furthermore, they are very helpful in HF research for estimation of sample sizes in the design of clinical trials.

Models for Inpatients

Commonly used models used for inpatients are listed in Table 3.4. Using the ADHERE database of more than 33,000 patients hospitalized for HF, Fonarow and coworkers[11] created a simple bedside tool for risk stratification of individuals hospitalized with ADHF. The value of 39 clinical predictors of HF death was evaluated during the period 2001–2003. More than 40% of patients had HFpEF, and patients were, on average, 73 years. Although the overall in-hospital mortality was only 4%, the risk stratification model could differentiate individuals at very low risk (mortality 2.1%), low-intermediate risk (5.5% and 6.4%), intermediate-high risk (12.4%), and very high risk for in-hospital death (21.9%). When the model was applied to more than 33,000 patient hospitalizations in a validation cohort, the model's predictive ability was well maintained.

Another predictive model of mortality in acute HF was derived from a retrospective analysis of data obtained from the Canadian Enhanced Feedback for Effective Cardiac Treatment (EFFECT) study, which included more than 4000 individuals admitted with the primary diagnosis of HF.[82] In hospital, 30-day, and 1-year mortality rates were 9%, 11%, and 33%. A multivariable risk score for predicting 30-day and 1-year mortality was derived from independent predictors of mortality and was calculated according to specific point allotments. The 30-day and 1-year mortality rates were similar in a validation group of 1400 inpatients with HF. The discriminative ability of the model to predict mortality was slightly higher for patients with HFrEF (receiver operating characteristic curve area of 0.81 at 30 days) than for all patients with HF (receiver operating characteristic curve area of 0.79 at 30 days). The model incorporates comorbidities that would be contraindicated in transplantation and does not include measures of functional capacity. These limitations render this model inapplicable for formal use in patients undergoing evaluation for transplantation or mechanical circulatory support until prospective validation studies for this population are performed. An online version of the EFFECT model can be found at http://www.ccort.ca/Research/CHFRiskModel.html.

The Get With Guidelines program is a large registry that provided a model for estimation of in-hospital mortality risk in 27,850 patients

TABLE 3.4 Inpatient Heart Failure Risk Prediction Models

Model	Derivation Cohort Size	Factors Associated With High Mortality Risk
OPTIMIZE-HF	48,612	Age Increased sCr Low p-sodium Increased HR Liver disease Prior CVA Peripheral vascular disease Caucasian LV systolic dysfunction COPD
EFFECT	4031	Age Increased respiratory rate Low plasma sodium Anemia Increased BUN Cerebrovascular disease Dementia Cancer COPD Liver cirrhosis
ADHERE	33,046	Elevated BUN Elevated sCr
GWTG program (in-hospital mortality)	27,850	Age Systolic BP COPD Hyponatremia Heart rate Non-black race BUN

ADHERE, acute decompensated heart failure national registry; *BUN,* blood urea nitrogen; *COPD,* chronic obstructive pulmonary disease; *CVA,* cerebrovascular accident; *EFFECT,* enhanced feedback for effective cardiac treatment; *GWTG,* get with the guidelines; *HR,* heart rate; *LV,* left ventricle.

and validated the model in more than 11,000 patients.[83] The group more recently has updated the model incorporating biomarkers, e.g., troponin and BNP.[84] A recent analysis compared the performance of the GWTG, EFFECT, and ADHERE models in more than 13,000 patients admitted with HF and found that they performed remarkably similar with C-statistics values between 0.68 and 0.70.[85]

It is important to recognize that the models apply only to populations similar to those in which the model was derived. All of the inpatient models include a much more heterogeneous sample than would be suitable for heart transplantation (especially with respect to age and comorbidity), and none of these models have been validated in a heart transplant candidate sample.

Models for Outpatients

The Heart Failure Survival Score (HFSS) was the first prospectively validated multivariable risk stratification model constructed to predict survival in patients with HF.[86] The score was derived from a cohort evaluated from 1986 to 1991 and subsequently validated in another cohort during the period 1993–1995. All patients were ambulatory, younger than 70 years, had an LVEF of 40% or less, and were able to perform cardiopulmonary exercise testing. Only 10% were receiving a beta-blocker. Independent predictors of mortality included an ischemic etiology for HF, resting heart rate, low ejection fraction, bundle branch block, low blood pressure, low peak VO_2, and serum sodium. Based on this, a risk score is calculated. Patients with high-risk and medium-risk HFSS were considered appropriate for cardiac transplant referral.

The HFSS tool was generated before the widespread use of many therapeutic interventions known to improve HF mortality, including beta-blockers, aldosterone inhibitors, ICDs, and biventricular pacemakers, but the model has subsequently been validated in more contemporary cohorts.[61,87]

The Seattle Heart Failure Model (SHFM) was developed by Levy and coworkers[88] to predict 1-year, 2-year, and 3-year survival in outpatients with HF. The SHFM is simple to use and employs variables that do not rely on a patient's ability to complete cardiopulmonary stress testing. Web-based SHFM calculators can be found at http://depts.washington.edu/shfm and an application for smartphone can be downloaded (Fig. 3.5). The model was partially derived from the patients in the PRAISE (Prospective Randomized Amlodipine Survival Evaluation) cohort, which included 1125 patients with an ejection fraction less than 30% and NYHA functional class IIIB and IV symptoms. Hazard ratios for certain HF medications and devices (defibrillators and biventricular pacemakers) were derived from published randomized trials or meta-analyses owing to low baseline rates of use (e.g., 0% were receiving a beta blocker and 0% had an implantable cardioverter-defibrillator) in the PRAISE derivation cohort.

The SHFM model has been validated in five independent samples. In addition to predicting survival, the model is useful for showing the expected mortality benefit of adding a medication or device to a patient's HF management. The SHFM has subsequently been investigated in a sample of patients presenting to an advanced HF clinic for transplant evaluation,[89] but it has been shown that the SHFM tends to underestimate mortality in patients with the greatest observed mortality.

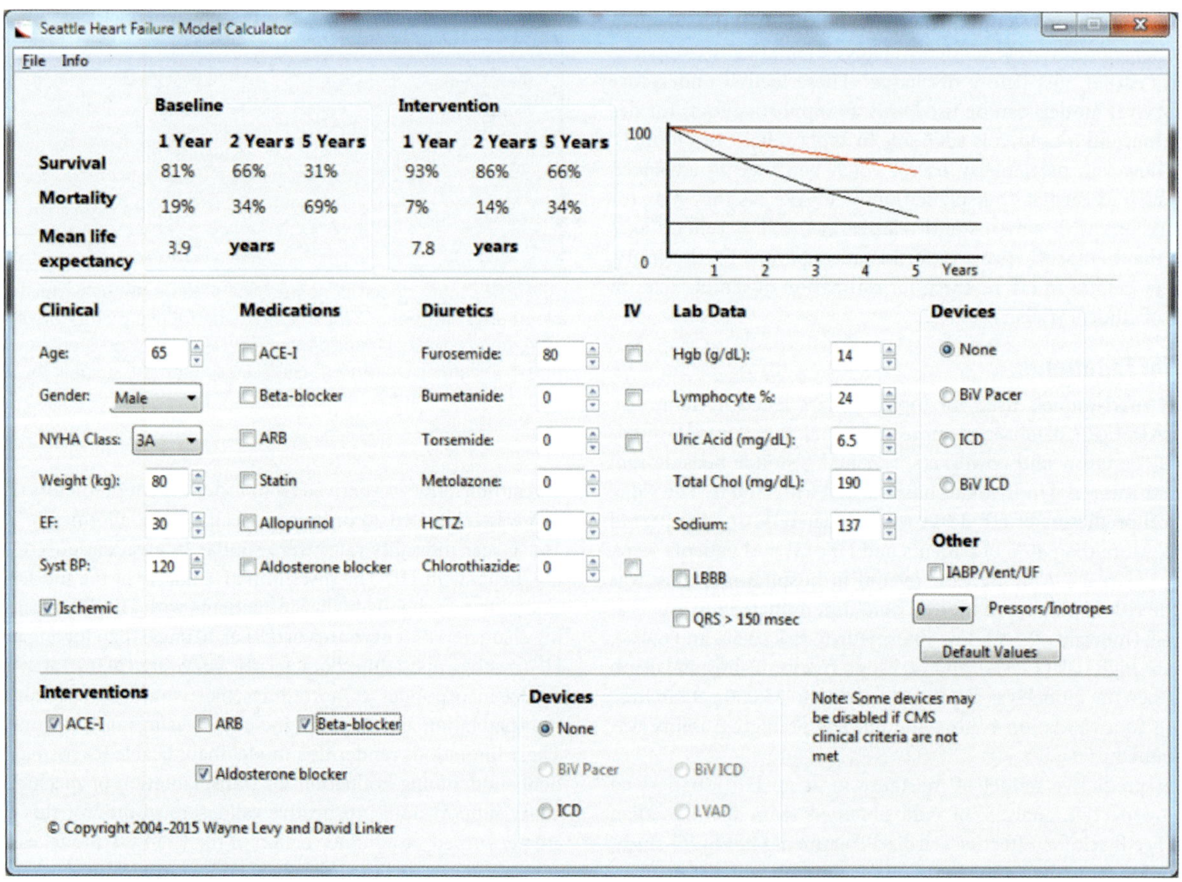

Fig. 3.5 Seattle Heart Failure Model Screen. Note the curve depicting the expected survival *(black)* and the curve showing the expected survival after the chosen intervention *(red)*.

Since the publication of these two first important survival models in HF outpatients, additional models have emerged, including the Gruppo Italiano per lo Studio della Sopravvivenza nell'Insufficienza Cardiaca Heart Failure (GISSI-HF) trial and the Meta-Analysis Global Group in Chronic Heart Failure (MAGICC HF) risk score.[90,91] The latter is based on data from 30 trials and registries and has gained widespread use. It can be calculated easily with an online calculator (www.heartfailurerisk.org). A review from 2014 identified more than 60 published models and concluded that the design of the models was very different but finally included a few common variables predictive of mortality: age, renal function, blood pressure, blood sodium level, LVEF, sex, natriuretic peptide, NYHA functional class, diabetes, body mass index, and exercise capacity.[92]

The clinical utility of the prediction models for outpatients is still under debate. In a recent analysis, the performance of MAGICC, GISSI-HF, SHFM, and the Candesartan in Heart Failure Assessment of Reduction in Mortality and morbidity (CHARM) model were applied to more than 6000 patients in the European Society of Cardiology (ESC) long-term HF registry. The models tended to overestimate mortality, but like previous analyses, the C-statistic was above 0.7 for all models.[93] The question remains whether this is sufficient for use in individual patients. Clearly, there is no evidence that one model is better than another, and great caution must be exercised when a model is applied to individual patients. Further, these models must be constantly updated as new outcome modifying interventions are implemented in clinical practice. Hopefully, future studies will evaluate use of these models as part of an HF management strategy and provide firm evidence for their utility.

CONCLUSION

Since the 1990s, a wealth of information on the prognosis and prognostic markers of HF has become available. Use of clinical data, measures of end-organ function, and powerful biomarkers such as natriuretic peptides has increased our ability to predict outcome in HF significantly, and the field continues to evolve. In chronic advanced HF, evaluation of physical and cardiovascular reserve using cardiopulmonary exercise test with measurement of oxygen uptake remains important in the prediction of long-term outcome and are a cornerstone in the selection of patients for heart transplantation and mechanical circulatory support. In recent years, multivariable risk models have been developed and validated, and they may assist in decision making owing to their objectivity. However, they all have limitations, and at the current time, therapeutic strategies cannot be based on these models alone. Hopefully, future work will refine the models, ensuring validity in broader HF cohorts and allowing for more dynamic changes in risk factors, so that they finally may be used safely in the individual patient.

REFERENCES

1. Khush KK, Tasissa G, Butler J, et al. Effect of pulmonary hypertension on clinical outcomes in advanced heart failure: analysis of the Evaluation Study of Congestive Heart Failure and Pulmonary Artery Catheterization Effectiveness (ESCAPE) database. *Am Heart J*. 2009;157:1026–1034.
2. Chen WC, Tran KD, Maisel AS. Biomarkers in heart failure. *Heart*. 2010;96:314–320.
3. Pocock WF 4th, De Marco T, Fonarow GC, et al. Cardiac troponin and outcome in acute heart failure. *N Engl J Med*. 2008;358:2117–2126.
4. Nieminen MS, Brutsaert D, Dickstein K, et al. EuroHeart Failure Survey II (EHFS II): a survey on hospitalized acute heart failure patients: description of population. *Euro Heart J*. 2006;27:2725–2736.
5. Akintoye E, Briasoulis A, Egbe A, et al. National Trends in Admission and In-Hospital Mortality of Patients With Heart Failure in the United States (2001–2014). *J Am Heart Assoc*. 2017;6(12).
6. Benjamin EJ, Virani SS, Callaway CW, et al. Heart Disease and Stroke Statistics—2018 Update: a report from the American Heart Association. *Circulation*. 2018;137:e67–e492.
7. Kociol RD, Hammill BG, Fonarow GC, et al. Generalizability and longitudinal outcomes of a national heart failure clinical registry: comparison of Acute Decompensated Heart Failure National Registry (ADHERE) and non-ADHERE Medicare beneficiaries. *Am Heart J*. 2010;160:885–892.
8. Maggioni AP, Dahlstrom U, Filippatos G, et al. EURObservational Research Programme: regional differences and 1-year follow-up results of the Heart Failure Pilot Survey (ESC-HF Pilot). *Eur J Heart Fail*. 2013;15:808–817.
9. Poss J, Koster J, Fuernau G, et al. Risk stratification for patients in cardiogenic shock after acute myocardial infarction. *J Am Coll Cardiol*. 2017;69:1913–1920.
10. Gheorghiade M, Abraham WT, Albert NM, et al. Systolic blood pressure at admission, clinical characteristics, and outcomes in patients hospitalized with acute heart failure. *JAMA*. 2006;296:2217–2226.
11. Fonarow GC, Adams KF, Abraham WT, et al. Risk stratification for in-hospital mortality in acutely decompensated heart failure: classification and regression tree analysis. *JAMA*. 2005;293:572–580.
12. Abraham WT, Adams KF, Fonarow GC, et al. In-hospital mortality in patients with acute decompensated heart failure requiring intravenous vasoactive medications: an analysis from the Acute Decompensated Heart Failure National Registry (ADHERE). *J Am Coll Cardiol*. 2005;46:57–64.
13. Mebazaa A, Parissis J, Porcher R, et al. Short-term survival by treatment among patients hospitalized with acute heart failure: the global ALARM-HF registry using propensity scoring methods. *Intensive Care Med*. 2011;37:290–301.
14. Fonarow GC, Stough WG, Abraham WT, et al. Characteristics, treatments, and outcomes of patients with preserved systolic function hospitalized for heart failure: a report from the OPTIMIZE-HF registry. *J Am Coll Cardiol*. 2007;50:768–777.
15. Stevenson LW, Couper G. On the fledgling field of mechanical circulatory support. *J Am Coll Cardiol*. 2007;50:748–751.
16. Stewart GC, Kittleson MM, Patel PC, et al. INTERMACS (Interagency Registry for Mechanically Assisted Circulatory Support) profiling identifies ambulatory patients at high risk on medical therapy after hospitalizations for heart failure. *Circ Heart Fail*. 2016;9(11).
17. Ahmed A, Allman RM, Fonarow GC, et al. Incident heart failure hospitalization and subsequent mortality in chronic heart failure: a propensity-matched study. *J Card Fail*. 2008;14:211–218.
18. Setoguchi S, Stevenson LW, Schneeweiss S. Repeated hospitalizations predict mortality in the community population with heart failure. *Am Heart J*. 2007;154:260–266.
19. Gustafsson F, Schou M, Videbaek L, et al. Incidence and predictors of hospitalization or death in patients managed in multidisciplinary heart failure clinics. *Eur J Heart Fail*. 2009;11:413–419.
20. Lauritsen J, Gustafsson F, Abdulla J. Characteristics and long-term prognosis of patients with heart failure and mid-range ejection fraction compared with reduced and preserved ejection fraction: a systematic review and meta-analysis. *ESC Heart Fail*. 2018;5:685–694.
21. The survival of patients with heart failure with preserved or reduced left ventricular ejection fraction. an individual patient data meta-analysis. *Euro Heart J*. 2012;33:1750–1757.
22. Owan TE, Hodge DO, Herges RM, et al. Trends in prevalence and outcome of heart failure with preserved ejection fraction. *N Engl J Med*. 2006;355:251–259.
23. Acikel S, Akdemir R, Kilic H, et al. Diastolic heart failure in elderly: the prognostic factors and interventions regarding heart failure with preserved ejection fraction. *Int J Cardiol*. 2010;138:311–313.
24. Gonzalez-Lopez E, Gallego-Delgado M, Guzzo-Merello G, et al. Wild-type transthyretin amyloidosis as a cause of heart failure with preserved ejection fraction. *Euro Heart J*. 2015;36:2585–2594.

25. Maurer MS, Schwartz JH, Gundapaneni B, et al. Tafamidis treatment for patients with transthyretin amyloid cardiomyopathy. *N Engl J Med.* 2018;379:1007–1016.
26. Damy T, Jaccard A, Guellich A, et al. Identification of prognostic markers in transthyretin and AL cardiac amyloidosis. *Amyloid.* 2016;23:194–202.
27. Shen L, Jhund PS, Petrie MC, et al. Declining risk of sudden death in heart failure. *N Engl J Med.* 2017;377:41–51.
28. Goldstein S. The changing epidemiology of sudden death in heart failure. *Curr Heart Fail Rep.* 2004;1:93–97.
29. Effect of metoprolol CR/XL in chronic heart failure. Metoprolol CR/XL Randomised Intervention Trial in Congestive Heart Failure (MERIT-HF). *Lancet.* 1999;353:2001–2007.
30. Olshansky B, Poole JE, Johnson G, et al. Syncope predicts the outcome of cardiomyopathy patients: analysis of the SCD-HeFT study. *J Am Coll Cardiol.* 2008;51:1277–1282.
31. Salerno-Uriarte JA, De Ferrari GM, Klersy C, et al. Prognostic value of T-wave alternans in patients with heart failure due to nonischemic cardiomyopathy: results of the ALPHA study. *J Am Coll Cardiol.* 2007;50:1896–1904.
32. Berger R, Huelsman M, Strecker K, et al. B-type natriuretic peptide predicts sudden death in patients with chronic heart failure. *Circulation.* 2002;105:2392–2397.
33. Pascual-Figal DA, Ordonez-Llanos J, Tornel PL, et al. Soluble ST2 for predicting sudden cardiac death in patients with chronic heart failure and left ventricular systolic dysfunction. *J Am Coll Cardiol.* 2009;54:2174–2179.
34. Almehmadi F, Joncas SX, Nevis I, et al. Prevalence of myocardial fibrosis patterns in patients with systolic dysfunction: prognostic significance for the prediction of sudden cardiac arrest or appropriate implantable cardiac defibrillator therapy. *Circ Cardiovasc Imaging.* 2014;7:593–600.
35. Perazzolo Marra M, De Lazzari M, Zorzi A, et al. Impact of the presence and amount of myocardial fibrosis by cardiac magnetic resonance on arrhythmic outcome and sudden cardiac death in nonischemic dilated cardiomyopathy. *Heart Rhythm.* 2014;11:856–863.
36. Chaudhry SI, Wang Y, Gill TM, et al. Geriatric conditions and subsequent mortality in older patients with heart failure. *J Am Coll Cardiol.* 2010;55:309–316.
37. Patel DB, Shah RM, Bhatt DL, et al. Guideline-appropriate care and in-hospital outcomes in patients with heart failure in teaching and nonteaching hospitals: findings from get with the guidelines-heart failure. *Circ Cardiovasc Qual Outcomes.* 2016;9:757–766.
38. Gustafsson F, Torp-Pedersen C, Brendorp B, et al. Long-term survival in patients hospitalized with congestive heart failure: relation to preserved and reduced left ventricular systolic function. *Eur Heart J.* 2003;24:863–870.
39. Hillege HL, Nitsch D, Pfeffer MA, et al. Renal function as a predictor of outcome in a broad spectrum of patients with heart failure. *Circulation.* 2006;113:671–678.
40. Rossignol P, Cleland JG, Bhandari S, et al. Determinants and consequences of renal function variations with aldosterone blocker therapy in heart failure patients after myocardial infarction: insights from the Eplerenone Post-Acute Myocardial Infarction Heart Failure Efficacy and Survival Study. *Circulation.* 2012;125:271–279.
41. Metra M, Davison B, Bettari L, et al. Is worsening renal function an ominous prognostic sign in patients with acute heart failure? The role of congestion and its interaction with renal function. *Circ Heart Fail.* 2012;5:54–62.
42. Gustafsson F, Steensgaard-Hansen F, Badskjaer J, et al. Diagnostic and prognostic performance of N-terminal ProBNP in primary care patients with suspected heart failure. *J Card Fail.* 2005;11:S15–S20.
43. Yancy CW, Jessup M, Bozkurt B, et al. ACC/AHA/HFSA focused update of the 2013 ACCF/AHA Guideline for the Management of Heart Failure: a report of the American College of Cardiology/American Heart Association Task Force on Clinical Practice Guidelines and the Heart Failure Society of America. *Circulation 2017.* 2017;136:e137–e161.
44. Maisel AS, Krishnaswamy P, Nowak RM, et al. Rapid measurement of B-type natriuretic peptide in the emergency diagnosis of heart failure. *N Engl J Med.* 2002;347:161–167.
45. Schou M, Gustafsson F, Corell P, et al. The relationship between N-terminal pro-brain natriuretic peptide and risk for hospitalization and mortality is curvilinear in patients with chronic heart failure. *Am Heart J.* 2007;154:123–129.
46. Solomon SD, Zile M, Pieske B, et al. The angiotensin receptor neprilysin inhibitor LCZ696 in heart failure with preserved ejection fraction: a phase 2 double-blind randomised controlled trial. *Lancet.* 2012;380:1387–1395.
47. Schou M, Gustafsson F, Videbaek L, et al. Adding serial N-terminal pro brain natriuretic peptide measurements to optimal clinical management in outpatients with systolic heart failure: a multicentre randomized clinical trial (NorthStar monitoring study). *Eur J Heart Fail.* 2013;15: 818–827.
48. Shah MR, Califf RM, Nohria A, et al. The STARBRITE trial: a randomized, pilot study of B-type natriuretic peptide-guided therapy in patients with advanced heart failure. *J Card Fail.* 2011;17:613–621.
49. Rauchhaus M, Clark AL, Doehner W, et al. The relationship between cholesterol and survival in patients with chronic heart failure. *J Am Coll Cardiol.* 2003;42:1933–1940.
50. Doehner W, Rauchhaus M, Ponikowski P, et al. Impaired insulin sensitivity as an independent risk factor for mortality in patients with stable chronic heart failure. *J Am Coll Cardiol.* 2005;46:1019–1026.
51. Shirazi LF, Bissett J, Romeo F, et al. Role of inflammation in heart failure. *Curr Atheroscler Rep.* 2017;19:27.
52. Russell SD, Saval MA, Robbins JL, et al. New York Heart Association functional class predicts exercise parameters in the current era. *Am Heart J.* 2009;158:S24–S30.
53. Bittner V, Weiner DH, Yusuf S, et al. Prediction of mortality and morbidity with a 6-minute walk test in patients with left ventricular dysfunction. SOLVD Investigators. *JAMA.* 1993;270:1702–1707.
54. Alahdab MT, Mansour IN, Napan S, et al. Six minute walk test predicts long-term all-cause mortality and heart failure rehospitalization in African-American patients hospitalized with acute decompensated heart failure. *J Card Fail.* 2009;15:130–135.
55. Guazzi M, Dickstein K, Vicenzi M, et al. Six-minute walk test and cardiopulmonary exercise testing in patients with chronic heart failure: a comparative analysis on clinical and prognostic insights. *Circ Heart Fail.* 2009;2:549–555.
56. Mehra MR, Canter CE, Hannan MM, et al. The 2016 International Society for Heart Lung Transplantation listing criteria for heart transplantation: a 10-year update. *J Heart Lung Transplant.* 2016;35:1–23.
57. Szlachcic J, Massie BM, Kramer BL, et al. Correlates and prognostic implication of exercise capacity in chronic congestive heart failure. *Am J Cardiol.* 1985;55:1037–1042.
58. Aaronson KD, Mancini DM. Is percentage of predicted maximal exercise oxygen consumption a better predictor of survival than peak exercise oxygen consumption for patients with severe heart failure? *J Heart Lung Transplant.* 1995;14:981–989.
59. Stelken AM, Younis LT, Jennison SH, et al. Prognostic value of cardiopulmonary exercise testing using percent achieved of predicted peak oxygen uptake for patients with ischemic and dilated cardiomyopathy. *J Am Coll Cardiol.* 1996;27:345–352.
60. Lund LH, Aaronson KD, Mancini DM. Validation of peak exercise oxygen consumption and the Heart Failure Survival Score for serial risk stratification in advanced heart failure. *Am J Cardiol.* 2005;95:734–741.
61. O'Neill JO, Young JB, Pothier CE, et al. Peak oxygen consumption as a predictor of death in patients with heart failure receiving beta-blockers. *Circulation.* 2005;111:2313–2318.
62. Lund LH, Aaronson KD, Mancini DM. Predicting survival in ambulatory patients with severe heart failure on beta-blocker therapy. *Am J Cardiol.* 2003;92:1350–1354.
63. Kleber FX, Vietzke G, Wernecke KD, et al. Impairment of ventilatory efficiency in heart failure: prognostic impact. *Circulation.* 2000;101: 2803–2809.
64. Balady GJ, Arena R, Sietsema K, et al. Clinician's guide to cardiopulmonary exercise testing in adults: a scientific statement from the American Heart Association. *Circulation.* 2010;122:191–225.
65. Farr MJ, Lang CC, Lamanca JJ, et al. Cardiopulmonary exercise variables in diastolic versus systolic heart failure. *Am J Cardiol.* 2008;102:203–206.
66. Sato T, Yoshihisa A, Kanno Y, et al. Cardiopulmonary exercise testing as prognostic indicators: comparisons among heart failure patients with reduced, mid-range and preserved ejection fraction. *Euro J Prev Cardiol.* 2017;24:1979–1987.

67. Shafiq A, Brawner CA, Aldred HA, et al. Prognostic value of cardiopulmonary exercise testing in heart failure with preserved ejection fraction. The Henry Ford HospITal CardioPulmonary EXercise Testing (FIT-CPX) project. *Am Heart J*. 2016;174:167–172.
68. Cooper LB, Mentz RJ, Stevens SR, et al. Hemodynamic predictors of heart failure morbidity and mortality: fluid or flow? *J Card Fail*. 2016;22:182–189.
69. Damman K, van Deursen VM, Navis G, et al. Increased central venous pressure is associated with impaired renal function and mortality in a broad spectrum of patients with cardiovascular disease. *J Am Coll Cardiol*. 2009;53:582–588.
70. Griffin BP, Shah PK, Ferguson J, et al. Incremental prognostic value of exercise hemodynamic variables in chronic congestive heart failure secondary to coronary artery disease or to dilated cardiomyopathy. *Am J Cardiol*. 1991;67:848–853.
71. Dorfs S, Zeh W, Hochholzer W, et al. Pulmonary capillary wedge pressure during exercise and long-term mortality in patients with suspected heart failure with preserved ejection fraction. *Euro Heart J*. 2014;35:3103–3112.
72. Afilalo J, Alexander KP, Mack MJ, et al. Frailty assessment in the cardiovascular care of older adults. *J Am Coll Cardiol*. 2014;63:747–762.
73. Fried LP, Tangen CM, Walston J, et al. Frailty in older adults: evidence for a phenotype. *J Gerontol A Biol Sci Med Sci*. 2001;56:M146–M156.
74. Jha SR, Hannu MK, Gore K, et al. Cognitive impairment improves the predictive validity of physical frailty for mortality in patients with advanced heart failure referred for heart transplantation. *J Heart Lung Transplant*. 2016;35:1092–1100.
75. Denfeld QE, Winters-Stone K, Mudd JO, et al. The prevalence of frailty in heart failure: a systematic review and meta-analysis. *Int J Cardiol*. 2017;236:283–289.
76. Jha SR, Hannu MK, Chang S, et al. The prevalence and prognostic significance of frailty in patients with advanced heart failure referred for heart transplantation. *Transplantation*. 2016;100:429–436.
77. Vidan MT, Blaya-Novakova V, Sanchez E, et al. Prevalence and prognostic impact of frailty and its components in non-dependent elderly patients with heart failure. *Eur J Heart Fail*. 2016;18:869–875.
78. Cacciatore F, Abete P, Mazzella F, et al. Frailty predicts long-term mortality in elderly subjects with chronic heart failure. *Eur J Clin Invest*. 2005;35:723–730.
79. Chung CJ, Wu C, Jones M, et al. Reduced handgrip strength as a marker of frailty predicts clinical outcomes in patients with heart failure undergoing ventricular assist device placement. *J Card Fail*. 2014;20:310–315.
80. Dunlay SM, Park SJ, Joyce LD, et al. Frailty and outcomes after implantation of left ventricular assist device as destination therapy. *J Heart Lung Transplant*. 2014;33:359–365.
81. Maurer MS, Horn E, Reyentovich A, et al. Can a left ventricular assist device in individuals with advanced systolic heart failure improve or reverse frailty? *J Am Geriatr Soc*. 2017;65:2383–2390.
82. Lee DS, Austin PC, Rouleau JL, et al. Predicting mortality among patients hospitalized for heart failure: derivation and validation of a clinical model. *Jama*. 2003;290:2581–2587.
83. Peterson PN, Rumsfeld JS, Liang L, et al. A validated risk score for in-hospital mortality in patients with heart failure from the American Heart Association Get With the Guidelines Program. *Circ Cardiovasc Qual Outcomes*. 2010;3:25–32.
84. Eapen ZJ, Liang L, Fonarow GC, et al. Validated, electronic health record deployable prediction models for assessing patient risk of 30-day rehospitalization and mortality in older heart failure patients. *JACC Heart Fail*. 2013;1:245–251.
85. Lagu T, Pekow PS, Shieh MS, et al. Validation and comparison of seven mortality prediction models for hospitalized patients with acute decompensated heart failure. *Circ Heart Fail*. 2016;9(8).
86. Aaronson KD, Schwartz JS, Chen TM, et al. Development and prospective validation of a clinical index to predict survival in ambulatory patients referred for cardiac transplant evaluation. *Circulation*. 1997;95:2660–2667.
87. Butler J, Khadim G, Paul KM, et al. Selection of patients for heart transplantation in the current era of heart failure therapy. *J Am Coll Cardiol*. 2004;43:787–793.
88. Levy WC, Mozaffarian D, Linker DT, et al. The Seattle Heart Failure Model: prediction of survival in heart failure. *Circulation*. 2006;113: 1424–1433.
89. Kalogeropoulos AP, Georgiopoulou VV, Giamouzis G, et al. Utility of the Seattle Heart Failure Model in patients with advanced heart failure. *J Am Coll Cardiol*. 2009;53:334–342.
90. Barlera S, Tavazzi L, Franzosi MG, et al. Predictors of mortality in 6975 patients with chronic heart failure in the Gruppo Italiano per lo Studio della Streptochinasi nell'Infarto Miocardico-Heart Failure trial: proposal for a nomogram. *Circ Heart Fail*. 2013;6:31–39.
91. Pocock SJ, Ariti CA, McMurray JJ, et al. Predicting survival in heart failure: a risk score based on 39, 372 patients from 30 studies. *Euro Heart J*. 2013;34:1404–1413.
92. Rahimi K, Bennett D, Conrad N, et al. Risk prediction in patients with heart failure: a systematic review and analysis. *JACC Heart Fail*. 2014;2:440–446.
93. Canepa M, Fonseca C, Chioncel O, et al. Performance of prognostic risk scores in chronic heart failure patients enrolled in the european society of cardiology heart failure long-term registry. *JACC Heart Fail*. 2018;6:452–462.

4

Candidate Selection and Decision Making in Mechanical Circulatory Support

Larry A. Allen, Randall C. Starling

KEY POINTS

INTRODUCTION

Deciding who should and who should not proceed with mechanical circulatory support (MCS)—including timing and device type—is one of the most difficult challenges in medicine. While there are now over 6 million people in the United States with heart failure (HF) and millions more worldwide, only a fraction of these patients will receive MCS. The reasons for this are multiple: patients die before MCS can be considered; cardiac anatomy and physiology limit the feasibility or effectiveness of MCS; complications during temporary MCS preclude longer-term durable MCS; patients have noncardiac comorbidity that makes MCS problematic or of minimal benefit to overall health; socioeconomic factors challenge the ability to manage MCS in the outpatient setting; and some patients simply do not wish to pursue MCS. Some of these decisions can be relatively straightforward, for example, a 30-year-old woman with left-ventricular-predominant peripartum cardiomyopathy rapidly failing medical therapy who "will do anything" to optimize her chances for survival or an 81-year-old man with severe HF with preserved ejection fraction and moderate dementia. However, countless factors go into appropriate decision making around MCS, creating a spectrum of eligibility further complicated by high levels of uncertainty. This all occurs within the context of patients often facing near-certain death without MCS or the premise of taking on major potential burdens with MCS. Although each case is unique and constantly evolving, approaching MCS candidate selection and decision making with clear principles and guidelines grounds this complex process. This chapter attempts to create a general framework from which clinicians can think through MCS candidacy for each individual patient. It is meant to be complementary to the 2013 International Society for Heart and Lung Transplantation (ISHLT) Guidelines on Mechanical Circulatory Support, which include multiple recommendations on MCS candidacy.[1] Much of the decision making for MCS candidacy has roots in processes developed for heart transplantation, and thus, a review of the 2016 ISHLT Listing Criteria for Heart Transplantation may provide further context.[2]

INDICATIONS FOR MECHANICAL CIRCULATORY SUPPORT

The role of MCS has evolved over time based on improving technology, increasing experience, and changes to the broader landscape of HF epidemiology and care. MCS was originally used for hours to days in patients who failed to wean from cardiopulmonary bypass after cardiotomy. With the development of pulsatile left ventricular assist devices (LVADs) designed to support patients for months, eligibility was widened, primarily to include bridge-to-transplant (BTT) patients with refractory HF or shock while on an active heart-transplant waiting list. With the relative success of these pulsatile devices and particularly with the improved durability of new-generation continuous-flow devices, longer-term durable MCS to include patients ineligible for transplantation has become possible as destination therapy (DT). Meanwhile, improvements in temporary external MCS—percutaneous ventricular assist devices and extracorporeal membranous oxygenation (ECMO)—have also expanded the ease and rapidity of supporting "crash and burn" Interagency Registry for Mechanically Assisted Circulatory Support (INTERMACS) 1 patients in frank cardiogenic shock with multiorgan failure,[3] which then facilitates refined assessment of eligibility and provides additional time for decision making. The result is that options for MCS have expanded greatly, broadening candidate selection across a greater range of disease (Fig. 4.1). However, given the surgical risks, frequent adverse events, patient and caregiver burdens, and the high costs of existing technologies, MCS will remain a "last resort" limited to certain patients with HF who have entered a severe end-stage phase of the disease. Use of MCS for "less ill" patients will necessitate improved technology with reduced adverse events and improvement in cost effectiveness.

Bridge to Transplant

Policies from the United Network for Organ Sharing (UNOS) and others have increasingly prioritized the use of donors for the sickest patients.[4] This has had a significant impact on the use of LVADs for BTT. With the ability to stabilize transplant-eligible patients with

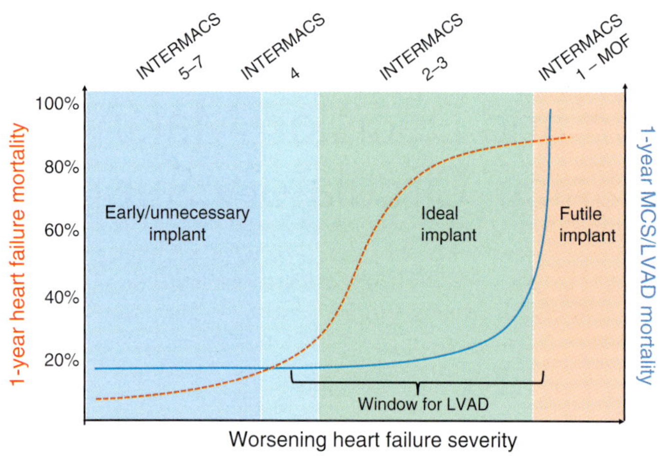

Fig. 4.1 INTERMACS clinical categories and mortality with ongoing medical therapy versus LVAD.[3] *HF*, Heart failure; *INTERMACS*, Interagency Registry for Mechanically Assisted Circulatory Support; *LVAD*, left ventricular assist device; *MCS*, mechanical circulatory support; *MOF*, multiorgan failure.

durable LVAD, thereby resulting in a higher transplant priority status for those MCS patients going forward, the remaining non-MCS patients at the lowest status now rarely undergo transplantation. This change toward performing transplantation on the sickest patients and continual increases in waiting time for non-MCS patients has contributed to pretransplant use of LVADs, now with more than half of patients having LVADs at the time of heart transplantation.[5] Further changes to the UNOS allocation system in 2018 promise to further increase the use of MCS prior to transplantation,[6] although further prioritization of the sickest patients may shift BTT MCS from durable LVAD to temporary forms of support.[7] Despite this growth in BTT MCS over time, the relatively fixed donor pool limits the number of transplants per year (~3000 annually in the United States) and caps the number of possible BTT LVADs.

Destination Therapy

Given the limited heart donor pool and complications related to transplantation, MCS has always been seen as a permanent alternative to transplantation, i.e., DT. However, not until the Randomized Evaluation of Mechanical Assistance for the Treatment of Congestive Heart Failure (REMATCH) study[8] in 2001 were MCS technologies and techniques advanced enough to consider LVAD as permanent therapy for large numbers of patients. Since REMATCH, and primarily driven by the increased durability of continuous-flow devices, DT LVAD outcomes have improved, and DT LVAD use has increased.[3] While BTT and DT LVADs tend to look essentially the same in terms of the devices and procedures involved, there are important differences. Patients considering DT have reasons they are not BTT candidates—e.g., advanced age, multiple comorbidities, or suboptimal social determinants of health—and these reasons can make living with the device more difficult, as well as worsen postimplantation survival and quality of life (QoL). Furthermore, the framework for decision making may be different, as DT LVAD patients do not have a "bail out option in the event of complications (e.g. recurrent gastrointestinal bleeding or infection) or dissatisfaction with the device.

Non-MCS Alternatives

Indications for MCS are framed by other available treatment options. There are relatively few alternative strategies to MCS for candidates who progress into irreversible cardiogenic shock. Intravenous inotropes can be used effectively in the short term for some patients awaiting transplant (either in hospital or at home). However, data from several studies have shown that the long-term outcome with LVAD is significantly better than continued use of intravenous inotropes.[9,10] Contemporary use of inotropes has seen improved outcomes, perhaps because of better patient selection.[11] Ongoing medical management with a shift to palliation is also an alternative[12] and remains the most common approach for the vast majority of patients dying from HF. Therefore, decisions about how to proceed with patients slipping into INTERMACS category 3 remain challenging and dependent on multiple patient factors. Recent evidence has also shown that both patient and physician perceptions of illness severity, risk of death, and need for advanced therapies in non–inotrope-dependent patients are likely underestimated.[13–15]

Timing

The most frequent question debated by MCS experts and industry is based on defining "ideal timing" for MCS therapy. Recent data suggest that there is a relatively narrow window for MCS. Clinical events can be useful as milestones marking the transition to end-stage disease and, thus, triggers for consideration of MCS (see the I-NEED-HELP mnemonic[16] in Table 4.1). That said, earlier LVAD implantation in patients not yet showing frank end-organ dysfunction while on oral therapies has not appeared to markedly improve post-LVAD survival compared with patients who continued with medical therapy with the potential for delayed LVAD implantation and exposes patients earlier to the operative and longer term risks of LVAD.[17] Thus, until patients have irreversible disease severity that markedly reduces quantity or quality of life, durable LVAD is generally delayed. This must be tailored to each patient; often, objective measures (6-minute walk and peak oxygen consumption) may meet MCS criteria, but the patient feels that his/her QoL is acceptable and must be balanced with the total burden

TABLE 4.1 The "I-NEED-HELP" Clinical Events That Suggest Transition to End-Stage Heart Failure (Stage D)[16]

I	Inotropes	Previous or ongoing requirement for dobutamine, milrinone, dopamine, norepinephrine, etc.
N	NYHA class/ natriuretic peptides	Persisting NYHA III or IV and/or persistently high BNP or NT-proBNP
E	End-organ dysfunction	Worsening renal or liver dysfunction in the setting of heart failure
E	Ejection fraction	Very low ejection fraction <20%
D	Defibrillator shocks	Recurrent appropriate defibrillator shocks
H	Hospitalizations >1	Hospitalizations with heart failure in last 12 months
E	Edema/escalating diuretics	Persisting fluid overload and/or increasing diuretic requirement
L	Low blood pressure	Consistently low BP with systolic <90–100 mm Hg
P	Prognostic medication	Inability to up-titrate (or particularly the need to decrease/cease) ACEI, ARB, ARNI, β-blocker, and MRA

ACEI, Angiotensin-converting enzyme inhibitor; *ARB*, angiotensin receptor blocker; *ARNI*, angiotensin receptor-neprilysin inhibitor; *BNP*, brain natriuretic peptide; *BP*, blood pressure; *MRA*, mineralocorticoid receptor antagonist; *NYHA*, New York Heart Association; *NT*, N-terminal pro B-type natriuretic peptide.

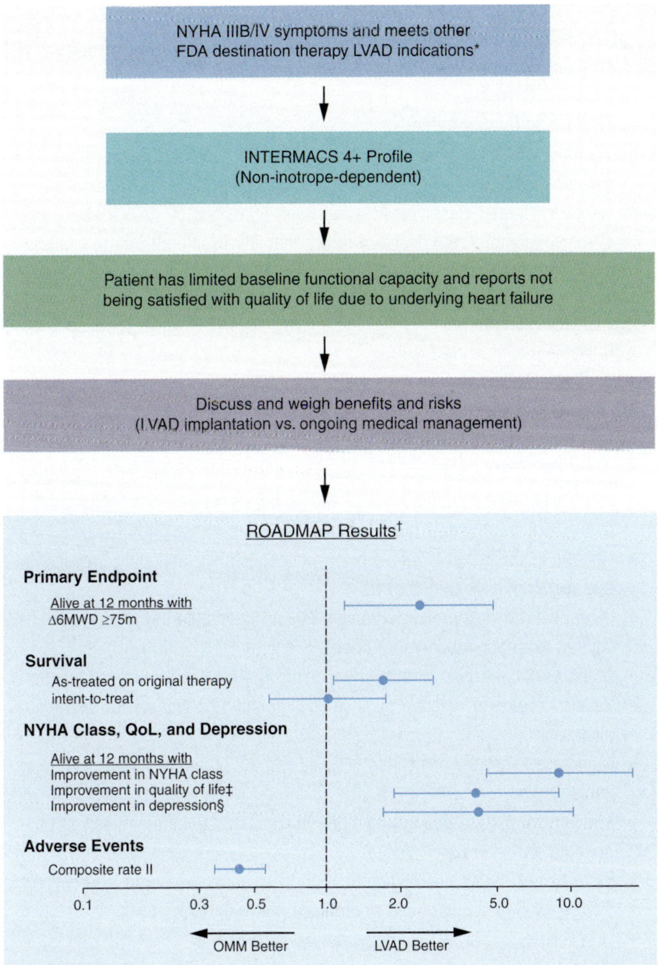

Fig. 4.2 Algorithm to guide decisions on non–inotrope dependent patients with advanced heart failure (INTERMACS 4–7). *6MWD*, 6-minute walk distance; *FDA*, Food and Drug Administration; *INTERMACS*, Interagency Registry for Mechanically Assisted Circulatory Support; *LVAD*, left ventricular assist device; *NYHA*, New York Heart Association; *OMM*, optimal medical management; *QoL*, quality of life. (From Estep JD, Starling RC, Horstmanshof DA, et al; ROADMAP Study Investigators. Risk assessment and comparative effectiveness of left ventricular assist device and medical management in ambulatory heart failure patients: results from the ROADMAP study. *J Am Coll Cardiol.* 2015;66:1747–1761.)

of MCS. INTERMACS 4 patients, but usually not INTERMACS 5–7 patients, are more likely to have significant improvements in QoL with LVAD (Fig. 4.2).[18,19]

Conversely, LVAD implantation too late puts cardiogenic shock patients at higher risk for postoperative complications and prolonged recovery. Even if such patients survive surgery, prolonged exposure to deranged hemodynamics may leave them with permanently impaired renal function, pulmonary hypertension, cardiac cirrhosis, and a very unsatisfactory post-MCS outcome.

Objective Measures of Disease Severity Warranting MCS

The generally accepted criteria for implantation of LVAD are based on parameters that indicate impaired systemic perfusion and end-organ function. These are discussed in detail in Chapter 3. Functional testing and hemodynamic measures are two of the most commonly employed methods. During cardiopulmonary stress testing, a peak oxygen consumption (VO_2) of <12–14 mL/kg/min with a respiratory exchange ratio (RER) >1.05 on optimal pharmacologic therapy suggests marked cardiac dysfunction; in the presence of a submaximal test (lower RER), a ventilation equivalent of carbon dioxide (VE/VCO_2) slope of >35 is also suggestive of poor prognosis. Similarly, right heart catheterization-derived invasive hemodynamics are useful to define advanced disease (as well as right ventricular [RV] function, discussed further in this chapter). Cardiogenic shock is suggested by the combination of (A) systolic blood pressure <90 mm Hg, (B) cardiac index less than 1.8 L/min/m^2 if the candidate is not supported by inotropes or <2.0 L/min/m^2 if the candidate is supported by at least one inotrope, and (C) pulmonary capillary wedge pressure greater than 15 mm Hg. The inability to improve these numbers without inotropic or mechanical support is a harbinger of severe progressive HF. That said, rarely should a single number be treated. Just as a VO_2 of <14 does not necessarily necessitate activation for advanced therapies, neither does a cardiac index <1.8 L/min/m^2 require initiation of inotropic support and movement toward MCS. Without end-organ dysfunction and manageable symptoms, many such patients—under close watch and with careful instructions to seek care for changes in clinical status—can do well for months to years.

Heart Failure Risk Scores

The totality of clinical information about a patient should be integrated to estimate prognosis and, thus, the need for MCS. However, with more than 100 variables known to be associated with mortality and rehospitalization in HF, appropriately prioritizing some information over others is important (see Chapter 3). Risk models work to narrow and weight prognostic information. Commonly used multivariable instruments for estimating prognosis in patients with symptomatic HF are the Heart Failure Survival Score,[20] the Seattle Heart Failure Model (SHFM) (https://depts.washington.edu/shfm/),[21] and the Meta-Analysis Global Group in Chronic Heart Failure (MAGGIC) risk calculator (http://www.heartfailurerisk.org/).[22] Because contemporary survival after LVAD implantation in carefully selected patients consistently caps out around 82% at 1 year, patients should generally not be considered for LVAD until their estimated mortality without LVAD meets or exceeds 18% in the coming year. The SHFM and MAGGIC online calculators can provide such tailored estimates for patients. However, application of these scores to individual patients should be interpreted with caution, as their miscalibration can lead to significant underestimation of risk in populations with particularly advanced HF.[23] Furthermore, most prognostic models in HF focus on mortality, whereas symptom relief and QoL also rank high in importance to individual patients. In addition, risk scores should be updated prospectively to account for the most recent clinical data.

Prediction of survival after LVAD implantation is even more difficult than prediction of survival with ongoing medical management of HF. A number of LVAD risk scores have been developed, only to be shown in validation testing to poorly predict whether patients will live well after device implantation. For example, the HeartMate II risk score[24] was found to have a *c* statistic of 0.64–0.71 in validation,[25,26] suggesting that, about one-third of the time, a randomly selected patient who survives will have a worse risk score than a randomly selected patient who dies. Calibration of these models has also been problematic when applied to different populations, with significant underestimation of survival when scores derived in largely INTERMACS 3 populations are applied in less sick populations being considered for LVAD.[26] The difficulty in predicting post-LVAD outcomes is likely not driven by failure to measure the right risk factors; post-LVAD mortality appears to be less dependent on preimplantation patient factors and more dependent upon operative and postimplantation events that are not present before surgery and thus cannot be measured before the decision to proceed with LVAD is made.

Despite the limitations of prognostic models, they are generally more accurate than clinical intuition, which is prone to bias. Therefore, clinicians treating patients with severe HF need to learn how to leverage objective risk models, while recognizing their limitations and adapting them based on unique clinical and psychosocial features and serial assessments not generally incorporated into such models. Furthermore, uncertainty should be actively recognized by clinicians in their approach to medical decision making and shared decision making (discussed further in the chapter).

CONTRAINDICATIONS TO MCS—MEDICAL, CARDIAC

The leading causes of morbidity and mortality with the use of ventricular assist devices (VADs) have not changed during the past 30 years and are the same regardless of indication (BTT or DT). These causes include infection, bleeding, renal failure, right heart failure, device malfunction requiring exchange, and stroke.[27] A need for rehospitalization post-MCS remains very common. Many of these complications can be traced to significant abnormalities in laboratory data, organ function, or clinical status before implantation that constitute significant risk factors for adverse outcome with MCS. A useful approach to deciding when not to initiate MCS in a patient who appears to be dying of HF is to systematically consider both cardiac and noncardiac reasons why patients are not likely to have a favorable outcome with MCS. With significant morbidity and high cost, contemporary MCS must be restricted to patients who have a high likelihood of realizing improved survival or QoL with LVAD implantation (Box 4.1).

BOX 4.1 Selection Guidelines for Durable Left Ventricular Assist Device[1]

Inclusion Criteria

- AHA Stage D heart failure
- VO_2 max <14 mL/kg/min or <50% predicted attainment of respiratory anaerobic threshold.
- NYHA functional class IIIB–IV for at least 45 of last 60 days, despite use of maximally tolerated doses of drugs. Inability to tolerate neurohormonal antagonist medications (e.g., β-blocker) may lead to earlier consideration.

Exclusion Criteria

- Reversible cardiac dysfunction
- Active uncontrolled coagulopathy
- Inability to tolerate anticoagulation mandated for the LVAD
- Active uncontrolled infection
- Renal disease that would significantly shorten life expectancy, including irreversible dysfunction not explained by HF; chronic hemodialysis is relatively incompatible with durable LVAD
- Hepatic disease that would shorten life expectancy, including irreversible dysfunction not explained by HF
- Lung disease that would negatively impact postimplantation survival, including recent pulmonary infarction
- Diabetes uncontrolled or with evidence of significant end-organ dysfunction
- Severe peripheral vascular disease accompanied by rest pain or extremity ulceration
- Moderate to severe aortic insufficiency without plans for correction during implantation
- Mechanical aortic valve that will not be converted to bioprosthesis at time of implantation or patch closed
- Severe right ventricular dysfunction requiring permanent right VAD support
- Severe cognitive impairment or organic brain syndrome
- Unresolved drug or alcohol dependency
- History of behavioral patterns or psychiatric illness likely to interfere with therapy compliance
- Unwillingness to accept blood or blood products
- Advanced age with frailty
- Insufficient financial means or insurance coverage
- Any other medical condition likely to limit short-term survival or quality of life following VAD implantation

AHA, American Heart Association; *HF*, heart failure; *LVAD*, left ventricular assist device; *NYHA*, New York Heart Association; *VAD*, ventricular assist device.

Right Ventricular Dysfunction

RV failure is one of the most important causes of mortality or morbidity after LVAD placement because contemporary durable MCS has evolved to devices implanted into the left ventricle (LV). Not only can RV failure leave patients with significant symptoms of HF that LVAD was supposed to treat (e.g., edema, fatigue, and orthostasis), but also RV failure contributes to bleeding, thrombosis, and renal failure. RV failure requiring prolonged inotropic support or RV mechanical support occurs in about 20% of patients undergoing LVAD placement. While some patients with limited pulmonary hypertension can get by for short periods of time on LVAD support alone (quasi-Fontan physiology), LVAD support alone does not produce adequate hemodynamic support in most patients absent significant RV function. Despite the development of numerous risk scores to predict RV failure post-LVAD, expert clinicians will need to synthesize important clinical information and use judgment to decide if RV function is appropriate for LVAD support. Another inherent vexing challenge is that RV function may deteriorate intraoperatively; hence, a "good" preoperative RV becomes prohibitively dysfunctional during surgery.[28,29] Device selection and types, including total artificial heart (TAH) and biventricular support, are addressed in Chapter 10.

Various information can be used to anticipate RV failure. RV failure after LVAD is most commonly due to preexisting RV failure. Patients with RV-predominant disease (e.g., arrhythmogenic RV cardiomyopathy or Ebstein anomaly) are obviously not candidates for LVAD. Patients with nonischemic etiology are more likely to present with biventricular failure and thus have a threefold to fourfold increased risk of needing RV support. Not surprisingly, patients with a chemotherapy-induced cardiomyopathy also experience increased RV failure post-MCS.[30] While a properly functioning LVAD tends to lower pulmonary venous pressures and thus improve RV afterload, LVADs can also cause the interventricular septum to shift leftward, potentially causing disadvantageous geometric changes in the right ventricle that reduce septal contribution to RV stroke volume and exacerbate tricuspid regurgitation.

Building on the risk model discussion from earlier, statistically derived models for the prediction of RV failure after LVAD implantation have been reported.[31,32] Dominant variables tend to include the inability of the RV to generate high pulmonary-artery pressures (e.g., RV stroke work index less than 300 mm Hg × mL/m^2) and maintain low central venous pressure (e.g., right atrial to post–capillary wedge pressure ratio >0.63 and elevated blood urea nitrogen >39 mg/dL), as well as lung disease at the time of surgery that is likely to create ongoing RV strain after implantation (e.g., preimplantation mechanical ventilator support). Predictive measurements made on echocardiogram before implantation include RV dimension, tricuspid annual plane systolic excursion, RV strain, and severe tricuspid regurgitation.[32,33] Some surgeons have advocated repair of tricuspid regurgitation at the time of LVAD implantation, but this added procedure increases cardiopulmonary bypass time and has not been clearly associated with reduced risks of RV failure.[34]

Pulmonary hypertension is generally not a contraindication to LVAD, in contrast to its relationship to heart transplant. The ability of the RV to generate high pulmonary-artery systolic pressures pre-LVAD is related to a high RV stroke work index and generally predicts a functioning RV. Because much pulmonary hypertension in patients being considered for LVAD is World Health Organization (WHO) group 2 (i.e., related to chronically elevated pulmonary venous pressures from LV dysfunction), these patients with higher pulmonary artery systolic pressures not only are at a lower risk of acute RV failure but also tend to see their pulmonary hypertension partially improve or reverse in the months after LVAD implantation.[35]

Ventricular Arrhythmia

Electrical abnormalities that affect RV function can also lead to poor outcome with LVAD. Therefore, patients with ventricular tachycardia and ventricular fibrillation that cannot be controlled are not candidates for LVAD; this is further complicated because intravenous inotropic support may also be contraindicated if it worsens the ventricular arrhythmia, leaving biventricular assist devices (BiVAD), veno-arterial ECMO, or TAH support to transplant as the only alternative to palliation and death in refractory cases. While some ventricular arrhythmias are driven by cardiac decompensation and can resolve with improved hemodynamic support, ventricular arrhythmias in patients being considered for LVAD support may be substrate/scar mediated and do not generally disappear postimplantation. Therefore, demonstration of rhythm control with antiarrhythmic or ablation preimplantation may be indicated prior to LVAD implantation. Concomitant intraoperative ventricular arrhythmia ablation at the time of LVAD surgery may be facilitated by epicardial access, but concerns about increased postoperative complications including LVAD thrombosis have been raised.[36] Post-LVAD implantation ablation may also be facilitated by LVAD hemodynamic support, but again may raise concerns about anticoagulation and thrombosis. Pre-MCS patients with complex ventricular arrhythmias require a collaborative management strategy developed by the electrophysiologist, HF cardiologist, and cardiac surgeon.

Cardiac Anatomy, Prior Surgery, and Valve Disease

Not all LV cardiac anatomy is amenable to LVAD (Special Populations, Chapter 17). The inflow cannula needs space in the left ventricle to avoid suction. Thus, patients with a nondilated LV—as seen in restrictive or hypertrophic cardiomyopathies—have often been excluded from LVAD and routed to consideration of TAH, ECMO, or continuous inotropic support as BTT (or palliation/hospice for non-transplant-eligible patients). LVAD registries show that relatively few patients with hypertrophic and restrictive cardiomyopathy undergo LVAD implantation, and most who do display some features of a dilated cardiomyopathy. The overall survival and adverse event profiles of these patients were similar to traditional dilated cardiomyopathy (DCM) patients; however, in those with very small ventricles, survival was inferior.[37]

Congenital heart disease may pose particular anatomic and physiologic problems for contemporary LVAD support. Additionally, chronic congestive hepatopathy can further complicate MCS in single-ventricle physiologies. A detailed discussion of the candidacy of various congenital heart diseases is provided in Chapter 18. Needless to say, teamwork among advanced HF, adult congenital, and pediatric cardiac surgery is vital.

Prior cardiac surgery, most commonly from coronary artery bypass grafting or valve replacement, raises operative risk and should be factored into decisions about candidacy and surgical approach. Fortunately, in carefully selected patients treated by skilled cardiac surgical teams, prior surgery does not appear to significantly raise risk.[38] All patients being considered for MCS, especially those who have a history of coronary artery bypass grafting, should have a chest computed tomography (CT) scan to define aortic calcification and provide the location and course of the bypass grafts to guide the surgical approach.

Valvular disease should also be factored into candidacy. See previous discussion for concerns about tricuspid regurgitation with RV dysfunction after LVAD. Mitral valve regurgitation does not appear to markedly affect LVAD outcomes, and repair at the time of LVAD placement also does not appear to offer a significant advantage.[39] In contrast, aortic regurgitation has significant adverse effects on LVAD function and typically progresses after LVAD implantation. Therefore, even mild degrees of aortic regurgitation should be addressed at the time of LVAD implantation, usually through repair or oversewing of the aortic valve, although the latter may create subsequent issues.[40] Transcatheter aortic valve replacement may be an option down the road after LVAD implantation, but there are concerns about anchoring of the device in noncalcified valves. Mechanical valves need to be addressed at the time of LVAD implantation, often through removal and replacement.

CONTRAINDICATIONS TO MCS—MEDICAL, NONCARDIAC

Hematologic, Gastrointestinal, and Anticoagulation Considerations

Thrombocytopenia and spontaneously elevated prothrombin time/international normalized ratio (PT/INR) are predictive of poor outcome after LVAD, likely due to their reflection of RV dysfunction with hepatic congestion, but also because persistently low platelets and coagulopathy exacerbate bleeding complications associated with LVAD. Conversely, hypercoagulability with recurrent thrombotic events may place patients at increased risk for device thrombosis and thus should be seriously considered in the evaluation process, potentially with hematology consultation.

Liver disease has long been shown to be associated with poor outcomes after cardiac surgery generally and LVAD specifically. Liver function and coagulopathy due to congestive hepatopathy often improve with MCS. However, frank cirrhosis is an absolute contraindication to LVAD. Therefore, careful hepatic evaluation in patients with evidence of chronic liver disease, including blood tests, imaging, transhepatic wedge pressure, and liver biopsy with hepatology consultation, is important. The Model for End-Stage Liver Disease score has been utilized to risk stratify patients with advanced HF and is discussed in Chapter 3.

Patients with a history of gastrointestinal bleeding should be carefully screened because all contemporary durable LVADs require systemic anticoagulation with warfarin and raise the risk of gastrointestinal bleeding. Documented current evidence of gastrointestinal blood loss should be assessed before LVAD implantation with both upper and lower endoscopy to define the cause and rule out malignancy. Patients who have been intolerant of oral anticoagulation require resolution of this issue prior to implantation or they may not be acceptable durable LVAD candidates.

Renal Dysfunction

Renal dysfunction is one of the most common comorbidities in patients with HF and has consistently been one of the strongest predictors of morbidity and mortality with ongoing medical management but also for poor outcome after LVAD (see HF Risk Scores, earlier).

Important to the evaluation of renal dysfunction pre-LVAD is the differentiation of hemodynamically mediated cardiorenal syndrome that may respond to LVAD (with improved hemodynamic environment) versus intrinsic renal disease[41] that is likely to remain or potentially worsen post-LVAD. The degree of renal dysfunction (i.e., worse estimated glomerular filtration rate), proteinuria,[42] and cortical thinning on renal ultrasound are all associated with persistent renal dysfunction after implantation. Acute kidney injury is frequent after LVAD implantation, particularly in those who go into surgery with impaired renal function, and more severe acute kidney injury is associated with higher mortality rates at 1 year after LVAD implantation.[43] Somewhat concerning, even in patients who receive LVAD and have temporary improvement in serum creatinine, creatinine frequently worsens again.[44] Therefore, pre-LVAD renal dysfunction of almost any type should be factored into decision making and expected outcomes.

The combination of LVAD and end-stage renal disease (ESRD) has been particularly problematic. In a study using the US Renal Data System, of the 155 Medicare beneficiaries with ESRD who underwent LVAD implantation between 2003 and 2013 (median time on dialysis, 1655 days preimplantation), the median survival was 16 days, and 52% died during the index hospitalization.[45] For those who stabilize, they remain at increased risk of device infection related to dialysis access; finding dialysis centers who will accept patients with an LVAD has been problematic in some areas. Therefore, preexisting ESRD is generally an absolute contraindication to durable LVAD. For patients in whom heart-kidney transplant is a consideration, in-hospital bridging with inotropes or temporary MCS should be considered. Even with avoidance of patients with preexisting chronic severe renal dysfunction, some patients will develop acute renal failure and need renal replacement therapy in the setting of critical illness. Many will recover renal function with adequate hemodynamic support, but this can take weeks, resulting in difficult medical decision making and management logistics.

Pulmonary Disease

Patients with severe obstructive or restrictive pulmonary disease are at increased risk related to LVAD therapy. Significant underlying pulmonary dysfunction or disease often leads to prolonged time in the intensive care unit and mechanical ventilation after implantation of an LVAD. There are no absolute pulmonary function criteria or limits for exclusion of use of an LVAD, but oxygen dependence at baseline should raise serious concerns.[1]

Accurate assessment of intrinsic pulmonary disease in the setting of severe cardiac dysfunction is challenging (similar to renal assessment above). The evaluation of a patient with underlying pulmonary disease or demonstrated hypoxemia may include chest x-ray, chest CT, pulmonary function testing, cardiopulmonary exercise testing, echocardiography with bubble study, right heart catheterization, and pulmonary consultation. Elevated left-sided filling pressures, causing pulmonary edema and pulmonary vasoconstriction, affect pulmonary test results. Mechanical ventilation before implantation has been shown to be one of the highest risk factors for a poor outcome.[24]

Peripheral Vascular Disease

The most common cause of consideration for LVAD is ischemic heart disease, and many patients with coronary artery disease also have atherosclerotic vascular disease elsewhere. Peripheral vascular disease can adversely affect outcomes after LVAD for multiple reasons. Aortic atheroma can increase surgical risk and chance of stroke. Claudication may limit postoperative ambulation and recovery.

Abdominal ultrasound, measurement of the ankle-brachial index, and carotid ultrasounds are warranted in patients with coronary disease, diabetes, a history of smoking, and advanced age. Echocardiogram assesses the proximal aorta, but a chest CT should be considered to evaluate the thoracic aorta for surgical planning.

Cancer

Many patients who receive an LVAD, especially as DT, are of an age at which malignancy is increasingly common. Preoperative screening for cancer should be determined by age and gender, as defined by the American Cancer Society[46] and US Preventative Services Task Force,[47] or as a result of abnormal findings. Given the frequency of gastrointestinal bleeding after durable LVAD implantation, patients with guaiac-positive stool specimen or iron-deficiency anemia should be thoroughly evaluated.

MCS should be avoided in patients who have an expected survival of less than 2 years.[1] Therefore, patients with active or previously treated malignancy that is associated with significant reduction in expected survival should be excluded from durable LVAD. Consultation with oncology to determine risk is often indicated. Additionally, cancer therapies that put patients at significant risk for thrombocytopenia, colitis, and infection may develop complex and problematic complications post-MCS. In contrast, patients with a malignancy that is considered to have a good prognosis may be acceptable candidates for LVAD support.

Infection

Infection and sepsis have been a leading cause of mortality and morbidity since the beginning of MCS use.[48] Therefore, additional risks for infection should be considered carefully prior to durable LVAD. Such risks include the presence of indwelling catheters, which have been in place for several days before the time of surgery; renal failure; mechanical ventilation; poorly controlled diabetes; vascular ulcers; and generalized debilitation with pressure ulcers.[49] Correcting as many of these factors as possible before device implantation can minimize the risk of infection and optimize long-term outcomes. Many patients are hospitalized for days to weeks for evaluation and optimization before implantation of the LVAD, which leads to changes in skin flora and significantly increases the risk of nosocomial infection after LVAD. Preoperative blood stream infections, especially associated with prosthetic valves and intracardiac devices, require sterilization, potential extraction, and consultation and planning with an infectious disease expert. Generalized markers of immunosuppression increase risk of infection and should be optimized when feasible.[50] Patients with active systemic infection should have durable LVAD support delayed.

Diabetes

Diabetes can indirectly raise the risk of MCS through a number of mechanisms, including peripheral vascular disease and infection risk.[51] Additionally, glucose control has similarities to anticoagulation and drive line care, such that demonstration of the ability to manage diabetes is a good barometer of how patients will engage MCS after implantation. Therefore, patients with long-standing diabetes should generally be able to show activities of good self-care and generally be able to maintain their hemoglobin A1c <9%.

Malnutrition and Obesity

Nutritional status strongly reflects underlying disease severity before LVAD and relates to healing and functional status after LVAD. The majority of patients with chronic HF have a serum albumin less than 3.2 mg/dL, despite a relatively high rate of obesity in this population. The cause of malnutrition in HF patients is multifactorial and includes poor appetite, elevated inflammatory cytokines, work of breathing, nausea, and early satiety in patients with significant hepatomegaly. As with non-VAD cardiac surgery data, the risk of operative death, but not infection, is correlated with cachexia and a low body mass index (BMI).[52] There is an "obesity paradox," where obesity is not associated with increased mortality risk until very high BMI, although morbid obesity does carry significant risk of wound and other postoperative infections. Providing hemodynamic support with an LVAD as a means for weight loss should be undertaken with a multidisciplinary team approach that includes physicians, nurses, dietitians, exercise physiologists, and, potentially, bariatric surgeons; significant weight loss after LVAD placement is rarely achieved.[53]

Neurologic Disease

Stroke is a devastating complication of MCS and occurs in ~10% of patients in the first year.[54a] Careful risk assessment preoperative is imperative (see Chapter 13).[54b] Stroke, dementia, and neuromuscular diseases (e.g., Duchenne muscular dystrophy) may be contraindications to LVAD if they significantly impair survival or QoL, but also if they impair the ability of a patient to ambulate after surgery or take care of his or her device. Evaluation by occupational and physical therapy is appropriate for many patients. Use of formal assessments of cognitive function, such as the Montreal Cognitive Assessment, may help standardize the process.[55] A patient who is blind and/or lacks the manual dexterity to change batteries, power connections, etc., may have a relative contraindication to MCS.

Frailty

Frailty is the aggregation of subclinical physiologic insults across many organ systems, resulting in a syndrome of heightened vulnerability in the face of stress. Patients with severe HF being considered for LVAD often also have advanced age or noncardiac morbidity, particularly in the DT setting, such that many such patients have significant degrees of frailty. Formal measures of frailty (e.g., Fried criteria) are highly predictive of adverse outcomes in many medical and surgical populations, including patients undergoing LVAD placement. Unfortunately, current assessments of frailty do not distinguish frailty that is a manifestation of severe cardiac disease (and thus which may reverse with MCS, i.e., LVAD sensitive) from frailty that is due to advanced age and other comorbidity (i.e., LVAD resistant).[56] About half of frail patients undergoing LVAD see their frailty assessments significantly improve, and half do not.[57]

CONTRAINDICATIONS TO MCS—NONMEDICAL

Psychosocial Considerations

Patients with psychiatric diseases that compromise their ability to engage the medical team, consistently follow medical advice, adhere to anticoagulation, and use and care for external system components are poor candidates for durable LVAD (and transplant). Guidelines stipulate that all patients considered for MCS should have a formal mental health evaluation by a trained health care professional.[1,2]

Unfortunately, substance abuse is a common aspect of MCS evaluation, as it predicts worse outcomes after LVAD placement. While tobacco use has generally been a contraindication to heart transplant, in the absence of significant lung or vascular disease, it has not been an absolute contraindication to MCS; tobacco use may prompt DT status with counseling and documentation of negative serum cotinine for future heart transplant consideration. Alcohol is ubiquitous in use but can lead to serious health problems (see Liver Disease, earlier) and suboptimal behaviors. Therefore, assessment of frequency of use, adverse consequences (e.g., loss of job and driving under the influence), and objective testing of serum phosphatidylethanol levels is warranted.[58] Marijuana is increasingly used as medical treatment and legally for recreation, such that it is becoming more like alcohol in how it factors into evaluation.[59] Active use of other substances of abuse, including narcotics and methamphetamines, is generally an absolute contraindication to durable LVAD and transplantation.

Adequate family or caregiver support, housing, consistent access to electricity, and community infrastructure are additional requirements for long term MCS. Most programs require a caregiver (dedicated family or friend) to provide supportive care when necessary. Patients must have a reliable means of transportation for follow-up visits and a convenient, reliable telephone service to call for medical help in an emergency.

The 2018 ISHLT/APM/AST/ICCAC/STSW Recommendations for the Psychosocial Evaluation of Adult Cardiothoracic Transplant Candidates and Candidates for Long-Term Mechanical Circulator Support provide specific guidance on the content and process of such aspects of evaluation.[60]

TEMPORARY SUPPORT TO ASSESS CANDIDACY

Short-term percutaneous circulatory support—intraaortic balloon pumps, Impella, ECMO, or other devices—may be initiated when acute or acute-on-chronic hemodynamic instability requires urgent intervention to avoid permanent end-organ dysfunction or death.[61] It may be instituted with the hope of supporting a reversible underlying condition, such as fulminate myocarditis or right HF after acute myocardial infarction. It may also be initiated in patients who might be potential candidates for transplantation or permanent circulatory support, in whom (1) there has not been opportunity to appropriately evaluate a patient's candidacy for more definitive high-dependence therapies, (2) reversibility of end-organ dysfunction is uncertain, or (3) contraindications to more definitive therapies may, or may not, resolve in the near future. If end-organ dysfunction or contraindications do not resolve, a decision will need to be made about discontinuation. A therapeutic plan and strategy, including the sequence of temporary and durable devices, should be discussed by the entire HF multidisciplinary team, when feasible, prior to initiation of temporary support. Details related to temporary support are reviewed in Chapters 4 and 5.

FORMAL EVALUATION PROTOCOLS

A systematic, multidisciplinary approach to candidacy evaluation is required to optimally address the litany of complex considerations. Professional studies have created guidelines outlining the process.[1] Medicare has defined criteria for what constitutes an adequate MCS program, including surgical, medical, social work, and palliative care specialists.[62] Yet individual programs must still develop their own internal protocols and standard order sets (e.g., Box 4.2; box is available online at expertconsult.inkling.com). All advanced HF therapeutic recommendations should be evaluated and adjudicated by a center-specific HF "heart team" whose members have specialized expertise with MCS.

SHARED DECISION MAKING

Advanced HF—with its high degree of prognostic uncertainty and complex tradeoffs in the choice of medical care—demands a thoughtful approach to communication and decision making, in addition to diagnosis and management. While MCS is often life-saving and, on average, significantly improves QoL, it also comes with significant risks for burdens. This is particularly true in older patients with multimorbidity. Therefore, decisions about MCS are relatively preference sensitive and should be mapped to patients' values and goals. Ideally, interactions with patients and families about MCS do not occur as one-time events but rather are anticipated and evolve as a series of discussions over time. Such interactions may be difficult and time consuming, and they often require planning in order to create a supportive environment for effective communication. Clinicians must determine how much quantitative information patients want about prognosis, comparative risks, and benefits for both length and QoL with available options. At the same time, clinicians must attend to the emotional nature of conversations with patients to build trust, clarify core values, and allow for sharper focus on the information. These challenges and suggestions for how to approach them have been outlined in a statement from the American Heart Association on Decision Making in Advanced Heart Failure.[12]

Shared decision making for MCS can be facilitated through the use of formal patient decision aids.[63] In a six-center stepped-wedge trial of 248 patients being considered for DT LVAD, patients enrolled in the intervention period—consisting of clinician education and use of DT LVAD pamphlet and video patient decision aids—had significantly better knowledge and higher concordance between stated values and patient-reported treatment choice (https://patientdecisionaid.org/lvad/).[64]

SUMMARY

The use of MCS is an important treatment option for management of patients with advanced HF. However, because of the complexity, burdens, and costs of the therapy, MCS should be carefully restricted to patients for whom MCS is likely to provide significant benefit, including expected survival with reasonable QoL beyond 2 years. Multidisciplinary teams must work together efficiency and quickly, following thoughtful, systematic protocols, to evaluate the multitude of factors that have been shown to have an adverse impact on outcomes. The engagement of patients and their caregivers is also critical in fully addressing candidacy. Only through such a careful approach to candidacy can MCS be a success.

REFERENCES

1. Feldman D, Pamboukian SV, Teuteberg JJ, et al. International Society for H and Lung T. The 2013 International Society for Heart and Lung Transplantation Guidelines for mechanical circulatory support: executive summary. *J Heart Lung Transplant*. 2013;32:157–187.
2. Mehra MR, Canter CE, Hannan MM, et al. International Society for Heart Lung Transplantation Infectious Diseases C, International Society for Heart Lung Transplantation Pediatric Transplantation C, International Society for Heart Lung Transplantation Heart F and Transplantation C. The 2016 International Society for Heart Lung Transplantation listing criteria for heart transplantation: A 10-year update. *J Heart Lung Transplant*. 2016;35:1–23.
3. Kirklin JK, Pagani FD, Kormos RL, et al. Eight annual INTERMACS report: special focus on framing the impact of adverse events. *J Heart Lung Transplant*. 2017;36:1080–1086.
4. https://unos.org/policy/
5. Chambers DC, Yusen RD, Cherikh WS, et al. International Society for H and Lung T. The Registry of the International Society for Heart and Lung Transplantation: Thirty-Fourth Adult Lung and Heart-Lung Transplantation Report-2017; Focus Theme: Allograft ischemic time. *J Heart Lung Transplant*. 2017;36:1047–1059.
6. Davies RR, Farr M, Silvestry S et al. The new United States heart allocation policy: progress through collaborative revision. *J Heart Lung Transplant*. 2017;36:595–596.
7. OPTN/UNOS Policy Notice Proposal to Modify the Adult Heart Allocation System. https://optn.transplant.hrsa.gov/media/2028/thoracic_policynotice_201612.pdf. Accessed December 6, 2017.
8. Rose EA, Gelijns AC, Moskowitz AJ, et al. Poirier VL and Randomized Evaluation of Mechanical Assistance for the Treatment of Congestive Heart Failure Study G. Long-term use of a left ventricular assist device for end-stage heart failure. *N Engl J Med*. 2001;345:1435–1443.
9. Rogers JG, Butler J, Lansman SL, et al; INTrEPID Investigators. Chronic mechanical circulatory support for inotrope-dependent heart failure patients who are not transplant candidates: results of the INTrEPID trial. *J Am Coll Cardiol*. 2007;50:741-7.
10. Stevenson LW, Miller LW, Desvigne-Nickens P, et al. Left ventricular assist device as destination for patients undergoing intravenous inotropic therapy: a subset analysis from REMATCH (Randomized Evaluation of Mechanical Assistance in Treatment of Chronic Heart Failure). *Circulation*. 2004;110:975–981.
11. Hashim T, Sanam K, Revilla-Martinez M, et al. Clinical characteristics and outcomes of intravenous inotropic therapy in advanced heart failure. *Circ Heart Fail*. 2015;8:880–886.
12. Allen LA, Stevenson LW, Grady KL, et al. American Heart Association; Council on Quality of Care and Outcomes Research; Council on Cardiovascular Nursing; Council on Clinical Cardiology; Council on Cardiovascular Radiology and Intervention; Council on Cardiovascular Surgery and Anesthesia. Decision making in advanced heart failure: a scientific statement from the American Heart Association. *Circulation*. 2012;125:1928–1952.
13. Stewart GC, Ambardekar AV, Kittleson MM. Defining ambulatory advanced heart failure: MedaMACS and beyond. *Curr Heart Fail Rep*. 2017;14:498–506.
14. Ambardekar AV, Thibodeau JT, DeVore AD, et al. Discordant perceptions of prognosis and treatment options between physicians and patients with advanced heart failure. *JACC Heart Fail*. 2017;5:663–671.
15. Stewart GC, Kittleson MM, Patel PC, et al. INTERMACS (Interagency Registry for Mechanically Assisted Circulatory Support) profiling identifies ambulatory patients at high risk on medical therapy after hospitalizations for heart failure. *Circ Heart Fail*. 2016;9:.
16. Baumwol J. "I Need Help"—a mnemonic to aid timely referral in advanced heart failure. *J Heart Lung Transplant*. 2017;36:593–594.
17. Starling RC, Estep JD, Horstmanshof DA, et al; ROADMAP Study Investigators. Risk assessment and comparative effectiveness of left ventricular assist device and medical management in ambulatory heart failure patients: the ROADMAP study 2 year results. *JACC Heart Fail*. 2017;5:518–527.
18. Shah KB, Starling RC, Rogers JG, et al; ROADMAP Investigators. Left ventricular assist devices versus medical management in ambulatory heart failure patients: An analysis of INTERMACS Profiles 4 and 5 to 7 from the ROADMAP study. *J Heart Lung Transplant*. 2017.
19. Estep JD, Starling RC, Horstmanshof DA, et al; ROADMAP Study Investigators. Risk assessment and comparative effectiveness of left ventricular assist device and medical management in ambulatory heart failure patients: results from the ROADMAP study. *J Am Coll Cardiol*. 2015;66:1747–1761.
20. Aaronson KD, Schwartz JS, Chen TM, Wong KL, Goin JE, Mancini DM. Development and prospective validation of a clinical index to predict survival in ambulatory patients referred for cardiac transplant evaluation. *Circulation*. 1997;95:2660–2667.
21. Levy WC, Mozaffarian D, Linker DT, et al. The Seattle Heart Failure Model: prediction of survival in heart failure. *Circulation*. 2006;113:1424–1433.
22. Pocock SJ, Ariti CA, McMurray JJ, et al; Meta-Analysis Global Group in Chronic Heart Failure. Predicting survival in heart failure: a risk score based on 39 372 patients from 30 studies. *Eur Heart J*. 2013;34:1404–1413.
23. Gorodeski EZ, Chu EC, Chow CH, Levy WC, Hsich E, Starling RC. Application of the Seattle Heart Failure Model in ambulatory patients presented to an advanced heart failure therapeutics committee. *Circ Heart Fail*. 2010;3:706–714.
24. Cowger J, Sundareswaran K, Rogers JG, et al. Predicting survival in patients receiving continuous flow left ventricular assist devices: the HeartMate II risk score. *J Am Coll Cardiol*. 2013;61:313–321.
25. Levy WC. Potential clinical applications of the HeartMate II risk score. *J Am Coll Cardiol*. 2013;61:322–324.
26. Lanfear DE, Levy WC, Stehlik J, et al. Accuracy of Seattle Heart Failure Model and HeartMate II Risk Score in non-inotrope-dependent advanced heart failure patients: insights from the ROADMAP study (Risk Assessment and Comparative Effectiveness of Left Ventricular Assist Device and Medical Management in Ambulatory Heart Failure Patients). *Circ Heart Fail*. 2017;10.
27. McIlvennan CK, Magid KH, Ambardekar AV, Thompson JS, Matlock DD, Allen LA. Clinical outcomes after continuous-flow left ventricular assist device: a systematic review. *Circ Heart Fail*. 2014;7:1003–1013.

28. Loghmanpour NA, Kormos RL, Kanwar MK, Teuteberg JJ, Murali S, Antaki JF. A Bayesian model to predict right ventricular failure following left ventricular assist device therapy. *JACC Heart Fail.* 2016;4:711–721.
29. Kormos RL. The right heart failure dilemma in the era of left ventricular assist devices. *J Heart Lung Transplant.* 2014;33:134–135.
30. Oliveira GH, Dupont M, Naftel D, et al. Increased need for right ventricular support in patients with chemotherapy-induced cardiomyopathy undergoing mechanical circulatory support: outcomes from the INTERMACS Registry (Interagency Registry for Mechanically Assisted Circulatory Support). *J Am Coll Cardiol.* 2014;63:240–248.
31. Kormos RL, Teuteberg JJ, Pagani FD, et al; HeartMate II Clinical Investigators. Right ventricular failure in patients with the HeartMate II continuous-flow left ventricular assist device: incidence, risk factors, and effect on outcomes. *J Thorac Cardiovasc Surg.* 2010;139:1316–1324.
32. Lampert BC, Teuteberg JJ. Right ventricular failure after left ventricular assist devices. *J Heart Lung Transplant.* 2015;34:1123–1130.
33. Grant AD, Smedira NG, Starling RC, Marwick TH. Independent and incremental role of quantitative right ventricular evaluation for the prediction of right ventricular failure after left ventricular assist device implantation. *J Am Coll Cardiol.* 2012;60:521–528.
34. Song HK, Gelow JM, Mudd J, et al. Limited utility of tricuspid valve repair at the time of left ventricular assist device implantation. *Ann Thorac Surg.* 2016;101:2168–2174.
35. Lim HS, Howell N, Ranasinghe A. The effect of left ventricular assist device therapy in patients with heart failure and mixed pulmonary hypertension. *Int J Artif Organs.* 2017;40:67–73.
36. McIlvennan CK, Babu AN, Brieke A, Ambardekar AV. Concomitant surgical cryoablation for refractory ventricular tachycardia and left ventricular assist device placement: a dual remedy but a recipe for thrombosis? *J Cardiothorac Surg.* 2016;11:53.
37. Patel SR, Saeed O, Naftel D, et al. Outcomes of restrictive and hypertrophic cardiomyopathies after LVAD: an INTERMACS analysis. *J Card Fail.* 2017;23:859–867.
38. Gaffey AC, Phillips EC, Howard J, et al. Prior sternotomy and ventricular assist device implantation do not adversely impact survival or allograft function after heart transplantation. *Ann Thorac Surg.* 2015;100: 542–549.
39. Stulak JM, Tchantchaleishvili V, Haglund NA, et al. Uncorrected pre-operative mitral valve regurgitation is not associated with adverse outcomes after continuous-flow left ventricular assist device implantation. *J Heart Lung Transplant.* 2015;34:718–723.
40. Robertson JO, Naftel DC, Myers SL, et al. Concomitant aortic valve procedures in patients undergoing implantation of continuous-flow left ventricular assist devices: an INTERMACS database analysis. *J Heart Lung Transplant.* 2015;34:797–805.
41. Hasin T, Topilsky Y, Schirger JA, et al. Changes in renal function after implantation of continuous-flow left ventricular assist devices. *J Am Coll Cardiol.* 2012;59:26–36.
42. Muslem R, Caliskan K, Akin S, et al. Pre-operative proteinuria in left ventricular assist devices and clinical outcome. *J Heart Lung Transplant.* 2017.
43. Muslem R, Caliskan K, Akin S, et al. Acute kidney injury and 1-year mortality after left ventricular assist device implantation. *J Heart Lung Transplant.* 2017.
44. Hasin T, Grupper A, Dillon JJ, et al. Early gains in renal function following implantation of HeartMate II left ventricular assist devices may not persist to one year. *ASAIO J.* 2017;63:401–407.
45. Bansal N, Hailpern SM, Katz R, et al. Outcomes associated with left ventricular assist devices among recipients with and without end-stage renal disease. *JAMA Intern Med.* 2017.
46. American Cancer Society, Cancer Screening Guidelines. https://www.cancer.org/healthy/find-cancer-early/cancer-screening-guidelines.html. Accessed December 24, 2017.
47. United States Preventative Services Task Force. Recommendations to primary care. https://www.uspreventiveservicestaskforce.org/Page/Name/recommendations. Accessed December 24, 2017.
48. Kusne S, Mooney M, Danziger-Isakov L, et al. An ISHLT consensus document for prevention and management strategies for mechanical circulatory support infection. *J Heart Lung Transplant.* 2017;36:1137–1153.
49. Schaffer JM, Allen JG, Weiss ES, et al. Infectious complications after pulsatile-flow and continuous-flow left ventricular assist device implantation. *J Heart Lung Transplant.* 2011;30:164–174.
50. Yamani MH, Chuang HH, Ozduran V, et al. The impact of hypogammaglobulinemia on infection outcome in patients undergoing ventricular assist device implantation. *J Heart Lung Transplant.* 2006;25:820–824.
51. Asleh R, Briasoulis A, Schettle SD, et al. Impact of diabetes mellitus on outcomes in patients supported with left ventricular assist devices: a single institutional 9-year experience. *Circ Heart Fail.* 2017;10:.
52. Mano A, Fujita K, Uenomachi K, et al. Body mass index is a useful predictor of prognosis after left ventricular assist system implantation. *J Heart Lung Transplant.* 2009;28:428–433.
53. Clerkin KJ, Naka Y, Mancini DM, Colombo PC, Topkara VK. The impact of obesity on patients bridged to transplantation with continuous-flow left ventricular assist devices. *JACC Heart Fail.* 2016;4:761–768.
54a. Goldstein DJ, Meyns B, Xie R, et al. Third annual report from the ISHLT mechanically assisted circulatory support registry: a comparison of centrifugal and axial continuous-flow left ventricular assist devices. *J Heart Lung Transplant.* 2019;38(4):352–363. https://doi.org/10.1016/j.healun.2019.02.004.
54b. Cho SM, Moazami N, Frontera JA. Stroke and intracranial hemorrhage in HeartMate II and HeartWare left ventricular assist devices: a systematic review. *Neurocrit Care.* 2017;27:17–25.
55. Bhat G, Yost G, Mahoney E. Cognitive function and left ventricular assist device implantation. *J Heart Lung Transplant.* 2015;34:1398–1405.
56. Flint KM, Matlock DD, Lindenfeld J, Allen LA. Frailty and the selection of patients for destination therapy left ventricular assist device. *Circ Heart Fail.* 2012;5:286–293.
57. Maurer MS, Horn E, Reyentovich A, et al. Can a left ventricular assist device in individuals with advanced systolic heart failure improve or reverse frailty? *J Am Geriatr Soc.* 2017;65:2383–2390.
58. Andresen-Streichert H, Beres Y, Weinmann W, et al. Improved detection of alcohol consumption using the novel marker phosphatidylethanol in the transplant setting: results of a prospective study. *Transpl Int.* 2017;30:611–620.
59. Allen LA, Ambardekar AV. Hashing It Out Over Cannabis: Moving Toward a Standard Guideline on Substance Use for Cardiac Transplantation Eligibility That Includes Marijuana. *Circ Heart Fail.* 2016;9.
60. Dew MA. DiMartini AF, Dobbels F. 2018 ISHLT/APM/AST/ICCAC/STSW recommendations for the psychosocial evaluation of adult cardiothoracic transplant candidates and candidates for long-term mechanical circulatory support. https://www.jhltonline.org/article/S1053-2498(18)31390-1/fulltext. Accessed December 24, 2017.
61. Rihal CS, Naidu SS, Givertz MM, et al; Society for Cardiovascular Angiography and Interventions (SCAI); Heart Failure Society of America (HFSA); Society of Thoracic Surgeons (STS); American Heart Association (AHA), and American College of Cardiology (ACC). 2015 SCAI/ACC/HFSA/STS clinical expert consensus statement on the use of percutaneous mechanical circulatory support devices in cardiovascular care: endorsed by the American Heart Association, the Cardiological Society of India, and Sociedad Latino Americana de Cardiologia Intervencion; Affirmation of Value by the Canadian Association of Interventional Cardiology—Association Canadienne de Cardiologie d'intervention. *J Am Coll Cardiol.* 2015;65:e7–e26.
62. National Coverage Determination for Ventricular Assist Devices. Medicare. https://www.cms.gov/medicare-coverage-database/details/ncd-detailsaspx?NCDId=360&ver=1. Accessed December 24, 2017.
63. Thompson JS, Matlock DD, McIlvennan CK, Jenkins AR, Allen LA. Development of a decision aid for patients with advanced heart failure considering a destination therapy left ventricular assist device. *JACC Heart Fail.* 2015;3:965–976.
64. Allen LA, McIlvennan CK, Matlock DD. Effectiveness of an intervention supporting shared decision making for destination therapy left ventricular assist device: the DECIDE-LVAD randomized stepped-wedge trial (in press). *JAMA Intern Med.* 2018.

5

Acute Circulatory Support

Jennifer Cowger, Daniel J. Goldstein

KEY POINTS

INTRODUCTION

Cardiogenic shock (CS) is a state of insufficient cardiac output and end-organ perfusion that can be the terminal phase of many different cardiac conditions, including acute coronary syndromes, arrhythmias, progression of chronic cardiomyopathy, and acute cardiac dysfunction in the setting of idiopathic, traumatic, or inflammatory cardiomyopathies. This shock state is characterized by pathologic systemic vasoconstriction, impairment of tissue microcirculation, release of proinflammatory cytokines, and alterations in nitric oxide synthase activity.[1] Subsequently, even with restoration of normal cardiac output, microcirculatory dysfunction can ensue, leading to loss of peripheral vasomotor tone, coagulopathy, and multisystem organ failure.[1,2]

According to data from the Nationwide Inpatient Sample (NIS), the number of hospital discharges of patients with a complication of CS has doubled over a decade (from 55,123 in 2004 to 126,555 in 2014).[3,4] Acute myocardial infarction is the most common precipitant of CS in the United States, and the incidence of CS complicating ST elevation myocardial infarction (STEMI) has increased from 6.5% in 2003 to 10% in 2010.[3] In patients enrolled into the Interagency Registry for Mechanically Assisted Circulatory Support (INTERMACS), fewer patients undergoing durable left ventricular assist device (LVAD) implantation in 2012–2014 were classified as INTERMACS Profile 1 ("critical CS"; 14%) or 2 ("decompensating on inotropes"; 36%) compared with those undergoing implantation between 2008 and 2011 (16% and 43%, respectively).[5] The decrement in shock phenotype is likely due to changes in patient selection. Nonetheless, CS or progressive decompensation (INTERMACS Profile 1–2 status) is present preoperatively in 50% of patients, and ~26% of ventricular assist device (VAD) patients are on some sort of temporary circulatory support prior to durable VAD intervention.[6]

Patients with CS have other high-risk factors for mortality upon presentation. While patients presenting with STEMI are getting younger (mean age has dropped from 70 years in 2004 to 68 years in 2010), they have higher burdens of comorbidities, including diabetes, obesity, peripheral vascular disease, and chronic kidney disease.[3] While both sexes have had an increase in CS frequency over the past decade, the incidence of CS complicating STEMI is overall higher in women (11%) than in men (9.7%).[3] In INTERMACS, patients requiring temporary mechanical circulatory support (TCS) for CS stabilization prior to durable VAD support are older, with greater evidence of malnutrition and renal dysfunction, and they are more likely to have suffered a preoperative cardiac arrest, with greater requirements for preoperative vasopressor and ventilator support than those who are more stable.[6]

Survival in patients with CS, regardless of management strategy, remains universally poor, and complication burdens are high. In patients with a global discharge diagnosis of CS, inpatient mortality ranges from 32% to 58%.[4] Those patients presenting with STEMI as the etiology for CS have demonstrated an improvement in survival with time, but inpatient mortality is still approximately 34%.[3,4] Durable LVAD patients with preoperative CS have a 1-year survival of 69%–80% compared with 83%–84% in those who are more stable, and 1-year mortality after durable VAD is highest (29%–43%) in those patients who need TCS in the form of extracorporeal membrane oxygenation (ECMO) or percutaneous circulatory support[6–8] (Fig. 5.1). Patients with preoperative CS also have longer lengths of stay and greater needs for postoperative right ventricular (RV) support, inotropes, and hemodialysis after durable VAD implantation.[7,8]

The advent of percutaneous TCS technologies and the creation of multidisciplinary teams trained in the management of CS have contributed to small gains in patient outcomes. However, as outlined in this chapter, survival is largely driven by the severity of shock at presentation, the ability to reverse the instigator of CS, the complication burdens encountered during CS resuscitation, and the opportunity for durable VAD support in those with ongoing cardiac failure.

THE SPECTRUM OF CARDIOGENIC SHOCK

CS is best identified using both hemodynamic criteria and clinical signs/symptoms. While various definitions are used in the literature, evidences of persistent hypotension (systolic blood pressure <80–90 mm Hg or a mean arterial pressure 30 mm Hg below baseline) with a low cardiac index (<1.8 L/min/m^2 without support or <2.0–2.2 L/min/m^2 with support), reduced cardiac power output (<0.6 W), and elevated filling pressures (left ventricular end-diastolic pressure >18 mm Hg or right atrial pressure >10–15 mm Hg), along with cool

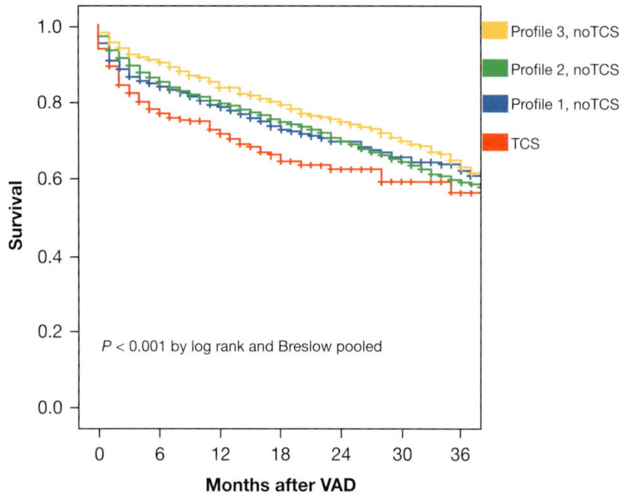

Fig. 5.1 Impact of preoperative cardiogenic shock and/or temporary circulatory support requirements on survival after durable ventricular assist device *(VAD)*. Survival in patients with preoperative cardiogenic shock (INTERMACS Profiles 1–2, *red*, *blue*, and *green lines*) is inferior to that in patients without shock (INTERMACS Profile 3, *orange line*). For those in shock, requirement for temporary circulatory support *(red line)* in the form of extracorporeal membrane oxygenation or percutaneous circulatory support portends worst survival. *INTERMACS*, Interagency Registry for Mechanically Assisted Circulatory Support; *TCS*, temporary mechanical circulatory support. (Reproduced with permission from Cowger J, Shah P, Stulak J, et al. INTERMACS profiles and modifiers: heterogeneity of patient classification and the impact of modifiers on predicting patient outcome. *J Heart Lung Transplant*. 2016;35:440–448.)

extremities, lactic acidosis, and/or evidence of end-organ dysfunction, are signs of CS.[4,9] CS presents on a wide continuum, and patient phenotypes can vary based on underlying cardiac etiology and the presence or absence of preexisting systolic dysfunction (Fig. 5.2). Compared to patients presenting with acute myocardial infarction and previously normal hearts, CS patients with longstanding HF, for example, tend to have worse hypochloremia, lower oxygen delivery and lower oxygen carrying capacity due to chronic anemia, greater peripheral extraction from chronically low cardiac output (lower mixed venous pulmonary artery saturations), greater degrees of anaerobic metabolism, and greater degrees of biventricular volume overload.[10] In a study of 64 patients undergoing ECMO for management of CS, recovery of cardiac function allowing support wean was achieved in 49% of those with acute primary CS compared with 0% of patients with chronic heart failure due to ischemic or nonischemic etiologies.[11]

Many risk factors for mortality in CS have been identified. In patients with acute coronary syndromes, the speed and success of reperfusion and the number of vessels requiring percutaneous intervention are correlated with mortality.[12,13] Other markers of mortality in CS of any etiology include advanced age, preoperative cardiac arrest, higher Acute Physiology and Chronic Health Evaluation II (APACHE II) score,[14] higher serum lactate and creatinine, altered mentation, need for ventilator support, and the number of inotropes/vasopressors required for support.[15–18] Because many of these risk factors are also markers of risk for RV failure and/or death after durable VAD, fewer patients with critical CS are undergoing VAD implant in the United States.[19,20]

The management of CS has evolved greatly over the last two decades. Options for temporary support devices have expanded beyond the intraaortic balloon pump (IABP) and ECMO to include percutaneously

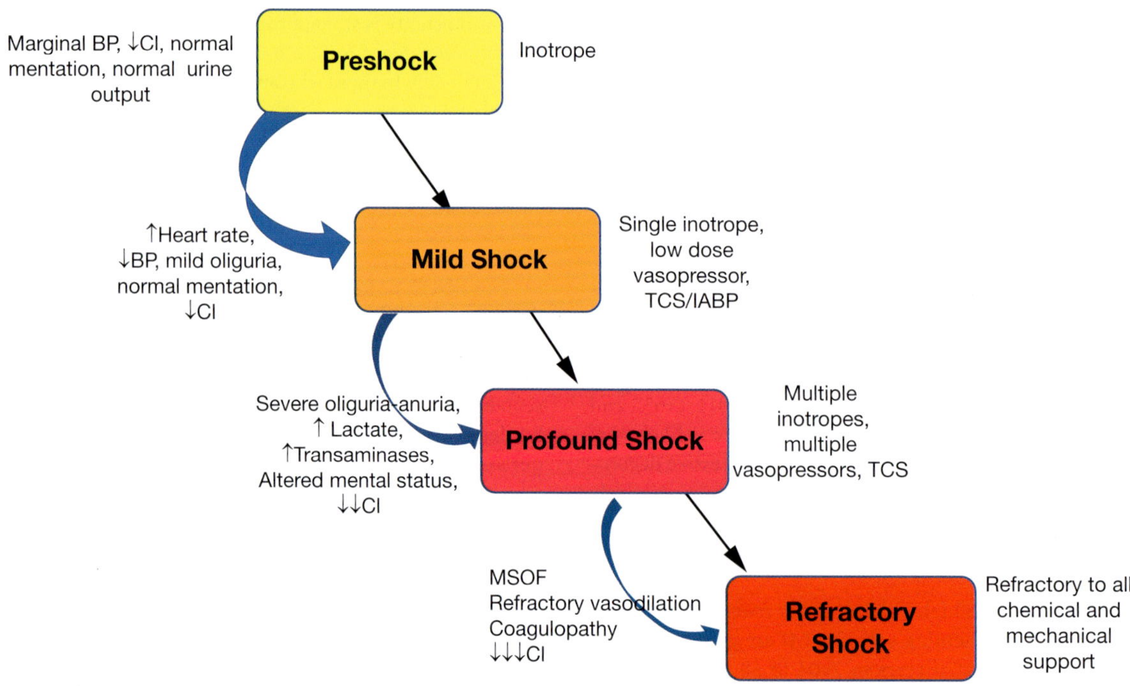

Fig. 5.2 The spectrum of cardiogenic shock. The cardiogenic shock phenotype varies based on patient end-organ function, degree of inotropic/vasopressor support requirements, and physiologic response to support. *BP*, Blood pressure; *CI*, cardiac index; *IABP*, intraaortic balloon pump; *MSOF*, multisystem organ failure; *TCS*, temporary circulatory support.

placed continuous-flow support devices and surgically placed paracorporeal pumps (discussed in detail later in this chapter). The clinical impact of CS and advanced heart failure has spurred the growth of the Advanced Heart Failure surgical and medical specialties and the development of institutional CS protocols dedicated to rapid patient resuscitation. In an analysis of 287 consecutive CS patients with acute coronary syndromes enrolled into the national cVAD registry, early initiation of Impella (Abiomed Inc., Danvers, MA) TCS before escalation of inotropes was associated with improved survival.[21] In the cohort, overall survival to discharge was 44%. While survivors had similar hemodynamics prior to the initiation of mechanical circulation support (MCS), survivors of CS were more likely to have received TCS prior to percutaneous intervention and had shorter times from the onset of CS to TCS initiation. Patients who received TCS within 1.3 hours of CS presentation had a 66% survival to discharge, compared with 37% and 26% in those who received TCS at 1.3–4.3 and >4.3 hours after CS presentation, respectively.[21] The frequency of survival was also inversely proportional to the number of inotropes required prior to the initiation of MCS. Results from the latter trial and others led to the development of CS teams across the United States. The Detroit CS Initiative, for example, is a multicenter consortium examining outcomes in patients presenting with acute myocardial infarctions and evidence of CS at four Detroit, MI, medical centers.[9] Using a protocolized management plan, survival to TCS explant improved from 51% prior to initiation of the shock protocol to 85% after.[9] In a similar analysis by the Inova Heart and Vascular Institute, survival improved from 47% prior to the initiation of a formal shock team to 81% within 2 years of shock protocol implementation.[22]

SHORT-TERM MECHANICAL CIRCULATORY SUPPORT DEVICES

Temporary circulatory support is increasingly being utilized in the management of CS and is best categorized by the method of device placement (surgical vs. percutaneous). Presently available percutaneous TCS devices include the IABP, ECMO, the Impella system, and the TandemHeart (TH) system (LivaNova, London, England) (Tables 5.1 and 5.2, Fig. 5.3). The CentriMag (Abbott, St. Paul, MN) and the CardioHelp (Maquet, Rasttat, Germany) are the main devices used for surgical paracorporeal support alone or as a driver during central or peripherally cannulated ECMO. These devices can be used in various configurations, in isolation or in conjunction with other devices, providing right and/or left ventricular support. For patients on ECMO, left ventricular TH, Impella, or IABP may be applied to assist in venting the left ventricle (LV). A comprehensive characterization of available TCS devices is depicted in Table 5.2, and clinical trial outcomes are summarized in Table 5.1. Patient support requirements, anatomy and size of available vasculature access, and institutional preference and expertise are all integral to selecting the optimal support for the patient in shock. A detailed discussion of each device is outlined in the following.

Intraaortic Balloon Pump Support

The most widely used percutaneous TCS device is the IABP (see Fig. 5.3A). An IABP can be implanted via the femoral artery or by means of percutaneous or axillary artery cut-down in a retrograde configuration, allowing for monitored patient ambulation. The IABP provides benefit during the entire cardiac cycle by inflating during early diastole to improve coronary arterial perfusion and deflating during systole to provide assistance with afterload reduction. The net benefit is a reduction in LV cardiac work and myocardial oxygen consumption. Volume shifting from IABP support is about 40 cc per beat, and this translates to only about 1 L/min of cardiac output.[1] In addition, IABP support can also improve RV hemodynamics, possibly related to ventricular interdependence. The reduction in LV filling pressures promotes more physiologic interventricular positioning, thereby improving the septal contribution to RV function.[23] In addition, IABP support is believed to augment RV function in those with high right-sided filling pressures by increasing flow (diastolic > systolic) through the right coronary artery.

Three studies evaluating the impact of IABP versus medical therapy in patients with acute myocardial infarction and CS (see Table 5.1) failed to show an improvement in survival.[24–26] The largest of these, the Intra-aortic Balloon Pump in Cardiogenic Shock (IABP-SHOCK II) trial, was a 1:1 randomized trial of usual care versus IABP support applied to 600 patients presenting with CS due to acute coronary syndromes.[24] At 30 days, mortality was 40% in the IABP arm and 41% in the controls.[24] IABP support provided no improvement in serum lactate levels, renal function, or inotrope-pressor dose.[24]

TABLE 5.1 Clinical Trials or Cohort Studies of Cardiogenic Shock and Use of Temporary Circulatory Support

Author	Year	Population	TCS Randomization	Primary Endpoint	Mortality
Thiele et al.[30]	2005	Acute MI/CS	IABP vs. TH	Cardiac power index	30 day: 45% IABP vs. 43% TH
Ohman et al.[26]	2005	Acute MI/CS	IABP vs. fibrinolytic medical therapy	30-day mortality	6 month: 39% IABP vs. 80% medical
Burkhoff et al.[27]	2006	Acute MI/CS or ADHF	IABP vs. TH	Improvement in hemodynamics	30 day: 36% IABP vs. 47% TH
Seyfarth et al.[29]	2008	Acute MI/CS	IABP vs. Impella 2.5	Cardiac index	30 day: 46% in both groups
Prodzinksky et al.[25]	2010	Acute MI/CS	IABP vs. medical therapy	APACHE II score	N/A
Thiele et al.[24]	2012	Acute MI/CS	IABP vs. medical therapy	30-day mortality	30 day: 40% IABP vs. 41% medical
Ouweneel et al.[28]	2017	Acute MI/CS	IABP vs. Impella CP	30-day mortality	6 month: 50% both groups

CS, Cardiogenic shock; *IABP*, intraaortic balloon pump; *MI*, myocardial infarction; *N/A*, not applicable; *TH*, TandemHeart.

TABLE 5.2 Temporary Circulatory Support Options for Managing Left or Right Ventricular Failure

	LEFT VENTRICULAR TEMPORARY MECHANICAL SUPPORT							RIGHT VENTRICULAR SUPPORT			BIVENTRICULAR SUPPORT
	IABP	**Impella 2.5**	**Impella CP**	**Impella 5.0**	**Impella LD**	**TandemHeart**	**CentriMag**	**ProTek DUO**	**Impella RP**	**CentriMag**	**Veno-Arterial ECMO**
Pump mechanism	Pneumatic	Axial flow	Axial flow	Axial flow	Axial flow	Centrifugal flow	Centrifugal flow	Centrifugal flow	Axial flow	Centrifugal flow	Centrifugal flow
Pump location	Extracorporeal	Intracorporeal	Intracorporeal	Intracorporeal	Intracorporeal	Paracorporeal	Paracorporeal	Paracorporeal	Intracorporeal	Paracorporeal	Paracorporeal
Cannula size	8 Fr	13 Fr	14 Fr	22 Fr	22 Fr	21 Fr inflow/var. outflow	Variable	21 Fr Inflow	23 Fr	Variable	Var inflow/outflow
Placement	Perc	Perc	Perc	Perc	Sternotomy	Perc	Perc/ Sternotomy	Perc	Perc	Perc/ sternotomy	Perc/sternotomy
Inflow	N/A	LV	LV	LV	LV	LA	LA or LV	RA	IVC	RA	RA
Outflow	N/A	Aorta	Aorta	Aorta	Aorta	FA	Aorta	PA	PA	PA	FA or aorta
Effect on LV afterload	Reduce	Reduce	Reduce	Reduce	Reduce	Increase	Increase	None	None	None	Increase
Max flow (L/min)	1	2.5	3.5	5	5	4	>5	4	4.5	>5	>5
Intensity of anticoagulation	Low	Low	Low	Low	Low	High	Moderate	High	Low	Moderate	High
Duration of support	Hours to days	Hours to days	Days	Days to weeks	Days to weeks	Days to weeks	Days to weeks	Days to weeks	Days	Days to weeks	Days to weeks
Hemolysis	Rare	Low–mod	Low–mod	Low	Low	Low	Low	Low	Low–mod	Low	Low
Risk of limb ischemia	Low	Low	Low	Low	None	High	Low–high[a]	None	None	None	Low–high[a]

[a]Degree of risk depends on whether outflow cannula is in the ascending aorta (low) or femoral artery (high).

IABP, Intraaortic balloon pump; *Fr*, French; *IVC*, inferior vena cava; *LA*, left atrium; *LV*, left ventricle; *Mod*, moderate; *NA*, not applicable; *PA*, pulmonary artery; *Perc*, percutaneous; *RA*, right atrium.

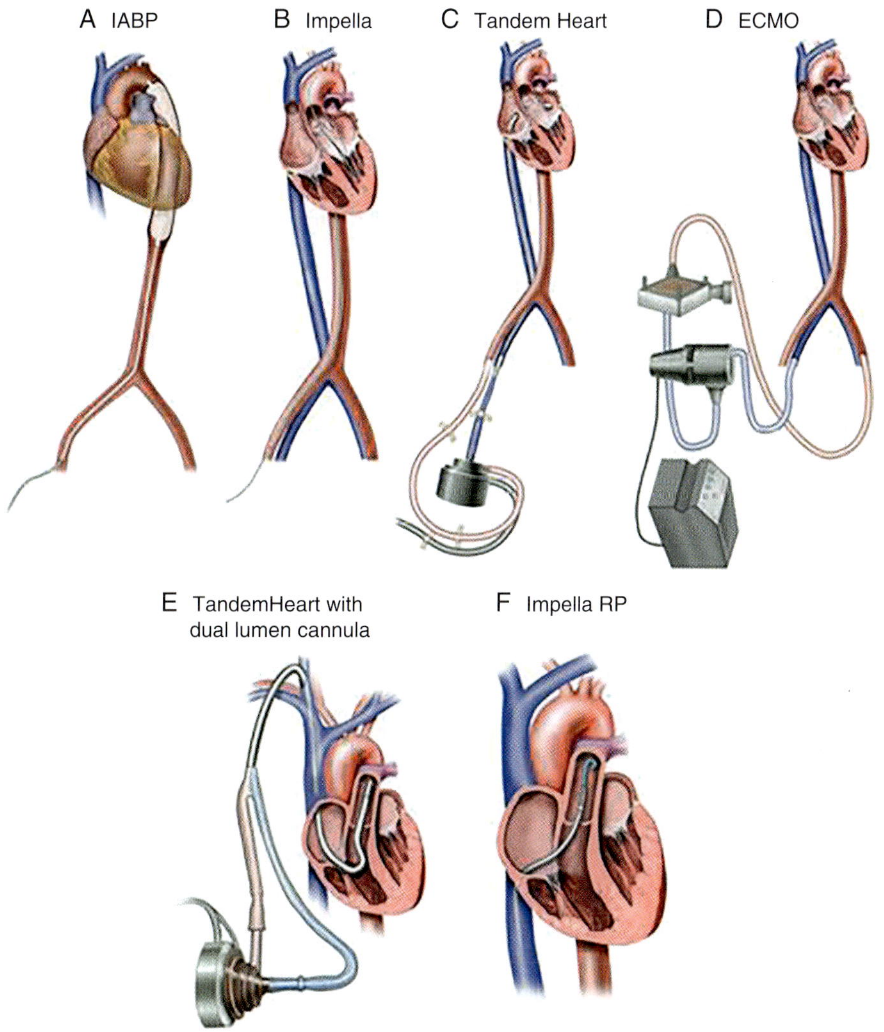

Fig. 5.3 Percutaneous and surgical temporary circulatory support options for management of cardiogenic shock. The upper row depicts common configurations for left sided support devices including (A) the intraaortic balloon pump, (B) the Impella, (C) the TandemHeart, and (D) extracorporeal membrane oxygenation *(ECMO)*. The bottom row shows right-sided circulatory support devices, including the (E) Protek-Duo TandemHeart and the (F) Impella RP. (Reproduced with permission from Mandawat A, Rao SV. Percutaneous mechanical circulatory support devices in cardiogenic shock. *Circ Cardiovasc Interv*. 2017;10.)

Four small trials (totaling 148 patients) have examined the use of IABP versus various percutaneous cardiac support technologies.[27–30] In the Impella Versus IABP Reduces Mortality in STEMI Patients Treated With Primary PCI in Severe Cardiogenic SHOCK (IMPRESS) trial, the 30-day mortality in patients (n = 48) treated with either an IABP or the Impella 3.7 L percutaneous TCS device was 50% and 46%, respectively.[28] Taken as a whole, data from randomized clinical studies examining IABP versus standard medical therapy or IABP versus other percutaneous temporary circulatory support devices have failed to show a beneficial impact on survival despite some improvement in hemodynamics. This observation has led the European Society of Cardiology to recommend against routine use of IABP support in CS.[31] Similarly, the American College of Cardiology Foundation/American Heart Association STEMI Guidelines have downgraded the use of IABP in patients failing pharmacologic therapy from a class I to IIa indication.[32]

Percutaneous Ventricular Assist Devices: Left Ventricular Support

The TandemHeart Left Ventricular Support System

The TH (see Fig. 5.3C) is a left atrial-to-femoral artery bypass system consisting of a proprietary trans-septal cannula, an arterial cannula (typically placed into the femoral artery), and an extracorporeal centrifugal blood pump. When placed percutaneously, the pump can deliver flow rates up to 5.0 L/min at a maximum speed of 7500 rpm. Placement of the left atrial cannula requires fluoroscopic and/or echocardiographic guidance, femoral venous advancement, and trans-septal puncture. The device has been used for the management of CS complicating myocardial infarction as well as in the setting of acute decompensation of other heart failure pathologics.[27,33,34] As a whole, this therapy is associated with significant improvements in hemodynamics, but at the expense of frequent bleeding complications. In randomized trails, survival using the TH mimics that achieved with IABP alone.[27,33]

Impella Left Ventricular Support System

The Impella family of devices (see Fig. 5.3B) includes three transfemoral artery devices (2.5, CP, 5.0), one transaxillary artery device (5.0L), and one transaortic device (LD) for support of the failing LV. These microaxial flow pumps are placed fluoroscopically in retrograde fashion through the femoral artery, axillary artery, or ascending aorta. The distal portion of the Impella is a pigtail configuration that is meant to reside in the mid LV approximately 3.5 cm below the aortic annulus. Blood is suctioned from an inlet (located just superior to the catheter's pigtail in the LV cavity) and then delivered through the Impella outlet, which is seated just above the aortic valve.

The Impella devices have been used in diverse clinical scenarios, including high-risk percutaneous interventions,[35,36–38] post-myocardial infarction shock,[17,28,29] acute decompensated heart failure,[39] and post-cardiotomy shock.[40] Complications include hemolysis and pigment-induced nephropathy, vascular access complications (e.g., limb ischemia and major bleeding), pericardial tamponade, mitral valve impingement with mitral regurgitation, and device failure due to thrombosis.

The limited clinical data collected from randomized clinical trials examining IABP, Impella, and TH suggest that while hemodynamics are improved, survival benefits are not seen. Thus, while tempting to summarily label these temporary options as unwarranted, several caveats must be underscored. First, most TCS trials included a small number of patients. Second, the timing of TCS initiation—perhaps one of the most important factors determining outcome—was not clearly described or predefined in these clinical trials. Moreover, and as discussed earlier, CS exists on a continuum. Depending on the stage of shock, different approaches may be required to achieve optimal outcomes.[41] Finally, and perhaps most critical, is the advent of more powerful percutaneous technologies (e.g., the Impella 5.0 [AbioMed Inc.] and the percutaneous heart pump [Abbott, Abbott Park, IL]) that can provide superior LV unloading and higher flows; these have yet to be examined within the context of prospective randomized trials. With regard to the former device, a recent meta-analysis examining the outcome of Impella 5.0 among a total of 163 patients in shock demonstrated 73.5% survival to discharge and a high rate of myocardial recovery among those explanted.[39] While data from the NIS suggest that mortality from CS is improving,[3,4] it is unknown if the improved outcomes are related to rapid intervention from advent of institutional shock protocols, greater application of TCS, improved TCS, or differences in baseline patient characteristics across the eras. Answers to these questions await future randomized clinical trials.

Percutaneous Ventricular Assist Devices: Right Ventricular Support

At present, only two percutaneous systems are commercially available for isolated RV support—the Impella RP pump and the TH Protek Duo system (see Fig. 5.3, bottom panel). The systems can aid in the management of acute RV failure of diverse etiologies, including myocardial infarction, acute pulmonary embolism, and isolated RV failure complicating LVAD implantation or orthotopic heart transplantation, among others. Both devices can be used in isolation or in conjunction with percutaneous or implantable left ventricular support.

Impella RP Right Ventricular Support Device

This particular device is the most recent addition to the Abiomed Impella device family and was the first percutaneous, single-access pump designed specifically for right heart support. The Impella RP heart pump, like all others in this family, rests entirely in an intracardiac position and delivers blood from the cannula inlet seated in the inferior vena cava to the outlet located above the pulmonic valve within the proximal pulmonary artery. The pump is inserted under fluoroscopic guidance via the femoral vein into the right atrium, across the tricuspid and pulmonic valves, and then into the pulmonary artery. Because access is presently available only via the femoral vein, patients are not able to ambulate. The device also cannot be configured for respiratory support.

The initial clinical experience with the Impella RA included 30 patients with either primary right heart failure or right heart failure following LVAD implantation.[42] Right-sided hemodynamics improved markedly. Duration of support averaged 3 days, and overall survival at 30 days was 73.3%.[42] With increasing availability and use of this technology, initial reports of biventricular percutaneous support (so called BiPELLA) are also now surfacing.[43,44] The benefit of this TCS configuration on short- and long-term patient outcomes remains unknown.

Protek Duo Right Ventricular Support Device

The Protek Duo RV support device (LivaNova, London, England) consists of a percutaneously placed dual lumen cannula that is inserted through the right internal jugular vein and advanced over a stiff wire into the main pulmonary artery. The system can be employed as isolated RV support or as a veno-venous ECMO respiratory support system. The actual pump is the same TH driver used in the LV configuration (see previous discussion). In addition, an oxygenator can easily be spliced into the system, all of which can be carried in a vest designed by the manufacturer to facilitate monitored patient mobilization.

Biventricular Support/Venoarterial Extracorporeal Membrane Oxygenation

In patients with advanced CS, biventricular failure is the norm. Multiple temporary circulatory support configurations with aforementioned pumps can be employed to achieve support of both ventricles. Moreover, in the event of coexisting respiratory failure, venoarterial (VA) ECMO support can be secured with many alternative combinations. A list of possible configurations is depicted in Table 5.3.

TABLE 5.3 Configurations for Venoarterial ECMO

Percutaneous Biventricular Support	
Left Ventricle	***Right Ventricle***
Impella CP	Impella RP
TandemHeart	Protek Duo
Impella 5.0 ax1	Impella RP
Surgically Placed Biventricular Support	
Left Ventricle	***Right Ventricle***
CentriMag	CentriMag
Impella LD	CentriMag
Percutaneous Venoarterial ECMO	
TandemHeart + Protek Duo-Oxygenator	
Any FV/FA3 cannulae attached to any centrifugal pump-oxygenator	
Surgically Placed Venoarterial ECMO	
Any RA/Ao4 cannulae attached to any centrifugal pump-oxygenator	

ECMO, Extracorporeal membrane oxygenation.

Venoarterial Extracorporeal Membrane Oxygenation

VA-ECMO represents the most comprehensive mechanical support of the circulation available, as it assists both ventricles and the respiratory system. It is comprised of a right-sided cannula(s) for venous drainage, a centrifugal pump, an oxygenator, and an arterial cannula (typically located in the aorta, axillary artery, or femoral artery) for arterial return. In essence, a VA-ECMO circuit is equivalent to the cardiopulmonary bypass circuit used routinely for cardiac operations except that it lacks a reservoir and cardiotomy suckers. Since 2010, VA-ECMO has witnessed expanded growth owing to the rapidity of deployment, improved cannula and oxygenator technologies, greater portability, attractive reimbursement, and recognition of the importance of rapid resuscitation in shock states. In many centers, institution of VA-ECMO (which was once a procedure relegated to cardiovascular surgeons) is now frequently performed by interventional cardiologists, critical care physicians, and even emergency room personnel. VA ECMO can be established percutaneously via cannulation of femoral vein and ipsilateral or contralateral femoral artery or centrally with transthoracic cannulas placed directly into the right atrium and aorta. Optimal flows of over 5 L can be easily achieved, particularly via the central route.

Certain issues unique to peripheral VA-ECMO deserve special consideration. First, this configuration leads to an increased afterload to the LV, which may impede aortic valve opening, thereby resulting in increased LV wall tension, myocardial ischemia, LV stasis, and thrombosis. Moreover, the elevated left-sided filling pressures often lead to an elevation in pulmonary capillary wedge pressure and development of pulmonary edema, which is associated with high mortality. Hence, in patients with akinetic LVs in which the aortic valve does not open, or opens infrequently, LV venting is mandated. Second, peripheral VA-ECMO can be fraught with unique complications that include local arterial injury (rupture and dissection), distal limb ischemia (from partial or complete occlusion of the ipsilateral distal femoral artery), and development of the harlequin syndrome. In the event of myocardial recovery with persistent respiratory failure, the cerebral and coronary circulations can be exposed to mixed saturated blood with an ensuing risk of ischemic events in these territories, all while the left upper extremity and lower body remain well saturated (hence harlequin). It is therefore recommended that in patients supported with peripheral VA-ECMO, a radial arterial line be used to monitor blood gases to allow for early detection of this syndrome. Distal limb ischemia can be mitigated by prophylactic placement of an antegrade or retrograde perfusion cannula in the femoral artery or pedal arteries, respectively.[45,46]

COMPLICATION OF TEMPORARY CIRCULATORY SUPPORT

The morbidity burden encountered by patients on TCS is very high. All devices require systemic therapeutic anticoagulation, making bleeding complications not infrequent. Hemolysis occurs due to shear stress on the red blood cells as they traverse the device and is exacerbated by device thrombus deposition or ingestion. Hemolysis can become severe and often presents with hemoglobinuria and elevated serum free hemoglobin and lactate dehydrogenase, with the potential for acute kidney injury due to pigment nephropathy. Thrombus deposition within pump lumens or impeller can lead to inadequate cardiac support and the potential for end-organ deterioration. Peripheral embolism can also complicate any form of TCS. For those on VA-ECMO support, the incidence of peripheral embolic complications during VA ECMO support is higher. In addition to an increased hemorrhagic stroke risk on anticoagulation, VA-ECMO leads to greater blood stasis within the LV or the aortic root, which can be a nidus for LV cavity and/or aortic root thrombosis, both with devastating results. Peripheral cannulation of VA-ECMO is inherently accompanied by retrograde blood flow from the femoral artery to the upper extremities and brain, increasing risks for atheroma embolization. In the event of myocardial recovery with persistent respiratory failure, the cerebral and coronary circulations can be exposed to mixed saturated blood and ensuing risk of ischemic events in these territories. Finally, local vascular complications can arise, especially in those with preexisting vascular disease or small vessels. The use of distal perfusion catheters to maintain antegrade or retrograde flow during femoral cannulation with any form of TCS is becoming more commonplace.[47,48]

One of the most poorly understood and potentially harmful complications of TCS is the activation of the systemic inflammatory response syndrome (SIRS). SIRS is believed to arise from shock-related hypoperfusion with subsequent microcirculatory dysfunction.[1] Studies have demonstrated higher levels of compliment activation, cytokines, and reactive oxygen species, along with evidence of endothelial cell breakdown, in CS patients.[49–51] Activation of the SIRS is believed to be one reason why end-organ dysfunction and hypotension can persist even after cardiac output is normalized (Fig. 5.4).[1] In fact, the severity of multisystem dysfunction (assessed by the APACHE II) and levels of SIRS biomarkers (including interleukin 6) are more predictive of mortality with CS than hemodynamic measures are (including cardiac power and cardiac index).[1] SIRS activation highlights the Achilles' heel of CS resuscitation and the dichotomy between achieving technical success with improved cardiac output and impacting morbidity and mortality.

CLINICAL OUTCOMES IN SHOCK PATIENTS SUPPORTED WITH SHORT-TERM MECHANICAL CIRCULATORY SUPPORT

Temporary circulatory support can provide a stable hemodynamic platform that allows medical and surgical teams the opportunity to decide on the best next step in management. As such, TCS can serve as a bridge to recovery and explantation, a bridge to transplant, a bridge to a durable LVAD, or as a bridge to palliation.

The aim of TCS prior to durable LVAD implant is to restore cardiac output and improve end-organ function with the ultimate goal of reducing LVAD operative mortality. Studies have shown that hemodynamic improvements are gained with TCS support, and for these reasons, patients requiring TCS can presently be categorized into INTERMACS Profiles 1–3 prior to durable LVAD implantation.[52] Data would suggest, however, that all patients requiring non-IABP forms of TCS be categorized as INTERMACS Profile 1 given the high associated morbidity and mortality despite improvements gained in hemodynamics and end-organ function immediately prior to durable LVAD placement.[6–8] In a multicenter study of 804 patients undergoing continuous flow LVAD placement, 68 were supported preoperatively with a non-IABP TCS device.[7] Patients requiring TCS were sicker than other Profile 1 patients who did not require TCS, demonstrating higher right atrial pressures, lower cardiac output, higher creatinine, and higher hepatic aspartate aminotransferase (AST).[7] After TCS placement, a significant improvement in cardiopulmonary hemodynamics (lower filling pressures and higher cardiac output then during pre-TCS), creatinine, and AST levels were achieved, and these levels were comparable or better than those of CS patients who were not supported with TCS. However, survival at 180 days after durable VAD

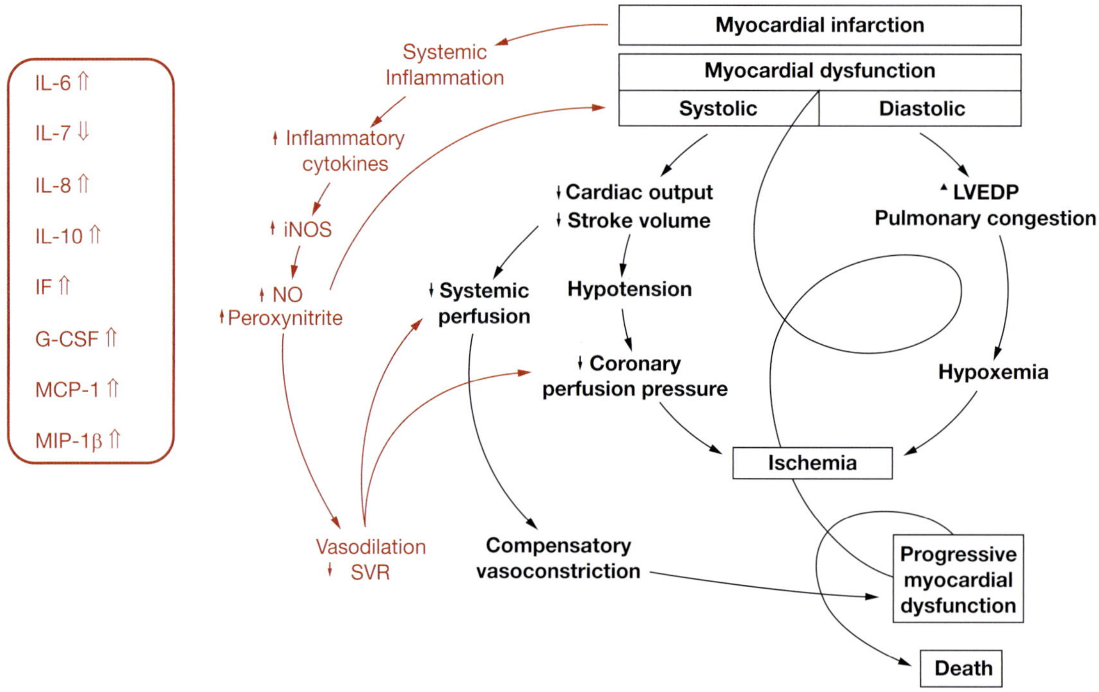

Fig. 5.4 Activation of cytokines and the systemic inflammatory response system during temporary circulatory support. Elevations in proinflammatory cytokines and oxidative stress markers and reduction in antiinflammatory mediators can contribute to macrocirculatory and microcirculatory dysfunction and subsequent systemic inflammatory response syndrome or sepsis in patients with cardiogenic shock. *G-CSF*, Granulocyte colony stimulating factor; *IF*, interferon; *iNO*, myo-inositol-phosphate synthase; *IL*, interleukin; *LVEDP*, left ventricular end diastolic pressure; *MCP*, monocyte-chemotactic protein; *MIP*, macrophage inflammatory protein; *NO*, nitric oxide; *SVR*, systemic vascular resistance. (Reproduced with permission from Werdan K, Gielen S, Ebelt H, Hochman JS. Mechanical circulatory support in cardiogenic shock. *Eur Heart J.* 2014;35:156–167.)

was 70% in patients requiring preoperative TCS compared with 79% and 88% in patients categorized as Profile 1 and Profile 2–3 without TCS, respectively.[7] In a separate analysis comparing outcomes in durable VAD patients supported preoperatively with either VA-ECMO or a left ventricular TH, patients requiring VA-ECMO (n = 14) had higher pulmonary wedge pressures, lower cardiac output, and greater needs for preoperative mechanical ventilation, inotropes, and vasopressors immediately prior to durable LVAD placement than did TH patients (n = 26).[8] After durable VAD implantation, patients requiring VA-ECMO had higher frequencies of post-LVAD RV failure and a twofold increase in renal failure requiring dialysis. Operative mortality in LVAD patients supported with preoperative VA-ECMO was 43%, compared with 12% in TH patients, 18% in non-TCS Profile 1 patients, and 8% in non-TCS Profile 2–3 patients.[8]

In an attempt to better characterize TCS use and outcomes nationally, an analysis of 8432 INTERMACS patients implanted between 2009 and 2014 was undertaken.[6] Of these patients, 26% (n = 2207) had a TCS requirement for management of CS, most commonly in the form of an IABP (80%).[6] ECMO and temporary percutaneous and/or paracorporeal VAD accounted for 11% and 7% of preoperative TCS use, respectively. Of the patients on TCS prior to LVAD, 44% were categorized as a Profile 1; 41%, as Profile 2; and 15%, as Profile 3. While use of the IABP for CS resuscitation was not associated with improved survival, patients with non-IABP TCS (redefined as ECMO, Impella, Tandem, or CentriMag device) upon entry into the operating room had a 72% 1-year survival, compared with 81% in INTERMACS patients without TCS.[6] Isolating outcomes to the cohort of INTERMACS patients categorized as having preoperative CS or rapid deterioration (INTERMACS Profiles 1–2), patients requiring TCS had a 40% higher mortality than did Profile 1–2 patients who did not require TCS. However, if a TCS patient survived the operative period, long-term survival was similar to those who did not receive TCS prior to LVAD.[6] Finally, a single-center cohort study of 58 patients undergoing Impella 5.0 placed as a bridge to candidacy demonstrated successful bridging in 67%, with 1-year survival rates of 87% and 65% in patients receiving transplant and VAD, respectively.[53] These data, in totality, suggest that VAD candidates with preoperative non-IABP TCS requirements represent a higher level of illness, even within the same INTERMACS Profile. The likely increased severity of illness in patients receiving non-IABP TCS confounds the interpretation of many of these comparative studies. While mortality and RV and renal failure rates are higher than those of more stable LVAD candidates, long-term survival gains can be achieved in carefully selected patients.[7,8,42,53–55]

CONCLUSIONS/SUMMARY

CS is associated with an in-hospital mortality of 20%–55%. Percutaneous and surgical options for managing CS patients with temporary circulatory support are growing, and national survival from CS is improving. Improvement in cardiopulmonary hemodynamics and end-organ function with use of TCS in CS does not necessarily translate into lower surgical durable VAD risk. While long-term survival may be improved with TCS and subsequent durable mechanical support, morbidity and mortality in this cohort of patients are much higher than in the general VAD population.

DISCLOSURES

Dr. Cowger is a consultant for Medtronic and Procyrion and a speaker for Abbott. Dr. Cowger works at Henry Ford. The Henry Ford Hospital receives institutional research grant funding from Medtronic and Abbott. Dr. Goldstein is National Principal Investigator for the MOMENTUM 3 Clinical trial. He receives fees as an educator and surgical proctor for Abbott Inc.

REFERENCES

1. Werdan K, Gielen S, Ebelt H, Hochman JS. Mechanical circulatory support in cardiogenic shock. *Eur Heart J.* 2014;35:156–167.
2. van Diepen S, Katz JN, Albert NM, Henry TD, Jacobs AK, Kapur NK, Kilic A, Menon V, Ohman EM, Sweitzer NK, Thiele H, Washam JB, Cohen MG. Contemporary management of cardiogenic shock: a scientific statement from the American Heart Association. *Circulation.* 2017;136:e232–e268.
3. Kolte D, Khera S, Aronow WS, Mujib M, Palaniswamy C, Sule S, Jain D, Gotsis W, Ahmed A, Frishman WH, Fonarow GC. Trends in incidence, management, and outcomes of cardiogenic shock complicating ST-elevation myocardial infarction in the United States. *J Am Heart Assoc.* 2014;3:e000590.
4. Mandawat A, Rao SV. Percutaneous mechanical circulatory support devices in cardiogenic shock. *Circ Cardiovasc Interv.* 2017;10.
5. Kirklin JK, Naftel DC, Pagani FD, Kormos RL, Stevenson LW, Blume ED, Myers SL, Miller MA, Baldwin JT, Young JB. Seventh INTERMACS annual report: 15,000 patients and counting. *J Heart Lung Transplant.* 2015;34:1495–1504.
6. Cowger J, Shah P, Stulak J, Maltais S, Aaronson KD, Kirklin JK, Pagani FD, Salerno C. INTERMACS profiles and modifiers: heterogeneity of patient classification and the impact of modifiers on predicting patient outcome. *J Heart Lung Transplant.* 2016;35:440–448.
7. Shah P, Pagani FD, Desai SS, Rongione AJ, Maltais S, Haglund NA, Dunlay SM, Aaronson KD, Stulak JM, Davis MB, Salerno CT, Cowger JA, Mechanical Circulatory Support Research Network. Outcomes of patients receiving temporary circulatory support before durable ventricular assist device. *Ann Thorac Surg.* 2017;103(1):106–112.
8. Shah P, Smith S, Haft JW, Desai SS, Burton NA, Romano MA, Aaronson KD, Pagani FD, Cowger JA. Clinical outcomes of advanced heart failure patients with cardiogenic shock treated with temporary circulatory support before durable LVAD implant. *ASAIO J.* 2016;62:20–27.
9. Basir MB, Schreiber T, Dixon S, Alaswad K, Patel K, Almany S, Khandelwal A, Hanson I, George A, Ashbrook M, Blank N, Abdelsalam M, Sareen N, Timmis SBH, O'Neill Md WW. Feasibility of early mechanical circulatory support in acute myocardial infarction complicated by cardiogenic shock: the Detroit cardiogenic shock initiative. *Catheter Cardiovasc Interv.* 2018;91:454–461.
10. Lim HS, Howell N. Cardiogenic shock due to end-stage heart failure and acute myocardial infarction: characteristics and outcome of temporary mechanical circulatory support. *Shock.* 2018;50:167–172.
11. Tarzia V, Bortolussi G, Bianco R, Buratto E, Bejko J, Carrozzini M, De Franceschi M, Gregori D, Fichera D, Zanella F, Bottio T, Gerosa G. Extracorporeal life support in cardiogenic shock: impact of acute versus chronic etiology on outcome. *J Thorac Cardiovasc Surg.* 2015;150:333–340.
12. Zeymer U, Vogt A, Zahn R, Weber MA, Tebbe U, Gottwik M, Bonzel T, Senges J, Neuhaus KL. Predictors of in-hospital mortality in 1333 patients with acute myocardial infarction complicated by cardiogenic shock treated with primary percutaneous coronary intervention (PCI); results of the primary PCI registry of the Arbeitsgemeinschaft Leitende Kardiologische Krankenhausarzte (ALKK). *Eur Heart J.* 2004;25:322–328.
13. Poss J, Koster J, Fuernau G, Eitel I, de Waha S, Ouarrak T, Lassus J, Harjola VP, Zeymer U, Thiele H, Desch S. Risk stratification for patients in cardiogenic shock after acute myocardial infarction. *J Am Coll Cardiol.* 2017;69:1913–1920.
14. Shah M, Patel B, Tripathi B, Agarwal M, Patnaik S, Ram P, Patil S, Shin J, Jorde UP. Hospital mortality and thirty day readmission among patients with non-acute myocardial infarction related cardiogenic shock. *Int J Cardiol.* 2018;270:60–67.
15. Thiele H, Zeymer U, Neumann FJ, Ferenc M, Olbrich HG, Hausleiter J, de Waha A, Richardt G, Hennersdorf M, Empen K, Fuernau G, Desch S, Eitel I, Hambrecht R, Lauer B, Bohm M, Ebelt H, Schneider S, Werdan K, Schuler G. and Intraaortic Balloon Pump in Cardiogenic Shock II Trial Investigators. Intra-aortic balloon counterpulsation in acute myocardial infarction complicated by cardiogenic shock (IABP-SHOCK II): final 12 month results of a randomised, open-label trial. *Lancet.* 2013;382:1638–1645.
16. Haft JW, Pagani FD, Romano MA, Leventhal CL, Dyke DB, Matthews JC. Short- and long-term survival of patients transferred to a tertiary care center on temporary extracorporeal circulatory support. *Ann Thorac Surg.* 2009;88:711–717, discussion 717–718.
17. Lauten A, Engstrom AE, Jung C, Empen K, Erne P, Cook S, Windecker S, Bergmann MW, Klingenberg R, Luscher TF, Haude M, Rulands D, Butter C, Ullman B, Hellgren L, Modena MG, Pedrazzini G, Henriques JP, Figulla HR, Ferrari M. Percutaneous left-ventricular support with the Impella-2.5-assist device in acute cardiogenic shock: results of the Impella-EUROSHOCK-registry. *Circ Heart Fail.* 2013;6:23–30.
18. Sieweke JT, Berliner D, Tongers J, Napp LC, Flierl U, Zauner F, Bauersachs J, Schafer A. Mortality in patients with cardiogenic shock treated with the Impella CP microaxial pump for isolated left ventricular failure. *Eur Heart J Acute Cardiovasc Care.* 2018;2048872618757393.
19. Kirklin JK, Pagani FD, Kormos RL, Stevenson LW, Blume ED, Myers SL, Miller MA, Baldwin JT, Young JB, Naftel DC. Eighth annual INTERMACS report: special focus on framing the impact of adverse events. *J Heart Lung Transplant.* 2017;36:1080–1086.
20. Ravichandran AK, Cowger J. Left ventricular assist device patient selection: do risk scores help? *J Thorac Dis.* 2015;7:2080–2087.
21. Basir MB, Schreiber TL, Grines CL, Dixon SR, Moses JW, Maini BS, Khandelwal AK, Ohman EM, O'Neill WW. Effect of early initiation of mechanical circulatory support on survival in cardiogenic shock. *Am J Cardiol.* 2017;119:845–851.
22. Tehrani B, Truesdell A, Singh R, Murphy C, Saulino P. Implementation of a cardiogenic shock team and clinical outcomes (INOVA-SHOCK Registry): observational and retrospective study. *JMIR Res Protoc.* 2018;7:e160.
23. Ntalianis A, Kapelios CJ, Kanakakis J, Repasos E, Pantsios C, Nana E, Kontogiannis C, Malliaras K, Tsamatsoulis M, Kaldara E, Charitos C, Nanas JN. Prolonged intra-aortic balloon pump support in biventricular heart failure induces right ventricular reverse remodeling. *Int J Cardiol.* 2015;192:3–8.
24. Thiele H, Zeymer U, Neumann FJ, Ferenc M, Olbrich HG, Hausleiter J, Richardt G, Hennersdorf M, Empen K, Fuernau G, Desch S, Eitel I, Hambrecht R, Fuhrmann J, Bohm M, Ebelt H, Schneider S, Schuler G, Werdan K. Intraaortic balloon support for myocardial infarction with cardiogenic shock. *N Engl J Med.* 2012;367:1287–1296.
25. Prondzinsky R, Unverzagt S, Russ M, Lemm H, Swyter M, Wegener N, Buerke U, Raaz U, Ebelt H, Schlitt A, Heinroth K, Haerting J, Werdan K, Buerke M. Hemodynamic effects of intra-aortic balloon counterpulsation in patients with acute myocardial infarction complicated by cardiogenic shock: the prospective, randomized IABP shock trial. *Shock.* 2012;37:378–384.
26. Ohman EM, Nanas J, Stomel RJ, Leesar MA, Nielsen DW, O'Dea D, Rogers FJ, Harber D, Hudson MP, Fraulo E, Shaw LK, Lee KL. Thrombolysis and counterpulsation to improve survival in myocardial infarction complicated by hypotension and suspected cardiogenic shock

or heart failure: results of the TACTICS Trial. *J Thromb Thrombolysis.* 2005;19:33–39.

27. Burkhoff D, Cohen H, Brunckhorst C, O'Neill WW. A randomized multicenter clinical study to evaluate the safety and efficacy of the TandemHeart percutaneous ventricular assist device versus conventional therapy with intraaortic balloon pumping for treatment of cardiogenic shock. *Am Heart J.* 2006;152:469.e1–469.e8.
28. Ouweneel DM, Eriksen E, Seyfarth M, Henriques JP. Percutaneous mechanical circulatory support versus intra-aortic balloon pump for treating cardiogenic shock: meta-analysis. *J Am Coll Cardiol.* 2017;69: 358–360.
29. Seyfarth M, Sibbing D, Bauer I, Frohlich G, Bott-Flugel L, Byrne R, Dirschinger J, Kastrati A, Schomig A. A randomized clinical trial to evaluate the safety and efficacy of a percutaneous left ventricular assist device versus intra-aortic balloon pumping for treatment of cardiogenic shock caused by myocardial infarction. *J Am Coll Cardiol.* 2008;52: 1584–1588.
30. Thiele H, Sick P, Boudriot E, Diederich KW, Hambrecht R, Niebauer J, Schuler G. Randomized comparison of intra-aortic balloon support with a percutaneous left ventricular assist device in patients with revascularized acute myocardial infarction complicated by cardiogenic shock. *Eur Heart J.* 2005;26:1276–1283.
31. Ponikowski P, Voors AA, Anker SD, Bueno H, Cleland JGF, Coats AJS, Falk V, Gonzalez-Juanatey JR, Harjola VP, Jankowska EA, Jessup M, Linde C, Nihoyannopoulos P, Parissis JT, Pieske B, Riley JP, Rosano GMC, Ruilope LM, Ruschitzka F, Rutten FH, van der Meer P. 2016 ESC guidelines for the diagnosis and treatment of acute and chronic heart failure: the task force for the diagnosis and treatment of acute and chronic heart failure of the European Society of Cardiology (ESC) developed with the special contribution of the Heart Failure Association (HFA) of the ESC. *Eur Heart J.* 2016;37:2129–2200.
32. O'Gara PT, Kushner FG, Ascheim DD, Casey Jr DE, Chung MK, de Lemos JA, Ettinger SM, Fang JC, Fesmire FM, Franklin BA, Granger CB, Krumholz HM, Linderbaum JA, Morrow DA, Newby LK, Ornato JP, Ou N, Radford MJ, Tamis-Holland JE, Tommaso CL, Tracy CM, Woo YJ, Zhao DX, Anderson JL, Jacobs AK, Halperin JL, Albert NM, Brindis RG, Creager MA, DeMets D, Guyton RA, Hochman JS, Kovacs RJ, Kushner FG, Ohman EM, Stevenson WG, Yancy CW. 2013 ACCF/AHA guideline for the management of ST-elevation myocardial infarction: a report of the American College of Cardiology Foundation/American Heart Association Task Force on Practice Guidelines. *Circulation.* 2013;127:e362–425.
33. Thiele H, Ohman EM, Desch S, Eitel I, de Waha S. Management of cardiogenic shock. *Eur Heart J.* 2015;36:1223–1230.
34. Kar B, Gregoric ID, Basra SS, Idelchik GM, Loyalka P. The percutaneous ventricular assist device in severe refractory cardiogenic shock. *J Am Coll Cardiol.* 2011;57:688–696.
35. Danek BA, Basir MB, O'Neill WW, Alqarqaz M, Karatasakis A, Karmpaliotis D, Jaffer FA, Yeh RW, Wyman M, Lombardi WL, Kandzari D, Lembo N, Doing A, Patel M, Mahmud E, Choi JW, Toma C, Moses JW, Kirtane A, Parikh M, Ali ZA, Garcia S, Karacsonyi J, Rangan BV, Thompson CA, Banerjee S, Brilakis ES, Alaswad K. Mechanical circulatory support in chronic total occlusion percutaneous coronary intervention: insights from a multicenter U.S. registry. *J Invasive Cardiol.* 2018;30:81–87.
36. O'Neill WW, Kleiman NS, Moses J, Henriques JP, Dixon S, Massaro J, Palacios I, Maini B, Mulukutla S, Dzavik V, Popma J, Douglas PS, Ohman M. A prospective, randomized clinical trial of hemodynamic support with Impella 2.5 versus intra-aortic balloon pump in patients undergoing high-risk percutaneous coronary intervention: the PROTECT II study. *Circulation.* 2012;126:1717–1727.
37. Cohen MG, Matthews R, Maini B, Dixon S, Vetrovec G, Wohns D, Palacios I, Popma J, Ohman EM, Schreiber T, O'Neill WW. Percutaneous left ventricular assist device for high-risk percutaneous coronary interventions: real-world versus clinical trial experience. *Am Heart J.* 2015;170:872–879.
38. Dixon SR, Henriques JP, Mauri L, Sjauw K, Civitello A, Kar B, Loyalka P, Resnic FS, Teirstein P, Makkar R, Palacios IF, Collins M, Moses J, Benali K, O'Neill WW. A prospective feasibility trial investigating the use of the Impella 2.5 system in patients undergoing high-risk percutaneous coronary intervention (The PROTECT I Trial): initial U.S. experience. *JACC Cardiovasc Interv.* 2009;2:91–96.
39. Batsides G, Massaro J, Cheung A, Soltesz E, Ramzy D, Anderson MB. Outcomes of Impella 5.0 in cardiogenic shock: a systematic review and meta-analysis. *Innovations (Philadelphia, Pa).* 2018;13:254–260.
40. Griffith BP, Anderson MB, Samuels LE, Pae WE Jr, Naka Y, Frazier OH. The RECOVER I: a multicenter prospective study of Impella 5.0/LD for postcardiotomy circulatory support. *J Thorac Cardiovasc Surg.* 2013;145:548–554.
41. Bellumkonda L, Gul B, Masri SC. Evolving concepts in diagnosis and management of cardiogenic shock. *Am J Cardiol.* 2018;122:1104–1110.
42. Anderson MB, Goldstein J, Milano C, Morris LD, Kormos RL, Bhama J, Kapur NK, Bansal A, Garcia J, Baker JN, Silvestry S, Holman WL, Douglas PS, O'Neill W. Benefits of a novel percutaneous ventricular assist device for right heart failure: the prospective RECOVER RIGHT study of the Impella RP device. *J Heart Lung Transplant.* 2015;34:1549–1560.
43. Kuchibhotla S, Esposito ML, Breton C, Pedicini R, Mullin A, O'Kelly R, Anderson M, Morris DL, Batsides G, Ramzy D, Grise M, Pham DT, Kapur NK. Acute biventricular mechanical circulatory support for cardiogenic shock. *J Am Heart Assoc.* 2017;6.
44. Pappalardo F, Schulte C, Pieri M, Schrage B, Contri R, Soeffker G, Greco T, Lembo R, Mullerleile K, Colombo A, Sydow K, De Bonis M, Wagner F, Reichenspurner H, Blankenberg S, Zangrillo A, Westermann D. Concomitant implantation of Impella((R)) on top of veno-arterial extracorporeal membrane oxygenation may improve survival of patients with cardiogenic shock. *Eur J Heart Fail.* 2017;19:404–412.
45. Juo YY, Skancke M, Sanaiha Y, Mantha A, Jimenez JC, Benharash P. Efficacy of distal perfusion cannulae in preventing limb ischemia during extracorporeal membrane oxygenation: a systematic review and meta-analysis. *Artificial organs.* 2017;41:E263–e273.
46. Ranney DN, Benrashid E, Meza JM, Keenan JE, Bonadonna D, Mureebe L, Cox MW, Daneshmand MA. Vascular complications and use of a distal perfusion cannula in femorally cannulated patients on extracorporeal membrane oxygenation. *ASAIO J.* 2018;64:328–333.
47. Kizner L, Flottmann C, Horstkotte D, Gummert J. Bilateral antegrade perfusion of the superficial femoral artery to prevent limb ischaemia during combined use of Impella CP left ventricular assist device and extracorporeal life support. *Interact Cardiovasc Thorac Surg.* 2016;23:335–337.
48. Makdisi G, Makdisi T, Wang IW. Use of distal perfusion in peripheral extracorporeal membrane oxygenation. *Ann Transl Med.* 2017;5:103.
49. Frydland M, Ostrowski SR, Moller JE, Hadziselimovic E, Holmvang L, Ravn HB, Jensen LO, Pettersson AS, Kjaergaard J, Lindholm MG, Johansson PI, Hassager C. Plasma concentration of biomarkers reflecting endothelial cell- and glycocalyx damage are increased in patients with suspected ST-elevation myocardial infarction complicated by cardiogenic shock. *Shock.* 2018;50:538–544.
50. Orrem HL, Nilsson PH, Pischke SE, Grindheim G, Garred P, Seljeflot I, Husebye T, Aukrust P, Yndestad A, Andersen GO, Barratt-Due A, Mollnes TE. Acute heart failure following myocardial infarction: complement activation correlates with the severity of heart failure in patients developing cardiogenic shock. *ESC Heart Fail.* 2018;5:292–301.
51. Parenica J, Jarkovsky J, Malaska J, Mebazaa A, Gottwaldova J, Helanova K, Litzman J, Dastych M, Tomandl J, Spinar J, Dostalova L, Lokaj P, Tomandlova M, Pavkova MG, Sevcik P, Legrand M. Infectious complications and immune/inflammatory response in cardiogenic shock patients: a prospective observational study. *Shock.* 2017;47:165–174.
52. Stevenson LW, Pagani FD, Young JB, Jessup M, Miller L, Kormos RL, Naftel DC, Ulisney K, Desvigne-Nickens P, Kirklin JK. INTERMACS

profiles of advanced heart failure: the current picture. *J Heart Lung Transplant*. 2009;28:535–541.

53. Hall SA, Uriel N, Carey SA, Edens M, Gong G, Esposito M, O'Kelly R, Annamalai S, Aghili N, Adatya S, Kapur NK. Use of a percutaneous temporary circulatory support device as a bridge to decision during acute decompensation of advanced heart failure. *J Heart Lung Transplant*. 2018;37:100–106.
54. Brown JL, Estep JD. Temporary percutaneous mechanical circulatory support in advanced heart failure. *Heart Fail Clin*. 2016;12:385–398.
55. Ravichandran AK, Baran DA, Stelling K, Cowger JA, Salerno CT. Outcomes with the Tandem Protek Duo Dual-Lumen Percutaneous Right Ventricular Assist Device. *ASAIO J*. 2018;64:570–572.

6

The Role of Extracorporeal Membrane Oxygenation in Cardiac Support

Christian A. Bermudez, Mani A. Daneshmand

KEY POINTS

BACKGROUND

The modern era of extracorporeal circulation began in the early 1950s, with cardiopulmonary bypass (CPB) used to support patients during open-heart operations for the repair of congenital heart defects. Over the course of the next two decades, improvements to the CPB circuits and oxygenator technology, especially the advent of the membrane oxygenator in the early 1970s, led to the development of extracorporeal membrane oxygenation (ECMO).[1] This new technology allowed for efficient shunting of blood between the venous and arterial systems while actively oxygenating the blood, thus providing cardiac and respiratory support. While the original CPB technology achieved the same goal, the advent of the membrane oxygenator allowed this technology to be used in the intensive care unit. As extracorporeal circulatory support technology continues to improve and evolve (Fig. 6.1), its use is more prevalent than ever.

The first report of successful ECMO support was in 1972 in an adult patient with advanced respiratory failure as a consequence of severe pulmonary contusion.[2] This success resulted in a fervor of enthusiasm for the therapy, which was abruptly stunted 2 years later when a clinical trial only had 2 survivors out of 17 patients supported with ECMO.[3] In the decades that followed, ECMO was rarely utilized in adults, but ECMO use was rapidly expanded to pediatric patients with congenital heart disease, meconium aspiration, or diaphragmatic hernia when no other options were available. As a therapy for adult patients, ECMO use was limited to acute cardiogenic shock refractory to medical therapy or to patients with inability to come off CPB after complex cardiac operations.[4] Limitations of the pump and oxygenator technology limited prolonged and stable support. Adults who were supported with ECMO had high rates of associated complications, including bleeding, thromboembolism, early oxygenator failure, disseminated intravascular coagulopathy, and systemic inflammatory response syndrome. These complications, coupled with the availability of other circulatory support options, limited the use of ECMO, such that it was considered only occasionally as a salvage option in patients with very advanced cardiopulmonary failure.

Fortunately, with the development of polymethylpentene (PMP) oxygenators, bearing-less centrifugal pumps, and better cannula technology, there has been a rapid increase in the use of ECMO for cardiac support since 2009 (Fig. 6.2).[5,6] ECMO has been successfully used as a bridge to cardiac recovery, a bridge to heart transplantation (BTT), a bridge to a more permanent left ventricular assist device (LVAD), a or as bridge-to-bridge (BTB). The indications for adult ECMO have also expanded to include patients with various etiologies of cardiac failure, including acute myocardial infarction (AMI), end-stage dilated cardiomyopathy, refractory ventricular arrhythmias, acute myocarditis, the inability to wean from bypass after cardiac surgery, and cardiac arrest.[7] The ability of ECMO to provide complete cardiac support (left and right ventricle) as well as oxygenation has several advantages over some other percutaneous and surgically implanted temporary devices. Its ease of implantation and versatility have made ECMO the most widely used circulatory support system, with close to 2500 implants per year in the United States for cardiac support (Fig. 6.2).

CURRENT ECMO TECHNOLOGIES USED IN CARDIAC SUPPORT

ECMO combines the use of a pump (ideally a centrifugal pump) for blood propulsion and a membrane oxygenator for gas exchange. Other components include the pump electrical drive unit (controller), tubing, cannulas, and a heat exchanger to prevent temperature loss (Fig. 6.3). A venous cannula is used to drain deoxygenated blood into the pump. This pump then pushes the blood through a membrane oxygenator for gas exchange, and then the oxygenated blood is returned to the patient via an arterial cannula, resulting in complete respiratory and hemodynamic support. The amount of blood flow through the circuit and the fraction of oxygen delivered through the oxygenator are the main determinants of blood oxygenation and circulatory support. The rate of gas flow through the oxygenator, known as the sweep gas flow rate, and the blood flow rate are the major determinants of carbon dioxide removal. In other words, as the flow of sweep gas through the oxygenator increases relative to the flow of blood through the oxygenator, the CO_2 content of the blood leaving the oxygenator and returning to the body decreases. Currently, there are no US Food and Drug Administration–approved devices for ECMO. The current systems have all been approved through the 510K device approval pathway for a 6-hour extracorporeal life support indication. However,

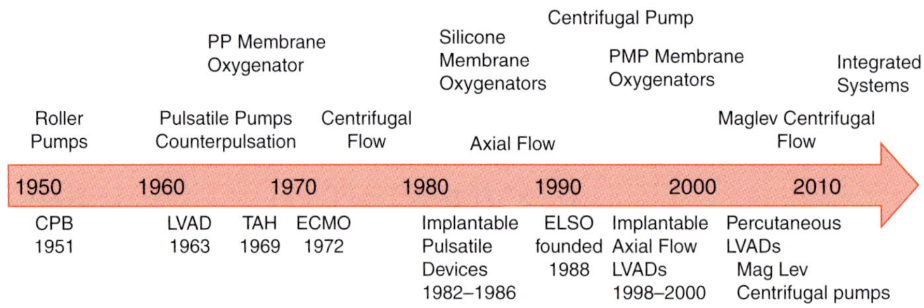

Fig. 6.1 Timeline of the evolution of blood pumps for mechanical circulatory support. *CPB*, Cardiopulmonary bypass; *ECMO*, extracorporeal membrane oxygenation; *ELSO*, Extracorporeal Life Support Organization; *LVAD*, left ventricular assist device; *PMP*, polymethylpentene; *PP*, polypropylene; *Mag Lev*, magnetic levitation; *TAH*, total artificial heart.

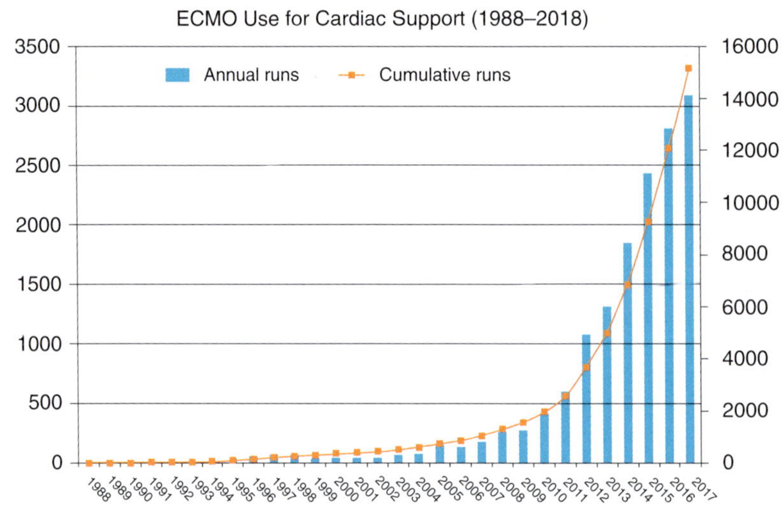

Fig. 6.2 Extracorporeal membrane oxygenation *(ECMO)* use by year, as documented in the Extracorporeal Life Support Organization registry in January 2018.

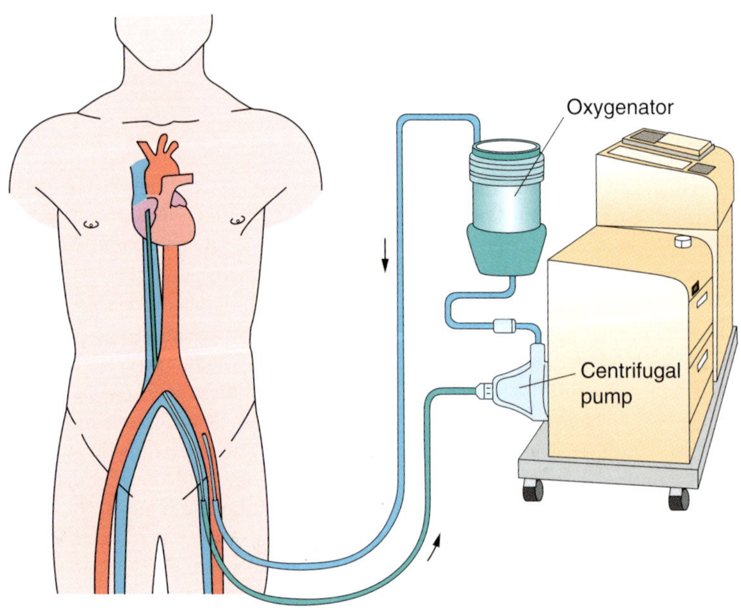

Fig. 6.3 Percutaneous extracorporeal membrane oxygenation (ECMO) circuit. A peripheral venoarterial ECMO configuration is depicted. Right atrial blood is removed via a catheter inserted into the femoral vein and advanced to the right atrium. Oxygenated blood is delivered via the femoral artery.

in practice, the use of this technology has been extended far beyond those limits, with an average cardiac ECMO support time of 166 hours as per the 2017 Extracorporeal Life Support Organization (ELSO) annual report.

Initially, roller pumps were used for blood propulsion in ECMO circuits. These pumps work by squeezing tubing carrying the blood to cause forward flow; with prolonged use, they result in significant blood trauma. Centrifugal pumps, on the other hand, have theoretically less associated blood trauma and have essentially replaced roller pumps in adult ECMO. The use of centrifugal pumps has been frequently associated with significantly decreased blood trauma, thrombus formation, secondary hemolysis, and acute pump failure, although some controversy still exists.[8–10] Centrifugal pumps are preload dependent, meaning that their flow rates are sensitive to the volume available to the pump inlet. They generate a negative inlet pressure, allowing for kinetic drainage. Centrifugal pumps are also after load sensitive, meaning that their flow rates are inversely responsive to the pressure at the pump outlet. For this reason, if the patient's blood pressure is abnormally elevated, ECMO flow decreases. This is a significant advantage relative to roller pumps because kinks in the tubing after the centrifugal pump can result in decreased flow, but not the catastrophic tubing ruptures that have happened with roller pumps. These properties also allow the centrifugal pump to be closer to the patient resulting in shorter lines, smaller priming volume, decreased surface area of blood exposure, and decreased blood transit time.

First-generation centrifugal pumps had a constrained vortex design with a closed center, a mechanical bearing, and a direct coupling of the pump rotor to drive motor. This design resulted in significant blood stagnation potential at various locations within the pump. To combat this stagnation potential, second-generation pumps used an impeller with an open-center "Mendler" design. Additionally, these pumps are magnetically coupled to the drive motor and use a pivot bearing. Third-generation pumps share similar bloodflow design, but with a "bearing-less" fully magnetically levitated impeller. This decreases heat generation and the likelihood of pump thrombosis. The pumps most frequently used for ECMO support in the United States include the Maquet Rotaflow (Getinge), the Sorin Revolution (LivaNova), and the St Jude Centrimag (Abbott) (Fig. 6.4). Newer centrifugal pump technologies (which are not approved for use in the United States) are commercially available in the European Union with CE Mark approval, including the Medos Deltastream DP3, which boasts minimal priming volume and the ability for pulsatile flow.

Improvements in oxygenator technology have been even more important than pump improvements for the recent success of ECMO support in treating cardiopulmonary disease. The advent of membrane oxygenation made ECMO possible, because all previous oxygenator technologies caused too much blood trauma. The first membrane oxygenators used solid silicone membranes for oxygen exchange.[1] These oxygenators were limited by a high rate of platelet deposition and thrombus formation that affected the durability and functionality of the oxygenators and resulted in early failure. Subsequently, the development of microporous, hollow-fiber (polypropylene) membranes allowed for better oxygen transfer with decreased membrane oxygenator size. Since the mid-2000s, the use of nanoporous hollow fibers with PMP has revolutionized oxygenator technology, allowing for prolonged support with decreased blood component trauma, decreased platelet activation, lower thromboembolism, and decreased device-related bleeding complications.[5,11,12] These PMP membranes have a compressed (skinned) surface, reduced pore size (<0.03 μm), high gas permeability, and infrequent plasma leakage. The PMP oxygenators most often used in the United States are the Quadrox D (Maquet/Getinge) and the EOS ECMO (Sorin/LivaNova) (Fig. 6.5), but the HiLiteLT (Xenios) and Novalung (Xenios) have also been available. Additionally, the newest oxygenators have integrated connections for heat exchange, which facilitate patient temperature control. More recently, integrated ECMO systems have been developed that couple a second-generation centrifugal pump with a PMP oxygenator, allowing for a decrease in the overall ECMO system size and increased portability. In general, while the "a la carte" combination of second- and third-generation pumps with PMP nanoporous oxygenators has been quite successful (Rotaflow/Centrimag pumps and Quadrox D oxygenator or Sorin Revolution or EOS Oxygenator), the use of integrated systems (Maquet CardioHelp or Tandem Lung) has become increasingly popular due to decreased size and improved portability (Fig. 6.6). Despite a multitude of available ECMO systems, there is no scientific evidence supporting the superiority of any of the modern technologies in patients supported with either venoarterial (VA) or venovenous (VV) ECMO.

Unlike pumps and oxygenators, there has been less innovation to cannula technologies for cardiac support. The current cannula designs have been borrowed from peripheral CPB systems. They are tapered, which facilitates peripheral (percutaneous or direct) cannulation as well as direct central cannulation, but they lack modifications for long-term use. While the cannulas have excellent flow

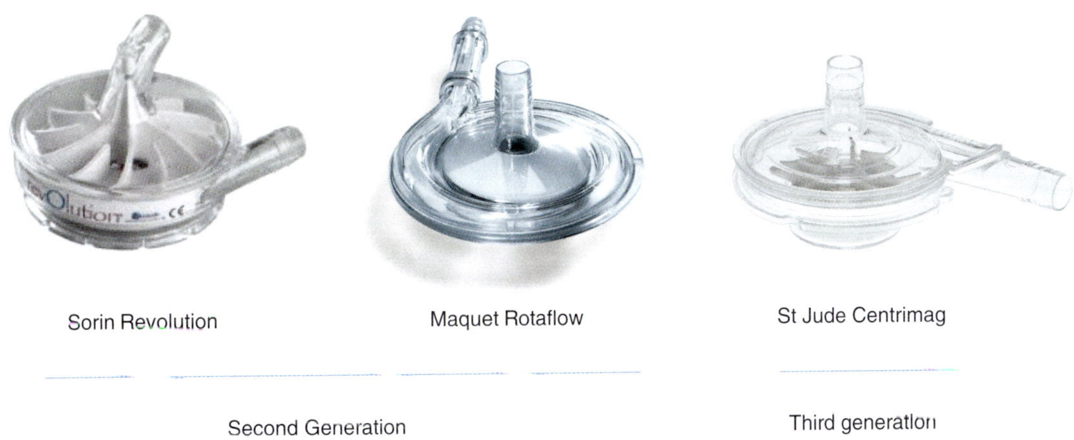

Fig. 6.4 Pumps used for extracorporeal membrane oxygenation support in the United States. (Used with kind permission from LivaNova, Getingo, and Abbott. Permission for use does not imply that any device is currently approved for prolonged support in the United States.)

PMP fibers

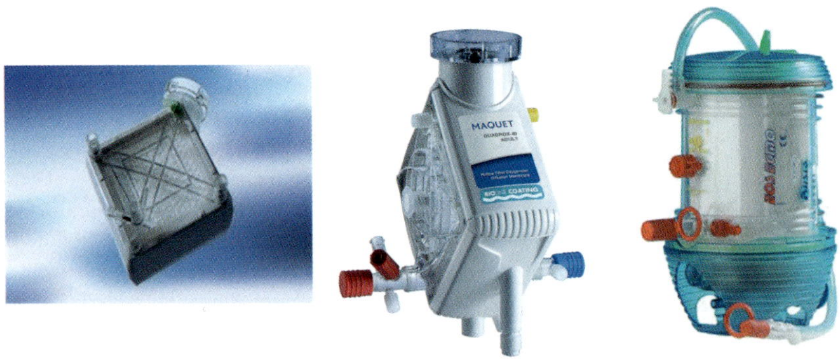

QUADROX D and QUADROX i(D) (Maquet) EOS ECMO (Sorin)

Fig. 6.5 Oxygenators used for ECMO support in the United States. *ECMO*, Extracorporeal membrane oxygenation; *PMP*, polymethylpentene. (Used with kind permission from Getinge and LivaNova. Permission for use does not imply that any device is currently approved for prolonged support in the United States.)

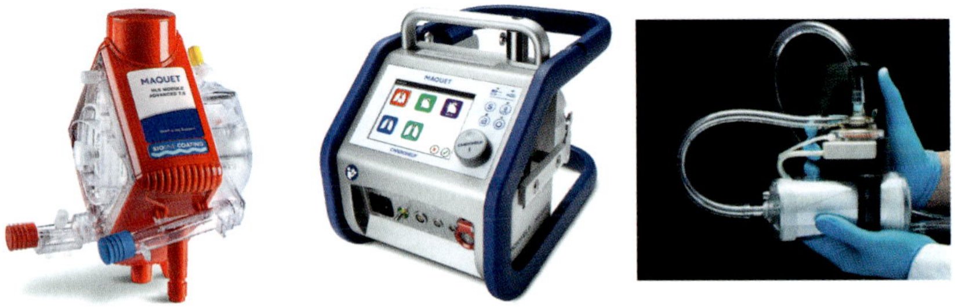

CardioHelp Tandem Lung

Fig. 6.6 Integrated systems for extracorporeal membrane oxygenation support. (Used with kind permission from Getinge and LivaNova/Tandem Life. Permission for use does not imply that any device is currently approved for prolonged support in the United States.)

characteristics (many achieve up to 6 L/min with minimal pressure gradient), they lack innovations that facilitate distal perfusion of peripheral vessels or enable easy percutaneous removal. Most of the innovation in tubing and cannula design has been focused on improving biocompatibility. Most tubing, cannulas, and other circuit components have a proprietary biocompatible surface coating (heparin, phosphorylcholine, poly-2-methoxy-ethyl acrylate (PMEA), and others) to decrease blood component activation, platelet deposition, and thrombus formation.[13]

While there have been significant advancements in ECMO technology over the years, there is still significant room for improvement. ECMO system designs currently under development and in the early phases of clinical use may allow further decreases in pump and oxygenator size, improved portability, and even the ability to provide counter pulsation through pump speed changes. Ultimately, the goal of any innovation in ECMO technology will be to improve biocompatibility, safety, and clinical outcomes.

ECMO CONFIGURATIONS AND CANNULATION STRATEGIES FOR CARDIAC SUPPORT

ECMO can be configured for either primarily respiratory support, VV-ECMO, or circulatory support, VA-ECMO. In VV-ECMO, deoxygenated blood is withdrawn from the venous system and oxygenated blood is returned to the venous system, effectively scrubbing CO_2 and preoxygenating blood before it is pumped to the lungs by the heart. During VA-ECMO, deoxygenated blood is withdrawn from the venous system and oxygenated blood is returned to the arterial system providing circulatory support. Occasionally, a hybrid technique where oxygenated blood is returned to the venous system and the arterial system simultaneously (known as veno-arterio-venous [VAV] or veno-veno-arterial [VVA] ECMO) is used, usually in patients with severely decreased pulmonary function or significant pulmonary shunt.

Cannulation techniques for VA-ECMO depend on the clinical condition of the patient and the available vascular access.[14–16] In patients with nonoperative cardiogenic shock (e.g., AMI, myocarditis, and decompensated chronic heart failure), percutaneous peripheral cannulation of the femoral artery and femoral vein is the most frequently used technique in adults (Fig. 6.7A). In the presence of femoral-iliac vascular disease, peripheral open subclavian artery cannulation is a useful option. This technique requires the creation of an end-to-side "chimney graft" with a Dacron graft to prevent subclavian arterial damage (see Fig. 6.7B). In these patients, the venous drainage cannulation can be placed in the femoral vein or the internal jugular (IJ) vein. Patients who have shock during or after cardiac surgery (through a sternotomy) can be supported with central cannulation, typically achieved with direct cannulation of the right atrium and aorta (Fig. 6.8).

For percutaneous femoral cannulation, the femoral artery is usually located by ultrasound and accessed using the modified

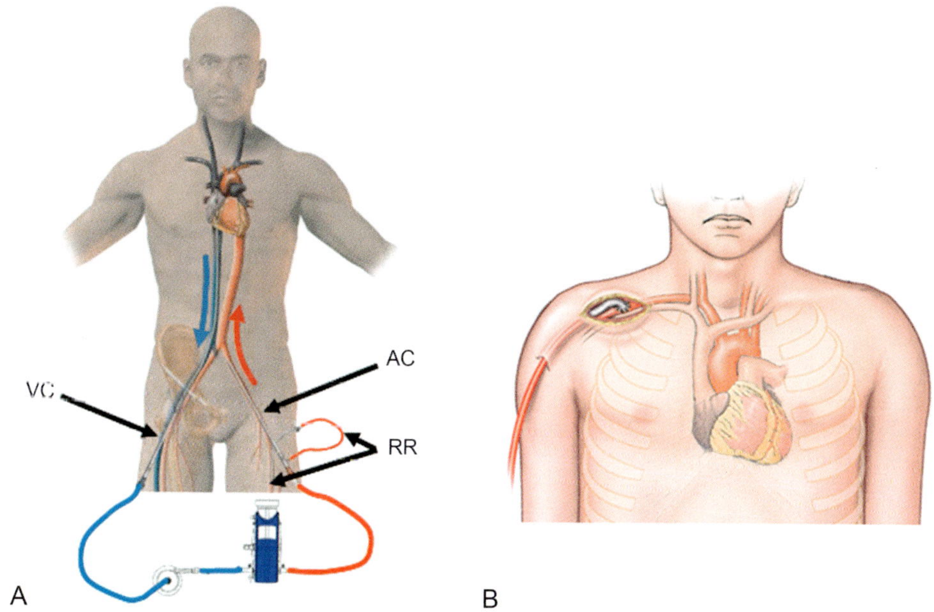

Fig. 6.7 Cannulation approaches for peripheral venoarterial extracorporeal membrane oxygenation (VA-ECMO). (A) Peripheral femoral VA-ECMO. (From Banfi C, Pozzi M, Brunner ME, et al. Veno-arterial extracorporeal membrane oxygenation: an overview of different cannulation techniques. Journal of thoracic disease. 2016;8(9):E875-E885.) (B) Peripheral subclavian VA-ECMO. *AC*, Arterial cannula; *RR*, distal perfusion catheter; *VC*, venous cannula.

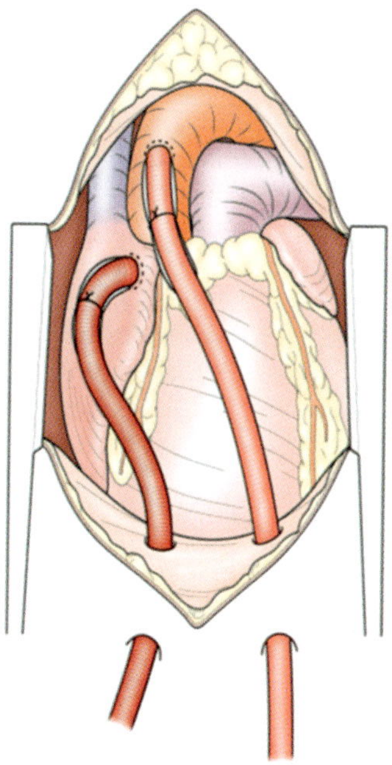

Fig. 6.8 Atrial-to-aorta cannulation for central venoarterial extracorporeal membrane oxygenation. (From Bermudez C, Poynter J. ECMO and Temporary Mechanical Circulatory Assistance. In Spray TL, Acker MA, eds. *Operative Cardiac Surgery*. 6th ed. 2018. CRC Press, Boca Raton.)

Seldinger technique. After progressive arterial dilation is performed using tapered dilators, the arterial cannula is then inserted over the guidewire and its tip is positioned in the distal abdominal aorta or proximal common iliac artery. Peripheral arterial cannulas sized 15–16 Fr are used for smaller patients (<60 kg), and 17–21 Fr cannulas are used for larger patients. A similar technique is used for the cannulation of the femoral vein, with the goal of placing the cannula tip in the body of the right atrium. When patients are cannulated emergently, arterial and venous cannulation occurs on whichever side is accessed first. In patients in more stable condition, the authors prefer to cannulate the right femoral vein and the contralateral femoral artery. This theoretically facilitates venous return in the leg with arterial cannulation and decreases the risk of limb ischemia. In the absence of image guidance (fluoroscopy or transesophageal echocardiography), secondary signs of wire placement must be used for venous cannulation, including ventricular ectopy and the "feel" of the wire. Generally, adequate venous drainage can be achieved with a 22 Fr multi-fenestrated venous cannula in smaller patients (<60 kg) and a 25 Fr multi-fenestrated venous cannula in larger patients; the target ECMO flow rate is 2.0–2.2 LPM/m^2. When ECMO cannulation is placed during cardiopulmonary resuscitation (CPR) in patients with small femoral vessels or patients whose vessels cannot be easily located on ultrasound, an open technique can be utilized. After the vessels are exposed surgically, cannulation is performed either directly through a purse string, over the wire through a purse string ("semi-Seldinger"), or through an end-to-side Dacron graft sewn to the artery.

Femoral arterial cannulation can jeopardize perfusion of the distal femoral artery and can be abated with a distal perfusion catheter (Fig. 6.7A). The use of distal arterial perfusion catheters is recommended in all patients undergoing peripheral VA-ECMO because there is increasing evidence that distal perfusion decreases the rate of serious vascular complications.[17,18] If the patient is relatively stable, inserting the distal perfusion cannula prior to femoral arterial cannulation is preferred; this facilitates identification of the distal superficial femoral artery. Then, using the modified Seldinger technique, a 5–10 Fr cannula or sheath is introduced in the superficial femoral artery and connected to the arterial limb of the circuit (Fig. 6.9). It is important to confirm the passage of the wire with ease into the distal part of the artery as the guide wire and cannula can easily be positioned in the profunda femoris artery, leading to subsequent ischemia of the lower extremity. If the procedure is performed in the operating room or if there is a specific concern regarding distal lower extremity

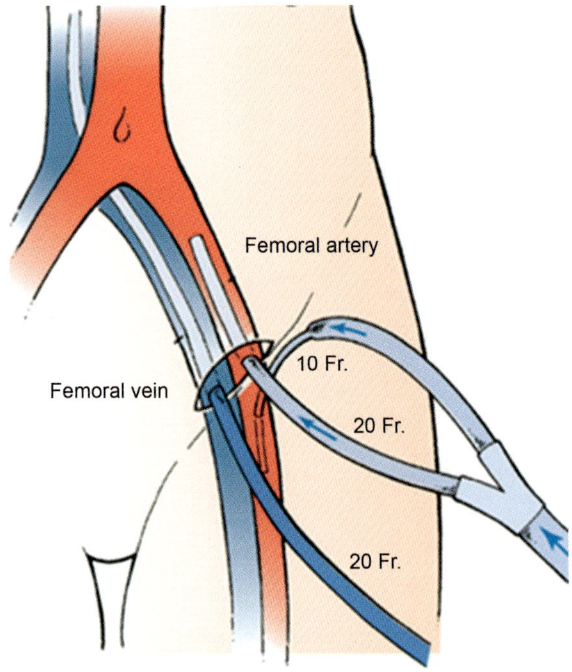

Fig. 6.9 Distal arterial perfusion. (Reprinted from McGee JEC, Moazami N. Temporary mechanical circulatory support. In Cohn LH, Adams DH, eds. *Cardiac Surgery in the Adult.* 5th ed. 2017. McGraw-Hill Education, New York. pp. 429-452.)

perfusion, angiography should be performed to confirm proper positioning.[19] Some clinicians routinely confirm positioning using angiography. There is recent evidence that near-infrared spectroscopy may identify limb ischemia, and advocates recommend monitoring both limbs for the duration of ECMO support as ischemia may occur in up to 30% of ECMO patients.[20,21]

Peripheral VA-ECMO support will increase mean arterial pressure and, in turn, increase left ventricular (LV) afterload. In some patients, this may cause an increase in LV end-diastolic pressure, leading to pulmonary injury and severe pulmonary congestion/edema.[22] The resulting pulmonary shunt will fill the LV with poorly oxygenated blood that may be ejected every cardiac cycle. If patients are femorally cannulated, this deoxygenated blood can fill the root of the aorta and head vessels, resulting in central hypoxia, known as North-South syndrome (Fig. 6.10). If the ventricle does not eject while on VA-ECMO, there can be intraventricular, LV outflow tract, or sinus of Valsalva thrombus formation, as well as severe LV distention, resulting in coronary ischemia, arrhythmias, or cerebrovascular thromboembolism.[23] Animal studies have demonstrated that peripheral VA-ECMO can cause pressure-volume curve dissociation, decreased coronary perfusion, and poor LV unloading when compared with devices that directly drain the LV.[24] To minimize the risks associated with femoral ECMO, patients should be monitored closely, and proactive steps should be taken to prevent complications. Specifically, it is important to prevent LV distention, LV thrombosis, and lung injury. This can be achieved either by placing an axial blood pump across the aortic valve to decompress the LV or by direct venting of the LV with a cannula placed either in the LV apex or in the right superior pulmonary vein, diverting blood into the venous limb of the ECMO circuit. LV unloading has been associated with improved survival and decreased pulmonary congestion and may facilitate myocardial recovery.[25]

In patients with North-South syndrome, VAV-ECMO (Fig. 6.11) has been used to improve oxygenation of blood that is ejected by the

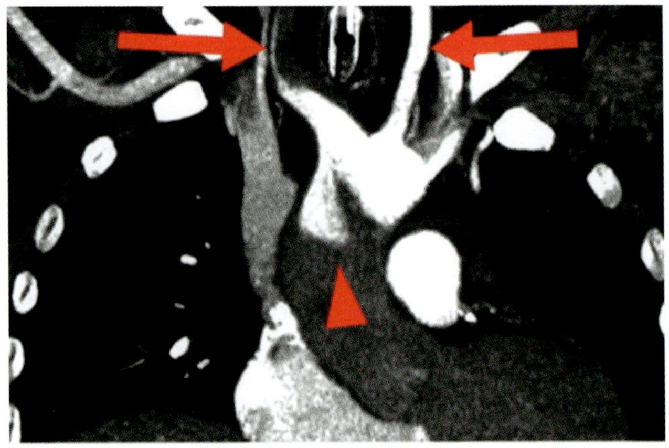

Fig. 6.10 Central hypoxia (North-South syndrome) due to increased pulmonary shunting in the presence of primary or secondary lung injury in patients on peripheral venoarterial extracorporeal membrane oxygenation. (From Napp LC, Kühn C, Hoeper MM, et al. Cannulation strategies for percutaneous extracorporeal membrane oxygenation in adults. *Clin Res Cardiol.* 2016;105(4):283–296.)

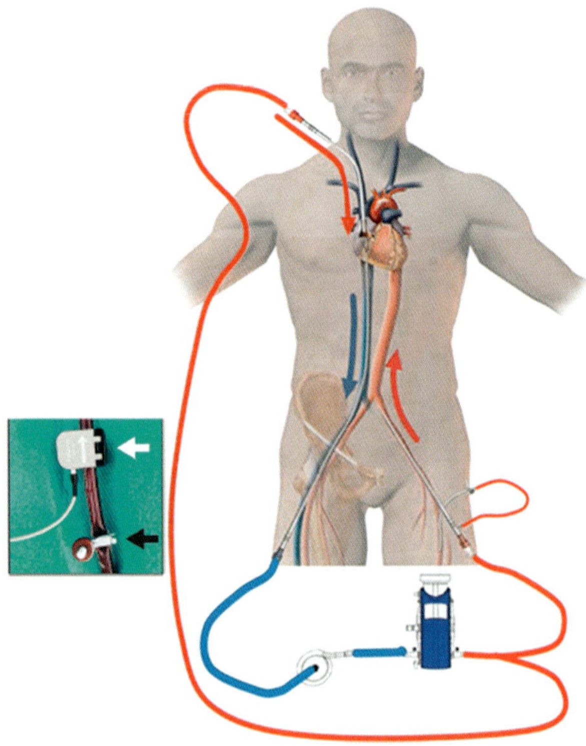

Fig. 6.11 Veno-arterial-venous extracorporeal membrane oxygenation. Cannulation of the femoral artery and vein and the addition of a right internal jugular venous cannula providing arterial blood. This cannulation is usually percutaneous. Flow through the inferior jugular cannula should be monitored with a flow probe and adjusted with a vascular clamp. (From Banfi C, Pozzi M, Siegenthaler N, et al. Veno-venous extracorporeal membrane oxygenation: cannulation techniques. *J Thorac Dise.* 2016;8(12):3762-3773.)

LV. This is achieved with the placement of a second cannula (16–18 Fr) in the right IJ vein. The insertion of this IJ cannula is similar to femoral venous cannulation using the modified Seldinger technique. The cannula is connected to the arterial limb of the ECMO circuit, in addition to the existing cannula in the arterial system. Oxygenated blood returns to the patient from both the femoral artery, providing circulatory support), and the right IJ vein, providing pulmonary support. Because of the compliance difference between the venous and arterial vascular trees, it is important to monitor and regulate flow between these "oxygenated" limbs. Flow is monitored using an ultrasonic flow probe and can be diverted from the right IJ cannula to the femoral cannula by partially occluding the right IJ cannula using a Hoffman clamp.

The most definitive technique for preventing LV thrombus formation is venting the LV, either with a surgically placed cannula or with a transvalvular axial pump.[26] In the absence of an LV vent, maintaining contractility to allow LV ejection and adequate anticoagulation will minimize the risk of thrombus formation. Typically, partial thromboplastin time is maintained at 50–70 seconds with intravenous heparin, if there is no concern for bleeding. LV ejection can be maintained by providing inotropic medications, reducing afterload (with medicines or an intra-aortic balloon pump), and optimizing volume status. A recent study compared the use of ECMO vs. ECMO and Impella for LV drainage. The findings suggested a survival benefit and improved ability to wean ECMO in patients whose LV was unloaded, suggesting that active venting may be beneficial.[27]

VA-ECMO using central cannulation is used frequently in patients presenting with cardiogenic shock after cardiac operations or in cases where peripheral access is not an option (e.g., femoral-iliac occlusive disease). Due to the antegrade flow in the aorta, central VA-ECMO is generally not associated with North-South syndrome and, may provide better unloading of the left and right ventricles than peripheral femoral ECMO, due to the larger drainage cannulas. After exposure of the heart via sternotomy or right anterior thoracotomy, purse-string sutures are placed in the ascending aorta and right atrium; the sutures are captured with tourniquets. Although standard CPB cannulas can be used for central ECMO, the authors prefer to use tapered percutaneous cannulas. This allows for exteriorization through the abdominal wall (Fig. 6.8) and, potentially, complete closure of the chest. For venous drainage, typically a large venous cannula (>28 Fr) is selected. Once on support, the LV is evaluated for distention and stasis. If there is any concern, a surgical vent is placed using purse-string sutures in the pulmonary artery, in the right superior pulmonary vein, or at the LV apex. Typically, temporary closure of the sternotomy is achieved by approximating the skin with a continuous suture without approximation of the sternal bone. If the skin cannot be approximated, an Esmarch bandage can be used. It is advisable to only temporarily close the median sternotomy to facilitate reexploration for postoperative bleeding, which is common.

CHARACTERISTICS OF ECMO VS OTHER TEMPORARY MECHANICAL CIRCULATORY SUPPORT SYSTEMS

In addition to ECMO, there are an increasing number of options for percutaneous circulatory support (Table 6.1). Catheter- or cannula-based vascular access with mechanical pumps can be used as first-line rescue therapy in patients with refractory cardiogenic shock (e.g., percutaneous LVADs).[28] Additionally, surgically implanted temporary ventricular assist devices (VAD) (e.g., Centrimag) have been used for many years in this patient population.[29] While VA-ECMO is still the only percutaneous circulatory support that can be implanted emergently at the bedside, there are now other options for percutaneous left, right, and biventricular support. Most notably, percutaneous right ventricular support can be provided with the Impella RP device (AbioMed) or with the ProTek Duo cannula (LivaNova) coupled with a centrifugal pump.[30,31] These devices can be used in combination with Impella devices (2.5, CP, 5.0, LD) for LV support or the Tandem Heart LVAD to provide percutaneous biventricular support.[32] Most commonly, these devices are used along with ECMO support to stabilize a patient waiting for recovery or definitive therapy.

INDICATIONS FOR ECMO IN PATIENTS WITH CARDIAC DISEASE

Box 6.1 summarizes the most frequent indications for ECMO use in patients with cardiac disease and contraindications to VA-ECMO. The indications for ECMO for cardiac support fall broadly into the following categories:

1. Cardiogenic shock refractory to multiple vasoactive medications or an existing mechanical circulatory support (MCS) device, such as an intraaortic balloon pump
2. Cardiac arrest unresponsive to conventional CPR (extracorporeal CPR, commonly known as ECPR)
3. Refractory ventricular arrhythmias
4. Acute or decompensated right heart failure in the context of pulmonary vascular disease (e.g., pulmonary hypertension or pulmonary embolism)

Unfortunately, unlike studies on ECMO for respiratory failure, there is an absence of randomized controlled trials examining the efficacy of ECMO for the treatment of cardiogenic shock. The reports in the literature are limited to cohort studies, cases series, metaanalyses, and case reports.

TABLE 6.1 Characteristics of Short-Term Mechanical Circulatory Support Systems

Characteristic	Impella 2.5–3.5 CP/RP	Impella 5.0/5.5	TandemHeart LVAD–RVAD	ECMO	Centrimag Temporary VAD
Bedside implantation	No	No	No	Yes (peripheral ECMO)	No
Flow L/min	2.5–3.5	4.5–5	3–4.5	3–6	4–6
LV unloading	Yes	Yes	Yes	Partial	Yes
RV support	Yes	Yes	Yes	Yes	Yes
Pulmonary support	No	No	No	Yes	no
Duration of support	Days–weeks	Days–weeks	Days–weeks	Days–weeks	Weeks–months
Insertion	Percutaneous	Graft	Percutaneous	Percutaneous/surgical	Surgical
Cannula or catheter/pump size	9 Fr/12–14 Fr 22 Fr RP	9 Fr, 19–21 Fr	17-21 Fr LVAD 29–31 Fr RVAD (Protek)	15-17 Fr arterial 22–25 Fr ven.	

ECMO, Extracorporeal membrane oxygenation; *LV*, left ventricular; *LVAD*, left ventricular assist device; *RV*, right ventricular; *RVAD*, right ventricular assist device *VAD*, ventricular assist device.

BOX 6.1 Indications and Contraindications for ECMO in Patients With Cardiac Disease

Indications

- Myocardial infarction–associated cardiogenic shock
- Fulminant myocarditis
- Sepsis-associated cardiomyopathy
- Adult congenital heart disease with acute decompensated heart failure
- Postcardiotomy cardiogenic shock
- RV support during LVAD implantation
- Bridge to VAD or heart transplantation
- Posttransplantation graft failure
- ECPR
- Cardiogenic shock post–cardiac arrest
- Refractory ventricular arrhythmia
- Pulmonary hypertension with RV failure
- Massive pulmonary embolism

Contraindications

Absolute

- Severe irreversible noncardiac organ failure limiting survival (e.g., severe anoxic brain injury)
- Irreversible cardiac failure if transplantation or long-term VAD will not be considered
- Severe aortic insufficiency
- Aortic dissection

Relative

- Severe coagulopathy or contraindication to anticoagulation
- Limited vascular access
- Severe peripheral arterial disease
- Age >75 years

ECMO, Extracorporeal membrane oxygenation; *ECPR*, extracorporeal cardiopulmonary resuscitation; *LVAD*, left ventricular assist device; *RV*, right ventricle; *VAD*, ventricular assist device.
Modified from Abrams D, Garan AR, Abdelbary A, et al. Position paper for the organization of ECMO programs for cardiac failure in adults. *Intensive Care Med.* 2018;44(6):717–729.

Heart Failure and Cardiogenic Shock

There are a broad range of therapies for patients with decompensated acute or chronic heart failure who present in cardiogenic shock. These include intravenous inotropes, intraaortic balloon pumps, peripherally inserted VADs, surgically implanted short-term extracorporeal VADs, VA-ECMO, and durable VADs. Despite a paucity of data supporting ECMO as a superior therapy, the utilization of ECMO in patients with heart failure is increasing, likely due to the ease of ECMO implantation and its ability to provide biventricular support. Based on expert consensus, ECMO can be considered in patients with cardiogenic shock due to (1) myocarditis, (2) cardiomyopathy, (3) myocardial infarction, (4) refractory malignant arrhythmia, (5) pulmonary embolism, (6) pulmonary hypertensive crisis, or (7) posttransplantation graft dysfunction.[28,33] While the indications for cardiac ECMO support are broad, the contraindications are consistent across etiologies. ECMO should be avoided in patients who have severe and irreversible neurological injury, irreversible cardiac failure without candidacy for transplant or LVAD placement, aortic dissection, severe aortic valve insufficiency, or any noncardiac comorbid condition that limits their life expectancy to less than 1 year.

Frequently, the call to consider a patient for ECMO support is done when the patient exhibits advanced stages of shock with limited time to define the most appropriate treatment option, and ECMO is generally considered as a bridge to decision. Once the clinical condition of the patient has been stabilized and the treatment course established using a multidisciplinary team approach, a destination therapy can be defined, including bridge to recovery, a durable VAD (BTB), or heart transplantation. If none of these options is viable due to progressive deterioration of multiorgan failure, preexisting conditions that preclude further therapy (e.g., advanced cancer), or a major life-threatening complication (e.g., intracranial bleeding), early palliative care referral and withdrawal of support should be considered.

According to the 2018 international summary report of the ELSO, based on >15,000 ECMO runs for cardiac failure, overall survival is 55%.[34] This survival varies considerably based on the indication for support. A recent metaanalysis by Cheng and colleagues of published cohort studies, including those that studied mixed causes of cardiogenic shock, showed that survival to discharge varies from 20% to 65%, with 5%–52% of the patients bridged from ECMO to a VAD and 4%–21% bridged to heart transplant, depending on the series (Table 6.2).[35] Among patients with cardiogenic shock secondary to an AMI, survival has increased to approximately 59% in specialized centers, and the strongest predictors of mortality are age older than 65 years, body mass index greater than 32 kg/m^2, and international normalized ratio (in the absence of warfarin) of greater than 2 at the time of cannulation.[36] The benefits of ECMO use in patients with AMI are likely due to an early stabilization of the patient, allowing early revascularization. In an observational study of patients with ST-segment elevation myocardial infarction and cardiogenic shock who underwent percutaneous coronary intervention (PCI) with or without ECMO support, those receiving ECMO had significantly lower 30-day mortality (39.1% vs. 72%; $P = 0.008$).[37] The interpretation of these data is limited, however, by an era effect and possible confounding variability in coronary stent use among the groups. In a recent analysis by Esper and colleagues of patients in the catheterization lab supported with ECMO for acute coronary syndrome complicated by cardiogenic shock, 83% underwent successful percutaneous revascularization, with a 67% survival to discharge and 55% survival at 6 months. Interestingly, close to 20% of these patients required support with a durable VAD during their original hospitalization.[38]

Similarly, ECMO has been applied to rescue patients with cardiogenic shock of nonischemic etiology, including fulminant myocarditis. Patients with fulminant myocarditis who are successfully bridged with ECMO have an acceptable weaning rate, comparable with patients requiring ECMO support for myocarditis presenting in milder forms.[39] In a recent cohort of patients who received either a biventricular assist device ($n = 6$) or ECMO ($n = 35$) for fulminant myocarditis with refractory cardiogenic shock, overall intensive care unit survival was 68%, with higher severity of illness and elevated cardiac biomarkers serving as independent predictors of mortality and an inability to wean from ECMO.[40] In a study comparing ECMO with biventricular assist device support for fulminant myocarditis, patients receiving ECMO had comparable rates of weaning from device therapy and survival to hospital discharge without the need for transplantation (83% vs. 80%) and more rapid improvement in renal and hepatic laboratory profiles, despite having a higher severity of illness and worse LV function before device implantation.[41] A large study by Liao and colleagues demonstrated a survival to discharge rate of 78% in patients presenting with acute fulminant myocarditis requiring ECMO support; acute renal failure (49%) and sepsis (21%) were the most frequent complications.[42]

Although ECMO has become a useful salvage option in patients presenting in advanced stages of refractory shock, it is important to

TABLE 6.2 Studies Included in the Metaanalysis by Cheng and Colleagues of Patients Undergoing ECMO for Cardiogenic Shock

Study	Number of Patients	Patient Type	Age (years)	Peripheral ECMO, *n* (%)	IABP, *n* (%)	Average Time on ECMO (hours)	Survival to Hospital Discharge, *n* (%)	Bridged to VAD/ Survival to Discharge, *n* (%)	Bridged to HTx/ Survival to Discharge, *n* (%)
Bakhtiary et al.[66]	45	PCCS	60.1 ± 13.6	29 (64)	30 (67)	153.6	13 (28.9)	5 (11.1)/3 (60)	2 (4.4)/1 (50)
Belle et al.[67]	51	Mixed	51 ± 15	51 (100)	5 (10)	—	14 (27.5)	—	—
Bermudez et al.[68]	42	Mixed	53.5	37 (88)	37 (88)	67.1	—	22 (52.4)/–	—
Elsharkawy et al.[69]	233	PCCS	57	156 (67)	22 (9.4)	—	84 (36.1)	—	—
Hei et al.[70]	68	PCCS	49.2 ± 13.3	67 (99)	11 (16)	114.6	43 (63.2)	—	8 (11.8)/6 (75)
Hsu et al.[71]	51	PCCS	63 ± 15.7	51 (100)	—	180	17 (33.3)	—	3 (5.9)/3 (100)
Kagawa et al.[72]	77	CA	61.9	77 (100)	52 (68)	—	16 (20.8)	4 (5.2)/–	—
Kim et al.[73]	27	AMI	63.7 ± 11	27 (100)	2 (7)	30.2	16 (59.3)	—	—
Loforte et al.[74]	73	Mixed	60.3 ± 11.6	73 (100)	73 (100)	261.6	33 (45.2)	3 (4.1)/2 (66.7)	0 (0)/N/A
Moraca et al.[75]	26	Mixed	57	24 (92)	21 (80)	72	17 (65.4)	9 (34.6)/6 (66.7)	1 (3.8)/1 (100)
Pagani et al.[76]	33	Mixed	47 ± 11	22 (67)	20 (61)	65	12 (36.4)	10 (30.3)/8 (80)	7 (21.2)/7 (100)
Rastan et al.[77]	517	PCCS	63.5 ± 11.2	141 (27)	383 (74)	78.7	128 (24.8)	15 (2.9)/3 (20)	5 (1)/2 (40)
Schmidt et al.[78]	220	Mixed	49 ± 16	—	—	320.9	—	—	—
Slottosch et al.[79]	77	Mixed	60 ± 13	—	72 (94)	79	—	—	—
Smith et al.[80]	17	PCCS	66.6 ± 13.6	11 (65)	14 (82)	86	7 (41.2)	—	—
Unosawa et al.[81]	47	PCCS	64.4 ± 12.5	32 (68)	39 (83)	63.5	14 (29.8)	—	—
Wang et al.[82]	62	PCCS	51 ± 15	—	19 (31)	61	34 (54.8)	—	—
Wu et al.[83]	110	PCCS	60 ± 14	—	—	143.3	46 (41.8)	—	—
Wu et al.[84]	60	Mixed	51.33	—	44 (73)	97.3	32 (53.3)	—	3 (5)/2 (66.7)
Zhang et al.[85]	32	PCCS	55.4 ± 11.9	17 (53)	—	64.8	8 (25.0)	—	—

AMI, Acute myocardial infarction; *CA*, cardiac arrest; *ECMO*, extracorporeal membrane oxygenation; *HTx*, heart transplant; *IABP*, intraaortic balloon pump; *Mixed*, mixed population; *PCCS*, postcardiotomy cardiogenic shock; *VAD*, ventricular assist device.
Modified from Cheng R, Hachamovitch R, Kittleson M, et al. Complications of extracorporeal membrane oxygenation for treatment of cardiogenic shock and cardiac arrest: a meta-analysis of 1,866 adult patients. *Ann Thorac Surg*. 2014;97(2):610–616.

note that other percutaneous options are also frequently considered in the presence of predominantly LV dysfunction. Percutaneous VADs are associated with improved ability to unload the LV and decreased infarct size in animal models of AMI when compared with peripheral VA-ECMO.[24,25] Percutaneous VADs can also be useful in reducing LV afterload in patients supported with ECMO. Combining either a percutaneous axial flow pump or direct LV venting through minimally invasive thoracotomy with peripheral VA-ECMO unloads the LV with similar therapeutic efficacy.[26] In a recent cohort study by Pappalardo and colleagues, the use of ECMO in combination with an axial flow percutaneous LVAD (the Impella 2.5 or CP) was associated with improved survival (74% vs. 48%) and a higher rate of bridging to either recovery or further therapy (62% vs. 36%) as compared with VA-ECMO alone in 63 propensity-matched patients presenting with cardiogenic shock.[32]

Postcardiotomy Shock

Patients who fail to wean from CPB exhibit significant morbidity. Historically, mortality in these patients exceeds 50%.[43] Despite significant advancements in both ECMO and MCS and a rapid increase in the number of patients supported, survival rates have decreased (Fig. 6.12).[44] Unfortunately, a consensus definition of postcardiotomy shock is lacking, and because of this, it is difficult to compare studies on ECMO use for postcardiotomy shock. Additionally, there are no standard guidelines for treatment of postcardiotomy shock, including when to initiate MCS or ECMO. In our practice, we have protocolized our response to postcardiotomy shock (Fig. 6.13). This has allowed us to standardize our care across the institution while still allowing us to provide tailored support to the patient. Ultimately, despite the low survival with ECMO, it is likely that all the patients would have died without ECMO therapy; therefore, even 15% survival is a drastic improvement as compared with the alternative. Predictors of mortality included (1) VA-ECMO support exceeding 7 days, (2) a lack of lactate clearance within the first 12 hours, and (3) the development of renal failure requiring renal replacement therapy while on ECMO support.[45,46]

Septic Shock

Despite the promising survival rates for neonates and children in septic shock supported with ECMO, survival in the adult population has been quite varied (Table 6.3). Some authors report survival rates as low as 7%.[47] Although others have reported much higher survival (up to 75%), many of those reports included patients who have cardiomyopathy and sepsis concomitantly.[48,49] Predictors of survival in patients with septic shock include the ability to identify a distinct causative pathogen, a lack of overt disseminated intravascular coagulopathy, and early lactate clearance.[50]

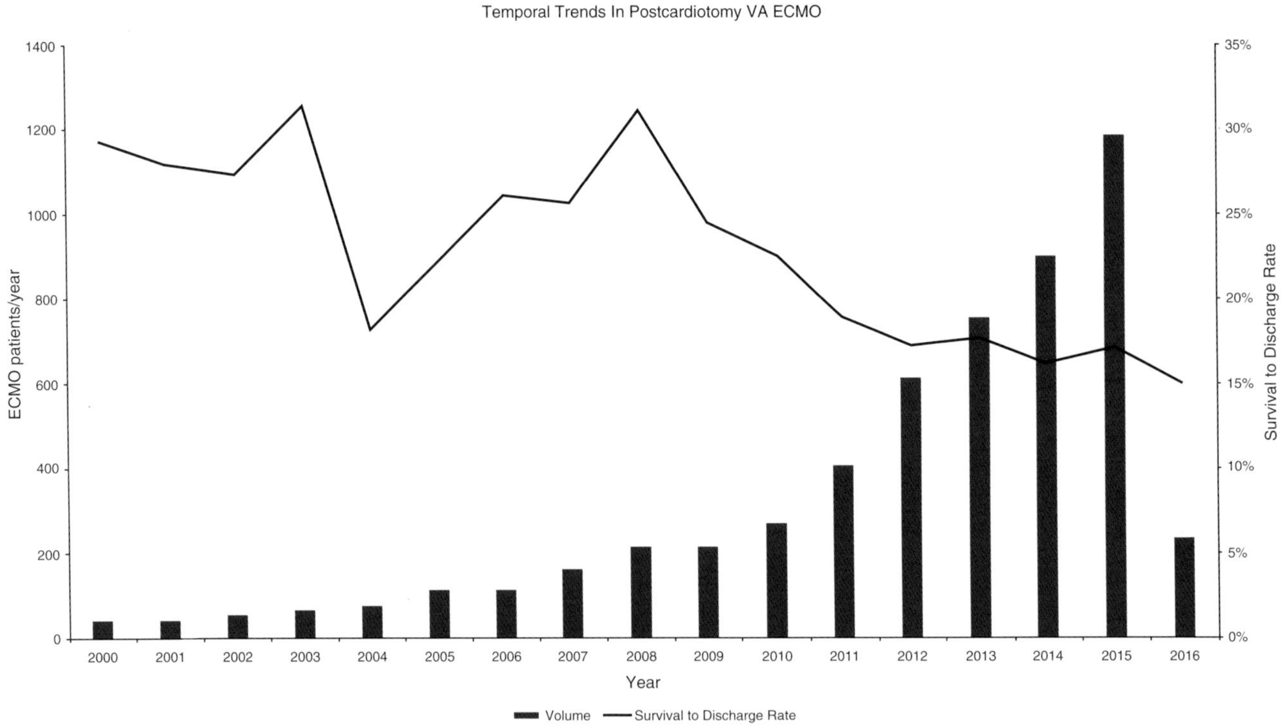

Fig. 6.12 Extracorporeal Life Support Organization data comparing the number of patients supported with ECMO for postcardiotomy shock with survival over time. *VA-ECMO*, Venoarterial extracorporeal membrane oxygenation. (From Whitman GJ. Extracorporeal membrane oxygenation for the treatment of postcardiotomy shock. *J Thorac Cardiovasc Surg.* 2017;153(1):95–101.)

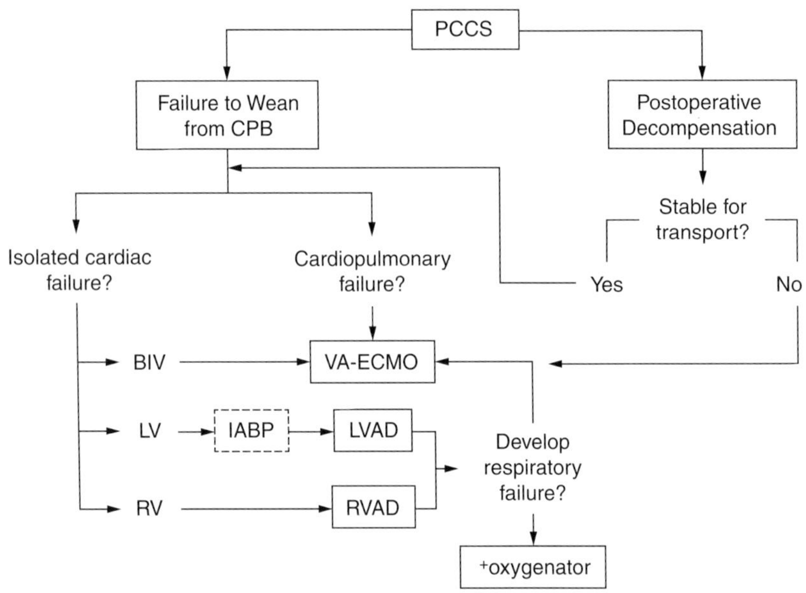

Fig. 6.13 The Duke algorithm for management of postcardiotomy shock. *BIV*, Biventricular; *CPB*, cardiopulmonary bypass; *IABP*, intraaortic balloon pump; *LV*, left ventricular; *LVAD*, left ventricular assist device; *PCCS*, postcardiotomy cardiogenic shock; *RV*, right ventricular; *RVAD*, right ventricular assist device; *VA-ECMO*, venoarterial extracorporeal membrane oxygenation.

Extracorporeal CPR

In general, survival of patients who receive CPR, either in hospital or out of hospital, is very low, ranging from 5% to 15%.[51] The use of ECMO as an adjuvant to CPR, eCPR, has been associated with improved survival and improved neurological function in patients undergoing CPR for an in-hospital witnessed cardiac arrest (Table 6.4).[52] The ELSO registry reports that 38% of patients who receive eCPR survive to decannulation and 29% survive to discharge.[34] The strongest predictors of survival among patients receiving eCPR for either in-hospital or out-of-hospital cardiac arrest are the time from arrest to the initiation of ECMO and the presence of even a transient return of spontaneous circulation.[53,54] A recent study of patients presenting

TABLE 6.3 Key Studies of ECMO Support of Patients With Septic Shock and Cardiopulmonary Failure

Author (year)	Study Dates	Study Comparisons	*n*	Post-ECMO Survival Outcomes	Other Findings/Notes	Type of Study
Brechot 2013[86]	2008–2011		14 patients	Twelve patients (86%) could be weaned off VA ECMO after 5.5 days (2–12 days) of support and 10 patients (71%) were discharged to home and were alive after a median follow-up of 13 months (3–43).	Myocardial function was recovered rapidly on support. 60% of patients experienced a major ECMO-related complication.	Single-institution, retrospective series
Cheng 2013[87]	2001–2009	Patients on VA-ECMO for cardiopulmonary failure with septic shock vs. patients on VA-ECMO for cardiopulmonary failure without septic shock	216 patients 108 with sepsis; 108 without	24.4% of patients with sepsis survived to discharge. 34.9% of patients w/o sepsis survived to discharge.	There was an increased risk of mortality in septic adults receiving VA-ECMO (hazard ratio, 2.54; 95% confidence intervals, 1.75–3.70; $P < 0.01$).	Propensity-matched cohort study using a single-institution registry
Huang 2013[88]	2005–2010		52 patients	15.0% survived to hospital discharge.	All patients older than 60 years died (20 patients).	Retrospective study of prospectively maintained institutional database
Park 2015[89]	2005–2013	Survivors and nonsurvivors	32 patients	ECMO was weaned successfully in 13 patients (40.6%) and 7 patients (21.9%) survived to hospital discharge.	Survivors had lower peak lactate (4.5 vs. 15.1 mmol/L, $P = 0.03$), lower SOFA day 3 score (15 vs. 18, $P = 0.01$) and higher peak troponin I (32.8 vs. 3.7 ng/mL, $P = 0.02$) than the nonsurvivors.	Retrospective study of prospectively maintained institutional database
Cheng 2016[90]	2001–2011	Survivors vs. nonsurvivors	151 patients VA-ECMO = 101 VV-ECMO = 50	Survival to discharge was 51% in patients who received ECMO within 4 days of hospitalization. Survival to discharge was 14% in patients who received ECMO >4 days after hospitalization. In patients <75 years of age and without immunocompromising conditions, 42% survived to discharge.	There were significantly more survivors among patients with Gram-positive cocci infections or viral infections (57.7%) than among those with fungal or Gram-negative infections (15.8%).	Retrospective study of a prospectively maintained institutional database
Choi 2017[91]	2007–2013	Survivors vs. nonsurvivors	28 patients VA-ECMO = 21 VV-ECMO = 4 VAV-ECMO = 3	Survival to discharge was 35.7% overall. For the VA-ECMO group, survival was 28.6%.	There was no statistical difference in ECMO-related complications between survivors and nonsurvivors.	Single-institution, retrospective series
Kim 2018[50]	2007–2015	Coagulation and lactate profiles in survivors and nonsurvivors	37 patients VA-ECMO = 26 VV-ECMO = 8 VAV-ECMO = 3	40.5% (15) of the patients survived.	Higher pre-ECMO DIC scores were associated with death. Lower lactate levels during support were associated with survival.	Single-institution, retrospective review of medical records
Ro 2018[47]	2005–2012	Patients on VA-ECMO for septic shock vs. patients on VA-ECMO for cardiogenic shock	71 patients with septic shock 253 patients with cardiogenic shock	11 patients with septic shock were weaned from ECMO (15.5%); 5 patients survived to discharge (7%).	In patients receiving VA-ECMO for septic shock, higher lactate levels were associated with decreased survival. Rates of successful weaning from VA-ECMO (15.5% vs. 45.5%) and survival to hospital discharge (7.0% vs. 28.9%) were significantly lower in patients with septic shock than in patients with cardiogenic shock ($P < 0.001$).	Retrospective study of a prospectively maintained institutional database

DIC, Disseminated intravascular coagulation; *ECMO*, extracorporeal membrane oxygenation; *SOFA*, sequential organ failure assessment; *VA*, venoarterial; *VAV*, veno-arterio-venous; *VV*, venovenous.

TABLE 6.4 **Summary of Metaanalyses of ECPR for Cardiac Arrest**

Author (year)	Publication Dates	Study Comparisons	*n*	Location of Patient During Cardiac Arrest	Post-ECMO Survival Outcomes	Other Findings/Notes	Type of Study
Xie 2015[92]	2000–Jan 2014	N/A	277 patients in 10 studies	NR	The weighted survival to discharge was 35.9% (95% CI, 28.1%–44%; $P = 0.37$; $I^2 = 0\%$). 30-day survival was 36.2% (95% CI, 23.1%–50.4%; $P = 0.093$; $I^2 = 58\%$), and 6-month survival was estimated to be 32.5% (95% CI, 25.2%–40.1%; $P = 0.317$; $I^2 = 13\%$).		MA
Ahn 2016[93]	2008–2015	ECPR vs. CCPR	38,160 patients in seven studies	Both	The overall survival rate was higher in ECPR than CCPR (OR, 2.29; 95% CI, 1.07–4.87). ECPR showed significantly better survival compared with CCPR in IHCA patients (OR, 2.40; 95% CI, 1.44–3.98; $I^2 = 0\%$). The survival rate in ECPR recipients was similar to that of CCPR recipients among OHCA patients (OR, 2.26; 95% CI, 0.45–11.20; $I^2 = 93\%$).	The overall neurologic outcome in ECPR patients was better than in CCPR patients (OR, 2.82; 95% CI, 1.36–5.82). ECPR showed similar neurologic outcome to CCPR in OHCA patients (OR, 3.14, 95% CI, 0.66–14.85; $I^2 = 80\%$), ECPR was associated with better neurologic outcome than CCPR in IHCA patients (OR, 2.63; 95% CI, 1.38–5.02; $I^2 = 3\%$).	SR and MA Five studies classified as high quality and two classified as low quality.
Kim 2016[94]	1965–2015	ECPR vs. CCPR	2280 patients in 10 studies 641 ECPR; 1639 CCPR	Both	Survival and good neurologic outcome tended to be superior in the ECPR group at 3–6 months after arrest.	ECPR showed higher survival rate at 3–6 months after arrest in OHCA patients There were no statistical differences among subgroups of OHCA and IHCA for survival to discharge and at 3–6 months. In both OHCA and IHCA groups, ECPR showed better neurologic outcomes at discharge and at 3–6 months.	MA
Ortega-Deballon 2016[95]	2005–2015	N/A	833 patients in 20 studies	OHCA	Overall reported survival rate was 22%; 13% had a good neurological recovery. Three studies reported patient outcomes at 3 months, with an overall survival rate of 21%, including 15% with good neurological function. Five studies reported patient outcomes at 6 months, with an overall survival rate of 16%, including 9% having good neurological function.		SR Quality of included studies was rated as good to fair.

Ouweneel 2016[96]	?–2015	ECMO group vs. control (no ECMO) group	3098 patients in nine studies 708 patients on ECMO 2390 patients with no ECMO support	Both	ECMO for refractory CA was associated with increased survival at 30 days (absolute risk difference, 13%; 95% CI, 6%–20%; *P*< 0.001; NNT, 7.7). The long-term difference in survival was 15% in favor of the ECMO-treated patients.	Secondary outcomes were long-term survival and 30-day and long-term favorable neurological outcome. The use of ECLS was associated with a higher rate of favorable neurological outcome at both 30 days (risk difference, 14%; 95% CI, 7%–20%; *P*< 0.0001; NNT, 7.1) and during long-term follow-up (risk difference, 11%; 95% CI, 6%–16%; *P*< 0.0001; NNT, 9.1).	SR and MA Quality of evidence in included studies was low.
D'Arrigo 2017[97]	?–March 2017	N/A	856 patients in 11 studies	IHCA	37.9% survived to discharge. Neurological outcomes were good in 84.4% of survivors.	Shockable initial rhythm, a shorter low-flow duration, lower blood lactate levels before ECPR start or on ICU admission, and a lower SOFA score or creatinine levels in the first 24 h after ICU admission were associated with a higher likelihood of survival.	SR and MA All studies included were classified as low or very low quality evidence.
Debaty 2017[98]	NR	N/A	841 patients in 15 studies	OHCA	Predictors of survival to discharge. 15% of patients had a favorable outcome (good neurologic status postsupport in 10 studies, survival in 5 studies).	Shorter low-flow duration, shockable cardiac rhythm, higher arterial pH value, and lower serum lactate concentration on hospital admission were associated with better outcomes for ECPR recipients after OHCA.	SR and MA Quality of evidence in included studies was classified as low.
Wang 2017[99]	2000–2015	ECPR vs. CCPR	2260 patients in six studies 376 ECPR 1884 CCPR	Both	There was a significant beneficial effect of ECPR on survival rate to discharge compared with CCPR in CA patients (RR, 2.37; 95% CI, 1.63–3.45; *P*< 0.001). Survival rate overall was 25.5%. In a subgroup analysis, there was a significant difference in survival to discharge favoring ECPR over CCPR group in OHCA patients (RR, 2.69; 95% CI, 1.48–4.91; *P*= 0.001), but no different in survival to discharge in IHCA patients (RR, 1.84; 95% CI, 0.91–3.73; *P*= 0.09).	Patients who underwent ECPR had a significantly better long-term neurological outcome than those who received CCPR (RR, 2.79; 95% CI, 1.96–3.97; *P*< 0.001). 19.4% of patients had good neurological outcome.	MA Studies needed to compare ECPR and CCPR and have ≥15 patients to be included. All included studies determined to be of high methodological quality by NOS scale.

CA, Cardiac arrest; *CCPR*, conventional cardiopulmonary resuscitation; *CI*, confidence interval; *ECMO*, extracorporeal membrane oxygenation; *ECPR*, ECMO for cardiopulmonary resuscitation; *ICU*, intensive care unit; *IHCA*, in-hospital cardiac arrest; *MA*, metaanalysis; *N/A*, not applicable; *NNT*, number needed to treat; *NOS*, Newcastle-Ottawa Scale; *NR*, not reported; *OHCA*, out-of-hospital cardiac arrest; *OR*, odds ratio; *RR*, relative risk; *SOFA*, sequential organ failure assessment; *SR*, systematic review.

with cardiac arrest requiring ECMO support and undergoing left heart catheterization, per protocol, confirmed the presence of significant coronary disease in a high percentage (40%–50%), suggesting that an early coronary angiogram and PCI may improve survival in the patient presenting with fibrillatory arrest.[55] Although ECMO has rapidly gained popularity as a resuscitation platform, the need for a coordinated and trained rapid response team is crucial to improve survival and quality of life after discharge. Among survivors, a German study found that health-related quality of life was, in general, inferior to a general sampling of patients, but it was similar to the quality of life seen in patients with chronic renal failure (Fig. 6.14).[56]

Bridge to Heart Transplantation or Durable LVAD

ECMO as a BTT is only selectively utilized, and less than 1% of heart transplant recipients in the United States undergo transplant while on ECMO.[57] Patients on ECMO are successfully bridged to transplant only 50%–70% of the time, with 1-year posttransplantation survival ranging from 50% to 75% in the largest available series in the United States and Europe.[57–60] A UNOS analysis of 109 patients supported with ECMO as a BTT between 2003 and 2016 confirmed a 90-day mortality of 30%, with higher rates of postoperative cerebrovascular accident, need for renal replacement therapy, and worse early postoperative functional status as compared with patients who were bridged to heart transplantation with an LVAD.[57] A report of 169 patients from the Spanish Registry supported on ECMO as a BTT showed 67% survival to hospital discharge, with a short time of support of only 6.5 days. Renal replacement therapy, age, and infections requiring intravenous antibiotics were associated with increased postoperative mortality.[58] Other predictors of mortality for patients bridged to heart transplantation with VA ECMO are age >50 years, Sequential Organ Failure Assessment (SOFA) score >10, and APACHE (Acute Physiology, Age, and Chronic Health Evaluation) IV score >47 (Table 6.5).[61,62] ECMO is more often used as a double bridge, or BTB, to a more durable VAD. Commonly, ECMO is used as a bridge to a durable LVAD, with transplantation reserved only for patients with LVADs whose clinical condition is appropriate or patients in whom LVADs are contraindicated. Since the first report of the use of ECMO as a BTB,[63] this application has rapidly gained popularity in patients presenting in advanced cardiogenic shock, instead of considering a high-risk transplant, when recovery of cardiac function is not an option. ECMO allows stabilization and improvement of end-organ function before LVAD placement. A recent study comparing ECMO used as a BTB in 49 patients with 48 patients who underwent direct LVAD implantation showed no difference in outcomes despite the fact that patients supported by ECMO were more decompensated (higher lactate and liver dysfunction). This suggests that ECMO as a BTB can be considered a reasonable strategy to optimize LVAD results in patients presenting in profound shock.[64] However, this is still a high-risk group, with high morbidity and mortality, even when ECMO is used as a bridge to an LVAD.[61,62,65]

CONCLUSION

ECMO therapy has evolved greatly since the first successful case in 1972. With significant innovations to improve pump function and oxygenator and circuit biocompatibility, ECMO is now a viable option for adult patients with heart failure. That said, ECMO therapy is resource intensive and requires significant expertise and clinical vigilance. Regardless of the indication, survival after ECMO for cardiac failure is dependent on (1) timely initiation of support, (2) prevention

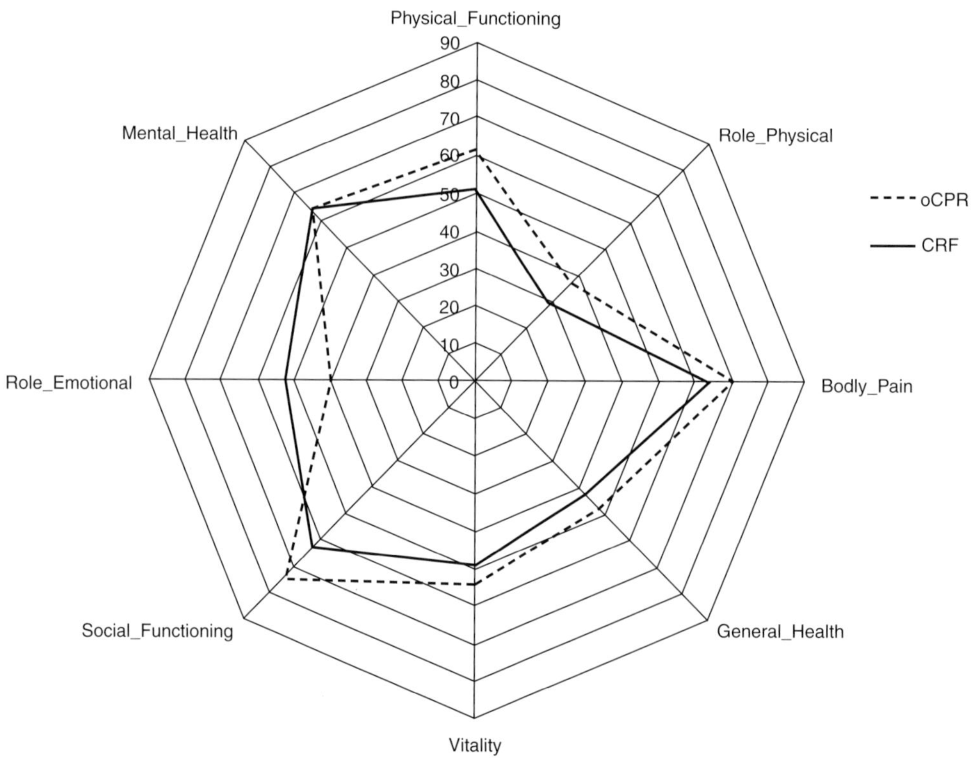

Fig. 6.14 Health-related quality of life using the SF-36 survey. In all areas, patients who required extracorporeal cardiopulmonary resuscitation (*eCPR*) assessed their quality of life similar to chronic renal failure (*CRF*) patients. (From Spangenberg T, Schewel J, Dreher A, et al. Health related quality of life after extracorporeal cardiopulmonary resuscitation in refractory cardiac arrest. *Resuscitation*. 2018;127:73–78.)

TABLE 6.5 Key Studies of ECMO as a Bridge to Heart Transplantation or a Durable VAD

Author (year)	Study Dates	Study Comparisons	*n*	Post-ECMO Survival Outcomes	Other Findings/Notes	Type of Study
Chung 2010[61]	1995–2007		70 patients	Bridging was successful in 31 patients (44%). 15 to HTx (11 survived to discharge and 1 year posttransplantation). 16 to VAD (8 survived to discharge and 1 year posttransplantation).	Age >50 years, pre-ECMO CPR, and SOFA score >10 at ECMO initiation were significant independent predictors of unsuccessful bridging.	Single-institution, retrospective series
Lebreton 2015[100]	2004–2010		49 patients with ECMO support before long-term MCS (BTB) 48 patients placed directly on long-term MCS	No difference in survival between patients assisted by long-term MCS after ECMO (BTB) and patients assisted by long-term MCS as a first-line therapeutic strategy.	Patients whose clinical condition improved while on ECMO support were more likely to survive than BTB patients whose condition did not improve.	Single-institution, retrospective series
Rousse 2015[101]	NR 3-year period	ECMO BTT vs. ECMO to recovery vs. ECMO to LVAD	13 patients ECMO BTT (98 patients total)	49 patients on ECMO survived to recovery, HTx, or LVAD implantation. After HTx, estimated 1-year survival was 51.0%.	Because most deaths occurred within the first 4 days of ECMO support, ~1 week of support prior to making further treatment decisions may be optimal.	Single-institution retrospective series
Jasseron 2016[59]	2010–2011	Adult patients on VA-ECMO at listing for HTx vs. all other patients listed for HTx, including those on other types of MCS	80 patients on VA-ECMO when listed for HT 786 patients in the control group	1-year overall survival of 52.2% for ECMO group (75.5% for comparison group). 55 patients survived to transplantation. 46 patients (83.6%) were transplanted directly from ECMO support. 1-year posttransplantation survival was 70% for the ECMO group (81% for comparison group).	Transplantation provides a survival benefit in listed patients on VA-ECMO even if posttransplantation survival remains inferior than for patients without VA-ECMO.	French national registry (CRISTAL) database study
Barge-Caballero 2018[58]	2010–2015	Patients bridged with ECMO vs. bridged with an LVAD or BiVAD	169 patients BTT with ECMO 70 patients BTT with LVAD 52 BTT with BiVAD	140 patients on ECMO survived to recovery, HTx, or LVAD implantation. Survival to hospital discharge was 54.4% with ECMO (78.6% with LVAD, 55.8% with BiVAD).	ECMO support was associated with a higher incidence of adverse clinical events than temporary LVAD or BiVAD support.	Spanish national registry database study
Fukuhara 2018[57]	2003–2016	Patients bridged with ECMO vs. bridged with an LVAD	107 patients BTT with ECMO 6148 patients BTT with LVAD	90-day survival: 73.1% ECMO (93.1%, LVAD). 3-year survival: 67.4%, ECMO (82.4%, LVAD) In propensity-matched cohort: 90-day survival: 74.8% ECMO (88.8% LVAD). 3-year survival: 69.3% ECMO (82.2% LVAD).	ECMO-supported patients were in worse clinical condition (sicker) than LVAD-supported patients as assessed by multiple criteria. A high MELD-XI score (>17) was associated with poor posttransplantation survival in ECMO-supported patients compared with those with a low MELD-XI score (<13).	UNOS database study
Lechiancole 2018[62]	2005–2017	Patients with APACHE IV score <47 and ≥47	32 patients	30-day survival was 81.3%	30-day survival was 40% in patients with APACHE IV score ≥47. In patients with APACHE IV score ≥47, 1-year and 5-year estimated survival was 26.6%. In patients with APACHE IV score <47, 1-year estimated survival was 89.7% and 5-year estimated survival was 81.5%.	Single-institution, retrospective series

APACHE IV score, Acute Physiology, Age, and Chronic Health Evaluation IV score; *BiVAD*, biventricular assist device; *BTB*, bridge-to-bridge; *BTT*, bridge to transplant; *CPR*, cardiopulmonary resuscitation; *ECMO*, extracorporeal membrane oxygenation; *HTx*, heart transplant; *LVAD*, left ventricular assist device; *MCS*, mechanical circulatory support; *MELD-XI* score, model for end-stage liver disease excluding international normalized ratio score; *NR*, not reported; *SOFA*, sequential organ failure assessment; *VA*, venoarterial; *UNOS*, United Network for Organ Sharing; *VAD*, ventricular assist device.

of end-organ failure, (3) the absence of neurological injury, (4) avoidance of LV distention, and (5) the ability to wean support (either due to recovery or to an alternative therapy) in a timely fashion. Given the complexity of care required for patients with heart failure requiring ECMO support, they are best served with rapid transfer to a quaternary care facility with the availability of multidisciplinary and multimodality care for end-stage heart failure.

REFERENCES

1. Bramson ML, Osborn JJ, Main FB, O'Brien MF, Wright JS, Gerbode F. A new disposable membrane oxygenator with integral heat exchange. *J Thorac Cardiovasc Surg*. 1965;50:391–400.
2. Hill JD, O'Brien TG, Murray JJ, et al. Prolonged extracorporeal oxygenation for acute post-traumatic respiratory failure (shock-lung syndrome). Use of the Bramson membrane lung. *N Engl J Med*. 1972;286(12):629–634.
3. Zapol WM, Snider MT, Hill JD, et al. Extracorporeal membrane oxygenation in severe acute respiratory failure. A randomized prospective study. *JAMA*. 1979;242(20):2193–2196.
4. Bartlett RH, Gazzaniga AB, Fong SW, Jefferies MR, Roohk HV, Haiduc N. Extracorporeal membrane oxygenator support for cardiopulmonary failure. Experience in 28 cases. *J Thorac Cardiovasc Surg*. 1977;73(3):375–386.
5. Khoshbin E, Roberts N, Harvey C, et al. Poly-methyl pentene oxygenators have improved gas exchange capability and reduced transfusion requirements in adult extracorporeal membrane oxygenation. *ASAIO J*. 2005;51(3):281–287.
6. Wang D, Zhou X, Liu X, Sidor B, Lynch J, Zwischenberger JB. Wang-Zwische double lumen cannula: toward a percutaneous and ambulatory paracorporeal artificial lung. *ASAIO J*. 2008;54(6):606–611.
7. Abrams D, Combes A, Brodie D. Extracorporeal membrane oxygenation in cardiopulmonary disease in adults. *J Am Coll Cardiol*. 2014;63 (25 Pt A):2769–2778.
8. Halaweish I, Cole A, Cooley E, Lynch WR, Haft JW. Roller and centrifugal pumps: a retrospective comparison of bleeding complications in extracorporeal membrane oxygenation. *ASAIO J*. 2015;61(5):496–501.
9. Thiara APS, Høyland V, Norum H, et al. Extracorporeal membrane oxygenation support for 59 days without changing the ECMO circuit: a case of *Legionella* pneumonia. *Perfusion*. 2009;24(1):45–47.
10. Toomasian JM, Bartlett RH. Hemolysis and ECMO pumps in the 21st Century. *Perfusion*. 2011;26(1):5–6.
11. Haines N, Wang S, Myers JL, Undar A. Comparison of two types of neonatal extracorporeal life support systems with pulsatile and nonpulsatile flow. *Artif Organs*. 2009;33(11):958–966.
12. Talor J, Yee S, Rider A, Kunselman AR, Guan Y, Undar A. Comparison of perfusion quality in hollow-fiber membrane oxygenators for neonatal extracorporeal life support. *Artif Organs*. 2010;34(4):E110–E116.
13. Maul TM, Massicotte MP, Wearden PD. ECMO Biocompatibility: surface coatings, anticoagulation, and coagulation monitoring. In: Firstenberg MS, ed. *Extracorporeal Membrane Oxygenation: Advances in Therapy*. InTech; 2016.
14. Napp LC, Kühn C, Hoeper MM, et al. Cannulation strategies for percutaneous extracorporeal membrane oxygenation in adults. *Clin Res Cardiol*. 2016;105(4):283–296.
15. Pavlushkov E, Berman M, Valchanov K. Cannulation techniques for extracorporeal life support. *Ann Transl Med*. 2017;5(4): 70.
16. Reeb J, Olland A, Renaud S, et al. Vascular access for extracorporeal life support: tips and tricks. *J Thorac Dise*. 2016;8(S4):S353–S363.
17. Rupprecht L, Lunz D, Philipp A, Lubnow M, Schmid C. Pitfalls in percutaneous ECMO cannulation. *Heart Lung Vessel*. 2015;7(4):320–326.
18. Tanaka D, Hirose H, Cavarocchi N, Entwistle JWC. The impact of vascular complications on survival of patients on venoarterial extracorporeal membrane oxygenation. *Ann Thorac Surg*. 2016;101(5):1729–1734.
19. Vallabhajosyula P, Kramer M, Lazar S, et al. Lower-extremity complications with femoral extracorporeal life support. *Thorac Cardiovasc Surg*. 2016;151(6):1738–1744.
20. Lamb KM, DiMuzio PJ, Johnson A, et al. Arterial protocol including prophylactic distal perfusion catheter decreases limb ischemia complications in patients undergoing extracorporeal membrane oxygenation. *J Vasc Surg*. 2017;65(4):1074–1079.
21. Steffen RJ, Sale S, Anandamurthy B, et al. Using near-infrared spectroscopy to monitor lower extremities in patients on venoarterial extracorporeal membrane oxygenation. *Ann Thorac Surg*. 2014;98(5):1853–1854.
22. Burkhoff D, Sayer G, Doshi D, Uriel N. Hemodynamics of mechanical circulatory support. *J Am Coll Cardiol*. 2015;66(23):2663–2674.
23. Napp LC, Kühn C, Bauersachs J. ECMO in cardiac arrest and cardiogenic shock. *Herz*. 2017;42(1):27–44.
24. Esposito ML, Shah N, Dow S, et al. Distinct effects of left or right atrial cannulation on left ventricular hemodynamics in a swine model of acute myocardial injury. *ASAIO J*. 2016;62(6):671–676.
25. Kapur NK, Paruchuri V, Urbano-Morales JA, et al. Mechanically unloading the left ventricle before coronary reperfusion reduces left ventricular wall stress and myocardial infarct size. *Circulation*. 2013;128(4):328–336.
26. Tepper S, Masood MF, Baltazar Garcia M, et al. Left ventricular unloading by Impella device versus surgical vent during extracorporeal life support. *Ann Thorac Surg*. 2017;104(3):861–867.
27. Pappalardo F, Schulte C, Pieri M, et al. Concomitant implantation of Impella® on top of veno-arterial extracorporeal membrane oxygenation may improve survival of patients with cardiogenic shock: Impella® improves survival in cardiogenic shock. *Eur Heart Fail*. 2017;19(3):404–412.
28. Rihal CS, Naidu SS, Givertz MM, et al. 2015 SCAI/ACC/HFSA/STS Clinical Expert Consensus Statement on the use of percutaneous mechanical circulatory support devices in cardiovascular care (Endorsed by the American Heart Association, the Cardiological Society of India, and Sociedad Latino Americana de Cardiologia Intervencion; Affirmation of Value by the Canadian Association of Interventional Cardiology–Association Canadienne de Cardiologie d'intervention)*. *J Card Fail*. 2015;21(6):499–518.
29. Takayama H, Soni L, Kalesan B, et al. Bridge-to-decision therapy with a continuous-flow external ventricular assist device in refractory cardiogenic shock of various causes. *Circ Heart Fail*. 2014;7(5):799–806.
30. Anderson MB, Goldstein J, Milano C, et al. Benefits of a novel percutaneous ventricular assist device for right heart failure: the prospective RECOVER RIGHT study of the Impella RP device. *J Heart Lung Transplant*. 2015;34(12):1549–1560.
31. Ravichandran A, Baran DA, Cowger JA, et al. Percutaneous right ventricular assist device outcomes: Protek Duo. *J Heart Lung Transplant*. 2017;36(4):S323.
32. Pappalardo F, Scandroglio AM, Latib A. Full percutaneous biventricular support with two Impella pumps: the Bi-Pella approach. *ESC Heart Fail*. 2018;5(3):368–371.
33. Abrams D, Garan AR, Abdelbary A, et al. Position paper for the organization of ECMO programs for cardiac failure in adults. *Intensive Care Med*. 2018;44(6):717–729.
34. ELSO. ELSO International Summary–July 2018. 2018; https://www.elso.org/Registry/Statistics.aspx. Accessed November 29, 2018.
35. Cheng R, Hachamovitch R, Kittleson M, et al. Complications of extracorporeal membrane oxygenation for treatment of cardiogenic shock and cardiac arrest: a meta-analysis of 1,866 adult patients. *Ann Thoracic Surg*. 2014;97(2):610–616.
36. Pabst D, Foy AJ, Peterson B, Soleimani B, Brehm CE. Predicting survival in patients treated with extracorporeal membrane oxygenation after myocardial infarction. *Crit Care Med*. 2018;46(5):e359–e363.
37. Sheu J-J, Tsai T-H, Lee F-Y, et al. Early extracorporeal membrane oxygenator-assisted primary percutaneous coronary intervention improved 30-day clinical outcomes in patients with ST-segment elevation myocardial infarction complicated with profound cardiogenic shock. *Crit Care Med*. 2010;38(9):1810–1817.
38. Esper SA, Bermudez C, Dueweke EJ, et al. Extracorporeal membrane oxygenation support in acute coronary syndromes complicated by cardiogenic shock. *Catheter Cardiovasc Interv*. 2015;86(suppl 1):S45–S50.

39. Asaumi Y, Yasuda S, Morii I, et al. Favourable clinical outcome in patients with cardiogenic shock due to fulminant myocarditis supported by percutaneous extracorporeal membrane oxygenation. *Eur Heart J.* 2005;26(20):2185–2192.
40. Mirabel M, Luyt C-E, Leprince P, et al. Outcomes, long-term quality of life, and psychologic assessment of fulminant myocarditis patients rescued by mechanical circulatory support. *Crit Care Med.* 2011;39(5):1029–1035.
41. Pages ON, Aubert S, Combes A, et al. Paracorporeal pulsatile biventricular assist device versus extracorporal membrane oxygenation-extracorporal life support in adult fulminant myocarditis. *J Thorac Cardiovasc Surg.* 2009;137(1):194–197.
42. Liao X, Li B, Cheng Z. Extracorporeal membrane oxygenation in adult patients with acute fulminant myocarditis: clinical outcomes and risk factor analysis. *Herz.* 2018(8); 728–732.
43. Chen SW, Tsai FC, Lin YS, et al. Long-term outcomes of extracorporeal membrane oxygenation support for postcardiotomy shock. *J Thorac Cardiovasc Surg.* 2017;154(2):469–477, e462.
44. Whitman GJ. Extracorporeal membrane oxygenation for the treatment of postcardiotomy shock. *J Thorac Cardiovasc Surg.* 2017;153(1):95–101.
45. Khorsandi M, Dougherty S, Bouamra O, et al. Extra-corporeal membrane oxygenation for refractory cardiogenic shock after adult cardiac surgery: a systematic review and meta-analysis. *J Cardiothorac Surg.* 2017;12(1):55.
46. Distelmaier K, Wiedemann D, Binder C, et al. Duration of extracorporeal membrane oxygenation support and survival in cardiovascular surgery patients. *J Thorac Cardiovasc Surg.* 2018;155(6):2471–2476.
47. Ro SK, Kim WK, Lim JY, Yoo JS, Hong SB, Kim JB. Extracorporeal life support for adults with refractory septic shock. *J Thorac Cardiovasc Surg.* 2018;156(3):1104–1109, e1101.
48. Perdue SM, Poore BJ, Babu AN, Stribling WK. Successful use of extracorporeal membrane oxygenation support in severe septic shock with associated acute cardiomyopathy. *J Card Surg.* 2018;33(1):50–52.
49. Vogel DJ, Murray J, Czapran AZ, et al. Veno-arterio-venous ECMO for septic cardiomyopathy: a single-centre experience. *Perfusion.* 2018;33(1 suppl):57–64.
50. Kim HS, Cheon DY, Ha SO, et al. Early changes in coagulation profiles and lactate levels in patients with septic shock undergoing extracorporeal membrane oxygenation. *J Thorac Dis.* 2018;10(3):1418–1430.
51. Grunau B, Hornby L, Singal RK, et al. Extracorporeal Cardiopulmonary Resuscitation for Refractory Out-of-Hospital Cardiac Arrest: The State of the Evidence and Framework for Application. *Can J Cardiol.* 2018;34(2):146–155.
52. Chen Y-S, Lin J-W, Yu H-Y, et al. Cardiopulmonary resuscitation with assisted extracorporeal life-support versus conventional cardiopulmonary resuscitation in adults with in-hospital cardiac arrest: an observational study and propensity analysis. *Lancet.* 2008;372(9638):554–561.
53. Yukawa T, Kashiura M, Sugiyama K, Tanabe T, Hamabe Y. Neurological outcomes and duration from cardiac arrest to the initiation of extracorporeal membrane oxygenation in patients with out-of-hospital cardiac arrest: a retrospective study. *Scand J Trauma Resusc Emerg Med.* 2017;25(1):95.
54. Chonde M, Sappington P, Kormos R, Althouse A, Boujoukos A. The use of ECMO for the treatment of refractory cardiac arrest or postarrest cardiogenic shock following in-hospital cardiac arrest: a 10 year experience. *J Intensive Care Med.* 2018. 885066617751398.
55. Yannopoulos D, Bartos JA, Raveendran G, et al. Coronary artery disease in patients with out-of-hospital refractory ventricular fibrillation cardiac arrest. *J Am Coll Cardiol.* 2017;70(9):1109–1117.
56. Spangenberg T, Schewel J, Dreher A, et al. Health related quality of life after extracorporeal cardiopulmonary resuscitation in refractory cardiac arrest. *Resuscitation.* 2018;127:73–78.
57. Fukuhara S, Takeda K, Kurlansky PA, Naka Y, Takayama H. Extracorporeal membrane oxygenation as a direct bridge to heart transplantation in adults. *J Thorac Cardiovasc Surg.* 2018;155(4):1607 1618, e1606.
58. Barge-Caballero E, Almenar-Bonet L, Gonzalez-Vilchez F, et al. Clinical outcomes of temporary mechanical circulatory support as a direct bridge to heart transplantation: a nationwide Spanish registry. *Eur J Heart Fail.* 2018;20(1):178–186.
59. Jasseron C, Lebreton G, Cantrelle C, et al. Impact of heart transplantation on survival in patients on venoarterial extracorporeal membrane oxygenation at listing in France. *Transplantation.* 2016;100(9):1979–1987.
60. Meyer DM, Rogers JG, Edwards LB, et al. The future direction of the adult heart allocation system in the United States: Heart Allocation in the United States. *Am J Transplant.* 2015;15(1):44 54.
61. Chung JC-Y, Tsai P-R, Chou N-K, Chi N-H, Wang S-S, Ko W-J. Extracorporeal membrane oxygenation bridge to adult heart transplantation. *Clin Transplant.* 2010;24(3):375–380.
62. Lechiancole A, Sponga S, Isola M, Vendramin I, Maiani M, Livi U. Heart transplantation in patients supported by ECMO: Is the APACHE IV score a predictor of survival? *Artif Organs.* 2018;42(6):670–673.
63. Pagani FD, Lynch W, Swaniker F, et al. Extracorporeal life support to left ventricular assist device bridge to heart transplant: a strategy to optimize survival and resource utilization. *Circulation.* 1999;100(19 suppl):II206–210.
64. Lebreton G, Pozzi M, Mastroianni C, Leger P, Pavie A, Leprince P. Extracorporeal life support as a bridge to bridge: a strategy to optimize ventricular assist device results. *Eur J Cardiothorac Surg.* 2015;48(5): 785–791.
65. Kurihara C, Kawabori M, Sugiura T, et al. Bridging to a long-term ventricular assist device with short-term mechanical circulatory support. *Artif Organs.* 2018;42(6):589–596.
66. Bakhtiary F, Keller H, Dogan S, et al. Venoarterial extracorporeal membrane oxygenation for treatment of cardiogenic shock: clinical experiences in 45 adult patients. *Thorac Cardiovasc Surg.* 2008;135(2):382–388.
67. Belle L, Mangin L, Bonnet H, et al. Emergency extracorporeal membrane oxygenation in a hospital without on-site cardiac surgical facilities. *EuroIntervention.* 2012;8(3):375–382.
68. Bermudez CA, Rocha RV, Toyoda Y, et al. Extracorporeal membrane oxygenation for advanced refractory shock in acute and chronic cardiomyopathy. *Ann Thorac Surg.* 2011;92(6):2125–2131.
69. Elsharkawy HA, Li L, Esa WA, Sessler DI, Bashour CA. Outcome in patients who require venoarterial extracorporeal membrane oxygenation support after cardiac surgery. *J Cardiothorac Vasc Anesth.* 2010;24(6):946–951.
70. Hei F, Lou S, Li J, et al. Five-year results of 121 consecutive patients treated with extracorporeal membrane oxygenation at Fu Wai Hospital. *Artif Organs.* 2011;35(6):572–578.
71. Hsu PS, Chen JL, Hong GJ, et al. Extracorporeal membrane oxygenation for refractory cardiogenic shock after cardiac surgery: predictors of early mortality and outcome from 51 adult patients. *Eur J Cardiothorac Surg.* 2010;37(2):328–333.
72. Kagawa E, Inoue I, Kawagoe T, et al. Assessment of outcomes and differences between in- and out-of-hospital cardiac arrest patients treated with cardiopulmonary resuscitation using extracorporeal life support. *Resuscitation.* 2010;81(8):968–973.
73. Kim H, Lim SH, Hong J, et al. Efficacy of veno-arterial extracorporeal membrane oxygenation in acute myocardial infarction with cardiogenic shock. *Resuscitation.* 2012;83(8):971–975.
74. Loforte A, Montalto A, Ranocchi F, et al. Peripheral extracorporeal membrane oxygenation system as salvage treatment of patients with refractory cardiogenic shock: preliminary outcome evaluation. *Artif Organs.* 2012;36(3):E53–E61.
75. Moraca RJ, Wanamaker KM, Bailey SH, et al. Salvage peripheral extracorporeal membrane oxygenation using Cobe Revolution(®) centrifugal pump as a bridge to decision for acute refractory cardiogenic shock. *J Card Surg.* 2012;27(4):521–527.
76. Pagani FD, Aaronson KD, Swaniker F, Bartlett RH. The use of extracorporeal life support in adult patients with primary cardiac failure as a bridge to implantable left ventricular assist device. *Ann Thorac Surg.* 2001;71(3 suppl):S77–S81, discussion S82-75.
77. Rastan AJ, Dege A, Mohr M, et al. Early and late outcomes of 517 consecutive adult patients treated with extracorporeal membrane oxygenation for refractory postcardiotomy cardiogenic shock. *Thorac Cardiovasc Surg.* 2010;139(2):302–311, 311, e301.

78. Schmidt M, Brechot N, Hariri S, et al. Nosocomial infections in adult cardiogenic shock patients supported by venoarterial extracorporeal membrane oxygenation. *Clin Infect Dis*. 2012;55(12):1633–1641.
79. Slottosch I, Liakopoulos O, Kuhn E, et al. Outcomes after peripheral extracorporeal membrane oxygenation therapy for postcardiotomy cardiogenic shock: a single-center experience. *J Surg Res*. 2013;181(2):e47–e55.
80. Smith C, Bellomo R, Raman JS, et al. An extracorporeal membrane oxygenation-based approach to cardiogenic shock in an older population. *Ann Thorac Surg*. 2001;71(5):1421–1427.
81. Unosawa S, Sezai A, Hata M, et al. Long-term outcomes of patients undergoing extracorporeal membrane oxygenation for refractory postcardiotomy cardiogenic shock. *Surg Today*. 2013;43(3):264–270.
82. Wang J, Han J, Jia Y, et al. Early and intermediate results of rescue extracorporeal membrane oxygenation in adult cardiogenic shock. *Ann Thorac Surg*. 2009;88(6):1897–1903.
83. Wu MY, Lin PJ, Lee MY, et al. Using extracorporeal life support to resuscitate adult postcardiotomy cardiogenic shock: treatment strategies and predictors of short-term and midterm survival. *Resuscitation*. 2010;81(9):1111–1116.
84. Wu MY, Lee MY, Lin CC, Chang YS, Tsai FC, Lin PJ. Resuscitation of non-postcardiotomy cardiogenic shock or cardiac arrest with extracorporeal life support: the role of bridging to intervention. *Resuscitation*. 2012;83(8):976–981.
85. Zhang R, Kofidis T, Kamiya H, et al. Creatine kinase isoenzyme MB relative index as predictor of mortality on extracorporeal membrane oxygenation support for postcardiotomy cardiogenic shock in adult patients. *Eur J Cardiothorac Surg*. 2006;30(4):617–620.
86. Brechot N, Luyt CE, Schmidt M, et al. Venoarterial extracorporeal membrane oxygenation support for refractory cardiovascular dysfunction during severe bacterial septic shock. *Crit Care Med*. 2013;41(7):1616–1626.
87. Cheng A, Sun HY, Lee CW, et al. Survival of septic adults compared with nonseptic adults receiving extracorporeal membrane oxygenation for cardiopulmonary failure: a propensity-matched analysis. *J Crit Care*. 2013;28(4). 532, e531-510.
88. Huang CT, Tsai YJ, Tsai PR, Ko WJ. Extracorporeal membrane oxygenation resuscitation in adult patients with refractory septic shock. *Thorac Cardiovasc Surg*. 2013;146(5):1041–1046.
89. Park TK, Yang JH, Jeon K, et al. Extracorporeal membrane oxygenation for refractory septic shock in adults. *Eur J Cardiothorac Surg*. 2015;47(2):e68–e74.
90. Cheng A, Sun HY, Tsai MS, et al. Predictors of survival in adults undergoing extracorporeal membrane oxygenation with severe infections. *Thorac Cardiovasc Surg*. 2016;152(6):1526–1536, e1521.
91. Choi MJ, Ha SO, Kim HS, Park S, Han SJ, Lee SH. The Simplified Acute Physiology Score II as a predictor of mortality in patients who underwent extracorporeal membrane oxygenation for septic shock. *Ann of Thorac Surg*. 2017;103(4):1246–1253.
92. Xie A, Phan K, Tsai YC, Yan TD, Forrest P. Venoarterial extracorporeal membrane oxygenation for cardiogenic shock and cardiac arrest: a meta-analysis. *J Cardiothorac Vasc Anesth*. 2015;29(3):637–645.
93. Ahn C, Kim W, Cho Y, Choi KS, Jang BH, Lim TH. Efficacy of extracorporeal cardiopulmonary resuscitation compared to conventional cardiopulmonary resuscitation for adult cardiac arrest patients: a systematic review and meta-analysis. *Sci Rep*. 2016;6:34208.
94. Kim SJ, Kim HJ, Lee HY, Ahn HS, Lee SW. Comparing extracorporeal cardiopulmonary resuscitation with conventional cardiopulmonary resuscitation: a meta-analysis. *Resuscitation*. 2016;103:106–116.
95. Ortega-Deballon I, Hornby L, Shemie SD, Bhanji F, Guadagno E. Extracorporeal resuscitation for refractory out-of-hospital cardiac arrest in adults: a systematic review of international practices and outcomes. *Resuscitation*. 2016;101:12–20.
96. Ouweneel DM, Schotborgh JV, Limpens J, et al. Extracorporeal life support during cardiac arrest and cardiogenic shock: a systematic review and meta-analysis. *Intensive Care Med*. 2016;42(12):1922–1934.
97. D'Arrigo S, Cacciola S, Dennis M, et al. Predictors of favourable outcome after in-hospital cardiac arrest treated with extracorporeal cardiopulmonary resuscitation: a systematic review and meta-analysis. *Resuscitation*. 2017;121:62–70.
98. Debaty G, Babaz V, Durand M, et al. Prognostic factors for extracorporeal cardiopulmonary resuscitation recipients following out-of-hospital refractory cardiac arrest. A systematic review and meta-analysis. *Resuscitation*. 2017;112:1–10.
99. Wang GN, Chen XF, Qiao L, et al. Comparison of extracorporeal and conventional cardiopulmonary resuscitation: a meta-analysis of 2 260 patients with cardiac arrest. *World J Emerg Med*. 2017;8(1):5–11.
100. Lebreton G, Pozzi M, Mastroianni C, Léger P, Pavie A, Leprince P. Extracorporeal life support as a bridge to bridge: a strategy to optimize ventricular assist device results. *Eur J Cardiothorac Surg*. 2015;48(5):785–791.
101. Rousse N, Juthier F, Pincon C, et al. ECMO as a bridge to decision: recovery, VAD, or heart transplantation? *Int J Cardiol*. 2015;187:620–627.

7

Understanding the Principles of Continuous-Flow Rotary Left Ventricular Assist Devices

Francis D. Pagani

KEY POINTS

Introduction
Historical Perspective
General Pump Design
CF Rotary Pump Design: Axial Versus Centrifugal Pumps
Bearing Design/Impeller Suspension
Hydrodynamic Performance of CF Pumps
Interaction of the CF Rotary Pump and Native Heart
Parallel and Series Circulation
Series Circulation Flow Estimation
Limitations in Flow Control With CF Rotary Pumps
Conclusion

INTRODUCTION

Mechanical circulatory support with durable left ventricular assist devices (LVADs) has become a mainstay therapy for treatment of advanced heart failure refractory to optimal medical management and has now surpassed cardiac transplantation as the most frequently utilized surgical therapy for treatment of end-stage heart failure. Important progress in the field has occurred with the introduction of continuous-flow (CF) rotary pump technology that has supplanted older pulsatile displacement pumps. CF rotary pump technology has afforded patients improved survival and reduced occurrence of major adverse events owing to the smaller size of these pumps, quieter operation, improved power efficiency, and greater reliability and durability. CF rotary pumps have significantly different flow characteristics compared to pulsatile pumps, and CF rotary pumps in clinical use have differing device designs that influence the flow properties of the pump and its interaction with the native heart. There are several important features of the CF rotary pump technology that permit characterization of the pumps based on axial versus centrifugal design, bearing design, hydrodynamic properties, and mode of pump speed operation. Despite the marked advantages of this technology, numerous challenges in the management of patients remain, related in part to limitations in the ability of CF rotary pumps to adapt to marked changes in preload and afterload conditions, reduced pulsatility, and lack of algorithms that provide physiologic input into pump speed control. A thorough understanding of the theory of operation and design features of the pumps is necessary to provide care for patients supported with this technology.

HISTORICAL PERSPECTIVE

Despite the controversies surrounding the issues of maintaining pulsatile or nonpulsatile circulation, the field of mechanical circulatory support (MCS) has significantly evolved from the use of volume displacement pulsatile pumps to CF rotary blood pumps.[1-5] CF rotary pumps now dominate the field of MCS, with nearly all LVAD implants in the United States representing CF rotary pump technology.[6,7] This trend has continued for both short-term (i.e., nonimplantable temporary devices) and implantable, durable MCS device designs.[6,8] CF rotary pumps offer several advantages over pulsatile, volume displacement pumps. These advantages include (1) a smaller pump size (due to the elimination of the displacement chamber required for a pulsatile pump), (2) fewer moving parts (limited to a single internal rotating impeller) resulting in greater durability and reliability, (3) limited blood contacting surfaces, (4) lower noise, and (5) reduced energy requirements that have translated into significantly improved clinical outcomes.[4,5] The small size of implantable CF rotary pumps has facilitated the expansion of the therapy into children or patients with small body habitus[9,10] and has promoted applications including implantable durable biventricular support,[11] total artificial heart support,[12] and minimally invasive surgical approaches.[13,14]

GENERAL PUMP DESIGN

A CF rotary pump consists of blood inlet and outlet ports and a single internal rotating element, that is, rotor or impeller, that is suspended within a pump housing that propels blood forward by spinning the impeller at high speeds, imparting significant kinetic energy to the blood that overcomes outflow resistance to the pump. The spinning of the impeller is accomplished by sequentially actuating an electrical current and creating a magnetic field that is coupled to the internal magnets within the impeller.[15,16] CF rotary pumps in clinical use today are powered by a brushless DC motor and currently require an external power source (most often provided by rechargeable batteries or an AC power cord) that is transmitted to the internal pump through a percutaneous cable or driveline. In the near future, wireless energy transfer systems should eliminate the need for the percutaneous lead to power implantable pumps.[15,16]

CF ROTARY PUMP DESIGN: AXIAL VERSUS CENTRIFUGAL PUMPS

There are essentially two types of CF rotary pumps in clinical use today: centrifugal flow pumps and axial flow pumps (Fig. 7.1).[15,16] The primary difference between centrifugal flow and axial flow pumps lies

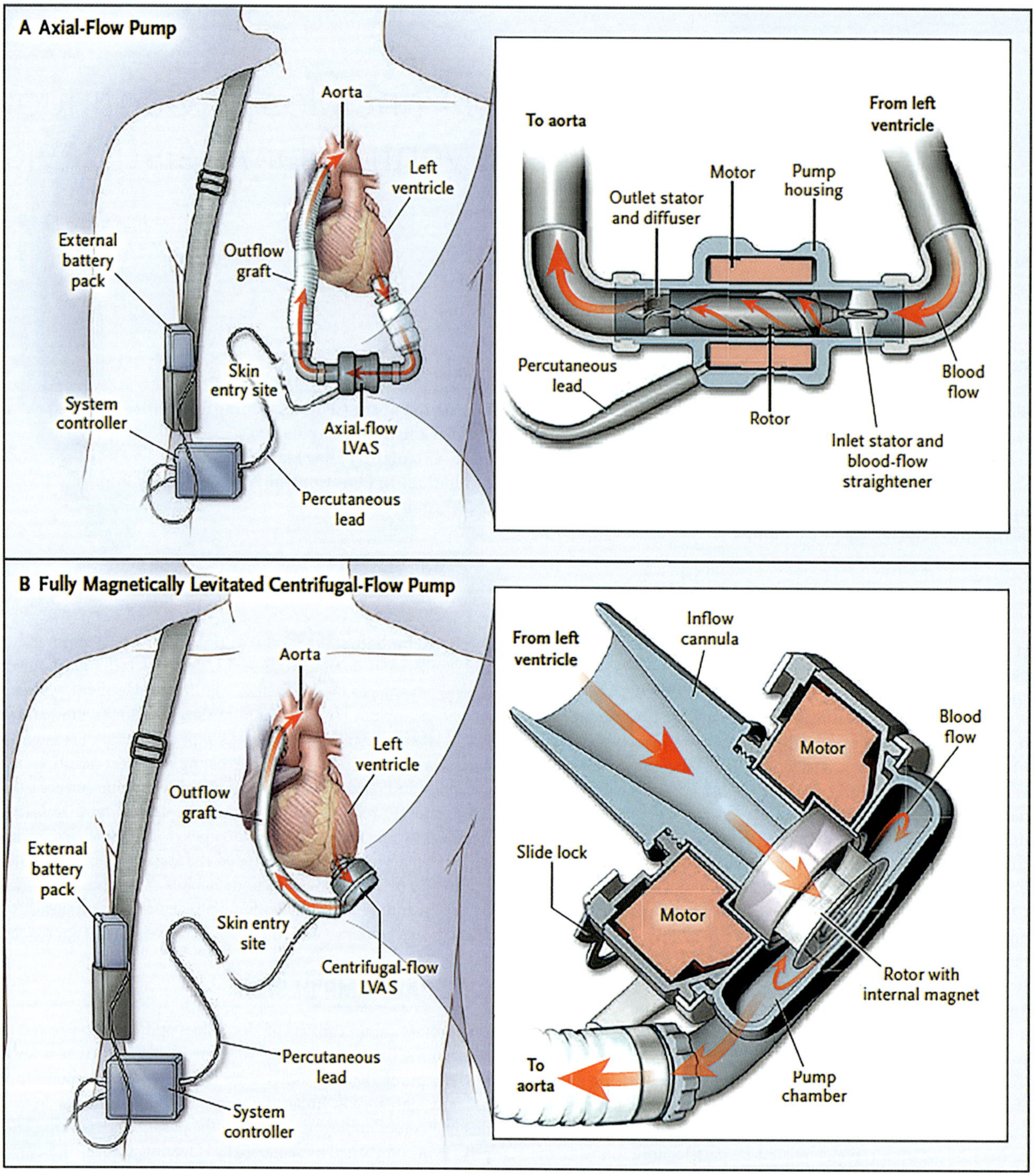

Fig. 7.1 (A) Diagram of the axial-flow pump. Blood enters at the inlet end of the rotor and is driven along the axis of rotation or centerline of the rotor to the out-flow end of the pump. (B). Diagram of a centrifugal blood pump where blood enters the pump inlet cannula along the axis of rotation or centerline of the impeller and is driven outward, tangentially to the outlet of the pump. (From Mehra MR, Naka Y, Uriel N, et al. A fully magnetically levitated circulatory pump for advanced heart failure. *N Engl J Med.* 2017;376:440–450.)[34]

in the design of their rotating element, or impeller. In a centrifugal pump, the outlet path is positioned 90 degrees relative to the axis of rotation or centerline of the impeller and the rotating element acts as a spinning disk with blades that capture fluid and propel the blood from impeller blades to the outflow cannula along a tangential course.[15,16] In an axial flow pump, the inlet and outlet blood paths are positioned parallel relative to the axis of rotation or centerline of the impeller and the rotating element operates like a propeller in a pipe that pushes fluid forward. In both cases, blood exits opposite to the direction of thrust generated by the pump motor.

Spinning of the impeller at high rotational speeds transfers significant kinetic energy to the blood and the blood leaves the pump at a higher pressure and velocity than at its entry. The rate at which a pump adds energy to a fluid is[17]:

$$W = \frac{dV}{dt} \times \Delta P = Q \times \Delta P$$

where $Q = \frac{dV}{dt}$ is the flow and ΔP is the difference in pressure between the inlet and outlet orifices of the pump. The efficiency of a pump is defined as the ratio of the power output to the required power input:

$$\eta_{pump} = \frac{Q \times \Delta P}{W_{input}}$$

Centrifugal devices generally have greater hydraulic efficiency at energy transfer and provide CF at rotational speeds that are much slower, approximately 2000 to 6000 rpm compared with 8000 to 15,000 rpm for pumps with axial flow designs.[15,16] This generally means that a lower shear stress is exerted on the blood elements and that there is a lower risk of hemolysis.[18] The hydraulic efficiency, defined previously as the ratio of power imparted to the fluid divided by the power input to the impeller, is related to the ability of a pump to transport fluid with minimal power loss over the blood flow path. Hydraulic efficiency is an important, but not sole, determinant of overall LVAD system efficiency. LVAD systems require power supplies and controllers that have unique methods of operating the pump. It is the sum of the efficiency of the motors and controllers and the hydraulic efficiency that contribute to the overall system efficiency.

BEARING DESIGN/IMPELLER SUSPENSION

CF rotary pump designs can be further distinguished by the mechanism of impeller suspension or levitation and include use of (1) mechanical bearings (Fig. 7.2), (2) hydrodynamic bearings (fluid forces), (3) hydrodynamic bearings working in synergy with magnetic suspension (Figs. 7.3 and 7.4), and (4) variations of active and/or passive magnetic suspension (Fig. 7.4).[15–19]

Mechanical Bearing

A mechanical pivot design or contact bearing utilizes mechanical bearings on spherical surfaces rotating in sockets (see Fig. 7.2). These bearings are made of ceramic components with low friction coefficient (i.e., ceramic or ruby). These bearings have long durability attributed, in part, to boundary lubrication from blood immersion.[15–20] Although simplistic in design, a major limitation of this mechanism of impeller support is that the point of contact of the mechanical bearings is a point of friction and heat generation that represent potential sites for fibrin deposition with thrombus formation.[21] Washing of these points by blood or fluid is necessary to provide adequate dissipation of heat. In addition, the concentration of hydrodynamic loads on these bearings, especially at stress concentration points, makes these contact points theoretically susceptible to wear and fatigue, particularly at the inlet bearing that receives a major component of the motor thrust.

Noncontact Bearing Designs

Noncontact bearing designs incorporate either hydrodynamic or magnetic forces or a combination of both to achieve suspension of the internal impeller without the use of mechanical contact supports.[15–19] Without the need for mechanical contacts, these suspension systems do not have points of friction and theoretically have an infinite or limitless lifespan. These levitation systems must control for six degrees of freedom of the impeller: three rotational movements (rotation around *x*, *y*, and *z* axis) and three translational movements (displacement without rotation; i.e., up, down, and sideways). Rotation around the axis of rotation or centerline of the pump is achieved by electromagnetic coupling of the motor stator and internal magnet of the impeller.

Hydrodynamic Bearing

Hydrodynamic bearings utilize pressure generated from a fluid film that acts to separate the rotating surfaces of the impeller from the stationary base of the pump (see Fig. 7.4).[15–19,22] However, in order to generate a hydrodynamic force, the surface of the impeller must be moving, and when the impeller is stationary, e.g., at pump startup or stop, impeller and stationary surfaces (such as the pump housing) will come into contact, which could result in damage to the surfaces of the

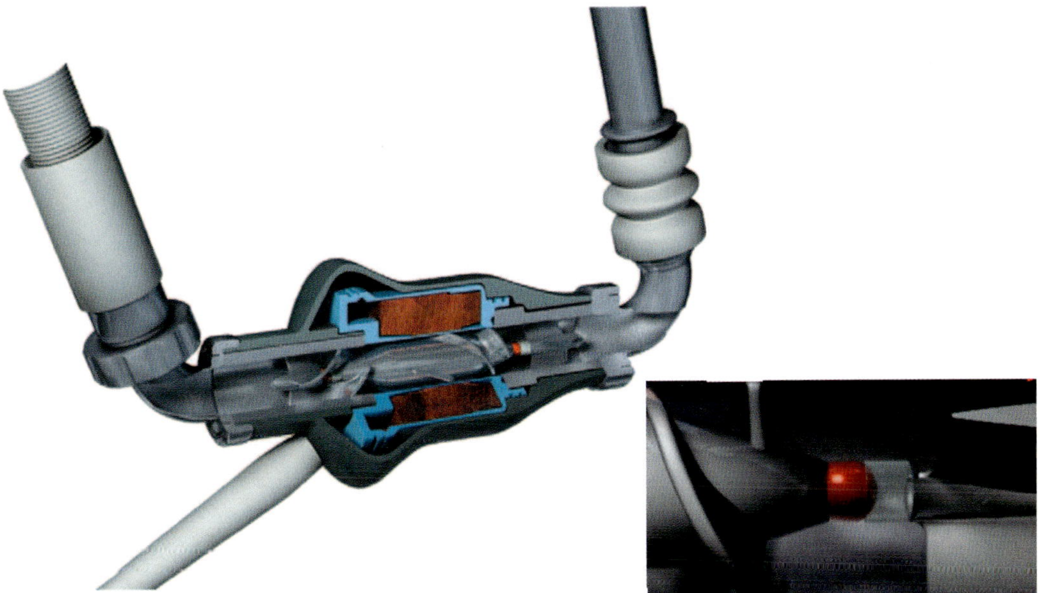

Fig. 7.2 Diagram of a continuous-flow rotary pump (axial pump) using a mechanical bearing or pivot design to suspend the internal rotor. The *insert* in the lower right hand corner of the figure demonstrates a "ball and socket" mechanical bearing design. The surfaces of the bearing are interspersed with a thin film of fluid to reduction friction and wear of the bearing. (Reproduced with permission of Abbott, © 2019.)

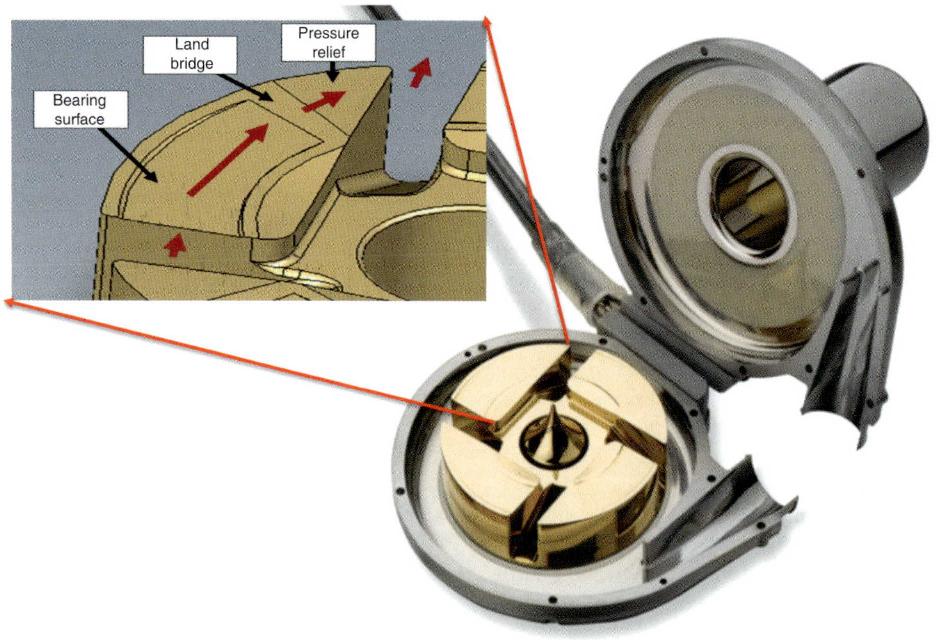

Fig. 7.3 Picture of a continuous-flow rotary pump (HVAD; Medtronic Inc., Minneapolis, MN) utilizing a combination of magnetic and hydrodynamic suspension of the internal rotor. The insert in the upper left hand corner of the picture details the hydrodynamic surface of the impeller that utilizes fluid forces to oppose magnetic forces generated from opposing magnets within the center post and impeller. (Courtesy Medtronic Inc., Minneapolis, MN, with permission.)

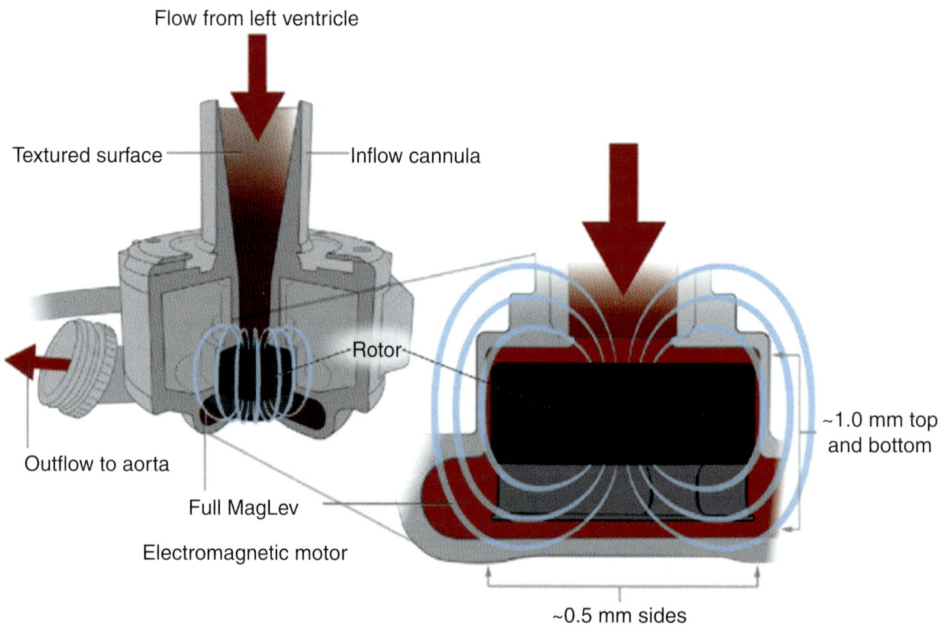

Fig. 7.4 Diagram of a continuous-flow rotary pump with total magnetic levitation of the internal impeller. (Courtesy Abbott Laboratories, Chicago, IL, with permission.)

impeller or pump housing, resulting in potential niduses for thrombus formation. Contact can also occur if rotating impeller speeds are not sufficient to overcome outflow pressures, resulting in impeller contact with the housing, or, even in the absence of contact, cause a significant decrease in the distance between impeller and pump housing, resulting in increased shear and friction of blood elements passing between the impeller and pump housing. Importantly, hydrodynamic forces dissipate quickly as a function of distance, thus limiting the distances between the stationary base (pump housing) and rotating impeller. As a result, the load-bearing fluid film is prone to higher shear stresses, which theoretically can result in more damage to blood elements with hemolysis. Hydrodynamic suspension systems do not utilize position sensors, resulting in a less complicated electronic design that enhances the ability to miniaturize pump sizes.

Magnet Bearing

Magnetic forces may be passive without the consumption of power (permanent magnet) or active (induction of magnetic field with electricity) in design (Fig. 7.5).[15–19] Passive magnets utilize rare earth magnets such as neodymium boron-iron magnets within the rotor and

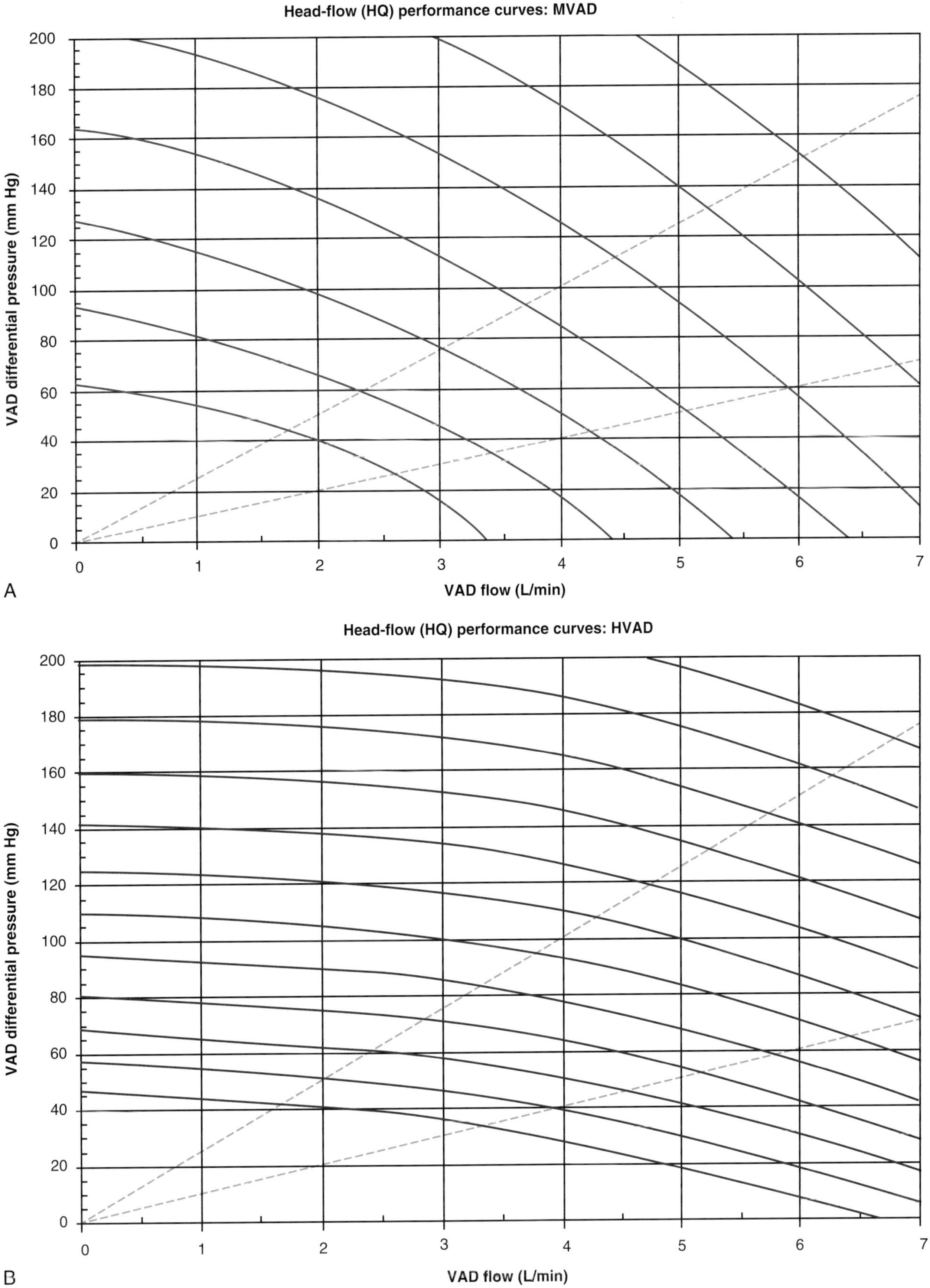

Fig. 7.5 (A) Diagram of a pressure-flow relationship or "head curve" for an axial flow rotary blood pump. The relationship between pressure and flow is nearly linear and represents a blood pump with a "steep" pressure-flow relationship. Each line on the graph represents differing pump speeds. (B) Diagram of a pressure-flow relationship or "head curve" for a centrifugal flow rotary blood pump. The relationship between pressure and flow is flat and represents a blood pump with greater sensitivity to changes in pressure. Each line on the graph represents differing pump speeds. *VAD*, Ventricular assist device. (Courtesy Medtronic Inc., Minneapolis, MN, with permission.)

along the housing to achieve suspension of the impeller. Permanent magnet bearings allow for a larger gap between the static motor armature and the rotor while eliminating the need for mechanical bearings, lubrication, sealing, or purging fluid. Magnetic forces are dependent on the instantaneous position of the rotor (i.e., magnetic forces are greater when magnets—impeller and pump housing—are at closer distances). Magnetic bearings are often used in conjunction with hydrodynamic or electromagnetic bearings. Control of any axis can be achieved with active or passive magnetic levitation. In an active mode, the repelling force is adjusted by changing the supplied current to the electromagnets based on the instantaneous position or other feedback. In a passive mode, the supplied current to the electromagnets is constant. The electromagnetic force adjusts automatically based on the position itself; i.e., as the impeller approaches the magnet in the pump housing, the repelling forces increase, and conversely, as the distance increases, the repelling forces decrease. However, active electromagnetic systems are complex and require position sensors, electromagnets and extra conductors, connector pins, and electronics to achieve the dedicated impeller position. In the event of an electrical contact failure in a connector pin or a momentary instability encountered in the control algorithm, pump failure can occur. Owing to the complexity of electromagnetic systems, electromagnetic bearing elements frequently utilize hydrodynamic bearings as a back-up mechanism to provide safe pump operation. The advantage of this approach is that the hydrodynamic bearing requires no additional controls. Distances between impeller and pump housing maintained by magnetic fields are a function of the strength of the magnetic field and, hence, a function of the size of the magnet. Thus, overall pump size and degree of miniaturization are a function of the size of the magnet needed to maintain the desired gap between the impeller and pump housing. Overall efficiencies of the pump are also determined, in part, by magnet strength. The major advantages of magnetic bearings are that distances between impeller and pump housing are generally larger and the degree of shear stresses on blood elements is less compared to mechanical contact bearings or hydrodynamic suspension systems. Theoretically, larger gaps with reduced shear on the blood elements may be associated with greater biocompatibility of the pump.

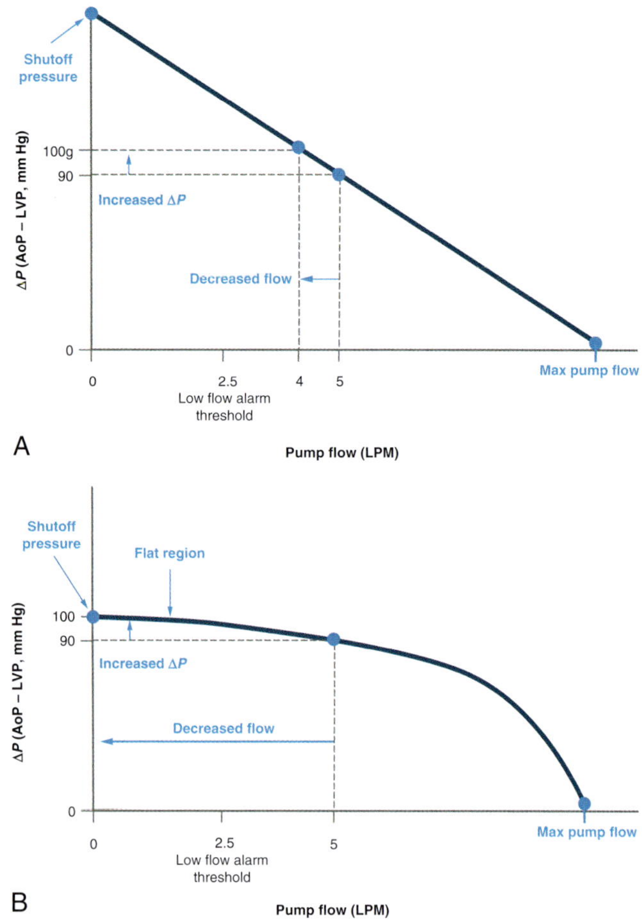

Fig. 7.6 (A) With a "steep" pressure-flow relationship, any given change in pressure is associated with a relatively small change in flow. (B) In a "flat" pressure-flow relationship, a small change in pressure is associated with a relatively larger change in flow. Pumps with a "flat" pressure-flow relationship are more sensitive to changes in preload and afterload conditions and in general, impart a greater degree of pulsatility to the systemic circulation. *AoP*, Aortic pressure; *LPM*, liters per minute; *LVP*, left ventricular pressure. (Courtesy Abbott Laboratories, Chicago, IL, with permission.)

HYDRODYNAMIC PERFORMANCE OF CF PUMPS

Blood flow through CF pumps, both axial and centrifugal, is directly proportional to pump speed and inversely proportional to the pressure difference across the inlet (e.g., left ventricular [LV] pressure) and outlet (e.g., aortic pressure) orifices of the pump.[15–19] This is referred to as the "ΔP" or "head pressure" and represents the work performed by the pump on the blood. A combination of torque and velocity allows the impeller to transfer energy to the blood and generate flow and pressure to overcome head pressure.

The relationship between ΔP and flow can be displayed in a series of curves reflecting blood flow over varying pressure gradients at differing pump speeds, i.e., the pressure-flow relationship or "head curve" (Figs. 7.5 and 7.6). This relationship between ΔP and flow is unique to each CF rotary pump, analogous to an individual's fingerprint. In general, most axial flow rotary pumps in clinical use to date have been designed with steeper pressure-flow relationships compared to centrifugal flow rotary pumps, but the generalizations do not hold for every pump design. A steep relationship between ΔP and flow is often represented by an almost linear relationship. A shallow or "flat" head curve represents greater sensitivity between the pressure-flow relationship such that small changes in pressure elicit greater changes in flow with any given change in pressure.

For a CF rotary pump with a flat head curve, the same ΔP will elicit a larger change in flow during systole relative to diastole compared to a CF rotary pump with a steep head curve. There are several important advantages of a flat head curve compared to a steep head curve. The more responsive pressure-flow relationship in CF rotary pumps with a flat head curve results in a greater degree of flow variability across the cardiac cycle (less flow in diastole and more flow in systole). In theory, the benefit of a rotary pump with a flat head curve versus that with a steep head curve is a greater aortic pulse pressure. Further, as ΔP increases in settings of lower preload, flow in a rotary pump with a flat head curve will decrease substantially more than in a rotary pump with a steep head curve. The ΔP at which zero flow occurs, i.e., shut off pressure, should generally be lower for pumps with a flat head curve compared to pumps with a steep head curve. Thus, there is theoretically less propensity to create ventricular collapse or a "suction event" resulting from the greater drop in pump flow as LV diastolic pressures decrease for pumps with a flat head pressure. Ventricular collapse or "suction" events elicited by a CF rotary pump may cause ventricular arrhythmias or increase the propensity for thrombus formation on bearings as a result of low flow or on the endocardium owing to trauma or increase the risk of damage to blood elements through generation of high negative pressures.

INTERACTION OF THE CF ROTARY PUMP AND NATIVE HEART

CF rotary pumps do not generate pulsation. However, CF rotary pumps operate in conjunction with the native ventricles and influence the hemodynamics and mechanics of the ventricle that alter ventricular function and geometry and systemic pulsatility. Flow through a CF rotary pump is continuous throughout the cardiac cycle but has superimposed phasic changes in pump flow caused by the interaction of the heart with the CF rotary pump.[15–19] Depending on hemodynamic conditions, the contractile state of the LV, pump speed, and the hydrodynamic properties of the pump, flow through a CF rotary pump may be more or less pulsatile. The hydrodynamic properties of the steepness of the head curve have important effects on the flow pattern of the CF rotary pump and its interaction with the native cardiac contraction. During the cardiac cycle, pump flow is greater during native cardiac systole because the native LV contraction raises intracardiac pressure, thereby lowering the ΔP (e.g., the difference between aortic and LV pressures) that the pump must overcome to generate forward flow. During diastole, the difference between LV pressure and aortic pressure is increased (i.e., ΔP is greater) and thus pump flow is less relative to systole (Fig. 7.7). These phasic changes in blood flow with a CF rotary pump impart a pulse to the native circulation. The magnitude of pulse pressure is typically diminished compared with the pulse pressure that is generated with a native heart contraction or a pulsatile flow pump. The magnitude of a pulse generated with a CF rotary pump is dependent on the relative differences in pressure changes during the cardiac cycle and the contributions of the native heart to the total cardiac output. Thus, conditions that create greater LV pressure generation (i.e., greater preload [Frank-Starling mechanism], inotrope therapy, and native LV recovery) will create a greater pulse pressure. Under normal circumstances (i.e., pump working in conjunction with the native heart contraction), the aortic flow pattern with a CF rotary pump is more accurately described as being continuous, rather than using the description of nonpulsatile flow. In circumstances in which there is absence of native heart contraction (e.g., ventricular fibrillation), the flow through a CF rotary pump is nonpulsatile. Importantly, CF rotary blood pumps do not contain unidirectional valves. In circumstances where afterload exceeds pressure generated by the pump and or if pump speed is inadequate, backflow through the pump may occur during portions of the cardiac cycle or throughout the entire cardiac cycle.

PARALLEL AND SERIES CIRCULATION

Depending on pump design and hemodynamic conditions, CF rotary pumps can provide either full support (pump responsible for all cardiac output) or partial support (pump supplies a portion of the total cardiac output). In circumstances of full pump support, the circulation is described as in "series" (Fig. 7.8). Conversely, in circumstances of partial pump support, the circulation is described as in "parallel." The presence of series or parallel circulations can vary during support. For example, a series circulation may exist early following pump

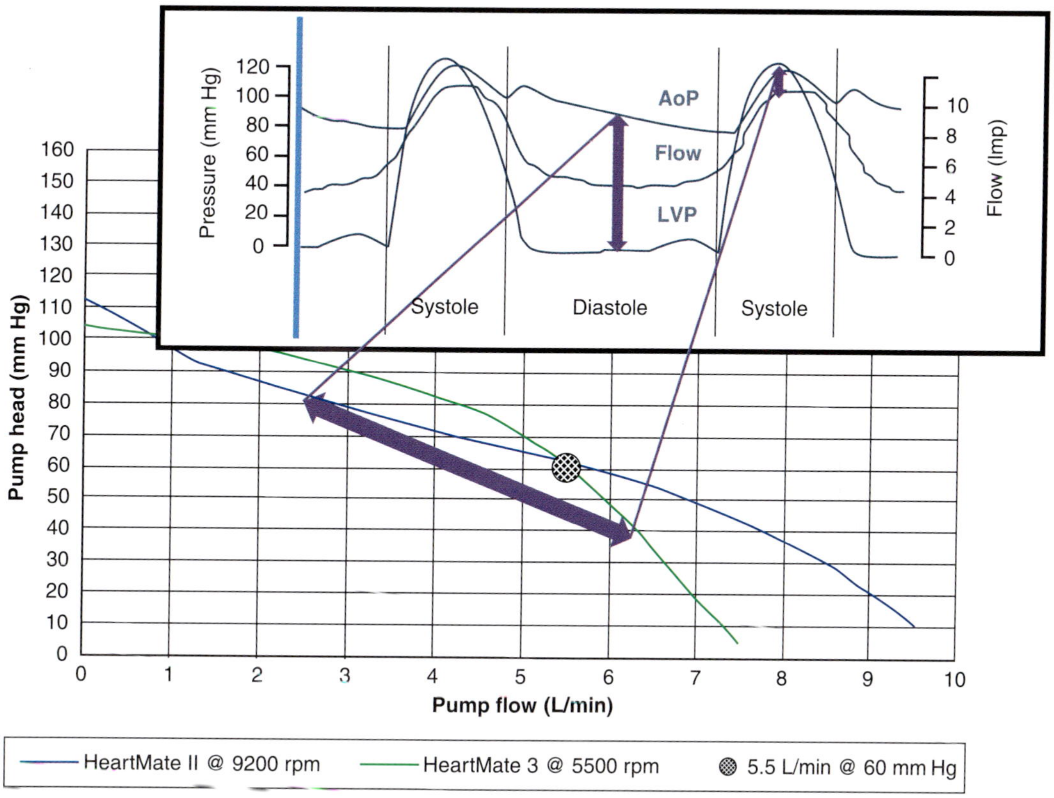

Fig. 7.7 Flow through a continuous-flow rotary pump varies with the cardiac cycle owing to the changes in head pressure during diastole and systole. During diastole, ΔP is greater and flow through the pump is less relative to systole where the difference in pressure between the left ventricle and aorta is less and ΔP is smaller. This flow variation across the cardiac cycle imparts a pulse to the systemic circulation. The size of the pulse imparted to the systemic circulation is dependent of the degree of flow variation during the cardiac cycle and dependent on contributions of the native heart to total cardiac output. The diagram shows two head curves, one for the HeartMate II pump (axial) and HeartMate 3 pump (centrifugal). *LVP*, Left ventricular pressure. (Courtesy Abbott Laboratories, Chicago, IL, with permission.)

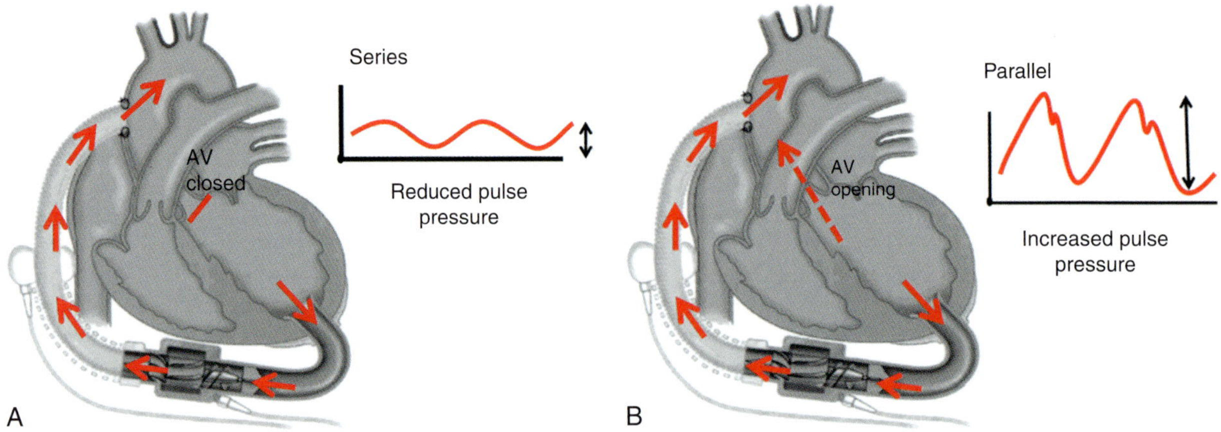

Fig. 7.8 (A) Circulation in "series" with the rotary pump. All cardiac output is delivered by the rotary pump and there is no native left ventricular ejection. In this circumstance, the systemic pulse pressure is significantly reduced compared to the native circulation. (B) Circulation in "parallel" with the rotary blood pump. In this circumstance, both rotary pump and native heart contractions contribute to total cardiac output. The systemic pulse pressure in these circumstances is generally greater owing to the contribution of the native heart ejection. *AV*, Aortic valve.

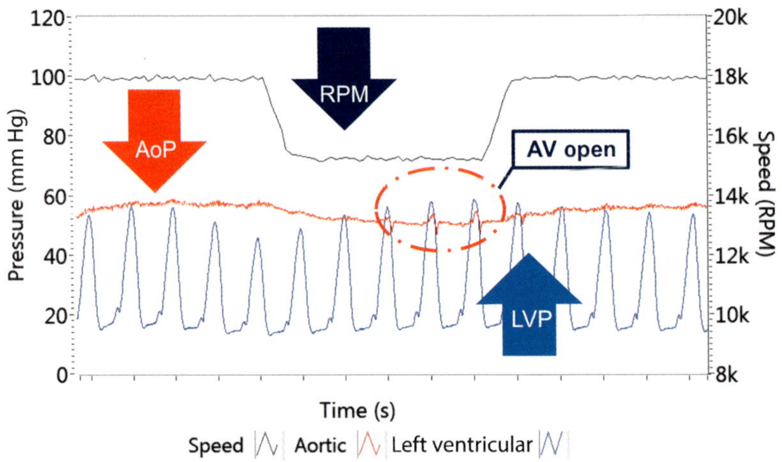

Fig. 7.9 Diagram demonstrating cycling between series and parallel circulations. As left ventricular pressure (*LVP*) exceeds aortic pressure, native ejection occurs, imparting contributions of the native heart to total cardiac output and imparting a greater pulse pressure to the systemic circulation. Native heart ejection depends on hemodynamic conditions, preload and afterload, state of contractility of the native heart, and pump speed. *AoP*, Aortic pressure; *AV*, aortic valve. (Courtesy Medtronic Inc., Minneapolis, MN, with permission.)

implantation, but as native LV function recovers, a parallel circulation may be created. Changes in a patient's preload caused by changes in volume status or activity could impart moment-to-moment cycling between series and parallel circulations (Fig. 7.9). With a series circulation, the aortic valve is continuously closed during the cardiac cycle. This phenomenon of continuous aortic valve closure has been associated with the development of physiologically important aortic insufficiency during pump support. Thus, there may be relative benefits of a parallel circulation compared to a series circulation to maintain aortic valve opening and native heart contributions to total cardiac output. Parallel circulation with maintenance of aortic valve opening has also been demonstrated to reduce platelet residence times and activation state characterized by shear stress accumulation in the LV, suggesting less risk of thrombogenesis within the LV cavity.[23]

FLOW ESTIMATION

Flow through a rotary blood pump is proportional to motor current or pump power, thus permitting motor current to be used as a sensorless index of pump flow and virtual index of LV pressure during the cardiac cycle. However, the relationship between motor current and pump flow is not linear throughout the entire range of flows and the relationship between motor current and flow differs between axial and centrifugal pumps. In addition, the point of power measurement may differ between different pump designs. Power output for centrifugal pumps tends to be more linear in the operating range of the pump compared to axial flow pumps, particularly at low flow rates. Thus, estimation of pump flow for centrifugal pumps tends to be more accurate as compared to axial flow pumps (Figs. 7.10 and 7.11).[15–19] In addition, viscosity has important effects on pump flow and power, with increasing hematocrit increasing motor current at any given flow. Incorporation of the hematocrit into the flow estimation thus increases the accuracy of the flow estimate.

LIMITATIONS IN FLOW CONTROL WITH CF ROTARY PUMPS

LVAD support with CF rotary pumps is associated with adverse physiologic sequelae that, in large part, represent the limitations of the current design of clinical LVADs operating in a "fixed speed"

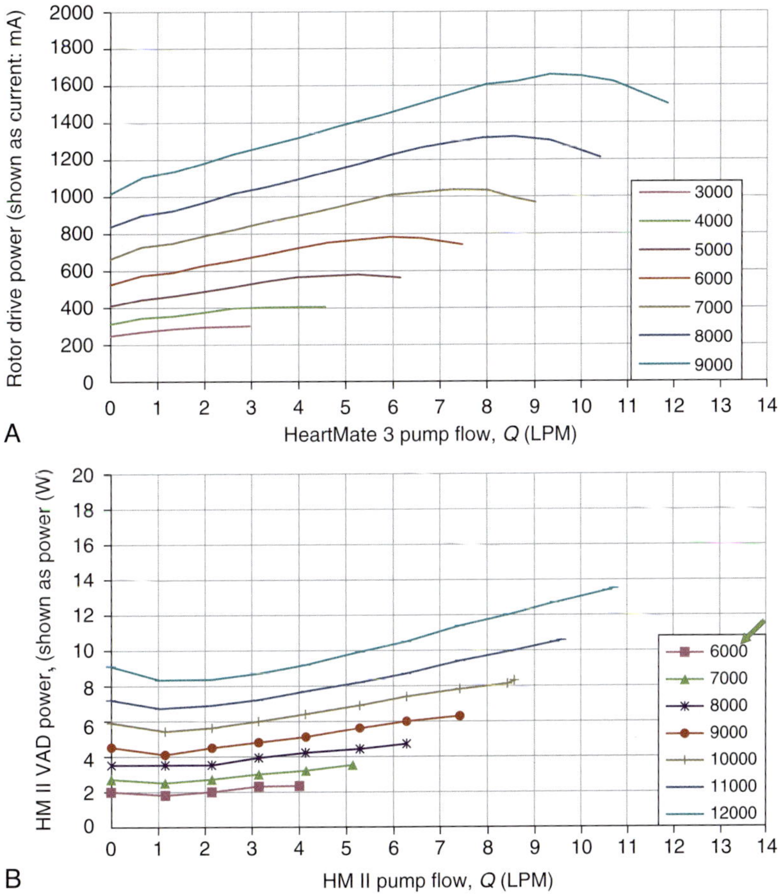

Fig. 7.10 (A) Diagram of the relationship between pump power (motor current) and flow for the HeartMate 3 pump (centrifugal). The relationship between power (motor current) and flow is nearly linear over the operating range of the pump. (B) Diagram of the relationship between pump power and flow for the HeartMate II pump (axial). The relationship between power and flow is not as linear over the operating range of the pump as compared to the HeartMate 3 pump (centrifugal), particularly at the lower ranges of flow. *HM*, HeartMate; *LPM*, liters per minute; *VAD*, ventricular assist device. (Courtesy Abbott Laboratories, Chicago, IL, with permission.)

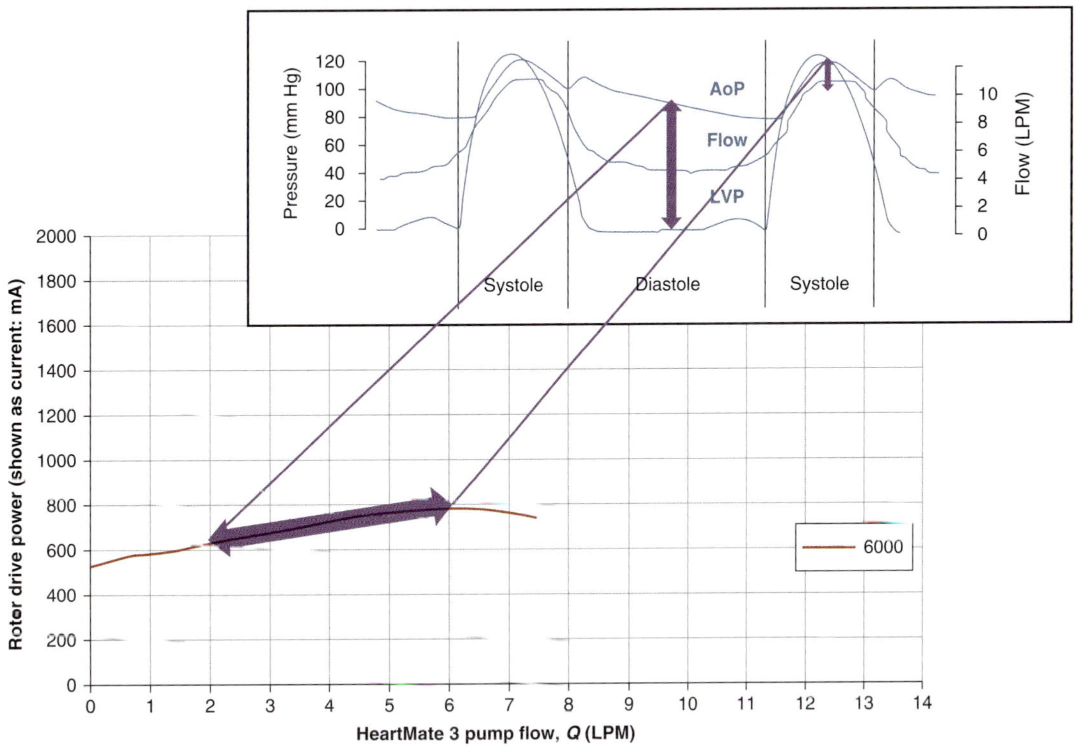

Fig. 7.11 Relationship between power (motor current) and flow over the operating ranges for the HeartMate 3 pump (centrifugal) is nearly linear. With correction for viscosity (hematocrit adjustment), flow estimations for the HeartMate 3 pump (centrifugal) are significantly more reliable as compared to the HeartMate II pump (axial). *AoP*, Aortic pressure; *LPM*, liters per minute; *LVP*, left ventricular pressure. (Courtesy Abbott Laboratories, Chicago, IL, with permission.)

mode algorithm that cause diminished arterial pulse pressure.[24–27] Further, this operating algorithm requires frequent provider interaction and assessment with clinical, echocardiographic, or right heart catheterization data to determine appropriate pump speeds necessary for clinical optimization. Changes in pump flow in CF rotary pumps can occur without changes in pump speed ("fixed speed" mode; reliance on the Starling mechanism to alter pump output) or as a consequence of changes in pump speed based upon an algorithm-based adjustment from a signal input (physiologic flow adjustments). The absence of autonomous speed control in LVADs eliminates the potential for creating pulsatility matching that of the normal physiologic state or significantly hinders the ability of current LVADs to respond to widely varying changes in preload and afterload conditions. Although current clinical LVADs possess hydrodynamic properties (Starling mechanism) that permit changes in pump output to altering preload and afterload conditions, this response under some circumstances is not appropriate, as the hydrodynamic properties of CF rotary pumps are less sensitive to changes in preload (i.e., small changes in pump output relative to large changes in preload) and more sensitive to changes in afterload (i.e., large changes in pump flow relative to small changes in afterload) compared to the native heart.[28] Thus, more appropriate changes in pump output are limited without alteration of pump speed. This "uninformed" mode of speed operation limits CF rotary pumps from autonomously and appropriately responding to widely varying changes in loading conditions and precludes (1) optimizing preload in the setting of increased physiologic demand, (2) maintenance of adequate pump flows in times of high afterload (i.e., hypertension), (3) maintenance of adequate LV volumes in times of low preload (i.e., prevention of "suction events"), and (4) appropriate flow balancing in applications with biventricular assist devices. Incorporation of physiologic pump speed adjustments based upon physiologic input (e.g., left atrial or LV pressure) to increase the safety of CF rotary pumps or to induce greater pulsatility to the systemic circulation has proved challenging.[24–32] Although CF rotary pumps in use today do not have speed algorithms to adjust flow to physiologic demand, systems do have speed adjustment algorithms to respond to "suction events" that utilize power assessments and the relationship between pump power and flow.

CONCLUSION

MCS with CF rotary blood pumps has demonstrated the feasibility of extended survival. Although current designs are associated with significant device-related adverse events, new technology has already overcome some of the major obstacles to date. Given the improvement in clinical outcomes with new device designs[33,34] and persistent limitations in heart transplantation as an alternative therapy, MCS with CF rotary pumps is likely to remain the dominant surgical treatment strategy for patients with advanced heart failure.

REFERENCES

1. Wesolowski SA, Fisher JH, Welsh CS. Perfusion of the pulmonary circulation by nonpulsatile flow. *Surgery*. 1953;33:370–375.
2. Nose Y. Is a pulsatile cardiac prosthesis a dying dinosaur? *Artif Organs*. 1992;16:233–234.
3. Hindman BJ, Dexter F, Ryu KH, Smith T, Cutkomp J. Pulsatile versus nonpulsatile cardiopulmonary bypass: No difference in brain blood flow or metabolism at 27° C. *Anesthesiology*. 1994;80:1137–1147.
4. Pagani FD, Miller LW, Russell SD, et al. Extended mechanical circulatory support with a continuous-flow rotary LVAD. *J Am Coll Cardiol*. 2009;54:312–321.
5. Slaughter MS, Rogers JG, Milano CA, et al. Advanced heart failure treated with continuous-flow left ventricular assist device. *N Eng J Med*. 2009;361:2241–2251.
6. Kirklin JK, Naftel DC, Pagani FD, et al. Seventh INTERMACS annual report: 15,000 patients and counting. *J Heart Lung Transplant*. 2015;34:1495–1504.
7. Schumer EM, Black MC, Monreal G, et al. Left ventricular assist devices: current controversies and future directions. *Eur Heart J*. 2016;37:3434–3439.
8. Stretch R, Sauer CM, Bonde P. National trends in the utilization of short-term mechanical circulatory support: incidence, outcomes and cost analysis. *J Am Coll Cardiol*. 2014;64:1407–1415.
9. Baldwin JT, Adachi I, Teal J, et al. Closing in on the PumpKIN trial of the Jarvik 2015 ventricular assist device. *Semin Thorac Cardiovasc Surg: Pediatr Card Surg Annu*. 2017;20:9–15.
10. Rogers JG, Pagani FD, Tatooles AJ, et al. Intrapericardial left ventricular assist device for advanced heart failure. *N Eng J Med*. 2017;376:451–460.
11. Krabatsch T, Potapov E, Stepanenko A, et al. Biventricular circulatory support with two minaturized implantable assist devices. *Circulation*. 2011;124:S179–S186.
12. Strueber M, Schmitto JD, Kutschka I, et al. Placement of two implantable centrifugal pumps to serve as a total artificial heart after cardiectomy. *J Thorac Cardiovasc Surg*. 2012;143:507–509.
13. Maltais S, Davis ME, Haglund N. Minimally invasive and alternative approaches for long-term LVAD placement: the Vanderbilt strategy. *Ann Cardiothorac Surg*. 2014;3:563–569.
14. Schmitto JD, Mokashi SA, Cohn LH. Minimally invasive valve surgery. *J Am Coll Cardiol*. 2010;56:455–462.
15. Pagani FD. Continuous flow rotary left ventricular assist devices with "3rd generation" design. *Semin Thorac Cardiovasc Surg*. 2008;20:255–263.
16. Moazami N, Fukamachi K, Kobayashi M, et al. Axial and centrifugal continuous flow rotary pumps: a translation from pump mechanics to clinical practice. *J Heart Lung Transplant*. 2013;32:1–11.
17. Capoccia M. Mechanical circulatory support for advanced heart failure: are we about to witness a new "gold standard"? *J Cardiovasc Dev Des*. 2016;3(35):1–22. https://doi.org/10.3390/jcdd3040035.
18. Bottrell S, Bennett M, Augustin S, et al. A comparison study of haemolysis production in three contemporary centrifugal pumps. *Perfusion*. 2014;29(5):411–416.
19. Hosseinipour M, Gupta R, Bonnell M, Elahinia M. Rotary mechanical circulatory support systems. *J Rehab Ass Technol Eng*. 2017;4:1–24.
20. Sundareswaran KS, Reichenbach SH, Masterson KB, Butler KC, Farrar DJ. Low bearing wear in explanted HeartMate II left ventricular assist devices after chronic clinical support. *ASAIO J*. 2013;59:41–45.
21. Starling RC, Moazami N, Silvestry SC, et al. Unexpected abrupt increase in left ventricular assist device thrombosis. *N Eng J Med*. 2014;370:33–40.
22. LaRose JA, Tamez D, Ashenuga M, Reyes C. Design concepts and principle of operation of the HeartWare ventricular assist system. *ASAIO J*. 2010;56:285–289.
23. Mahr C, Chivukula VK, McGah P, et al. Intermittent aortic valve opening and risk of thrombosis in VAD patients. *ASAIO Journal*. 2017;63(4):425–432.
24. Salamonsen RF, Mason DG, Ayre PJ. Response of rotary blood pumps to changes in preload and afterload at a fixed speed setting are unphysiological when compared with the natural heart. *Artif Organs*. 2011;35:E47–E53.
25. Salamonsen RF, Pellegrino V, Fraser JF, et al. Exercise studies in patients with rotary blood pumps: cause, effects, and implications for starling-like control of changes in pump flow. *Artif Organs*. 2013;37:695–703.
26. Saeed O, Jermyn R, Kargoli F, et al. Blood pressure and adverse events during continuous flow left ventricular assist device support. *Circ Heart Fail*. 2015;8:551–556.

27. Ising MS, Sobieski MA, Slaughter MS, Koenig SC, Giridharan GA. Feasibility of pump speed modulation for restoring vascular pulsatility with rotary blood pumps. *ASAIO J.* 2015;61:526–532.
28. Tchantchaleishvili V, Luc JGY, Cohan CM, et al. Clinical implications of physiologic flow adjustment in continuous-flow left ventricular assist devices. *ASAIO J.* 2017;63:240–250.
29. Bertram CD. Measurement for implantable rotary blood pumps. *Physiol Meas.* 2005;26(4):R99–117.
30. Pektok E, Demirozu ZT, Arat N, et al. Remote monitoring of left ventricular assist device parameters after HeartAssist-5 implantation. *Artif Organs.* 2013;37(9):820–825.
31. Bullister E, Reich S, D'Entremont P, Silverman N, Sluetz J. A blood pressure sensor for long-term implantation. *Artif Organs.* 2001;25(5):376–379.
32. Zhou M-D, Yang C, Liu Z, Cysyk JP, Zheng S-Y. An implantable Fabry-Pérot pressure sensor fabricated on left ventricular assist device for heart failure. *Biomed Microdevices.* 2012;14(1):235–245.
33. Mehra M, Goldstein DJ, Uriel N, et al. Two-year outcomes with a magnetically levitated cardiac pump in heart failure. *N Eng J Med.* March 11, 2018. https://doi.org/10.1056/NEJMoa1800866.
34. Mehra MR, Naka Y, Uriel N, et al. A fully magnetically levitated circulatory pump for advanced heart failure. *N Eng J Med.* 2017;376:440–450.

8

Hemocompatibility in Mechanical Circulatory Support

Jeff Larose, Daniel Timms

KEY POINTS

Introduction
Biological Factors
Hemocompatibility-Related Engineering Aspects

INTRODUCTION

Understanding the hemocompatibility of mechanical circulatory support (MCS) devices requires insight into two scientific disciplines: biology and physics/engineering.

Biology related to MCS is only partially understood and at times seems unpredictable. Mother Nature is responsible for unleashing a variety of random and often chaotic situations in life, many of which are not well understood. Tissue and cells are living organisms that follow rules that are often beyond conventional wisdom.

Physics and engineering, however, are predictable. Laws of motion, for example, are repeatable and allow a degree of confidence in the output for a given input. This relationship is a powerful tool for engineers to design and accomplish monumental feats, often at the behest of Mother Nature. However, when combining these two disciplines to develop MCS devices, Mother Nature has the upper hand. The diversity of a patient population creates a conundrum when attempting to develop a single MCS device to serve them. The goal posts change from patient to patient and even change with time in the same patient.

Despite these challenges, significant advancements have been made with MCS development, on the back of an increased understanding of the biological factors that influence device hemocompatibility, as well as improvements in engineering designs and techniques available to combat the deleterious effects of poor blood handling.

This chapter discusses the biological factors that influence MCS hemocompatibility and physics/engineering techniques available to design and operate devices for short and long periods of time in this complex environment created by Mother Nature.

BIOLOGICAL FACTORS

The biological factors involved in MCS hemocompatibility are generally those provoked due to the nonphysiologic interaction between the device and the blood. The blood-to-device interaction opposes the most basic premises of the mammalian inflammation and coagulation cascade, a complex innate response designed to maintain stasis. Both intrinsic and extrinsic coagulation pathways are triggered as a response to mechanical loading on the blood and dynamic vascular endothelium. Interestingly, there are many different devices, grafts, and stents that are chronically instrumented yet do not have the same dramatic complications seen with long-term MCS.

In the native cardiovascular system, blood is exposed to shear stresses within a narrowly defined range as it circulates the body. However, when an MCS device assumes the blood pumping function of the heart, shear stresses in certain locations within the device may fall outside this range. This may be due to impeller blades producing nonphysiologic velocity profiles, small clearances between moving and stationary parts, or possibly inadequate surface washing of all regions inside the device. The MCS/cardiovascular system interface can also produce alterations in natural flow patterns within the ventricle and arteries. Some of these deviations from physiological conditions may be tolerated if the exposure time is below a threshold. Additionally, if the temperature of this material is elevated due to rubbing contact or heat dissipation of the device power components, further cellular damage may also occur. If blood is exposed to elevated shear stresses or heat for a certain period, cell lysis, platelet activation, and protein destruction may occur. In contrast, if shear stresses are too low and exposure time is too long, or inadequate washing of recirculation zones or vortices is achieved, localized coagulation of blood may result.

These effects may produce or lead to adverse events in patients receiving MCS therapy such as hemolysis, thrombosis (leading to stroke), and excessive bleeding. Along with infection, the conditions are considered important barriers to the widespread use of MCS therapy, since they increase the requirement for rehospitalization and increase therapy cost.

Hemolysis

Hemolysis relates to the destruction of red blood cells and release of hemoglobin into the plasma. This causes a drop in hematocrit levels leading to complications like those experienced with anemia, such as a reduction in the efficient transport of oxygen to cells, and may lead to a hypercoagulable state or a decrease in kidney function.[1] The reticuloendothelial system, however, works to clear damaged erythrocytes, mostly in the spleen. While blood transfusions can assist in replenishing blood cell levels, ultimately, the device is not considered acceptable for long-term use if levels of red cell destruction approach or exceed levels that the body can replenish.

The measure of hemolysis is in milligrams per deciliter of hemoglobin concentrated in plasma. Normal levels are below 2 mg/dL.[2] Serum concentrations of hemoglobin levels exceeding 20 mg/dL are considered significantly elevated.[3] Higher levels of 21 ± 15 mg/dL are tolerated by some patients,[4] while levels greater than 40 mg/dL constitute a hemolytic event.[5] Additionally, damaged red cells release lactate dehydrogenase (LDH), for which elevated levels are considered a marker for hemolysis.

However, while these levels of cell destruction may not lead to immediate clinical issues, any level of elevated hemolysis may unmask other conditions, such as increases in platelet activation and consequences from microparticle (MP) generation.[3,4]

Thrombosis

A major complicating factor for MCS device use is the development of thrombosis. Clots form in areas of stagnation and on foreign bodies or rough surfaces. Thrombosis is tolerable if small and contained but can manifest in adverse events if clots grow large enough to impede blood flow or the moving structures in the device. This situation can lead to a catastrophic adverse event, requiring attempts to pharmacologically lyse the clot or ultimately pump exchange. Additionally, strokes or infarcts in end organs may result if they break free and form emboli, which lodge in the brain or end organs, impeding blood supply.

Through the extrinsic pathway, tissue factors form active complexes with Factor VIIa, triggering Factor IX and X to convert prothrombin to thrombin. Thrombin not only exacerbates platelet activation but also speeds up the conversion of fibrinogen to strands of fibrin. Additionally, the intrinsic pathway promotes further fibrin formation via contact proteins, particularly high-molecular-weight kininogen. Fibrin strands capture erythrocytes into the platelet mass, inducing thrombus formation.[6]

The mechanism for thrombus formation is explained by Virchow's Triad. Essentially, the competing influences of high and low shear create a delicate environment for which shear levels must be maintained within a narrow range to avoid the creation of clots. Too high shear and white clots may form. These are predominantly composed of platelets and their formation is influenced by antiplatelet therapy. Too low shear and red clots may form due to recirculation and stasis. These are predominantly fibrin and their formation can be influenced by anticoagulant therapy.

The ability to control the clotting of blood is a feature of human circulation. The endothelial cells of arteries and veins secrete a variety of chemical substances, including thrombomodulin and heparin-like proteoglycans, that inhibit blood clotting on their walls.[7] Artificial materials used in MCS devices do not have this ability; therefore, the blood may clot when presented with a foreign surface. The HeartMate ventricular assist device (VAD) series employs a textured surface to promote the growth of a protein layer on the blood-contacting surfaces.[8] This technique aims to reduce levels of thrombosis formation and cell damage by attempting to recreate the arterial lining.

High Shear

Shear stress encountered by blood in transit through the pump system can affect both cells and large proteins in the plasma. Thrombosis at high shear rates depends primarily on activated platelets and the adhesion protein von Willebrand factor (vWF) and fibrinogen, with hemodynamics playing an important role in each stage of thrombus formation, including vWF binding, platelet adhesion, platelet activation, and rapid thrombus growth.[9]

Platelets have been long regarded as the prominent cells involved in physiologic hemostasis and pathologic thrombosis. The shear-induced platelet activation generally elevated with increasing shear stress magnitude and exposure time.[10] The areas of recirculation in a pump may trap platelets, increasing their exposure time to the artificial surface while also increasing the local concentrations of the procoagulant proteins adenosine diphosphate and thromboxane A2, continuing the self-perpetuating platelet aggregation. Also, high-shear regions in a pump may become problematic as passing platelets are transiently activated by the shear and deposit on pump seams and bearings that under low-shear flow may have been free from thrombus.

When blood experiences high shear stresses in VADs, the plasma protein vWF extends from a globular form to an elongated form and can theoretically form intertwining nets to form many bonds to platelets, capturing thousands of circulating platelets. The formation of vWF nets under high-shear conditions increases the contact area between platelets and vWF, like a catcher's mitt. The capture of circulating platelets at high shear is primarily due to the exposure of A1 binding sites on vWF nets to rapidly capture the circulating platelet glycoprotein 1b (Gp 1b). The positive feedback cycle of platelet activation, release of more vWF into vWF nets, and capture of new circulating platelets result in the explosive growth of high-shear, platelet-rich thrombus.[9]

Other than platelets and vWF, MCS devices expose blood cells to high shear stress, potentially resulting in the production of cell-derived MPs, which promote coagulation and inflammation.[11] MPs are small cell vesicles that can be released by a variety of cell types during cell activation and apoptosis, and they possess inflammatory and procoagulatory characteristics. Circulating levels of MPs from platelets, leukocytes, and endothelial cells are significantly higher in patients with left VADs (LVADs) than in healthy controls.[12] Tissue factor that rises during MCS may originate from platelet MPs, which contribute to the occurrence of thromboembolic complications, as described earlier.

Coagulation/Low Shear

Exposure of blood to implanted or temporary devices is known to be associated with coagulopathies, which historically have been managed with the administration of anticoagulants. The biological response with implanted devices is biphasic in nature. An acute fibrinolytic response preoperatively produces a high risk of bleeding. Secondary response ensures a procoagulant environment, exposing the recipient to risk of thrombus formation. This can cause catastrophic complications, including device thrombosis and stroke. MCS devices activate the coagulation system through blood contact with foreign surfaces and altered rheological conditions (blood flow or stasis in native heart).

Anticoagulants provide the pivotal therapy to avoid thrombosis formation. Anticoagulation regimes differ between institutions but typically include the use of antiplatelet therapy, vitamin K antagonists with an international normalized ratio (INR) can remain deranged for target anywhere from 1.5 to 3, with or without heparin bridging postoperatively. The coagulation system can remain deranged for up to 90 days and endothelial responses up to 180 days postimplantation. Health status, including active infection, can complicate drug effectiveness. Patient compliance can influence the levels of protection. Furthermore, patient diet (such as the ingestion of leafy greens high in vitamin K) can also lower the effectiveness of anticoagulation therapies.[1]

Gastrointestinal (GI) bleeding is a well-documented complication of MCS that can be exacerbated with anticoagulation therapy and whose etiology is complex. Another bleeding risk associated with mechanical devices is shear stress-induced acquired vWF disease. Destruction or alteration in the composition of the vWF molecule may inhibit its ability to take part in the coagulation process, leading to prolonged bleeding episodes. Emerging evidence shows that GI bleeding may in part be caused by angiogenesis induced through the neural hormone angiotensin II pathway and associated growth factors. The causative arteriovenous malformations may be reduced with antagonism of the angiotensin II pathway with angiotensin receptor blocker or angiotensin converting enzyme inhibitor therapy, which are commonly used antihypertensives.[13]

Considerable interpatient variability in anticoagulation substrate complicates management.[14] For example, blood type variability leads to variations in vWF factor levels, with lower levels in patients with O blood type.[15]

The thrombogenic environment initiated by MCS also increases the risk of venous thrombosis in an already at-risk patient cohort.[16] Comorbid conditions that promote venous stasis and thrombosis include heart failure and/or myocardial infarction, peripheral venous congestion and stasis, and decreased mobility due to poor exercise tolerance or prolonged hospital stay, increasing age, and infection. Optimal device performance can effectively reduce venous congestion in the absence of advanced right heart failure.

HEMOCOMPATIBILITY-RELATED ENGINEERING ASPECTS

MCS for left side support drains blood upstream of the aortic valve and discharges the blood downstream of the aortic valve. Right side circulatory support drains blood upstream of the pulmonary valve and discharges the blood downstream of the pulmonary valve. Draining blood from a reservoir requires careful inflow cannula placement to ensure sufficient patient support, minimize thrombosis potential in the reservoir due to the new flow patterns, and minimize cellular damage in the instance of reduced flow area due to the close proximity of the inflow cannula and any surrounding biologic structure. This can be further complicated as cardiac remodeling and/or unloading the reservoir can change the inflow cannula position relative to the surrounding structures. Thrombosis in the inflow cannula can cause reduced effective flow area into the device, leading to reduced flow capacity and possible embolization. The net effect can create nonphysiologic flow patterns and fluid stresses and associated thrombosis and cellular damage potentials.

Pump Configurations

Rotary pump technology has been incorporated commercially into implanted MCS devices since the mid-2000s. The delay in successful uptake often relates to the development of technology to minimize thrombosis and cellular damage. MCS requires a pumping mechanism, an electrical motor mechanism, a drive system connecting the pump to the motor, and an impeller suspension system to minimize or eliminate contact between the rotating pump impeller and the stationary housing.

There are three main types of rotary pumps that have been utilized in implanted MCS devices: axial flow, centrifugal flow, and mixed flow pumps. The first commercially viable rotary MCS device was the axial flow Thoratec HeartMate II long-term device.[17] First-generation axial flow devices utilized mechanical bearings with upstream and downstream support structures to hold the rotating impeller. The upstream support member is utilized as a flow straightener, and the downstream support structure, as a vanned diffuser. The diffuser efficiently converts the swirling flow, kinetic energy, downstream of the impeller into differential pressure. The first commercially viable and Food and Drug Administration–approved centrifugal long-term MCS device was the HeartWare HVAD.[18] This device utilized passive magnetic forces and hydrodynamic bearings to support the rotating impeller in a contactless manner. This device utilizes a traditional vaneless diffuser called a volute to collect the high-velocity blood from the impeller and efficiently direct it to the outflow cannula. The first commercially viable mixed-flow MCS device was the acute, percutaneous Abiomed Impella device.[19] This device utilizes a solid shaft and sealed bearing system, which is externally purged with saline, connecting the motor and the rotating impeller. The intended use requires that the outer diameter is minimized to facilitate percutaneous deployment, and since sufficient performance exists, an additional diffuser was not needed.

Pump Curves

The main performance curves for a rotary pump are called a Head-Flow or "H-Q" curves. The hemodynamic consequences of pump design are covered in Chapter 7. The characteristics of pump flow that are particularly relevant to pump thrombosis are discussed here.

Every pump rotational speed curve contains a singular differential pressure that will yield zero net flow through the device, also known as shut-off condition (Fig. 8.1). If the differential pressure is higher than the shut-off condition, which may occur if the rotational speed of the device is set low and the heart contractility is high, then the net flow rate becomes retrograde. Centrifugal pumps are more susceptible to retrograde flow than axial flow pumps, with the inflection in slope typically being in the retrograde region. Typically, the slope inflection for axial flow pumps is in the forward flow portion of the curve.

The average blood residence time can be calculated with the H-Q curves by dividing the pump priming volume by the flow rate through the device. An example centrifugal pump average residence time curve is shown in Fig. 8.2. The residence time increases exponentially as the flow rate approaches zero, thereby increasing the probability for cellular damage and thrombosis. Inefficiencies in the hydraulic design may have a portion of the flow rate, with residence times significantly longer than average. This needs to be minimized as much as possible. Note that several cardiac cycles are required to clear the pump and outflow graft, indicating that careful attention to thrombosis prevention is not limited to just the pump. Avoiding shut-off differential pressure and full or partial occlusion of either the inflow or outflow is important in maintaining reasonably short residence times and minimizing the risk for thrombus generation.

The primary design goals for the prevention of thrombosis are to ensure "sufficient" wall shear stress or "washing," to reduce the time that blood may react with the surface, and to eliminate or periodically relocate flow eddies. The angle between the impeller blade leading edge and the incoming flow must be reasonably small to ensure sufficient washing of the impeller surface and the surrounding casing. The notion of "sufficient" wall shear stress generally means that regions with higher wall shear stress may be more tolerant to rougher surfaces and geometric discontinuities. Flow eddies increase the amount of time blood constituents remain within the device, thereby increasing the probability of thrombosis and potentially increasing the time at nonphysiologic stresses. Macroaspects such as impeller blade, casing, and cannula design; microaspects such as surface finish and device part discontinuities; and blood-to-surface compatibility are particularly important design considerations. Machine marks, scratches, and other surface blemishes can become the nidus for thrombus formation. Surface finish requirements are required for all blood contacting surfaces.[20]

Surface Preparation/Roughness

Early input from manufacturing experts is important to ensure that the final product can be mass produced at a reasonable cost. To avoid compromised clinical performance, teamwork to coordinate where and how components are joined is critical and best decided early. This is

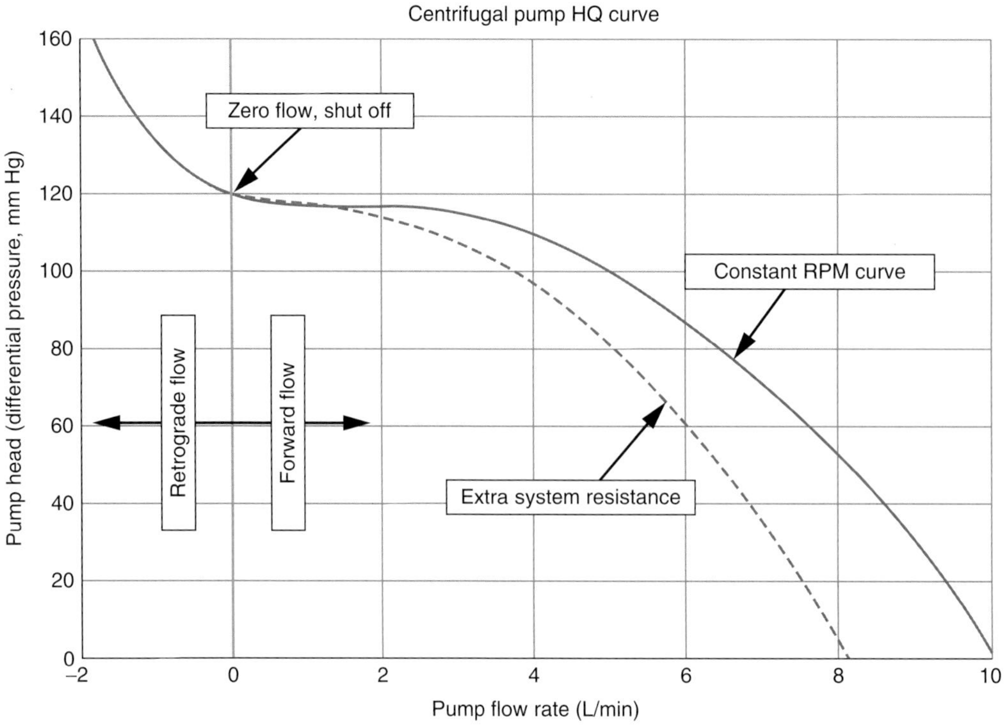

Fig. 8.1 Example centrifugal HQ curve. *HQ*, Head-flow; *RPM*, revolutions per minute.

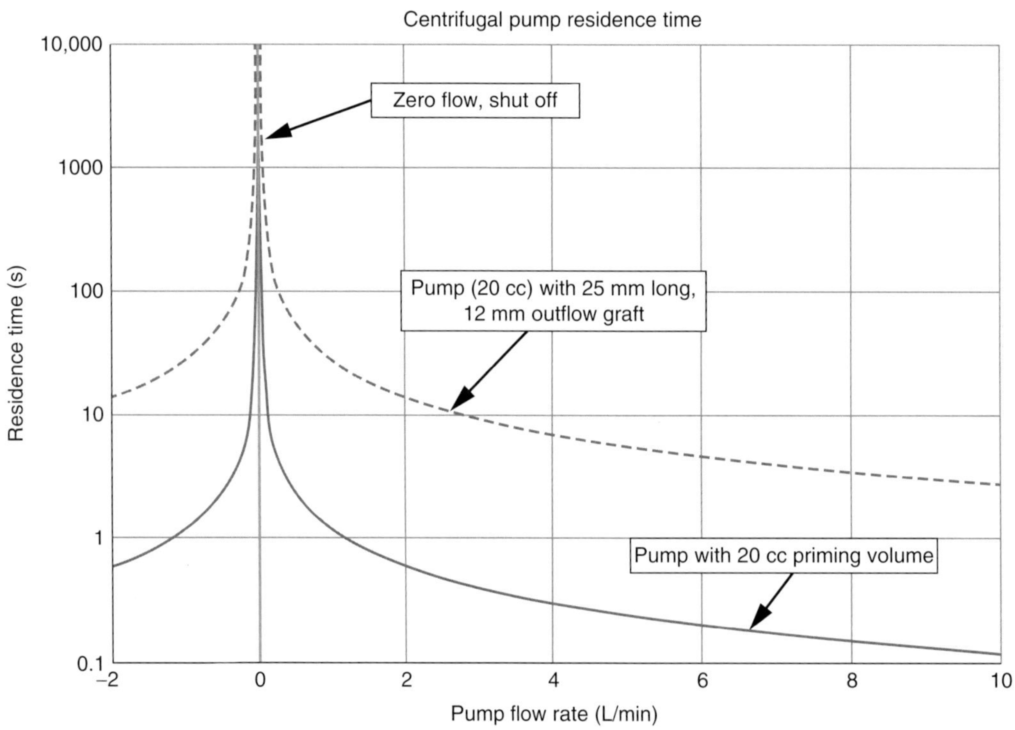

Fig. 8.2 Centrifugal pump residence time.

particularly important in setting average and maximum allowable surface roughness specifications and allowable component interface mismatch, as standards do not yet exist. There can be limitations with metrology capabilities as well, so understanding what is truly required is important prior to finalizing the product specifications. Allowable impeller mass imbalance and correction methods for adding/removing mass and in the process and any final functional testing need to be discussed with the manufacturing team.

Flow Analysis (Device/Ventricle)

Design tools for the prevention of thrombosis include, in order of increasing cost, computational fluid dynamics (CFD), particle image velocimetry (PIV), acute and chronic in vivo studies, and device initial clinical trials. CFD analysis tools and methods simulate the flow field within a device and within the circulatory system. The analyses are commonly either steady-state or "instant-in-time" analysis such as "stage" averaging methods or "frozen rotor" analysis. These methods provide useful design information, but micro fluid structures are more qualitative than quantitative. PIV studies can be either steady state or transient and may account for microaspects such as surface finish and device part discontinuities. In vivo studies are the initial biological environments that are much closer to actual human testing than CFD and PIV studies are. Human clinical trial testing is usually more confirmative than learning, but that is not always the case. There is still much to learn about patient-device interaction and adverse events such as thrombotic complications and the associated proper design and clinical management mitigations. This is further complicated by the variability in patient anatomies, comorbidities, and medical history.

Specific thrombosis considerations exist for each pump type. Axial-flow and mixed-flow pumps with mechanical bearings have the design challenge of getting "sufficient" wall shear stress near the contact bearing(s) due to centrifugal forces pushing the blood radially away from the bearing. If flow structures are required to support the bearings, then the challenges to reduce potential for thrombosis becomes harder due to the increased surface area. Centrifugal pumps have the complication of at least one additional flow path that needs to have "sufficient" wall shear stress. The additional flow path is on the impeller surface opposite the impeller blade defining primary flow path, that is, typically the bottom surface. This secondary flow path requires careful attention for "sufficient" surface washing throughout the operating range, as this flow rate is dependent upon the pressure difference between the impeller blade trailing edge and the leading edge. Additionally, all three pump types are subjected to ingested particles that can be captured within the device and increase the probability of thrombosis and embolization. Particle ingestion is more of a long-term MCS design consideration involving the interaction of the inflow cannula and the surface washing within the reservoir being drained.

Two other engineering aspects may adversely impact surface washing and thrombus potential. The first is impeller vibration due to mass imbalance, which can locally reduce fresh blood flow, thereby increasing the local residence times. The second is heat generation from the motor and/or impeller bearing system, which may adversely impact blood cells and cause proteins in the blood to denature. Proteins are sensitive to their environmental conditions; however, blood parameters do not appear to alter significantly when exposed to surface temperatures up to 45°C.[21] Blood through the pump is used as a coolant, so flow rates near shut-off must be avoided.

Material Science

Sometimes, a surface coating or treatment is used to improve hemocompatibility or protect the integrity of surface finish. One surface coating used in medical devices is the thromboresistant heparin codding, with product name Carmeda BioActive Surface by Gore (www.carmeda.se). Polished titanium is very soft and can be scratched easily, potentially lowering the threshold for a thrombosis event. The impeller in a wearless suspension system contacts the stationary housing when the device is unpowered. Protective coatings that have been used clinically include titanium nitride[18] or diamond-like carbon.[22]

Inflow/Outflow Cannula

Long-term MCS inflow cannulas have multiple layers of metal spheres metallurgically sintered to the cannula[23] to create a matrix structure that promotes ingrowth at the insertion site. This is utilized to reduce embolization potential caused by loose adjacent tissue. Besides sintering, there are two other design methods used to reduce the inflow cannula thrombosis potential. The first is the use of an impeller rotational speed modulation algorithm to momentarily increase biologic surface and inflow cannula surface washing.[18] The second is the ongoing development of an adjustable position sewing ring to fine tune each implant,[24] given the variability of patient anatomy.

The inflow cannula tip shape and diameter also impact the device susceptibility to inflow suction and occlusion events. These events can result in zero net flow, dramatically increasing the blood contact residence time, and must be avoided to minimize thrombotic potential. Larger-diameter inflows have smaller inflow velocities and may be less prone to suction. Contouring the inflow tip may increase the effective inflow surface area, thus reducing susceptibility to suction.[25] The fluid velocity exiting the inflow cannula and entering the impeller affects the angle at which blood enters the impeller blade leading edge. This forces a design tradeoff decision linking the impeller blade design and the inflow cannula inner diameter to minimize thrombosis potential. Software that detects the loss of flow to the MCS device due to inflow occlusion is also utilized[24] to avoid abnormally long residence times.

A similar design decision is related to the outflow cannula. The system performance is linked to the impeller blade design interaction with the diffuser and outflow cannula. Long-term implantable MCS devices use cardiovascular outflow grafts. This facilities tailoring the implant for the range of patient anatomies but results in variability of system losses and impacts the effective HQ capacity curves. Design margin on thrombosis protection is required to ensure adequate clinical performance for the inevitable off-label cases the medical community will encounter. Outflow graft kinking, even temporarily, can result in periods of zero net flow with the associated long residence times and high thrombosis potential.

Shear Stress

The primary design feature for the prevention of cellular damage is hydraulic design to minimize the fluid stress generated by the device while minimizing the duration of exposure to shear stress above the normal physiologic range. High-fluid-stress regions within a pump typically include an impeller and diffuser (if used) blade leading and trailing edges and blade tip clearance adjacent to stationary casing. These clearances typically range from 0.03 to 3 mm and should be optimized to produce the lowest levels of hemolysis while maintaining the highest possible hydraulic efficiency. The rotational speed of the impeller directly affects the level of shear stress encountered in the clearance gaps. A larger peripheral velocity results in larger shear stresses; therefore, the rotational speed of the impeller should be optimized through efficient hydraulic design.[26]

While it is generally considered that hemolysis will increase with a decreasing clearance below 0.5 mm, further reductions in clearance gaps below 0.1 mm may improve hemolysis levels. The majority of red blood cells are thought to avoid entering the gap, and when combined with a smaller fluidic volume and shorter residence time, fewer cells are damaged.[27–29]

Typically, cellular damage is greater at very low and very high flow rates, forcing numerous design iterations to ensure acceptable performance at all operating conditions. A Helium's fluid stress versus time analysis[30] is useful to evaluate design alternatives, as well as hemolysis index[30] and damage index[31] based upon CFD simulated fluid flow fields. Red blood cell damage may be more likely with short-duration high fluid stresses, whereas longer duration of lower fluid stresses promotes platelet activation. The calculation of fluid stress history based upon the numerous flow streamline paths through the device allows an aggregate "damage index" to be calculated, facilitating comparison of design configurations and operating conditions.

A threshold value of shear stress has been identified at 1500 dyne/cm^2 (150 Pa) for the start of red blood cell lysis, while the majority of red blood cell hemolysis occurs at shear stress values exceeding 3000 dyne/cm^2 (300 Pa). No appreciable damage is detected when exposure levels are limited to 1000 dyne/cm^2 (100 Pa).[32] However, exposure time is also critically important to determine the likelihood of red cell disruption. A threshold exists for elevated hemolysis above 425 Pa and 620 ms,[33] while shear stress levels of 842 Pa are tolerable at shorter exposure times of 54 ms.[34]

Current continuous-flow (CF) devices can elevate cellular damage as measured by LDH for hemolysis, D-dimer for platelet activation, and vWF for bleeding potential.[35] Fortunately, determination of the cellular damage profile of a device does not require a clinical trial. There are many established hematology in vitro tests for cell lysis, platelet activation and concentration, MP generation, and Western blot electrophoresis. A test plan may require multiple donors for increased sample size to adequately represent general clinical performance. These tests are very useful when used with a reference device that has known clinical performance.

Cavitation is another physical process associated with cellular damage,[36] particularly near the impeller inlet, where the lowest blood pressures exist. Use of CFD to develop hydraulically efficient pumps for use at physiologic pressures avoids this condition. The pressure drop with long inflow cannulas typically used in acute use systems can reduce the safety margin to cavitation.

These device-specific performance characteristics, thrombosis-resistant wall shear stress profiles, and cellular damage characteristics result in significant variability during the cardiac cycle and during acute patient hemodynamic changes. These important parameter variations usually change the traditional design philosophy from a "best variable point" to a "best variable operating range" strategy.

Speed Modulation

CF pumps have offered several advantages over pulsatile-flow (PF) pumps, including improved durability, less surgical trauma, greater reliability, and higher energy efficiency. These benefits translate into better survival, improved quality of life, and higher functional capacity of patients. However, concerns remain about the diminished arterial pressure and decreased flow pulsatility delivered by CF pumps. Mounting evidence shows unanticipated consequences of CF support, such as GI bleeding, arteriovenous malformations, pump thrombosis, aortic valve insufficiency, valve fusion, and acquired von Willebrand syndrome.[37–44] Different approaches have been proposed and used to produce a cyclic controlled speed change function or a pulsatility control algorithm in CF pumps during long-term support.[37,42] Various speed profiles, including the use of a trapezoidal, rectangular, or sinusoidal profile and a synchronous flow modulation strategy with an adaptive physiological controller, have been employed to generate pulsatility.[43–48]

A cyclic controlled speed change function (Lavare Cycle) incorporated in HVAD allows for changes in left ventricular filling and flow rate through the LVAD once per minute during a 3-second cycle.[18] The changes in ventricular volume and pump flow during the cyclic controlled speed change are intended to decrease potential areas of blood stasis. Another approach was incorporating with an intermittent low speed (ILS) controller in the Jarvik 2000. Operating an axial flow pump at ILS allows the aortic valve to open and the aortic root to be washed out even in states of low cardiac output and under CF conditions, thus preventing valvular thrombosis, fusion, or both.[49] An induced PF was created in HMIII by rapidly changing the pump operation from low to high speeds.[50] Latest clinical trials showed that no pump thrombosis occurred in patients with a fully magnetically levitated CF HeartMate 3 left ventricular assist system (St. Jude Medical Inc., St. Paul, MN), which is programmed to facilitate rapid changes in rotor speed to create an intrinsic artificial pulse.[51,52] However, bleeding including hemorrhagic strokes persisted in these studies. It is still unknown how much pulsatility is needed to normalize vascular responses and avoid pump-related bleeding. There are ongoing efforts to create an artificial pulse while preserving the advantages of the smaller continuous flow ventricular assist devices (CFVADs). The ultimate solution may be a return to recreating our natural physiology.

CONCLUSIONS

The industry has made great strides in understanding MCS device hemocompatibility and translating those findings into guiding engineering principles. Future prospective clinical trials that record system operating parameters, including measured and derived device flow rate, heart rate, and hopefully ventricular and arterial pressures, will expand the knowledge base on conditions prone to adverse events. Then, new engineering practices and clinical management practices can facilitate early intervention and reduce hemocompatibility-related adverse events.

REFERENCES

1. Tromp TR, de Jonge N, Joles JA. Left ventricular assist devices: a kidney's perspective. *Heart Fail Rev*. 2015;20(4):519–532.
2. Kazmierczak SC. *Hemolysis, Lipemia, and High Bilirubin: Effect on Laboratory Tests. Accurate Results in the Clinical Laboratory*. San Diego: Elsevier; 2013 [chapter 5:53–62].
3. Baskin L, Dias V, Chin A, Abdullah A, Naugler C. *Effect of Patient Preparation, Specimen Collection, Anticoagulants, and Preservatives on Laboratory Test Results. Accurate Results in the Clinical Laboratory*. San Diego: Elsevier; 2013 [chapter 3:19–34].
4. Mankad AK, Tang DG, Clark WB, Flattery M, Harton S, Katlaps GJ, et al. Persistent anemia after implantation of the total artificial heart. *J Card Fail*. 2012;18(6):433–438.
5. Katz JN, Jensen BC, Chang PP, Myers SL, Pagani FD, Kirklin JK. A multicenter analysis of clinical hemolysis in patients supported with durable, long-term left ventricular assist device therapy. *J Heart Lung Transplant*. 2015;34(5):701–709.
6. de Biasi AR, Manning KB, Salemi A. Science for surgeons: understanding pump thrombogenesis in continuous-flow left ventricular assist devices. *J Thorac Cardiovasc Surg*. 2015;149(3):667–673.
7. Yau JW, Teoh H, Verma S. Endothelial cell control of thrombosis. *BMC Cardiovasc Disord*. 2015;15(1):130.
8. Maher TR, Butler KC, Poirier VL, Gernes DB. HeartMate left ventricular assist devices: a multigeneration of implanted blood pumps. *Artif Organs*. 2001;25(5):422–426.
9. Casa LDC, Ku DN. Thrombus formation at high shear rates. *Annu Rev Biomed Eng*. 2017;19(1):415–433.
10. Ding J, Chen Z, Niu S, Zhang J, Mondal NK, Griffith BP, et al. Quantification shear-induced platelet activation: high shear stresses for short exposure time. *Artif Organs*. 2015;39(7):576–583.
11. Nascimbene A, Hernandez R, George JK, Parker A, Bergeron AL, Pradhan S, et al. Association between cell-derived microparticles and adverse events in patients with nonpulsatile left ventricular assist devices. *J Heart Lung Transplant*. 2014;33(5):470–477.
12. Diehl P, Aleker M, Helbing T, Sossong V, Beyersdorf F, Olschewski M, et al. Enhanced microparticles in ventricular assist device patients predict platelet, leukocyte and endothelial cell activation. *Interact Cardiovasc Thorac Surg*. 2010;11(2):133–137.
13. Houston BA, Schneider ALC, Vaishnav J, Cromwell DM, Miller PE, Faridi KF, et al. Angiotensin II antagonism is associated with reduced risk for gastrointestinal bleeding caused by arteriovenous malformations in patients with left ventricular assist devices. *J Heart Lung Transplant*. 2017;36(4):380–385.

14. Blitz A. Pump thrombosis—a riddle wrapped in a mystery inside an enigma. *Ann Cardiothorac Surg*. 2014;3(5):450–471.
15. Gastineau DA, Moore SB. How important are ABO-related variations in coagulation factor levels? *Transfusion*. 2001;41(1):4–5.
16. Office of the Surgeon General (US); National Heart, Lung, and Blood Institute (US). The Surgeon General's call to action to prevent deep vein thrombosis and pulmonary embolism. In: *SECTION I: Deep Vein Thrombosis and Pulmonary Embolism as Major Public Health Problems*. 2008.
17. Burke D, Burke E, Parsaie V, Butler K, Thomas D, Taylor L, et al. The Heartmate II: design and development of a fully sealed axial flow left ventricular assist system. *Artif Organs*. 2001;25(5):380–385.
18. LaRose JA, Tamez D, Ashenuga M, Reyes C. Design concepts and principle of operation of the HeartWare ventricular assist system. *ASAIO J*. 2010;56(4):285–289.
19. Weber DM, Raess DH, Henriques JPS, Siess T. *Principles of Impella Cardiac Support. SUPPLEMENT TO CARDIAC INTERVENTIONS TODAY*; 2009.
20. Linneweber J, Dohmen PM, Kerzscher U, Affeld K, Nose Y, Konertz W. The effect of surface roughness on activation of the coagulation system and platelet adhesion in rotary blood pumps. *Artif Organs*. 2007;31(5):345–351.
21. Hamilton KF, Schmidt VI, Mager I, Schmitz-Rode T, Steinseifer U. Consequences arising from elevated surface temperatures on human blood. *Artif Organs*. 2010;34(9):783–787.
22. Esmore D, Spratt P, Larbalestier R, et al. VentrAssist™ left ventricular assist device: clinical trial results and Clinical Development Plan update. *Eur J Cardiothorac Surg*. 2007;32(5):735–744.
23. Sin DC, Kei HL, Miao X. Surface coatings for ventricular assist devices. *Expert Rev Med Devices* 2009;6(1):51–60.
24. Cheung A, Chorpenning K, Tamez D, et al. Design concepts and preclinical results of a miniaturized HeartWare platform: the MVAD system. *Innovations (Phila)*. 2015:10(3):151–156.
25. Schmid C, Jurmann M, Birnbaum D, et al. Influence of inflow cannula length in axial-flow pumps on neurologic adverse event rate: results from a multi-center analysis. *J Heart Lung Transplant*. 2008;27(3):253–260.
26. Nishida M, Asztalos B, Yamane T, et al. Flow visualization study to improve hemocompatibility of a centrifugal blood pump. *Artif Organs*. 1999;23(8):697–703.
27. James NL, Wilkinson CM, Lingard NL, Van der Meer AL, Woodard JC. Evaluation of hemolysis in the VentrAssist implantable rotary blood pump. *Artif Organs*. 2003;27(1):108–113.
28. Kim NJ, Diao C, Ahn KH, Lee SJ, Kameneva MV, Antaki JF. Parametric study of blade tip clearance, flow rate, and impeller speed on blood damage in rotary blood pump. *Artif Organs*. 2009;33(6):468–474.
29. Leslie LJ, Marshall LJ, Devitt A, Hilton A, Tansley GD. Cell exclusion in Couette flow: evaluation through flow visualization and mechanical forces. *Artif Organs*. 2013;37(3):267–275.
30. Fraser KH, Zhang T, Taskin ME, Griffith BP, Wu ZJ. A quantitative comparison of mechanical blood damage parameters in rotary ventricular assist devices: shear stress, exposure time and hemolysis index. *J Biomech Eng*. 2012;134(8). 081002–11.
31. Fraser KH, Taskin ME, Griffith BP, Wu ZJ. The use of computational fluid dynamics in the development of ventricular assist devices. *Med Eng Phys*. 2011;33(3):263–280.
32. Nevrail. Physical effects in red blood cell trauma. *AICHE J*. 1969;15(5):707–711.
33. Paul R, Apel J, Klaus S, Schügner F, Schwindke P, Reul H. Shear stress related blood damage in laminar Couette flow. *Artif Organs*. 2003;27(6): 517–529.
34. Boehning F, Mejia T, Schmitz-Rode T, Steinseifer U. Hemolysis in a laminar flow-through Couette shearing device: an experimental study. *Artif Organs*. 2014;38(9):761–765.
35. Birschmann I, Dittrich M, Eller T, et al. Ambient hemolysis and activation of coagulation is different between HeartMate II and HeartWare left ventricular assist devices. *J Heart Lung Transplant*. 2014;33(1):80–87.
36. Sneckenberger DS, Stinebring DR, Deutsch S, Geselowitz DB, Tarbell JM. Mitral heart valve cavitation in an artificial heart environment. *J Heart Valve Dis*. 1996;5(2):216–227.
37. Cheng A, Williamitis CA, Slaughter MS. Comparison of continuous-flow and pulsatile-flow left ventricular assist devices: is there an advantage to pulsatility? *Ann Cardiothorac Surg*. 2014;3(6):573–581.
38. Crow S, John R, Boyle A, et al. Gastrointestinal bleeding rates in recipients of nonpulsatile and pulsatile left ventricular assist devices. *J Thorac Cardiovasc Surg*. 2009;137(1):208–215.
39. Heilmann C, Geisen U, Beyersdorf F, et al. Acquired von Willebrand syndrome in patients with ventricular assist device or total artificial heart. *Thromb Haemost*. 2010 22.11.2017;104(05):962-967.
40. Klovaite J, Gustafsson F, Mortensen SA, Sander K, Nielsen L. Severely impaired von Willebrand factor-dependent platelet aggregation in patients with a continuous-flow left ventricular assist device (HeartMate II). *J Am Coll Cardiol*. 2009;53(23):2162–2167.
41. Soucy KG, Koenig SC, Giridharan GA, Sobieski MA, Slaughter MS. Defining pulsatility during continuous-flow ventricular assist device support. *J Heart Lung Transplant*. 2013;32(6):581–587.
42. Barić D. Why pulsatility still matters: a review of current knowledge. *Croat Med J*. 2014;55(6):609–620.
43. Bearnson GB, Olsen DB, Khanwilkar PS, Long JW, Allaire PE, Maslen EH. Pulsatile operation of a centrifugal ventricular assist device with magnetic bearings. *ASAIO J*. 1996;42(5):M620–M624.
44. Cox LGE, Loerakker S, Rutten MC, de Mol BA, van de Vosse FN. A mathematical model to evaluate control strategies for mechanical circulatory support. *Artif Organs*. 2009;33(8):593–603.
45. Vandenberghe S, Segers P, Antaki JF, Meyns B, Verdonck PR. Hemodynamic modes of ventricular assist with a rotary blood pump: continuous, pulsatile, and failure. *ASAIO J*. 2005;51(6):711–718.
46. Gao B, Chang Y, Gu K, Zeng Y, Liu Y. A pulsatile control algorithm of continuous-flow pump for heart recovery. *ASAIO*. 2012;58(4):343–352.
47. Shiose A, Nowak K, Horvath DJ, Massiello AL, Golding LAR, Fukamachi K. Speed modulation of the continuous-flow total artificial heart to simulate a physiologic arterial pressure waveform. *ASAIO J*. 2010;56(5):403–409.
48. Kleinheyer M, Timms DL, Tansley GD, et al. Rapid speed modulation of a rotary total artificial heart impeller. *Artif Organs*. 2016;40(9):824–833.
49. Tuzun E, Gregoric ID, Conger JL, et al. The effect of intermittent low speed mode upon aortic valve opening in calves supported with a Jarvik 2000 axial flow device. *ASAIO J*. 2005;51(2):139–143.
50. Farrar DJ, Bourque K, Dague CP, Cotter CJ, Poirier VL. Design features, developmental status, and experimental results with the Heartmate III centrifugal left ventricular assist system with a magnetically levitated rotor. *ASAIO J*. 2007;53:310–315.
51. Mehra MR, Naka Y, Uriel N, et al. A fully magnetically levitated circulatory pump for advanced heart failure. *N Engl J Med*. 2017;376(5):440–450.
52. Krabatsch T, Netuka I, Schmitto JD, et al. Heartmate 3 fully magnetically levitated left ventricular assist device for the treatment of advanced heart failure–1 year results from the CE Mark trial. *J Cardiothorac Surg*. 2017;12(1):23. 2017/04/04.

9

The Biological Response to Ventricular Unloading

Stavros G. Drakos, Nir Uriel

KEY POINTS

INTRODUCTION

Heart failure (HF) is one of the major medical burdens in our society. Complete recovery of the heart after insult has been an attractive goal for many clinicians and scientists for long time. Mechanical circulatory support (MCS) devices, such as left ventricular assist devices (LVADs), effectively unload the heart by reducing the pressure overload/increased afterload, ultimately resulting in a degree of myocardial reverse remodeling. Currently, the predominantly used LVADs are continuous-flow devices, for patients suffering from end-stage HF.

The important research advantages of the VAD population are that they present us with a translational research medium through which investigations for new anti-remodeling and regenerative therapies for HF can be studied. Particularly, tissue specimens obtained from bridge to transplant (BTT) patients before LVAD implantation (referred to as "pre") and at the time of LVAD explantation (referred to as "post") provide a platform to perform molecular, structural, and functional studies. This in turn could pave the way for understanding the mechanisms behind progressive myocardial dysfunction during HF and the pathways that regulate reverse cardiac remodeling.[1]

A subset of patients who undergo LVAD-induced mechanical unloading show significant improvements in cardiac structure and function to the point where some of these patients can be weaned from the support and achieve sustained recovery (i.e., responders), while the others show no such sign of recovery (i.e., nonresponders). Comparing responders and nonresponders in several aspects such as cardiac hypertrophy regression, contractile dysfunction, metabolism, cell death, extracellular matrix remodeling, and others could be helpful in revealing signatures of myocardial recovery, which in turn could help design novel HF therapies. However, in order to unmask the mechanisms driving myocardial recovery, the fundamental biological effects on myocardial structure and function must be understood. This chapter attempts to compile the ongoing clinical, translational, and basic science research in the field of MCS and cardiovascular remodeling.

CARDIAC HYPERTROPHY-ATROPHY

Myocardial unloading with a pulsatile flow LVAD has been shown to induce regression of cardiac myocyte hypertrophy.[2–4] Animal models with prolonged unloading of nonfailing, nonhypertrophic myocardium (heterotopic transplantation,[5] LVAD,[6] or mitral regurgitation[7]) suggested that mechanical unloading could lead to cardiac myocyte atrophy. Based on these data it was postulated that this phenomenon may also apply to hypertrophic and failing myocardium.[8,9] This notion of prolonged LVAD unloading in HF patients causing regression of cardiac hypertrophy to the point of atrophy prevailed until structural, ultrastructural, microstructural, metabolic, molecular, and clinical functional data indicated that prolonged continuous-flow LVAD unloading does not induce myocardial atrophy and degeneration (Fig. 9.1).[10–15] Specifically, in two human HF studies, unloading by means of pulsatile flow LVAD support decreased cardiac myocyte size, but not to the levels below respective normal cardiac myocytes.[10,11] Furthermore, light (Fig. 9.2) and confocal (Fig. 9.3) microscopy findings complemented by ultrastructural, metabolic, and molecular data did not identify any evidence suggesting cardiac myocyte atrophy or degeneration during continuous-flow LVAD support.[11,15] These data support echocardiographic observations in LVAD patients that show regression of hypertrophy without atrophy.[12] Ongoing investigations have examined the roles of several complex regulatory pathways as critical components of these structural changes, including cyclooxygenase-2–induced Akt phosphorylation, mitogen activated protein kinase/Erk, and Akt kinase/glycogen synthase kinase 3β. Also, a recent study reported that Akt activation stimulates glucose utilization but impairs mitochondrial oxidative capacity independently of cardiac hypertrophy.[16] Whether the primary stimulus for the regression of hypertrophy is related

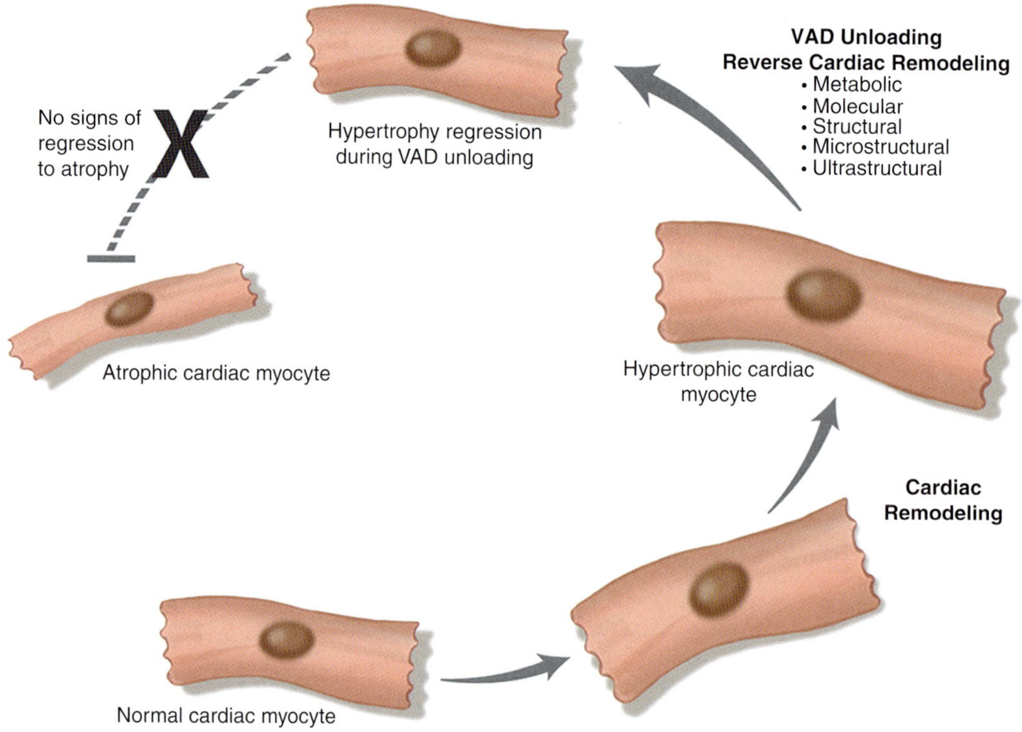

Fig. 9.1 Forward and reverse cardiac remodeling during mechanical unloading of the failing human heart induced by left ventricular assist devices *(VADs)* shows regression of cardiac hypertrophy with no signs of disuse myocardial atrophy. (From Diakos NA, et al. Myocardial atrophy and chronic mechanical unloading of the failing human heart: implications for cardiac assist device-induced myocardial recovery. *J Am Coll Cardiol.* 2014;64:1602–1612, doi:10.1016/j.jacc.2014.05.073.)

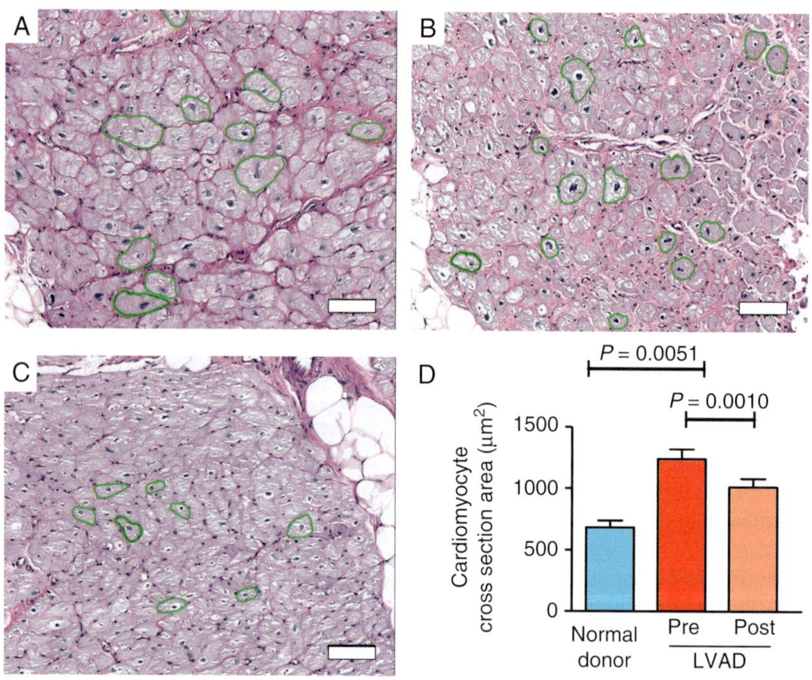

Fig. 9.2 Cardiomyocyte size evaluation. Representative photomicrographs of myocardial tissue stained with Periodic Acid Schiff histochemical stain before continuous-flow left ventricular assist device *(LVAD)* implantation (A), after LVAD support at the time of transplant (B), and from a normal heart (C). (D) Plots present the mean ± SEM of cardiomyocyte cross-sectional area (CSA) (n = 44 heart failure patients, 5 normal donors). CSA was significantly decreased after LVAD unloading (1238 ± 81 μm^2 vs. 1011 ± 68 μm^2, P=0.001). However, CSA was not decreased below that of a normal heart (682 ± 56 μm^2), a finding that would have suggested that LVAD unloading induces hypertrophy regression to the point of atrophy. The results were similar in the subgroup of patients with prolonged duration of mechanical unloading of more than 6 months. The *green circles* indicate the cardiac myocytes that were selected in order to have their CSA measured. (From Diakos NA, et al. Myocardial atrophy and chronic mechanical unloading of the failing human heart: implications for cardiac assist device-induced myocardial recovery. *J Am Coll Cardiol* 2014;64:1602–1612. doi:10.1016/j.jacc.2014.05.073.)

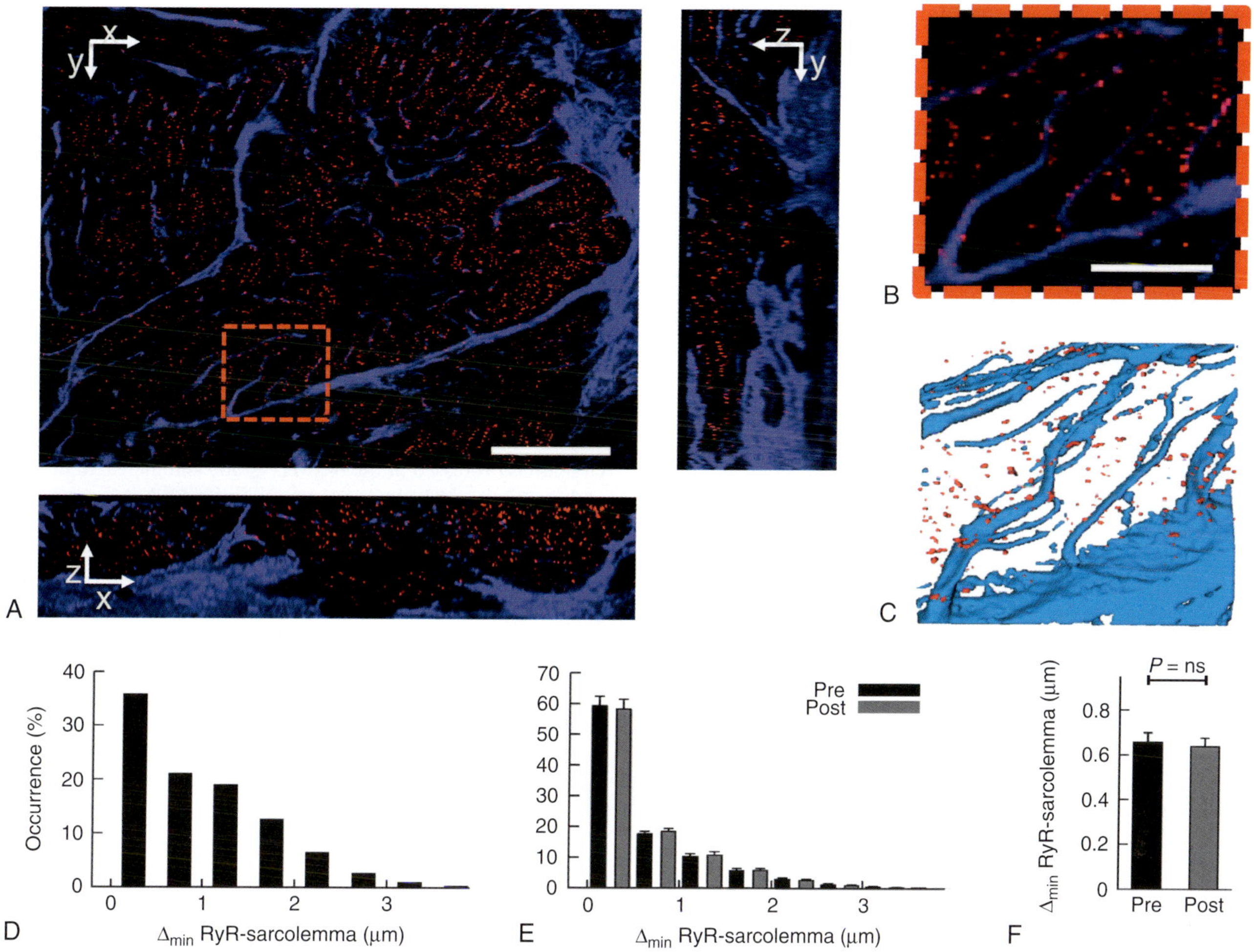

Fig. 9.3 Analysis of t-tubules and ryonadine receptor *(RyR)* clusters in tissue sections. (A) Cross-sections from image stack from confocal microscopy. Wheat germ agglutinin *(blue)* is used as a marker of sarcolemma and t-tubules. RyR clusters *(red)* were commonly close to the sarcolemma and t-tubules but were also found in some distance to the sarcolemma. Bar in (A): 20 μm. (B) Zoom into marked region in (A). Bar in (B): 5 μm. (C) Three-dimensional reconstruction of region marked in (A) with a thickness of 3 μm. (D) Summary RyR intensity grouped by sarcolemmal distance. The histogram was calculated for the tissue section presented in (A). (E) The histogram was calculated from tissues pre- and post-LVAD implantation. (F) Differences between RyR-sarcolemmal distance pre- and post-LVAD implantation were not significant (n = 11). All together, these findings are not suggestive of myocardial disuse atrophy. (From Diakos NA, et al. Myocardial atrophy and chronic mechanical unloading of the failing human heart: implications for cardiac assist device-induced myocardial recovery. *J Am Coll Cardiol.* 2014;64:1602–1612. doi:10.1016/j.jacc.2014.05.073.)

directly to mechanical unloading/stretch or to circulating systemic factors needs further investigation.

CONTRACTILE DYSFUNCTION, CALCIUM HANDLING, AND CYTOSKELETAL PROTEINS

Contractile function of the heart is conducted through composite processes such as sympathetic and parasympathetic heart rate control, core conduction system activities (thin [actin, tropomyosin, and troponin] and thick [myosin] filaments), calcium regulatory pathways that orchestrate shortening and relaxation, and humoral substances like catecholamines.[17] The failing heart has high energy demands that place considerable stress on the cardiac contractile machinery, which in turn diminishes myocardial contractility. The myocyte contractile defects observed in failing hearts were shown to be reversed after pulsatile-flow LVAD unloading, with improved shortening and relaxation in isolated myocytes and isolated strips of ventricular tissue.[18,19] Improvements in LVAD-induced contractile dysfunction can be partially explained by changes in Ca^{++} handling, such as faster sarcolemmal Ca^{++} entry and shorter action potential durations, higher sarcoplasmic reticulum Ca^{++} content, improved abundance of sarcoplasmic reticulum (SR)/endoplasmic reticulum calcium ATPase, decreased abundance of Na^{+}/Ca^{++} exchanger, and beneficial changes in L-type calcium channel and ryanodine receptor (RyR) function.[18,20–22] There is an increase in RyR clusters that are not near sarcolemmal L-type calcium channels due to reduced density of the tubular system (t-system); hence, they are not contained by couplons. This shift of RyR clusters away from sarcolemmal L-type calcium channels can affect the excitation-contraction coupling for two reasons: first, these nonjunctional RyR clusters can result in decreased calcium release from SR; and second, they create asynchronous calcium release due to a reduced open probability, which does not correlate with the quick opening of junctional RyR clusters. A recent study demonstrated a direct relationship linking the distance between nonjunctional RyR clusters and the change in left ventricular

(LV) ejection fraction (EF) in post-LVAD patients.[23] The authors reported that the EF improved when the distance was less than 1 μm, whereas a distance that exceeded 1 μm was not associated with improvement in EF. An intact t-system at the time of LVAD implantation may serve as a predictor for cardiac recovery induced through unloading (Fig. 9.4).[23]

The action potential initiates the excitation-contraction cycle in ventricular cardiomyocytes. Depolarization starts with sodium (Na^+) channels activating the L-type Ca^{++} current that causes local Ca^{++}-induced Ca^{++} release (CICR) in the SR. The increased cytosolic Ca^{++} binds to myofilaments, causing contraction followed by diastolic Ca^{++} elimination, i.e., dissociation of Ca^{++} from the contractile filaments and the excess cytosolic Ca^{++} extruded via SR-Ca^{++} ATPase, Na^+-Ca^{++} exchanger, and sarcolemmal Ca^{++} pump. Abnormalities in Ca^{++} regulation may lead to increased diastolic Ca^{++}, which is the hallmark of contractile dysfunction in end-stage chronic HF patients.[24] Therapeutic measures targeting Ca^{++} homeostasis may facilitate the reverse remodeling in HF patients. Fischer et al. recently showed that increased SR-Ca^{++} leak correlated with deteriorating LV function after LVAD implantation, and this SR-Ca^{++} leak was significantly reduced by Ca^{++} calmodulin-dependent protein kinase II (CaMKII) inhibition. CaMKII hyperphosphorylates RYR2, leading to disturbed diastolic closure of RYR2, and has a cascading effect on the Ca^{++} homeostasis in HF patients.[24] The observation that CaMKII inhibition reduces the SR-Ca^{++} leak in HF suggests that CaMKII inhibition may be a promising therapeutic target for cardiac remodeling after LVAD implantation.[25] Furthermore, CICR in rodent HF models suggests that the mechanical unloading by heterotopic abdominal heart transplantation increases calcium transient amplitude and normalizes the calcium spark frequencies and L-type calcium channel activity in cardiomyocytes.[26] The role of short-term continuous-flow LVAD unloading was studied in an ovine model of acute myocardial infarction (MI), where it was observed that mechanical unloading prevented cardiac remodeling and dysfunction. Compared to a non-LVAD control group, calcium handling proteins were not altered, thereby preserving calcium cycling and improving cardiac function.[27] These recent investigations demonstrate that extensive structural remodeling of the t-system, along with its depletion and change in orientation, plays an important role in the development and progression of ventricular dysfunction.

The effect of mechanical unloading on cytoskeletal proteins has been studied in LVAD clinical studies. Birks et al. showed significant differences (between the time of implantation and explantation/transplantation) in the regulation of nonsarcomeric proteins (lamin A/C, spectrin), integrins (β1, β5, β6, α5, and α7), and sarcomeric proteins that changed only in the recovered group (β-actin, α-tropomyosin, α1-actinin, and α-filament A).[28] They also reported that vinculin, Wiskott-Aldrich syndrome protein, p21-activated kinase, Rho, and Graf levels decreased in the recovery group and increased in the nonrecovery group.[28] These observations warrant further investigations on the role of the previously reported proteins in cardiac reverse remodeling.[29] Cardiac ankyrin repeat protein (CARP) has been associated with cardiac hypertrophy, acts as transcription cofactor under mechanical stress and pressure overload, and has a critical role in the Nkx2.5 transcriptional pathway that regulates the ventricular muscle gene expression in the developing heart.[30] A recent report on the CARP revealed increased levels in HF that eventually returned to normal levels after LVAD support. They also reported that CARP levels were increased after transaortic constriction in mice lacking βII spectrin, which the authors previously reported as an essential nodal protein following its significant alteration in their human and animal HF studies.[30,31] Together, these observations indicate the potentially important role of cytoskeletal proteins in the myocardial reverse remodeling processes and further investigations are warranted.

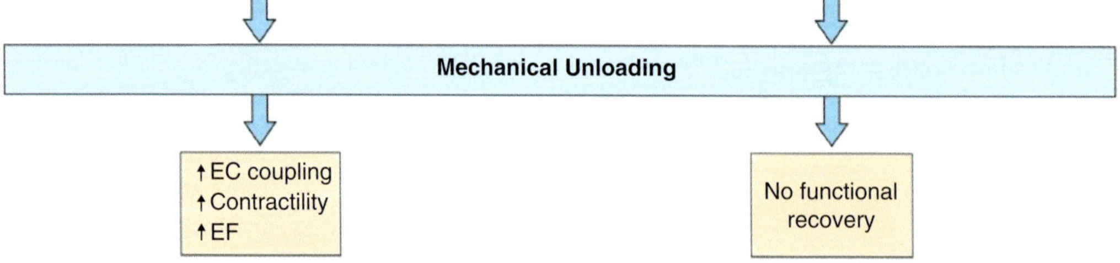

Fig. 9.4 Proposed role of the tubular-system (t-system) in functional cardiac recovery in chronic human heart failure. In some failing hearts, normal t-tubules remodel to t-sheets, t-system components that are significantly widened in the myocyte long axis direction, but still run transversely. Concomitantly, t-system density decreases, which causes a higher fraction of nonjunctional ryanodine receptor *(RyR)* clusters. As a result, triggering of calcium release from the sarcoplasmic reticulum *(SR)* becomes less efficient. Thus, excitation-contraction *(EC)* coupling can only recover in failing hearts with a preserved t-system, leading to improved contractility and left ventricular ejection fraction *(EF)* following unloading, but not in failing hearts with t-sheets and reduced t-system density. (From Seidel T, et al. Sheet-like remodeling of the transverse tubular system in human heart failure impairs excitation-contraction coupling and functional recovery by mechanical unloading. *Circulation.* 2017;135:1632–1645. doi:10.1161/CIRCULATIONAHA.116.024470.)

CARDIAC METABOLISM AND BIOENERGETICS

The heart utilizes multiple energy substrates like fatty acids, glucose, ketone bodies, lactate, and amino acids to meet its enormous energy demand for sustaining normal contractile function.[32] This versatile use of substrates to meet its metabolic demand (i.e., the metabolic flexibility of the heart) is impaired during HF. This metabolic remodeling is integral to HF development and progression, with the failing heart reverting to a fetal pattern of energy substrate metabolism, i.e., enhanced glycolysis with decrease in fatty acid oxidation.[33] This decrease in fatty acid metabolism seems beneficial in cardiac ischemic insults leading to hypoxic conditions, where anaerobic respiratory processes like glycolysis are beneficial, but may be deleterious in other cardiac conditions. Mechanical unloading with LVAD may reverse the maladaptive metabolic switches of the failing heart and even activate cellular pathways of cardioprotection and repair. Studies on LVAD-induced mechanical unloading have shown (1) improved respiratory capacity and augmented nitric oxide–dependent control of mitochondrial respiration[34,35]; (2) normalization of cardiolipin, a lipid component of the mitochondrial membrane important for adenosine triphosphate (ATP) formation and substrate transport, suggesting improved mitochondrial structure and function[36]; (3) depletion of long-chain acyl carnitine levels suggesting impairment of mitochondrial FA oxidation in failing hearts and substrate versatility of the mammalian heart[37]; (4) increased concentration of several amino acids, such as alanine, leucine/isoleucine, glutamine/glutamic acid and citrulline[38]; and (5) significant upsurge in the levels of total cholesterol, high-density lipoproteins, low-density lipoproteins, and triglycerides after LVAD implantation. Also, this increased level of total cholesterol from baseline to 3 months and a higher absolute cholesterol level postimplantation (at 3 months) were strongly associated with decreased mortality rate.[39] From all of the aforementioned studies, it is evident that LVAD unloading relieves a significant part of the metabolic distress in the failing heart.

One intriguing concept is that glycolysis, although less efficient in terms of generating ATP, could be a sufficient energy source due to the decreased myocardial energy demand during unloading. Recent investigations on metabolic changes during HF showed upregulation of glycolysis without a subsequent increase in pyruvate oxidation through the Krebs cycle. This mismatch between glycolysis upregulation and mitochondrial pyruvate oxidations was attributed to the impaired structure and function of mitochondria (Fig. 9.5).[40] These metabolic changes may also be associated with the shift toward ketone body metabolism during chronic HF.[41] The earlier observations, along with post-LVAD alterations in the expression of several metabolism-related genes and proteins,[19,22,42] require further investigation to elucidate the specific role of cardiac metabolic adaptations during myocardial reverse remodeling.[54,55]

CELL DEATH AND STRESS

Chronic HF is accompanied by loss of myocytes resulting in increased demand and stress. Cell death is mainly mediated by three processes, namely, apoptosis, necrosis, and autophagy. Apoptosis plays an important role in ventricular remodeling and contributes to the progressive impairment of contractile function.[43–45] Apoptosis is mostly mediated through extrinsic (death receptors) and intrinsic (mitochondrial pathways) pathways resulting in cell shrinkage, fragmentation, and phagocytosis of the fragmented particles by the macrophages or neighboring cells. Several studies demonstrating changes compatible with reduced apoptosis during LVAD unloading were reviewed in detail by Soppa et al., who suggested that LVAD unloading interrupts apoptosis, and the increased levels of apoptosis in HF might be reversible via LVAD support.[19] Correspondingly, a recent study showed that BCL2 associated X protein (Bax) and heat shock protein 72 (Hsp72) were significantly increased post-LVAD, suggesting a change in cardiac apoptotic environment and activation of antiapoptotic or protective factors.[46] In contrast, patients following continuous-flow LVAD implantation showed a slight increase in caspase-1 signaling along with an escalation in inflammation and other apoptotic markers.[47] Matrix metalloprotease-2 (MMP-2)/Janus kinase–mediated apoptotic and β1D-integrin/focal adhesion kinase–mediated survival pathways were reported to be activated in the nonischemic adjacent zone after MI in sheep, where LVAD unloading for 2 weeks attenuated remodeling, in part, by its negative effect on stretch-induced apoptosis and inhibition of MMP-2 activity.[48] All in all, the majority of studies reported decreased levels of apoptosis upon unloading, which likely plays a role in the reverse remodeling and subsequent improvement in cardiac function and structure.

Markers of autophagy have been shown to be downregulated after LVAD unloading of failing hearts.[49,50] Autophagy is a lysosome-mediated clean-up process, where damaged cytoplasmic organelles and proteins are digested through Beclin-1–initiated autophagocytosis to generate ATP. In cardiomyocytes, autophagy is also promoted via Fork-head box class O (FoxO) family transcription factors and plays a role in hypertrophy regression. Experimental studies have reported increased autophagy and levels of FoxO1 proteins after unloading.[51,52] Atg5 is an essential molecule in the autophagosome assembly and is crucial for autophagy-mediated degradation. *Atg5*-deficient mice showed significant decrease in cardiac contractility following mild transverse aortic constriction and angiotensin II treatment (known to induce hypertrophy). After the aortic constriction was removed (i.e., unloading), only controls showed signs of regression of hypertrophy, suggesting that autophagy also plays a role in the regression of LV hypertrophy.[53] Lastly, reports on cell stress during HF and with LVAD-unloading showed decreased mitochondrial reactive oxygen species production and increased mitochondrial coupling efficiency.[54] These favorable changes in myocyte attrition are complemented by data suggesting that LVAD unloading reduces myocardial stress, as indicated by reductions in the stress proteins metallothionein and hemeoxygenase-1.[55,56] The aforementioned studies reveal that cardiomyocytes modify cell death pathways during overload and might use them to renew the damaged organelles when unloaded via LVAD.

NATRIURETIC PEPTIDES AND NEUROHORMONES

Neurohormones drive survival and injury responses via several mechanisms. In chronic HF, neurohormonal responses are mostly triggered as a response to reduced myocardial contractility and hemodynamic overload, and levels of natriuretic peptides are used diagnostically.[57] The sympathetic nervous system and the renin-angiotensin-aldosterone system play a crucial role in vasculature, cardiac, and renal hypertrophy and progression of HF. Studies investigating β-adrenergic signaling and sympathetic innervation reported that pulsatile flow LVAD unloading improved (1) β-adrenergic receptor density, location and distribution pattern, contractile response to β adrenergic stimuli, and adenyl cyclase activity[18–20] and (2) sympathetic innervation in the failing heart accompanied by clinical, functional, and hemodynamic improvements.[58] Interestingly, continuous-flow LVADs are associated with higher muscle sympathetic nerve activity than pulsatile flow LVADs, suggesting that flow patterns and the degree of myocardial

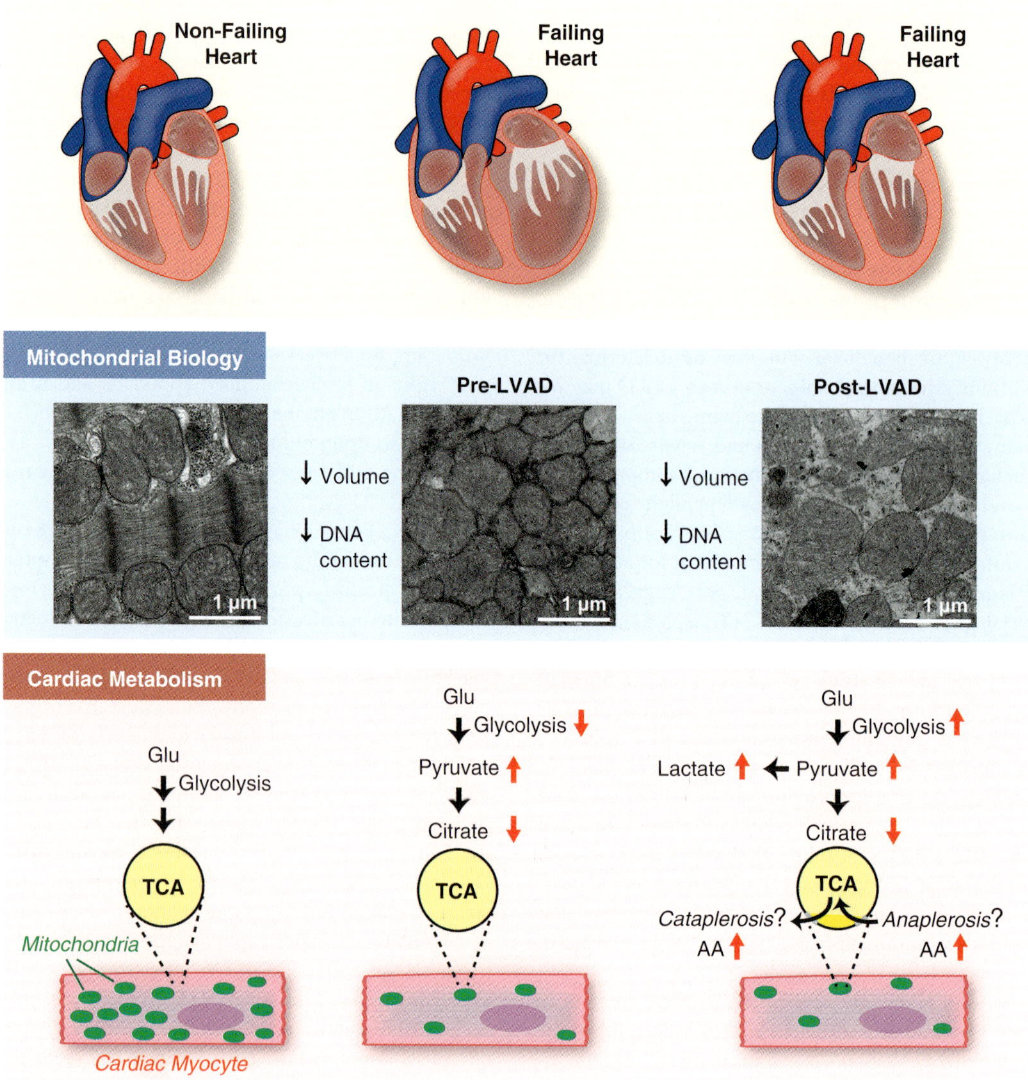

Fig. 9.5 Schematic model of the mitochondrial and metabolomics adaptation to heart failure and ventricular unloading. Glycolytic intermediates are induced following left ventricular assist device *(LVAD)* as exemplified by pyruvate, and also increased levels of lactate. These findings suggest that the increased pyruvate was not utilized by the mitochondria and the Krebs cycle for complete oxidation but instead is converted to lactate in the cytoplasm. Such a pyruvate mitochondrial oxidation "mismatch" correlates with the findings of altered mitochondrial function and structure specifically the lack of post-LVAD improvement in the impaired mitochondrial oxidative functional capacity of the failing human heart, and persistent reduction in mitochondrial volume density and DNA content. Therefore, therapeutic interventions, such as myocardial conditioning, that are known to improve mitochondrial biogenesis, structure, and function might be useful to further improve cardiac metabolism and energy production and thereby enhance myocardial reverse remodeling and cardiac recovery with LVAD-facilitated mechanical unloading. *AA*, Amino acids; *TCA*, tricarboxylic acid cycle. (From Diakos NA, et al. Evidence of glycolysis up-regulation and pyruvate mitochondrial oxidation mismatch during mechanical unloading of the failing human heart: implications for cardiac reloading and conditioning. *JACC Basic Transl Sci*. 2016;1:432–444. doi:10.1016/j.jacbts.2016.06.)

unloading may differ depending on the characteristics of a specific device.[59]

Studies on pulsatile-LVAD unloading have been associated with decreased levels of atrial and brain natriuretic peptides (BNP) and tumor necrosis factor-α (TNF-α) in serum and myocardial tissue.[12,60,61] Circulating levels of epinephrine, norepinephrine, renin, angiotensin II, and arginine vasopressin have been shown to decrease during pulsatile LVAD unloading, but the specific implications of these changes need to be further investigated.[62]

Recent studies involving patients with continuous-flow LVAD reported decreased NT-proBNP (N-terminal fragment in the prohormone BNP) levels consistent with low ventricular wall stress.[63,64] It was also proposed that postoperative improvement of BNP levels during LV unloading can be used as a predictive tool for postoperative outcomes such as length of stay, right ventricular failure, and postoperative survival.[63] NT-proBNP levels decreased by 40%–60% following LVAD support, with incremental decreases to 80% with neurohormonal blockade drug therapy.[65] Patients with lowest BNP levels 60 days postimplantation are more likely to experience functional recovery with the lowest risk of ventricular arrhythmia.[66,67] In summary, most studies suggest a significant reduction in neurohormonal activation with LVAD support. Future investigations should study whether this is an epiphenomenon of other benefits derived by the MCS or an active mechanism that can be further manipulated to improve cardiac reverse remodeling and, in general, the cardiovascular health of mechanically assisted patients.

INFLAMMATORY MARKERS

Inflammation is one of the most crucial biological processes implicated in several aspects of cardiovascular disease. There is mounting evidence of the effect of LVAD support on the inflammatory response; however, some of the reports are conflicting and the complete picture of the effect of ventricular unloading on the HF inflammatory response is unclear. Significant increases in interleukin (IL)-6 and IL-8 have been identified in LVAD patient samples when compared to other advanced HF patients, while TNF-α remained unchanged.[68] IL-33/suppression of tumorigenesis 2 (ST2) signaling in cardiac fibroblasts and cardiomyocytes is activated as a myocardial response to mechanical overload. A recent study showed that ST2 knockout mice exhibited increased LV hypertrophy, fibrosis, and apoptosis.[69] Furthermore, recombinant IL-33 treatment following transverse aortic constriction reduced hypertrophy and fibrosis in wild-type mice, but not in ST2 knockout mice, suggesting that the IL-33/ST2 pathway plays an important role during mechanical overload.[69] In addition, a recent study reported lower tissue expression of IL-33 and ST2 in LVAD patients compared to heart transplant patients. These investigators also observed that the levels of IL-33, ST2, IL-8, and TNF-α were low pre-LVAD and significantly increased after LVAD support.[70] All together, these studies suggest that the IL-33/ST2 pathway is involved in the decline of cardiac function in HF and in reverse cardiac remodeling following LVAD support and therefore may serve as a new therapeutic target for myocardial recovery.

In another study, inflammatory markers before LVAD implantation and 3, 6, and 9 months following LVAD implantation were compared to those of a healthy control group.[71] BNP levels and LV dimension by echocardiography dropped significantly after LVAD implantation (Fig. 9.6A). Advanced HF patients undergoing LVAD implantation had elevated C reactive protein (CRP), monocyte chemoattractant protein-1, and interferon γ-induced protein 10 prior to LVAD implantation and remained elevated thereafter (see Fig. 9.6B). However, levels of IL-8, TNF-α, macrophage inflammatory proteins-1β, and macrophage-derived chemokine significantly increased 9 months following LVAD implantation (see Fig. 9.6C).[71] These findings have been linked to LVAD-associated adverse events, and their full translational and clinical importance warrants further investigation.

EXTRACELLULAR MATRIX AND FIBROSIS

Investigations of the effect of LVAD unloading on extracellular matrix have shown conflicting results; a few studies reported decreased fibrosis, whereas other investigations found a significant increase in fibrosis.[4,19,72] The explanation for the contradictory observations is not clear, with some attributing the inconsistent results to the differences in background medications, patient-specific heterogeneity, and the variable fibrosis assessment methodologies employed in these studies.[4,19] A human myocardial tissue study addressed this controversial issue with the use of advanced image analysis techniques in whole-field digital microscopy, an approach that reduces observer bias, markedly increases the amount of myocardial tissue analyzed, and permits comprehensive endocardium-to-epicardium evaluation.[11] Myocardial tissue from HF patients pre-LVAD implantation had increased interstitial and total fibrosis as compared to normal myocardium.[11] The interstitial and total collagen content appeared to be further increased after pulsatile flow LVAD unloading in these patients.[11] The effects of pulsatile flow LVAD unloading on the myocardial tissue levels of the renin-angiotensin-aldosterone axis and matrix metalloproteinases supported the previous results.[73,74] Whether the observed increase in fibrosis is a manifestation of further progression of cardiac remodeling and HF (which LVAD support could not reverse) or a direct detrimental effect of MCS warrants further investigation.

In an attempt to identify novel biomarkers that regulate fibrosis during HF, Koshman et al. investigated the role of connective tissue growth factor (CTGF; a modulator of extracellular matrix production during inflammatory tissue injury) in the failing human heart and the response to mechanical unloading. While TGF-β1, CTGF, COL1-α1, and COL3-α1 mRNA levels were reduced by unloading, there was only a modest reduction in tissue fibrosis and no difference in protein-bound hydroxyproline concentration between pre- and post-LVAD tissue samples. They postulated that the persistent post-LVAD fibrosis may be related to a concomitant reduction in MMP-9 following unloading. They proposed that CTGF may be a key regulator of fibrosis during maladaptive remodeling and progression to HF, and although mechanical unloading normalizes most genotypic and functional abnormalities, its effect on extracellular matrix remodeling during HF appears to be incomplete.[75] Along the same lines, Galectin-3 was identified as a regulator of myocardial fibrosis and was found to be elevated in end-stage HF patients. Following LVAD implantation, Galectin-3 levels were found to increase during the period of LVAD support.[76] Lastly, Lok and colleagues found an increase in fibrosis as well as circulating profibrotic markers after continuous-flow LVAD support.[77] The same group investigated the role of growth differentiation factor-15 (GDF-15; a stress-responsive cytokine) during LVAD support and found that high circulating levels of GDF-15 correlate with myocardial fibrosis that decline after 1 month of mechanical unloading and subsequently remain stable. Furthermore, they observed that the cardiac mRNA and protein expressions of GDF-15 are very low, suggesting that the heart is not an important source of GDF-15 production in these patients.[78]

Several studies suggest that LVAD mechanical unloading is associated with altered extracellular matrix synthesis.[79] Recently, persistent myocardial fibrosis (but no further increase) has been demonstrated in patients with end-stage HF supported with LVAD.[80] Gene expression analysis on isolated cardiac macrophages revealed decreased Kruppel-like factor-4, transglutaminase-2, mannose receptor-1, and IL 10, along with reduced levels of metalloproteinase-2 and profibrotic M2 macrophage gene expression after LVAD unloading. These findings suggest persistence of inflammation-activated fibroblasts after LVAD unloading that might contribute to poor extracellular matrix turnover and impede the potential of myocardial recovery observed in a subset of these patients.[80] The same investigators aimed to test the hypothesis that bone marrow stem cells (CD34+) injected in the epicardium would improve histological measurements of vascularity, fibrosis, and inflammation in human subjects (n = 6) undergoing LVAD placement. They found no significant differences

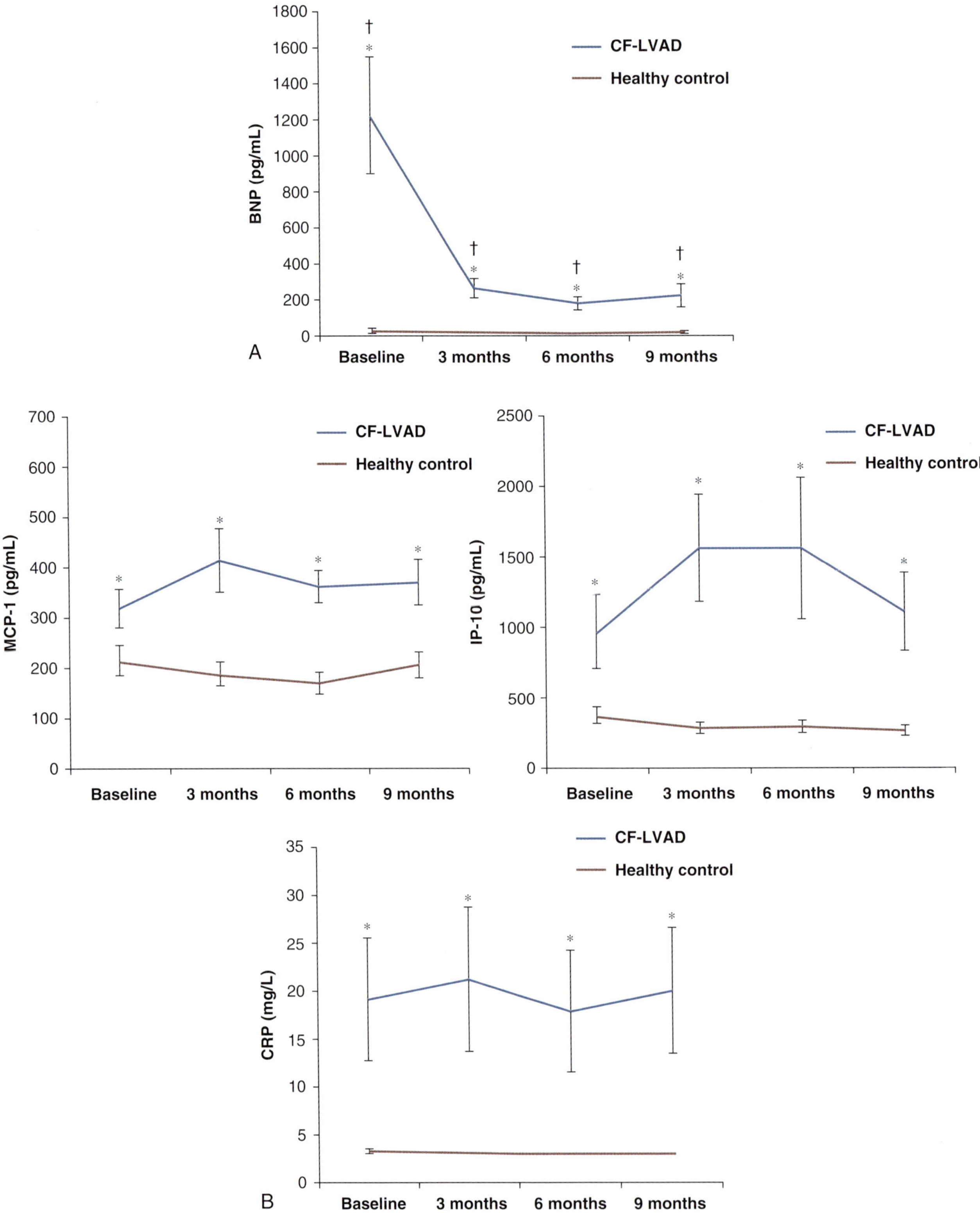

Fig. 9.6 (A) BNP levels in CF-LVAD patients before and after implantation compared with healthy controls. (B) MCP-1, CRP, and IP-10 levels in CF-LVAD patients before and after implantation compared to healthy controls.

(Continued)

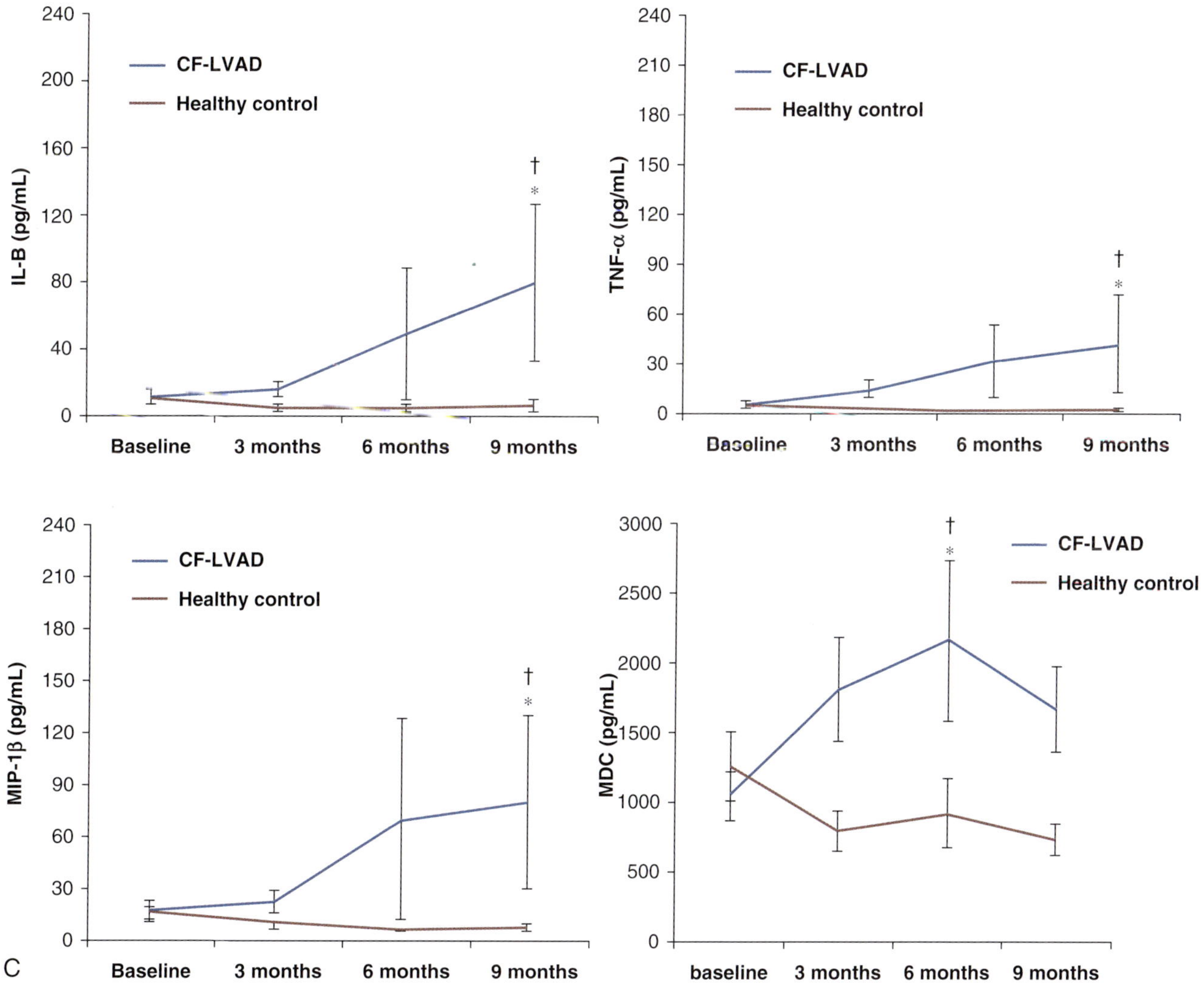

Fig. 9.6, Cont'd (C) IL-8, TNF-α, MIP-1β, and MDC levels in CF-LVAD patients before and after implantation compared to healthy controls. *BNP*, Brain natriuretic peptide; *CF*, Continuous flow; *LVAD*, left ventricular assist device; *CRP*, C reactive protein; *MCP-1*, monocyte chemoattractant protein-1; *ICP-10*, interferon γ–induced protein 10; *IL-8*, interleukin-8; *TNF-α*, tumor necrosis factor-α; *MIP-1β*, macrophage inflammatory proteins-1β; *MDC*, macrophage-derived chemokine. (Source: Grosman-Rimon L, Jacobs I, Tumiati LC, et al. Longitudinal assessment of inflammation in recipients of continuous-flow left ventricular assist devices. *Can J Cardiol*. 2015;31:348–56.)

in fibrosis or inflammation between groups; however, the density of activated fibroblasts was decreased in both CD34+- and CD34-injected areas.[81] These findings suggest that changes in myofibroblast numbers might be insufficient to alter myocardial fibrosis.[81] In tandem, Sakamuri et al. found that mechanical unloading can restore several components of the fibrillar extracellular matrix and the basement membrane but at the same time showed persistent elevation of adverse remodeling of the nonfibrillar extracellular matrix, which could contribute to disease progression and HF relapse after removal of LVAD support.[82,83]

Given the mixed results, further studies to determine the effects of MCS on extracellular matrix and identification of adjuvant therapies that could enhance the potential of myocardial recovery during LVAD support are needed.

GENE EXPRESSION, RNA, AND PROTEOMIC PROFILING

Biological perturbations in HF patients can be analyzed by means of combining -omics techniques. Several studies have analyzed mRNA expression, micro-RNA, long noncoding RNA, protein, and protein modifications in HF patients undergoing LVAD inplantation.[84–96] Such studies will become much more useful in our effort to better understand the molecular basis of reverse cardiac remodeling, particularly if comparisons are made between patients who have sustained recovery and those who do not recover. In such a study, Dhar et al. reported that myosin light chain kinase and IL 6 gene expression were significantly higher in LVAD responders (i.e., patients that showed myocardial functional improvement after LVAD support) compared to nonresponders.[89] Hopefully, future investigations using these technologies will consistently include in their study design the collection of functional myocardial recovery data and thus increase their potential to provide cardiac reverse remodeling mechanistic insights.

ENDOTHELIUM AND VASCULATURE

Chronic HF is accompanied by endothelial dysfunction and impaired vascular function.

Studies performed with pulsatile flow LVADs were associated with gene expression changes that regulate vascular organization and migration.[97] Furthermore, pulsatile flow LVAD unloading induced a significant increase in microvascular density.[11] The same study provided immunohistochemical and ultrastructural evidence of endothelial cell activation that was consistent with the observed increase in microvascular density.[11] Animal data have also shown that mechanical unloading by means of heterotopic transplantation increased microvascular density.[98]

Due to mainly bioengineering reasons, continuous-flow assist devices have become the predominant LVAD used clinically, and since then, several studies have demonstrated that the consequent nonphysiologic flow pattern negatively affects vascular health.[59,99,100] Specifically, patients who receive long-term support with continuous-flow LVADs have impaired endothelial cell function, increased adventitial fibrosis and collagen deposition, and collapse of elastic lamina along with increased vascular stiffness. This impairment might be an effect of decreased pulsatility, variations in laminar flow pattern in ascending aorta due to LVAD outflow graft, and changes in cytoskeletal and mitochondrial structures in endothelial cells due to oxidative stress. This increase in adventitial fibrosis and elastic remodeling of vessels may also negatively affect the potential for reverse remodeling and myocardial recovery.[101–106] Future investigations should explore these biological changes in the vasculature and deduce targets for developing novel therapies along with ways of introducing pulsatility in newer LVAD technologies, in order to prevent chronic adverse vascular remodeling and its associated side effects.

STUDIES ON ANGIOGENESIS

Angiogenesis, the formation of new blood vessels, is regulated by angiopoietins (Ang-1 and Ang-2)[112] (Fig. 9.7A). Ang-1 is produced by perivascular cells and, together with vascular endothelial growth factor (VEGF), promotes stable vessel development through its activation of the Tie-2 receptor, located on the endothelial cell surface (see Fig. 9.7B).[113] Ang-2 is synthesized by endothelial cells and stored in Weibel-Palade bodies along with von Willebrand factor.[107] Following its release into the plasma, Ang-2 interacts with VEGF and the Tie-2 receptor to cause unstable blood vessel formation and acts as an inhibitor of the activity of Ang-1 on the Tie-2 receptor.[108,109] Overexpression of Ang-2 with a corresponding decrease in Ang-1 is associated with vascular malformations[110] and gastrointestinal (GI) angiodysplasia.[111]

As discussed previously, LVAD patients have higher circulating levels of TNF-α leading to increased apoptosis and tissue factor expression in endothelial cells. Those tissue factors are strong activators of thrombin, and indeed, multiple studies have demonstrated elevated thrombin levels in patients with LVADs along with elevated TNF-α levels.[112–114] Furthermore, thrombin is known to stimulate Ang-2 overexpression, and a study that measured Ang-2 levels revealed that LVAD patients have elevated levels of Ang-2 in both the plasma and in endothelial cells (Fig. 9.8).[115] In addition, increased abnormal blood vessel formation is mediated by high Ang-2 levels and reversed by an Ang-2-blocking antibody or by the use of vorapaxar, a direct thrombin inhibitor (Fig. 9.9A and B).[115]

High TNF-α levels also induce apoptosis of pericytes and suppress Ang-1 expression in these cells, which may contribute to a decline in Ang-1 levels and thus stall normal blood vessel growth. In an in vitro study utilizing LVAD patients' blood, pericyte apoptosis was reduced by using TNF-α blockers, leading to a significant reduction in the formation of abnormal blood vessels (Fig. 9.10A and B).[116] The net result is a decrease in Ang-1, an increase in Ang-2, and a reduced Ang-1/Ang-2 ratio in LVAD patients (Fig. 9.11). Recent clinical studies have linked these abnormal angiogenesis mechanisms to increased nonsurgical bleeding in LVAD patients in general and more specifically to GI bleeding through increased formation of arteriovenous malformations. Blood analysis of patients enrolled in the Prevention of Recurrent Venous Thromboembolism (PREVENT) study showed that the rate of nonsurgical bleeding was significantly higher in patients with elevated TNF-α and Ang-2 both prior to device implantation and 3 months after.[117] This suggests that understanding these biological changes following ventricular unloading with LVAD implantation may help to reduce adverse events.

FUTURE DIRECTIONS

Understanding the mechanisms of cardiac recovery following LVAD support may be paramount to facilitating cardiac recovery in the broader HF population. As mentioned previously, a critical shortcoming in the field of the biological effects of LVAD unloading is failure to correlate functional outcomes with molecular, cellular, and histological findings.[4–6] As a result, earlier studies shed limited information on whether observed biological changes occurring during the period of MCS therapy could be associated with true cardiac recovery mechanisms or alternatively represented epiphenomena related to the MCS therapy, but not directly related to reverse cardiac remodeling. Examination of tissue from patients with various degrees of MCS-induced myocardial functional recovery (i.e., "responders") and from MCS patients without functional myocardial improvement (i.e., "nonresponders") is critical. Thus, combined functional and biological studies represent a sound approach to begin distinguishing between these two scenarios: true mechanistic insights versus epiphenomena. Future in-depth, investigational steps incorporating a rigorous basic science scientific approach could assign causality and lead to the discovery of novel therapeutic targets.

Extrapolating the lessons learned from the LVAD investigational setting to the broader HF population is the holy grail of this field. With the precedents set by the significant impact of studies of other well-controlled and tractable subsets on larger populations, such as the genetic work in both cancer and cardiovascular disease,[118–121] the work to improve our understanding of cardiac recovery and resilience in LVAD patients could be transformational for the greater HF population. Research in this field could be innovative in many ways, and such opportunities include genome-phenome systems biology approaches, genetic epidemiology, bioinformatics and precision medicine at the population level, advanced imaging modalities including molecular and metabolic imaging, and minimally invasive surgical and percutaneous bioengineering approaches. These new avenues of investigations could lead to new treatments that target phylogenetically conserved pathways involved in cardiac reparative mechanisms rather than perpetuating current approaches of targeting pathways that attenuate adverse remodeling. They also have the potential to change the paradigm

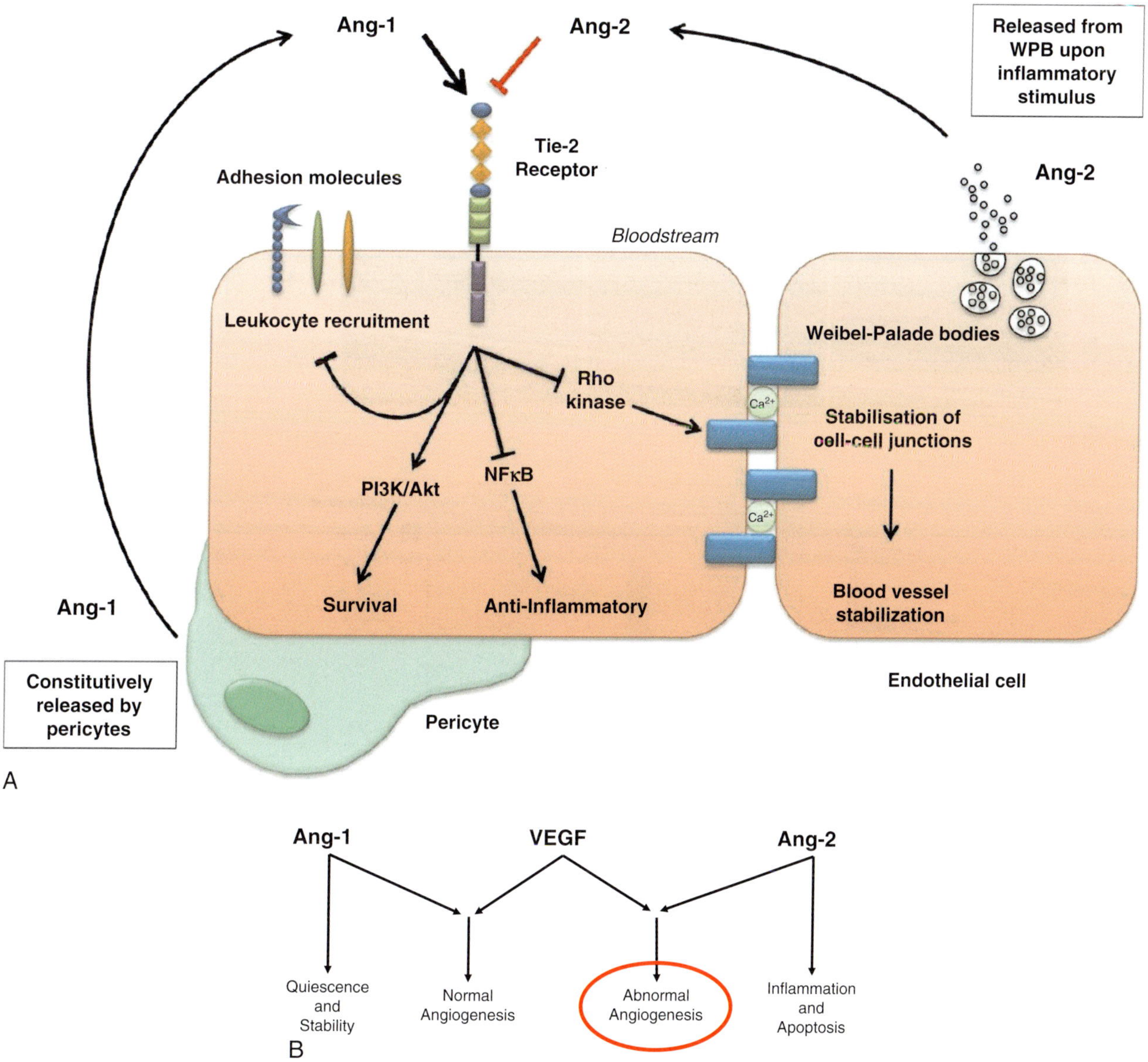

Fig. 9.7 (A) Role of Ang-1 and -2 in angiogensis. (From van Meurs M, Kümpers P, Ligtenberg JJ, Meertens JH, Molema G, Zijlstra JG. Bench-to-bedside review: angiopoietin signalling in critical illness—a future target? *Crit Care*. 2009;13:207.) (B) Role of VEGF in promoting stable vessel development through interaction with angiopoietins. *Ang-1*, Angiopoietin 1; *Ang-2*, angiopoietin 2; *NFkB*, nuclear factor kappa-light-chain-enhancer of activated B cells; *VEGF*, vascular endothelial growth factor; *WPB*, Weibel-Palade bodies.

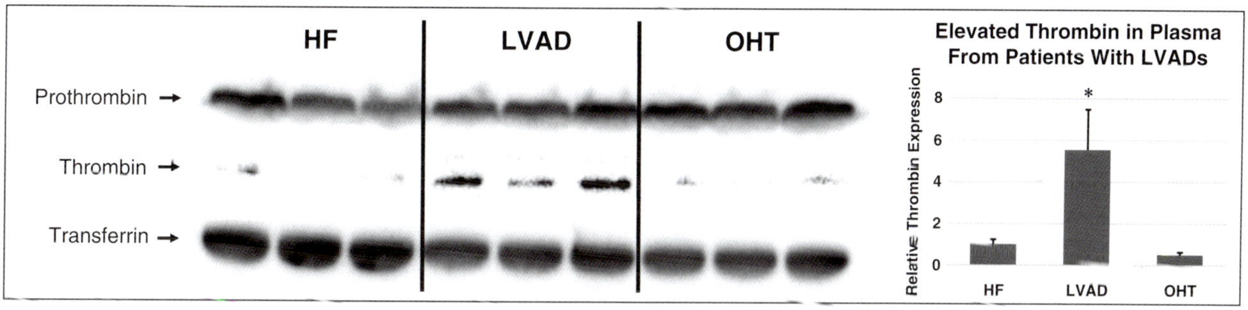

Fig. 9.8 Elevated thrombin levels seen in continuous flow-LVAD patients, leading to overexpression of Ang-2 *HF*, Heart failure; *LVAD*, left ventricular assist device; *OHT*, orthotopic heart transplantation. (From Tabit CE, Chen P, Kim GH, et al. Elevated angiopoietin-2 level in patients with continuous-flow left ventricular assist devices leads to altered angiogenesis and is associated with higher nonsurgical bleeding. *Circulation*. 2016;134:141–152.)

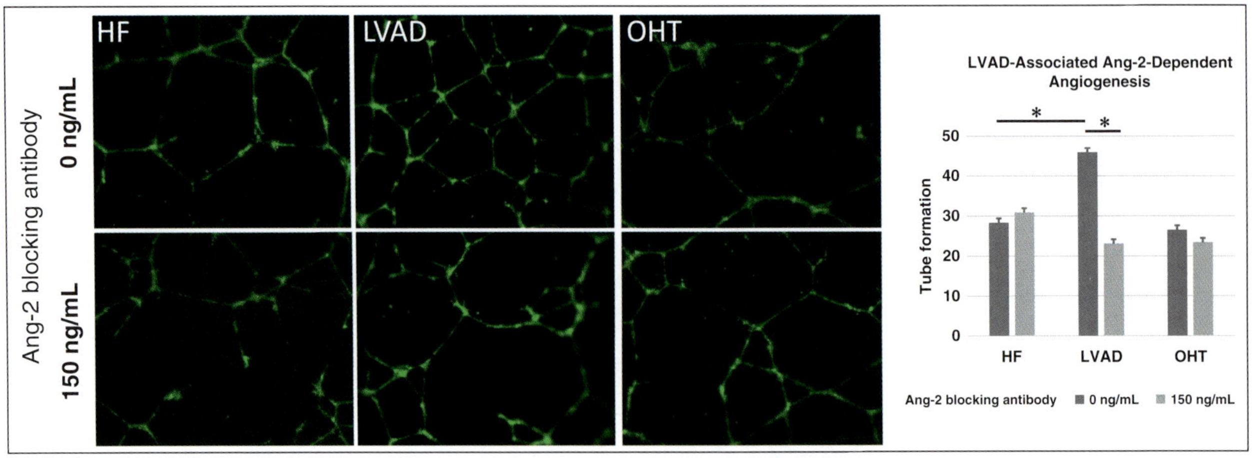

A

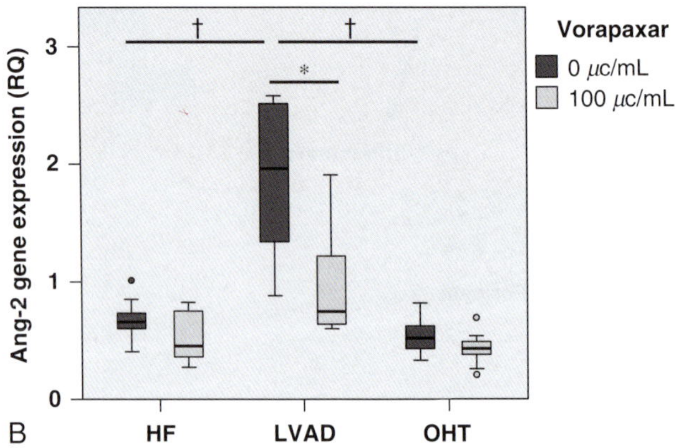

B

Fig. 9.9 (A) Increased abnormal blood vessel formation mediated by high Ang-2 levels reversed by Ang-2-blocking antibody or by the use of vorapaxar, a direct thrombin inhibitor. (B) Increased abnormal blood vessel formation mediated by high Ang-2 levels reversed by the use of vorapaxar, a direct thrombin inhibitor. *Ang-2*, Angiopoietin 2; *HF*, heart failure; *LVAD*, left ventricular assist device; *OHT*, orthotopic heart transplantation. (A and B from Tabit CE, Chen P, Kim GH, et al. Elevated angiopoietin-2 level in patients with continuous-flow left ventricular assist devices leads to altered angiogenesis and is associated with higher nonsurgical bleeding. *Circulation*. 2016;134:141–152.)

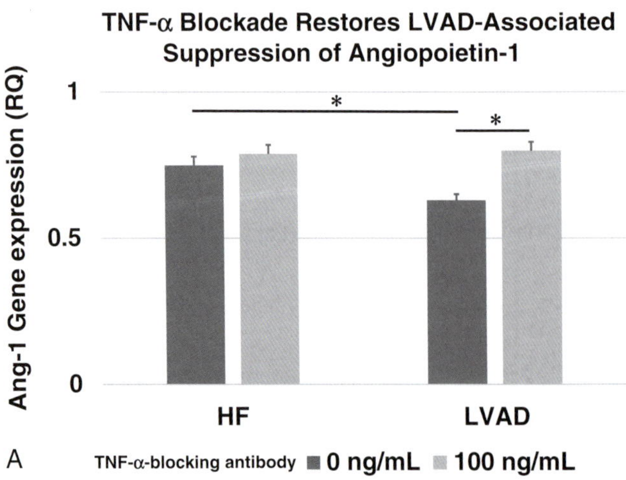

A

Fig. 9.10 (A) Blockade of TNF-α levels leads to increased Ang-1 gene expression in CF-LVAD patients.

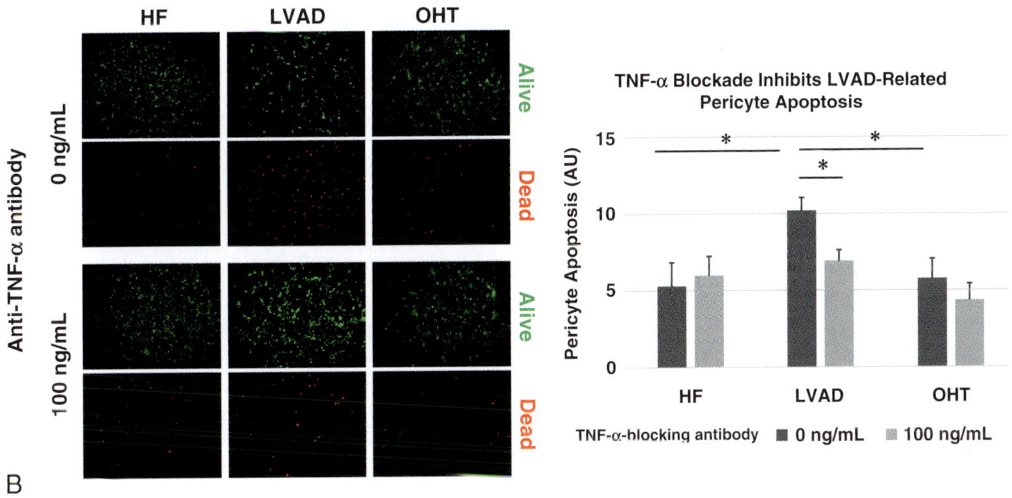

Fig. 9.10—Cont'd (B) TNF-α blockers in CF-LVAD patients lead to a significant reduction in the formation of abnormal blood vessels. *CF*, Continuous flow; *HF*, heart failure; *LVAD*, left ventricular assist device; *OHT*, orthotopic heart transplantation; *TNF-α*, tumor necrosis factor-α. (A and B from Tabit CE, Coplan MJ, Chen P, Jeevanandam V, Uriel N, Liao JK. Tumor necrosis factor-α levels and non-surgical bleeding in continuous-flow left ventricular assist devices. *J Heart Lung Transplant*. 2018;37:107–115.)

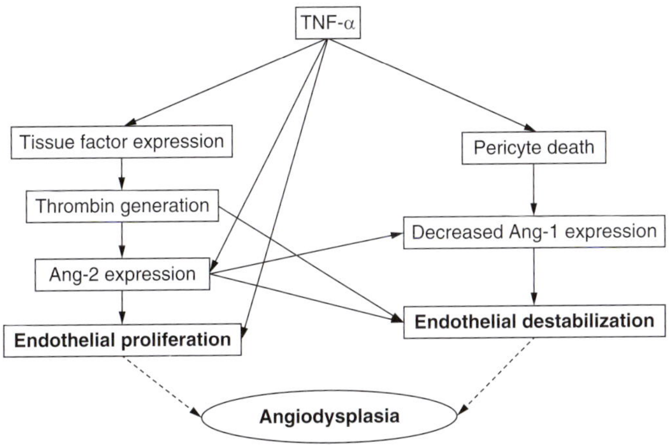

Fig. 9.11 TNF-α leads to a decrease in Ang-1, increase in Ang-2, and a reduced Ang-1/Ang-2 ratio, culminating in angiodysplasia seen in left ventricular assist device patients. *Ang-1*, Angiopoietin 1; *Ang-2*, angiopoietin 2; *TNF-α*, tumor necrosis factor-α. (From Tabit CE, Coplan MJ, Chen P, Jeevanandam V, Uriel N, Liao JK. Tumor necrosis factor-α levels and nonsurgical bleeding in continuous-flow left ventricular assist devices. *J Heart Lung Transplant*. 2018;37:107–115.)

in the treatment of chronic HF from one of attenuation of adverse cardiac remodeling to induction of self-repair mechanisms in specific patient populations.

Recently, the National Heart Lung Blood Institute convened a working group of experts to develop recommendations aimed at advancing the science of cardiac recovery in the setting of MCS.[122] The working group made the following recommendations[122]:

1. Explore mechanistic approaches at the genetic, molecular, cellular, microstructural, or physiological level to improve the understanding of myocardial recovery and develop novel interventions.
2. Utilize epidemiological approaches and population based studies to identify the associative host factors and LVAD device characteristics that influence the incidence and degree of myocardial recovery associated with LVAD.
3. Leverage innovative strategies and approaches to investigate the science and engineering of myocardial recovery with LVAD.

SUMMARY

HF is one of the major medical burdens in our society. MCSs such as LVADs are being used as a destination therapy or as a BTT for advanced HF patients in everyday clinical practice. This increasing clinical use of LVADs presents a key opportunity for in-depth investigations on the biology of the failing heart. LVAD-induced functional, structural, and molecular changes are helping us to begin understanding the specific biological signatures of myocardial recovery. In this chapter, the MCS-induced structural and functional effects on the vasculature and myocardium were reviewed, as well as how advanced technologies like RNA sequencing, tracer studies, and others may help us enhance the depth of our understanding of these phenomena. As the fundamental biological underpinnings of cardiovascular health and disease are increasingly elucidated, successful deduction of the mechanisms responsible for HF progression and regression will be within reach in the near future.

REFERENCES

1. Drakos SG, Pagani FD, Lundberg MS, Baldwin JT. Advancing the Science of Myocardial Recovery With Mechanical Circulatory Support: A Working Group of the National, Heart, Lung, and Blood Institute. *JACC Basic Transl Sci*. 2017;2:335–340. https://doi.org/10.1016/j.jacbts.2016.12.003.
2. Yacoub MH. A novel strategy to maximize the efficacy of left ventricular assist devices as a bridge to recovery. *Eur Heart J*. 2001;22:534–540. https://doi.org/10.1053/euhj.2001.2613.
3. Zafeiridis A, Jeevanandam V, Houser SR, Margulies KB. Regression of cellular hypertrophy after left ventricular assist device support. *Circulation*. 1998;98:656–662.
4. Baba HA, Wohlschlaeger J. Morphological and molecular changes of the myocardium after left ventricular mechanical support. *Curr Cardiol Rev*. 2008;4:157–169. https://doi.org/10.2174/157340308785160606.

5. Razeghi P, et al. Atrophic remodeling of the heart in vivo simultaneously activates pathways of protein synthesis and degradation. *Circulation*. 2003;108:2536–2541. https://doi.org/10.1161/01.CIR.0000096481.45105.13.
6. Kinoshita M, Takano H, Takaichi S, Taenaka Y, Nakatani T. Influence of prolonged ventricular assistance on myocardial histopathology in intact heart. *Ann Thorac Surg*. 1996;61:640–645. https://doi.org/10.1016/0003-4975(95)01087-4.
7. Thompson EW, Marino TA, Uboh CE, Kent RL, Cooper Gt. Atrophy reversal and cardiocyte redifferentiation in reloaded cat myocardium. *Circ Res*. 1984;54:367–377.
8. Hill JA, Olson EN. Cardiac plasticity. *N Engl J Med*. 2008;358:1370–1380. https://doi.org/10.1056/NEJMra072139.
9. Oriyanhan W, et al. Determination of optimal duration of mechanical unloading for failing hearts to achieve bridge to recovery in a rat heterotopic heart transplantation model. *J Heart Lung Transplant*. 2007;26:16–23. https://doi.org/10.1016/j.healun.2006.10.016.
10. Jacquet L, Zerbe T, Stein KL, Kormos RL, Griffith BP. Evolution of human cardiac myocyte dimension during prolonged mechanical support. *J Thorac Cardiovasc Surg*. 1991;101:256–259.
11. Drakos SG, et al. Impact of mechanical unloading on microvasculature and associated central remodeling features of the failing human heart. *J Am Coll Cardiol*. 2010;56:382–391. https://doi.org/10.1016/j.jacc.2010.04.019.
12. Maybaum S, et al. Cardiac improvement during mechanical circulatory support: a prospective multicenter study of the LVAD Working Group. *Circulation*. 2007;115:2497–2505. https://doi.org/10.1161/CIRCULATIONAHA.106.633180.
13. Cheng A, Williamitis CA, Slaughter MS. Comparison of continuous-flow and pulsatile-flow left ventricular assist devices: is there an advantage to pulsatility? *Ann Cardiothorac Surg*. 2014;3:573–581. https://doi.org/10.3978/j.issn.2225-319X.2014.08.24.
14. Ambardekar, A. V., Dorosz, J. L., Cleveland, J. C., Jr., Lindenfeld, J. & Buttrick, P. M. Longitudinal left ventricular structural and functional imaging during full support with continuous-flow ventricular assist devices: a retrospective, preliminary analysis. *J Heart Lung Transplant*. 2012;31:1311–1313. https://doi.org/10.1016/j.healun.2012.09.004.
15. Diakos NA, et al. Myocardial atrophy and chronic mechanical unloading of the failing human heart: implications for cardiac assist device-induced myocardial recovery. *J Am Coll Cardiol*. 2014;64:1602–1612. https://doi.org/10.1016/j.jacc.2014.05.073.
16. Wende AR, et al. Enhanced cardiac Akt/protein kinase B signaling contributes to pathological cardiac hypertrophy in part by impairing mitochondrial function via transcriptional repression of mitochondrion-targeted nuclear genes. *Mol Cell Biol*. 2015;35:831–846. https://doi.org/10.1128/MCB.01109-14.
17. Stienen GJ. Pathomechanisms in heart failure: the contractile connection. *J Muscle Res Cell Motil*. 2015;36:47–60. https://doi.org/10.1007/s10974-014-9395-8.
18. Ambardekar AV, Buttrick PM. Reverse remodeling with left ventricular assist devices: a review of clinical, cellular, and molecular effects. *Circ Heart Fail*. 2011;4:224–233. https://doi.org/10.1161/CIRCHEARTFAILURE.110.959684.
19. Soppa GK, Barton PJ, Terracciano CM, Yacoub MH. Left ventricular assist device-induced molecular changes in the failing myocardium. *Curr Opin Cardiol*. 2008;23:206–218. https://doi.org/10.1097/HCO.0b013e3282fc7010.
20. Hall JL, et al. Clinical, molecular, and genomic changes in response to a left ventricular assist device. *J Am Coll Cardiol*. 2011;57:641–652. https://doi.org/10.1016/j.jacc.2010.11.010.
21. Terracciano CM, et al. Clinical recovery from end-stage heart failure using left-ventricular assist device and pharmacological therapy correlates with increased sarcoplasmic reticulum calcium content but not with regression of cellular hypertrophy. *Circulation*. 2004;109:2263–2265. https://doi.org/10.1161/01.CIR.0000129233.51320.92.
22. Hall JL, et al. Molecular signature of recovery following combination left ventricular assist device (LVAD) support and pharmacologic therapy. *Eur Heart J*. 2007;28:613–627. https://doi.org/10.1093/eurheartj/ehl365.
23. Seidel T, et al. Sheet-like remodeling of the transverse tubular system in human heart failure impairs excitation-contraction coupling and functional recovery by mechanical unloading. *Circulation*. 2017;135:1632–1645. https://doi.org/10.1161/CIRCULATIONAHA.116.024470.
24. Wehrens XH, Lehnart SE, Reiken SR, Marks AR. Ca2+/calmodulin-dependent protein kinase II phosphorylation regulates the cardiac ryanodine receptor. *Circ Res*. 2004;94:e61–e70. https://doi.org/10.1161/01.RES.0000125626.33738.E2.
25. Fischer TH, et al. Inhibition of CaMKII attenuates progressing disruption of Ca(2+) homeostasis upon left ventricular assist device implantation in human heart failure. *Artif Organs*. 2016;40:719–726. https://doi.org/10.1111/aor.12677.
26. Ibrahim M, et al. Mechanical unloading reverses transverse tubule remodelling and normalizes local Ca(2+)-induced Ca(2+)release in a rodent model of heart failure. *Eur J Heart Fail*. 2012;14:571–580. https://doi.org/10.1093/eurjhf/hfs038.
27. Wei X, et al. Short-term mechanical unloading with left ventricular assist devices after acute myocardial infarction conserves calcium cycling and improves heart function. *JACC Cardiovasc Interv*. 2013;6:406–415. https://doi.org/10.1016/j.jcin.2012.12.122.
28. Birks EJ, et al. Gene profiling changes in cytoskeletal proteins during clinical recovery after left ventricular-assist device support. *Circulation*. 2005;112:I57–I64. https://doi.org/10.1161/CIRCULATIONAHA.104.526137.
29. Dullens HF, et al. Integrin expression during reverse remodeling in the myocardium of heart failure patients. *Cardiovasc Pathol*. 2012;21:291–298. https://doi.org/10.1016/j.carpath.2011.09.009.
30. Zou Y, et al. CARP, a cardiac ankyrin repeat protein, is downstream in the Nkx2-5 homeobox gene pathway. *Development*. 1997;124:793–804.
31. Kempton A, et al. Altered regulation of cardiac ankyrin repeat protein in heart failure. *Heliyon*. 2018;4:e00514. https://doi.org/10.1016/j.heliyon.2018.e00514.
32. Karwi QG, Uddin GM, Ho KL, Lopaschuk GD. Loss of metabolic flexibility in the failing heart. *Front Cardiovasc Med*. 2018;5:68. https://doi.org/10.3389/fcvm.2018.00068.
33. Jaswal JS, Keung W, Wang W, Ussher JR, Lopaschuk GD. Targeting fatty acid and carbohydrate oxidation–a novel therapeutic intervention in the ischemic and failing heart. *Biochim Biophys Acta*. 2011;1813:1333–1350. https://doi.org/10.1016/j.bbamcr.2011.01.015.
34. Lee SH, Doliba N, Osbakken M, Oz M, Mancini D. Improvement of myocardial mitochondrial function after hemodynamic support with left ventricular assist devices in patients with heart failure. *J Thorac Cardiovasc Surg*. 1998;116:344–349.
35. Mital S, Loke KE, Addonizio LJ, Oz MC, Hintze TH. Left ventricular assist device implantation augments nitric oxide dependent control of mitochondrial respiration in failing human hearts. *J Am Coll Cardiol*. 2000;36:1897–1902.
36. Heerdt PM, et al. Disease-specific remodeling of cardiac mitochondria after a left ventricular assist device. *Ann Thorac Surg*. 2002;73:1216–1221.
37. Ahmad T, et al. Prognostic implications of long-chain acylcarnitines in heart failure and reversibility with mechanical circulatory support. *J Am Coll Cardiol*. 2016;67:291–299. https://doi.org/10.1016/j.jacc.2015.10.079.
38. Gupte AA, et al. Mechanical unloading promotes myocardial energy recovery in human heart failure. *Circ Cardiovasc Genet*. 2014;7:266–276. https://doi.org/10.1161/CIRCGENETICS.113.000404.
39. Vest AR, et al. Recovery of serum cholesterol predicts survival after left ventricular assist device implantation. *Circ Heart Fail*. 2016;9:e002881. https://doi.org/10.1161/CIRCHEARTFAILURE.115.002881.
40. Diakos NA, et al. Evidence of glycolysis up-regulation and pyruvate mitochondrial oxidation mismatch during mechanical unloading of the failing human heart: implications for cardiac reloading and conditioning.

JACC Basic Transl Sci. 2016;1:432–444. https://doi.org/10.1016/j.jacbts.2016.06.009.
41. Aubert G, et al. The failing heart relies on ketone bodies as a fuel. *Circulation*. 2016;133:698–705. https://doi.org/10.1161/CIRCULATIONAHA.115.017355.
42. Cullen ME, et al. Myocardial expression of the arginine:glycine amidinotransferase gene is elevated in heart failure and normalized after recovery: potential implications for local creatine synthesis. *Circulation*. 2006;114:I16–I20. https://doi.org/10.1161/CIRCULATIONAHA.105.000448.
43. Moe GW, Marin-Garcia J. Role of cell death in the progression of heart failure. *Heart Fail Rev*. 2016;21:157–167. https://doi.org/10.1007/s10741-016-9532-0.
44. Kolwicz SC Jr, Purohit S, Tian, R. Cardiac metabolism and its interactions with contraction, growth, and survival of cardiomyocytes. *Circ Res* 2013;113:603–616. https://doi.org/10.1161/CIRCRESAHA.113.302095 (2013).
45. Orogo AM, Gustafsson AB. Cell death in the myocardium: my heart won't go on. *IUBMB Life*. 2013;65:651–656. https://doi.org/10.1002/iub.1180.
46. Prescimone T, et al. Cardiac molecular markers of programmed cell death are activated in end-stage heart failure patients supported by left ventricular assist device. *Cardiovasc Pathol*. 2014;23:272–282. https://doi.org/10.1016/j.carpath.2014.04.003.
47. Prescimone T, et al. Caspase-1 transcripts in failing human heart after mechanical unloading. *Cardiovasc Pathol*. 2015;24:11–18. https://doi.org/10.1016/j.carpath.2014.08.002.
48. Li T, et al. Left ventricular unloading after acute myocardial infarction reduces MMP/JNK associated apoptosis and promotes FAK cell-survival signaling. *Ann Thorac Surg*. 2016;102:1919–1924. https://doi.org/10.1016/j.athoracsur.2016.05.007.
49. Kassiotis C, et al. Markers of autophagy are downregulated in failing human heart after mechanical unloading. *Circulation*. 2009;120:S191–S197. https://doi.org/10.1161/CIRCULATIONAHA.108.842252.
50. Slaughter MS, et al. Advanced heart failure treated with continuous-flow left ventricular assist device. *N Engl J Med*. 2009;361:2241–2251. https://doi.org/10.1056/NEJMoa0909938.
51. Cao DJ, et al. Mechanical unloading activates FoxO3 to trigger Bnip3-dependent cardiomyocyte atrophy. *J Am Heart Assoc*. 2013;2:e000016. https://doi.org/10.1161/JAHA.113.000016.
52. Nishida K, Taneike M, Otsu K. The role of autophagic degradation in the heart. *J Mol Cell Cardiol*. 2015;78:73–79. https://doi.org/10.1016/j.yjmcc.2014.09.029.
53. Oyabu J, et al. Autophagy-mediated degradation is necessary for regression of cardiac hypertrophy during ventricular unloading. *Biochem Biophys Res Commun*. 2013;441:787–792. https://doi.org/10.1016/j.bbrc.2013.10.135.
54. Scheiber D, et al. Reduced myocardial mitochondrial ROS production in mechanically unloaded hearts. *J Cardiovasc Transl Res*. 2018;https://doi.org/10.1007/s12265-018-9803-3.
55. Baba HA, et al. Reversal of metallothionein expression is different throughout the human myocardium after prolonged left-ventricular mechanical support. *J Heart Lung Transplant*. 2000;19:668–674.
56. Grabellus F, et al. Reduction of hypoxia-inducible heme oxygenase-1 in the myocardium after left ventricular mechanical support. *J Pathol*. 2002;197:230–237. https://doi.org/10.1002/path.1106.
57. Ponikowski P, et al. 2016 ESC Guidelines for the diagnosis and treatment of acute and chronic heart failure: The Task Force for the diagnosis and treatment of acute and chronic heart failure of the European Society of Cardiology (ESC). Developed with the special contribution of the Heart Failure Association (HFA) of the ESC. *Eur J Heart Fail*. 2016;18:891–975. https://doi.org/10.1002/ejhf.592.
58. Drakos SG, et al. Myocardial sympathetic innervation and long-term left ventricular mechanical unloading. *JACC Cardiovasc Imaging*. 2010;3:64–70. https://doi.org/10.1016/j.jcmg.2009.10.008.
59. Witman MA, et al. Further peripheral vascular dysfunction in heart failure patients with a continuous-flow left ventricular assist device: the role of pulsatility. *JACC Heart Fail*. 2015;3:703–711. https://doi.org/10.1016/j.jchf.2015.04.012.
60. Bruggink AH, et al. Brain natriuretic peptide is produced both by cardiomyocytes and cells infiltrating the heart in patients with severe heart failure supported by a left ventricular assist device. *J Heart Lung Transplant*. 2006;25:174–180. https://doi.org/10.1016/j.healun.2005.09.007.
61. Torre-Amione G, et al. Decreased expression of tumor necrosis factor-alpha in failing human myocardium after mechanical circulatory support: a potential mechanism for cardiac recovery. *Circulation*. 1999;100:1189–1193.
62. James KB, et al. Effect of the implantable left ventricular assist device on neuroendocrine activation in heart failure. *Circulation*. 1995;92:II191–195.
63. Yost G, Bhat G, Pappas P, Tatooles A. Postoperative B-type natriuretic peptide as predictor for postoperative outcomes in patients implanted with left ventricular assist devices. *ASAIO J*. 2018;https://doi.org/10.1097/MAT.0000000000000797.
64. Muthiah K, et al. Longitudinal structural, functional, and cellular myocardial alterations with chronic centrifugal continuous-flow left ventricular assist device support. *J Heart Lung Transplant*. 2017;36:722–731. https://doi.org/10.1016/j.healun.2016.05.017.
65. Grupper A, et al. Effect of neurohormonal blockade drug therapy on outcomes and left ventricular function and structure after left ventricular assist device implantation. *Am J Cardiol*. 2016;117:1765–1770. https://doi.org/10.1016/j.amjcard.2016.03.011.
66. Sato T, et al. Serum brain natriuretic peptide concentration 60 days after surgery as a predictor of long-term prognosis in patients implanted with a left ventricular assist device. *ASAIO J*. 2015;61:373–378. https://doi.org/10.1097/MAT.0000000000000237.
67. Hellman Y, et al. B-type natriuretic peptide levels predict ventricular arrhythmia post left ventricular assist device implantation. *Artif Organs*. 2015;39:1051–1055. https://doi.org/10.1111/aor.12486.
68. Caselli C, et al. Impact of normalization strategy on cardiac expression of pro-inflammatory cytokines: evaluation of reference genes in different human myocardial regions after left ventricular assist device support. *Cytokine*. 2013;63:113–122. https://doi.org/10.1016/j.cyto.2013.04.021.
69. Sanada S, et al. IL-33 and ST2 comprise a critical biomechanically induced and cardioprotective signaling system. *J Clin Invest*. 2007;117:1538–1549. https://doi.org/10.1172/JCI30634.
70. Caselli, C. et al. IL-33/ST2 pathway and classical cytokines in end-stage heart failure patients submitted to left ventricular assist device support: a paradoxic role for inflammatory mediators? *Mediators Inflamm* 2013;498703. https://doi.org/10.1155/2013/498703.
71. Grosman-Rimon L, et al. Longitudinal assessment of inflammation in recipients of continuous-flow left ventricular assist devices. *Can J Cardiol*. 2015;31:348–356. https://doi.org/10.1016/j.cjca.2014.12.006.
72. Drakos SG, et al. Left ventricular assist device unloading effects on myocardial structure and function: current status of the field and call for action. *Curr Opin Cardiol*. 2011;26:245–255. https://doi.org/10.1097/HCO.0b013e328345af13.
73. Klotz S, Burkhoff D, Garrelds IM, Boomsma F, Danser AH. The impact of left ventricular assist device-induced left ventricular unloading on the myocardial renin-angiotensin-aldosterone system: therapeutic consequences? *Eur Heart J*. 2009;30:805–812. https://doi.org/10.1093/eurheartj/ehp012.
74. Klotz S, et al. Mechanical unloading during left ventricular assist device support increases left ventricular collagen cross-linking and myocardial stiffness. *Circulation*. 2005;112:364–374. https://doi.org/10.1161/CIRCULATIONAHA.104.515106.
75. Koshman YE, et al. Regulation of connective tissue growth factor gene expression and fibrosis in human heart failure. *J Card Fail*. 2013;19:283–294. https://doi.org/10.1016/j.cardfail.2013.01.013.
76. Coromilas E, et al. Dynamics and prognostic role of galectin-3 in patients with advanced heart failure, during left ventricular assist device

support and following heart transplantation. *BMC Cardiovasc Disord.* 2016;16:138https://doi.org/10.1186/s12872-016-0298-z.
77. Lok SI, et al. Myocardial fibrosis and pro-fibrotic markers in end-stage heart failure patients during continuous-flow left ventricular assist device support. *Eur J Cardiothorac Surg.* 2015;48:407–415. https://doi.org/10.1093/ejcts/ezu539.
78. Lok SI, et al. Circulating growth differentiation factor-15 correlates with myocardial fibrosis in patients with non-ischaemic dilated cardiomyopathy and decreases rapidly after left ventricular assist device support. *Eur J Heart Fail.* 2012;14:1249–1256. https://doi.org/10.1093/eurjhf/hfs120.
79. Humphrey JD, Dufresne ER, Schwartz MA. Mechanotransduction and extracellular matrix homeostasis. *Nat Rev Mol Cell Biol.* 2014;15:802–812. https://doi.org/10.1038/nrm3896.
80. Farris SD, et al. Cell-specific pathways supporting persistent fibrosis in heart failure. *J Am Coll Cardiol.* 2017;70:344–354. https://doi.org/10.1016/j.jacc.2017.05.040.
81. Stempien-Otero A, et al. Mechanisms of bone marrow-derived cell therapy in ischemic cardiomyopathy with left ventricular assist device bridge to transplant. *J Am Coll Cardiol.* 2015;65:1424–1434. https://doi.org/10.1016/j.jacc.2015.01.042.
82. Sakamuri SS, et al. Differential impact of mechanical unloading on structural and nonstructural components of the extracellular matrix in advanced human heart failure. *Transl Res.* 2016;172:30–44. https://doi.org/10.1016/j.trsl.2016.02.006.
83. Takawale A, Sakamuri SS, Kassiri Z. Extracellular matrix communication and turnover in cardiac physiology and pathology. *Compr Physiol.* 2015;5:687–719. https://doi.org/10.1002/cphy.c140045.
84. Blaxall BC, Tschannen-Moran BM, Milano CA, Koch WJ. Differential gene expression and genomic patient stratification following left ventricular assist device support. *J Am Coll Cardiol.* 2003;41:1096–1106.
85. Margulies KB, et al. Mixed messages: transcription patterns in failing and recovering human myocardium. *Circ Res.* 2005;96:592–599. https://doi.org/10.1161/01.RES.0000159390.03503.c3.
86. Matkovich SJ, et al. Reciprocal regulation of myocardial microRNAs and messenger RNA in human cardiomyopathy and reversal of the microRNA signature by biomechanical support. *Circulation.* 2009;119:1263–1271. https://doi.org/10.1161/CIRCULATIONAHA.108.813576.
87. de Weger RA, et al. Proteomic profiling of the human failing heart after left ventricular assist device support. *J Heart Lung Transplant.* 2011;30:497–506. https://doi.org/10.1016/j.healun.2010.11.011.
88. Ramani R, et al. A micro-ribonucleic acid signature associated with recovery from assist device support in 2 groups of patients with severe heart failure. *J Am Coll Cardiol.* 2011;58:2270–2278. https://doi.org/10.1016/j.jacc.2011.08.041.
89. Dhar K, et al. Targeted myocardial gene expression in failing hearts by RNA sequencing. *J Transl Med.* 2016;14:327https://doi.org/10.1186/s12967-016-1083-6.
90. D'Amico A, et al. Uncovering the cathepsin system in heart failure patients submitted to left ventricular assist device (LVAD) implantation. *J Transl Med.* 2014;12:350 https://doi.org/10.1186/s12967-014-0350-7.
91. Shahinian JH, et al. Proteomics highlights decrease of matricellular proteins in left ventricular assist device therapy. *Eur J Cardiothorac Surg.* 2017;51:1063–1071. https://doi.org/10.1093/ejcts/ezx023.
92. Barsanti C, et al. Differential regulation of microRNAs in end-stage failing hearts is associated with left ventricular assist device unloading. *Biomed Res Int.* 2015;2015:592512. https://doi.org/10.1155/2015/592512.
93. Akat KM, et al. Comparative RNA-sequencing analysis of myocardial and circulating small RNAs in human heart failure and their utility as biomarkers. *Proc Natl Acad Sci U S A.* 2014;111:11151–11156. https://doi.org/10.1073/pnas.1401724111.
94. Nandi SS, et al. Induction of autophagy markers is associated with attenuation of miR-133a in diabetic heart failure patients undergoing mechanical unloading. *Am J Transl Res.* 2015;7:683–696.
95. Yang KC, et al. Deep RNA sequencing reveals dynamic regulation of myocardial noncoding RNAs in failing human heart and remodeling with mechanical circulatory support. *Circulation.* 2014;129:1009–1021. https://doi.org/10.1161/CIRCULATIONAHA.113.003863.
96. Dangwal S, Schimmel K, Foinquinos A, Xiao K, Thum T. Noncoding RNAs in heart failure. *Handb Exp Pharmacol.* 2017;243:423–445. https://doi.org/10.1007/164_2016_99.
97. Hall JL, et al. Genomic profiling of the human heart before and after mechanical support with a ventricular assist device reveals alterations in vascular signaling networks. *Physiol Genomics.* 2004;17:283–291. https://doi.org/10.1152/physiolgenomics.00004.2004.
98. Rakusan K, Heron MI, Kolar F, Korecky B. Transplantation-induced atrophy of normal and hypertrophic rat hearts: effect on cardiac myocytes and capillaries. *J Mol Cell Cardiol.* 1997;29:1045–1054. https://doi.org/10.1006/jmcc.1996.0350.
99. Lou X, Templeton DL, John R, Dengel DR. Effects of continuous flow left ventricular assist device support on microvascular endothelial function. *J Cardiovasc Transl Res.* 2012;5:345–350. https://doi.org/10.1007/s12265-011-9321-z.
100. Sansone R, et al. Macrovascular and microvascular function after implantation of left ventricular assist devices in end-stage heart failure: role of microparticles. *J Heart Lung Transplant.* 2015;34:921–932. https://doi.org/10.1016/j.healun.2015.03.004.
101. Rogers JG. Changing the carburetor without changing the plugs: the intersection of stock car racing with mechanically assisted circulation. *JACC Heart Fail.* 2015;3:712–714. https://doi.org/10.1016/j.jchf.2015.07.001.
102. Ambardekar AV, et al. Changes in aortic wall structure, composition, and stiffness with continuous-flow left ventricular assist devices: a pilot study. *Circ Heart Fail.* 2015;8:944–952. https://doi.org/10.1161/CIRCHEARTFAILURE.114.001955.
103. Patel AC, et al. Dynamic Changes in Aortic Vascular Stiffness in Patients Bridged to Transplant With Continuous-Flow Left Ventricular Assist Devices. *JACC Heart Fail.* 2017;5:449–459. https://doi.org/10.1016/j.jchf.2016.12.009.
104. Patibandla PK, et al. Evaluation of the effect of diminished pulsatility as seen in continuous flow ventricular assist devices on arterial endothelial cell phenotype and function. *J Heart Lung Transplant.* 2016;35:930–932. https://doi.org/10.1016/j.healun.2016.03.008.
105. Ambardekar AV, et al. Coronary artery remodeling and fibrosis with continuous-flow left ventricular assist device support. *Circ Heart Fail.* 2018;11:e004491. https://doi.org/10.1161/CIRCHEARTFAILURE.117.004491.
106. Moulton KS, et al. PTEN deficiency promotes pathological vascular remodeling of human coronary arteries. *JCI Insight.* 2018;3:https://doi.org/10.1172/jci.insight.97228.
107. Metcalf DJ, Nightingale TD, Zenner HL, Lui-Roberts WW, Cutler DF. Formation and function of Weibel-Palade bodies. *J Cell Sci.* 2008;121:19–27. https://doi.org/10.1242/jcs.03494.
108. Cascone T, Heymach JV. Targeting the angiopoietin/Tie2 pathway: cutting tumor vessels with a double-edged sword? *J Clin Oncol.* 2012;30:441–444. https://doi.org/10.1200/JCO.2011.38.7621.
109. Randi AM, Laffan MA, Starke RD. Von Willebrand factor, angiodysplasia and angiogenesis. *Mediterr J Hematol Infect Dis.* 2013;5:e2013060. https://doi.org/10.4084/MJHID.2013.060.
110. Redondo P, et al. Angiogenic and prothrombotic markers in extensive slow-flow vascular malformations: implications for antiangiogenic/antithrombotic strategies. *Br J Dermatol.* 2010;162:350–356. https://doi.org/10.1111/j.1365-2133.2009.09513.x.
111. Holleran G, Hall B, O'Regan M, Smith S, McNamara D. Expression of Angiogenic Factors in Patients With Sporadic Small Bowel Angiodysplasia. *J Clin Gastroenterol.* 2015;49:831–836. https://doi.org/10.1097/MCG.0000000000000260.
112. Spanier T, et al. Activation of coagulation and fibrinolytic pathways in patients with left ventricular assist devices. *J Thorac Cardiovasc Surg.* 1996;112:1090–1097. https://doi.org/10.1016/S0022-5223(96)70111-3.
113. John R, et al. Activation of endothelial and coagulation systems in left ventricular assist device recipients. *Ann Thorac Surg.* 2009;88:1171–1179. https://doi.org/10.1016/j.athoracsur.2009.06.095.
114. Wagner WR, et al. Thrombin activity resides on LVAD Dacron inflow and outflow grafts. *ASAIO J.* 1992;38:M634–M637.
115. Tabit CE, et al. Elevated Angiopoietin-2 Level in Patients With Continuous-Flow Left Ventricular Assist Devices Leads to

Altered Angiogenesis and Is Associated With Higher Nonsurgical Bleeding. *Circulation*. 2016;134:141–152. https://doi.org/10.1161/CIRCULATIONAHA.115.019692.
116. Tabit CE, et al. Tumor necrosis factor-α levels and non-surgical bleeding in continuous-flow left ventricular assist devices. *J Heart Lung Transplant*. 2018;37:107–115. https://doi.org/10.1016/j.healun.2017.06.001.
117. Kim G, et al. *J Heart Lung Transplant*. 2018;37:S71.
118. Futreal PA, Liu Q, Shattuck-Eidens D, et al. BRCA1 mutations in primary breast and ovarian carcinomas. *Science*. 1994;266:120–122.
119. Miki Y, Swensen J, Shattuck-Eidens D, et al. A strong candidate for the breast and ovarian cancer susceptibility gene BRCA1. *Science*. 1994;266:66–71.
120. Goldgar DE, Cannon-Albright LA, Oliphant A, et al. Chromosome 17q linkage studies of 18 Utah breast cancer kindreds. *Am J Hum Genet*. 1993;52:743–748.
121. Keating M, Atkinson D, Dunn C, Timothy K, Vincent GM, Leppert M. Linkage of a cardiac arrhythmia, the long QT syndrome, and the Harvey ras-1 gene. *Science*. 1991;252:704–706.
122. Drakos SG, Pagani FD, Lundberg MS, Baldwin JT. Advancing the science of myocardial recovery with mechanical circulatory support: a working group of the National, Heart, Lung, and Blood Institute. *JACC Basic Transl Sci*. 2017;2:335–340.

10

Current Types of Devices for Durable Mechanical Circulatory Support

Igor D. Gregoric, Francisco A. Arabia

KEY POINTS

DEVELOPMENT OF MECHANICAL CIRCULATORY SUPPORT SYSTEMS

The methods for providing mechanical circulatory support (MCS) have varied greatly. The evolution of MCS technology has been gradual, as the biological barriers to progress have remained constant and difficult.[1] Clinicians and engineers have collaborated for many years to develop an array of devices that range from very small catheter-mounted devices to fully implantable total cardiac replacement systems (Table 10.1). This variety of device types is necessary to support the vast and complex needs of a heart failure population. Although considerable progress has been made in recent years with medical technology and medical care, the future of heart failure treatment remains complex and dynamic. MCS is increasingly a key component of heart failure management.

Various types of blood pumps have evolved as the development of smaller, biocompatible, and durable devices continue. Fig. 10.1 provides a concise timeline of MCS technology development. The modern era of MCS began in the early 1950s when cardiopulmonary bypass was first used to support patients during open heart operations for the repair of congenital heart defects.[2,3] As the field of cardiac surgery proliferated through the 1960s, it became apparent that there was a need for MCS beyond the operating room. Patients with cardiogenic shock needed temporary circulatory support to avoid organ failure and to allow time for recovery of myocardial function. Counterpulsation with the intraaortic balloon pump (IABP) was introduced in 1968 as a means to augment cardiac function by improving cardiac output and decreasing myocardial work.[4] Since that time, the IABP has supported large numbers of patients with heart failure. During this early era, it was also realized that some form of long-term circulatory support was necessary to treat the expanding heart failure population. Cardiac replacement with heart transplantation or a total artificial heart (TAH) and temporary support with a left ventricular assist device (LVAD) were attempted in a small number of cases during the 1960s,[5–7] but the dismal results led to a suspension of these treatments, and researchers continued developing MCS technologies.

Throughout the 1970s, researchers continued to work on developing artificial heart technology with the goal of providing near total circulatory support with an implantable device for durations of many years.[8] Because of immunologic barriers, a heart transplant was not an effective therapy; thus, developers believed that MCS systems must replace cardiac function and closely mimic the function of the natural heart. Therefore, early devices were large and bulky but could provide up to 10 L/min of cardiac output with a stroke volume and pump rate in the normal physiologic range. Early in the 1980s, heart transplantation was renewed with the development of effective immunosuppressive therapy, and MCS technology had undergone over a decade of research and development. Under the direction and funding support from the National Heart Lung and Blood Institute, pulsatile blood pumps for use as a TAH or ventricular assist device (VAD) were developed for clinical evaluation. Clinical trials for bridge to transplant (BTT) and bridge to recovery (BTR) with LVADs were initiated as a consequence of the limitations of heart transplantation. At the same time, the TAH was implanted in a small number of patients as destination therapy (DT) and for BTT, with mixed results.[9,10]

Axial flow blood pumps were first introduced in the late 1980s, with a catheter-mounted device that was inserted either percutaneously via the femoral artery or directly through an open chest to the left ventricle and across the aortic valve.[11] Clinical studies demonstrated that continuous blood flow generated by a miniature pump was feasible and that there may be a broader application of this type of pump.[12] The early concerns of excessive hemolysis from these small devices were eventually dispelled as clinical results indicated that this type of pump caused clinically tolerable damage to blood components. In the 1990s, implantable axial flow devices were developed due to the need for smaller and more reliable devices for long-term support. Having a single moving component and durable bearings, these devices have proven to provide long-term support with a low incidence of mechanical pump failure. The smaller size of these devices and their improved durability have contributed to a reduction in life-threatening complications and enhanced survival.[13,14] Recent LVAD designs have centrifugal flow pumps that utilize magnetic and/or hydrodynamic bearings to eliminate friction and wear of the rotating impeller. This type of pump design is used in both short- and long-term MCS systems. With the miniaturization of the centrifugal and axial flow blood pumps and improved catheter designs, LVADs that are inserted percutaneously are now being used for first-line support of patients with cardiogenic shock.

TABLE 10.1 Mechanical Circulatory Support Systems Currently for Chronic Support

Device Name	Manufacturer	Type of Pump	Type of Support	Pump Position
HeartMate II	Abbott, Chicago, IL	Axial flow, mechanical bearing	LVAD	Preperitoneal pocket
HeartMate 3	Abbott, Chicago, IL	Centrifugal flow, magnetic bearing	LVAD	Intrapericardial
HVAD	HeartWare Inc., Framingham, MA	Centrifugal flow; magnetic and hydrodynamic bearings	LVAD	Intrapericardial
Jarvik 2000	Jarvik Heart Inc., New York, NY	Axial flow with blood-immersed bearings	LVAD	Left Ventricle
InCor	Berlin Heart, Berlin, Germany	Axial flow with blood-immersed bearings	LVAD	Preperitoneal pocket
Evaheart	Evaheart Inc., Houston, TX	Centrifugal flow; hydrodynamic bearing	LVAD	Preperitoneal pocket
EXCOR	Berlin Heart, Woodlands, TX	Pneumatic, pulsatile, diaphragm	BiVAD	Paracorporeal
Syncardia TAH	Syncardia Inc., Tucson, AZ	Pneumatic, pulsatile, diaphragm	Biventricular replacement	Intrapercardial

BiVAD, Biventricular assist device; *LVAD*, left ventricular assist device; *TAH*, total artificial heart.

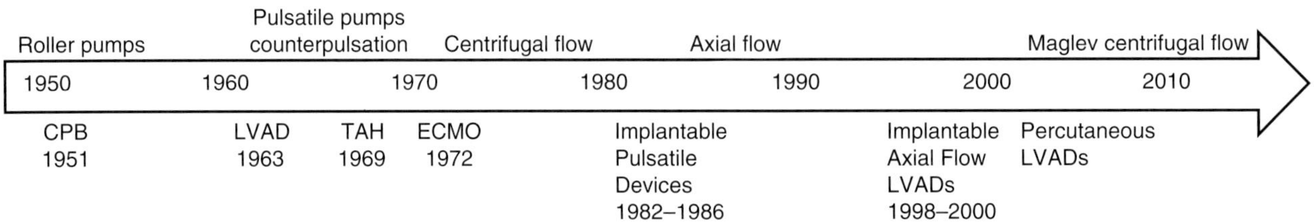

Fig. 10.1 Timeline showing the evolution of the various types of blood pumps used for mechanical circulatory support. *CPB*, Cardiopulmonary bypass; *ECMO*, extracorporeal membrane oxygenation; *LVAD*, left ventricular assist device; *TAH*, total artificial heart.

The best treatment option for patients with end-stage heart failure has been heart transplantation. However, the shortage of donor organs has encouraged the continued development of MCS systems for long-term use. Furthermore, the persistent high mortality rate of cardiogenic shock requires that MCS devices be inserted rapidly and with minimal invasiveness. Since their invention in the 1950s, MCS with VADs and artificial hearts has matured substantially, with outcomes approaching that of a heart transplant.

DURABLE LEFT VENTRICULAR ASSIST DEVICES

During the 1980s and 1990s, the efficacy of implantable pulsatile VADs as BTT, BTR, and DT was established in patients with severe acute and chronic heart failure. Also, in this era, although to a smaller degree, the TAH was used in some centers for BTT in patients with obvious biventricular failure when other treatment options were not suitable. The HeartMate IP-1000, VE, and XVE left ventricular assist system (LVAS) (Abbott Laboratories, formerly Thoratec Corp., Abbott Park, IL) and the Novacor LVAS (Baxter Healthcare Corporation, formerly Worldheart, Deerfield, IL) underwent clinical trials for BTT indication and received market approval based on improved survival.[15–18] The HeartMate XVE was then studied for DT in the Randomized Evaluation of Mechanical Assistance for the Treatment of Congestive Heart failure (REMATCH) trial, where it was demonstrated that device therapy was superior to medical therapy with regard to survival; however, adverse event rates were high, leading to low adoption of this therapy.[19] The Thoratec paracorporeal VAD (pVAD) system offered versatility for univentricular or biventricular support to a wide range of patient sizes due to positioning of the blood pumps on the anterior abdomen.[20,21] All of these devices saved many lives; however, bleeding, infection, pump thrombosis, and device failure were complications that limited the overall effectiveness of the therapy.[22] As the need for smaller and more durable devices became more apparent, manufacturers responded by developing continuous-flow pumps—the primary type of device used today.[23] Examples and descriptions of these devices follow.

HeartMate II LVAS

The HeartMate II (Abbott Laboratories) LVAD is an implantable, axial flow LVAD that is intended for long-term support for BTT and DT in patients with chronic heart failure. When implanted, the pump resides in a preperitoneal pocket below the left hemidiaphragm, with the inflow cannula in the left ventricle and the outflow graft anastomosed to the ascending aorta (Fig. 10.2). A percutaneous driveline from the pump exits the right upper quadrant of the abdomen. The system includes a controller, a power base unit, a system monitor, rechargeable batteries, and a battery clip. A microprocessor-based controller, worn by the patient, monitors and controls the pump's function. The device can provide up to 10 L/min of cardiac output support with a speed operating range of 6000 to 15,000 rpm. The usual operating speed range is 8000 to 10,000 rpm. Power is provided by both AC and DC power sources, with wearable batteries for ambulatory operation. A system monitor is used to make changes in pump speed, collect data on device function, and display pump parameters in the acute care setting.

This implantable LVAD device has been the most widely used in recent years. Clinical trials for BTT and DT have demonstrated that the use of this device is safe and effective when used for these indications.[13,24,25] The BTT clinical trial for the HeartMate II included 489 patients, with published results of the initial 133 patients,[24] and an 18-month follow-up analysis was completed on 281 patients.[13] The 1-year survival rate was 68% in the initial 133 patient cohort, increasing to 73% in the follow-up analysis that included a larger number of subjects (n = 281). The HeartMate II DT trial was a 2:1 randomized comparison against the HeartMate XVE LVAD in 200 patients (HeartMate II, n = 134, and HeartMate XVE LVAD, n = 66).[25] In this trial, the primary study endpoint was 2-year survival free of disabling stroke and reoperation for pump replacement. A significantly higher percentage of patients supported by the HeartMate II reached the primary endpoint as compared to the patients randomized to the HeartMate XVE LVAD. The actuarial 1- and 2-year survival rates of the HeartMate II were 68% and 58%, respectively and significantly, than the 1- and 2-year survival rates for the HeartMate XVE LVAD.

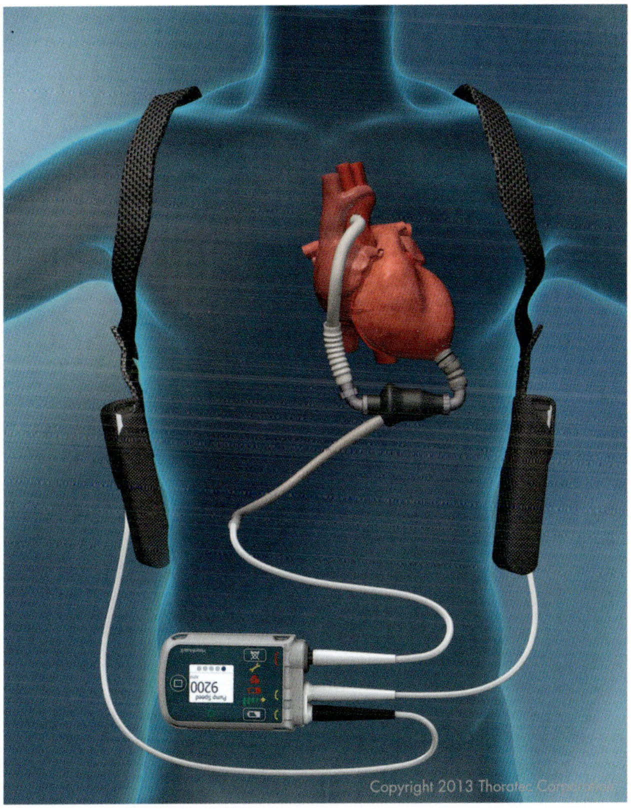

Fig. 10.2 The HeartMate II Left Ventricular Assist System. (HeartMate II is a trademark of Abbott or its related companies. Reproduced with permission of Abbott, © 2019. All rights reserved.)

Postmarket studies for the BTT indication showed that the overall 1-year survival rate increased from 76% during the clinical trial to 85% in the postmarket study.[26] This increase in survival rate was attributed to better patient selection and the timing of LVAD implant. Earlier use of the LVAD resulted in fewer adverse events during support.[27] Similarly, for DT patients supported by the HeartMate II, postmarket 2-year survival rates increased to 62% compared to 58% during the trial.[28] Again, the posttrial patients had fewer adverse events, most likely due to the better timing of implantation and improved patient management.

The Interagency Registry for Mechanically Assisted Circulatory Support (INTERMACS) maintains a database of patients implanted with durable MCS systems that have received market approval.[22] In 2012, the registry reported that a subset of patients, most of whom were implanted with the HeartMate II for DT, had early 1- to 2-year survival rates compared to that of heart transplantation.[29] The INTERMACS registry has also demonstrated that survival rates for patients with continuous-flow devices have continued to improve over time with recent 1- and 2-year survival rates of over 80% and 70%, respectively.

In addition to better survival rates for both BTT and DT indication, a number of postmarket clinical studies have demonstrated improved functional status and quality of life during support with the HeartMate II.[30–34] The Risk Assessment and Comparative Effectiveness of LVAD and Medical Management in Ambulatory Heart Failure Patients (ROADMAP) was a prospective, multicenter, nonrandomized, controlled observational trial of 200 patients with advanced New York Heart Association (NYHA) class III–IIIB or ambulatory NYHA class IV symptoms who received treatment with either optimal medical management or a HeartMate II.[35] The results of the ROADMAP study demonstrated that patients receiving the LVAD experienced higher rates of adverse events but had better functional status and 2-year survival rates as compared to patients maintained on optimal medical management.[36,37] However, overall survival was similar in both groups when patients in the medical arm of the study that subsequently received an LVAD were included in the follow-up analysis.

With improved outcomes, the rate of implants with the HeartMate II has increased considerably since market approval. However, in 2011, an increased rate of pump thrombosis was reported by Starling and colleagues.[38] These finding were corroborated in a subsequent national analysis through INTERMACS.[39] Pump thrombosis has an important effect on morbidity and cost due to the need for exchange of the device and subsequent recovery from the operation. The increase in pump thrombosis was believed to be multifactorial, including changes in anticoagulation therapy and lower pump speed.[40] Some studies indicated that a lower anticoagulation regimen than recommended in the pivotal clinical trials levels was safe; however, a widespread change in practice may have been detrimental, leading to a higher incidence of pump thrombosis.[41,42] In addition, gastrointestinal bleeding became a prominent complication that was often treated with lower anticoagulation therapy.[43–46] A set of pump thrombosis prevention guidelines was developed and then studied prospectively at 24 medical centers.[47] These prevention guidelines included surgical implant techniques to maintain unobstructed blood flow paths, an anticoagulation protocol that increased coagulation parameters, and pump speeds greater than 9000 rpm. With strict adherence to these prevention guidelines, the rate of pump thrombosis decreased.[47]

HeartMate 3 LVAS

The HeartMate 3 LVAS (Abbott Laboratories) is the most recent generation of HeartMate devices that is intended to support patients as BTT or for lifetime DT (Fig. 10.3). This system was designed for enhanced

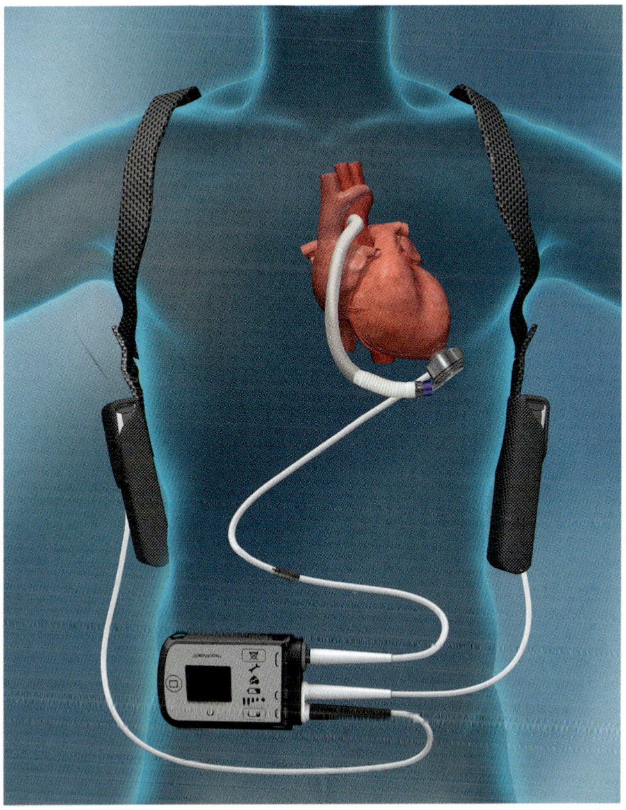

Fig. 10.3 HeartMate 3 Left Ventricular Assist System. (HeartMate 3 is a trademark of Abbott or its related companies. Reproduced with permission of Abbott, © 2019. All rights reserved.)

hemocompatibility to reduce thrombosis and hemolysis.[48] The centrifugal blood pump incorporates a fully magnetically levitated rotor with wide blood-flow gaps, which minimize shear forces on blood components, thereby possibly reducing damage to red blood cells and von Willebrand factor. The rotor is the single moving component that contains no mechanical bearings, thereby eliminating wear, friction, and heat generation within the pump, important for reduction of thrombogenicity. Less hemolysis is thought to minimize thrombosis within the pump and preserve von Willebrand factor, which may help to lower the incidence or severity of gastrointestinal bleeding during support. The blood contacting surfaces within the pump are textured to allow adhesion of circulating cells and the development of a nonthrombogenic tissue lining. The device can provide 2.5–10 L/min of cardiac output support with a speed operating range of 3000 to 9000 rpm. Importantly, the device can operate in an artificial-pulse mode, which enables the rotor to change speed every two seconds in order to generate a pulse wave.

The HeartMate 3 LVAS was first introduced in 2014 for short- or long-term support of patients with advanced stage heart failure.[49] The Conformité Europėene (CE) mark clinical study included 50 patients implanted with the HeartMate 3 at 10 centers in Australia, Austria, Canada, Czech Republic, Germany, and Kazakhstan.[50] Study inclusion criteria included adult heart failure patients with an ejection fraction ≤25%, cardiac index <2.2 L/min/m^2 while not taking inotropes, or inotrope-dependent status while on optimal medical management. This study did not use BTT or DT indications as criteria for inclusion. At the 6-month study endpoint, 92% of patients were alive, exceeding the 88% performance goal. Physical status and quality of life were improved for most patients, with 43 patients being discharged from the hospital. There were no instances of hemolysis, pump thrombosis, or device failure. The 1-year follow-up analysis demonstrated satisfactory survival with no new adverse events. These study data resulted in the device receiving the European Union's certification mark.

The Multicenter Study of MagLev Technology in Patients Undergoing Mechanical Circulatory Support Therapy With HeartMate 3 (MOMENTUM 3) clinical trial conducted in the United States was a randomized, controlled, noninferiority investigation comparing outcomes of the HeartMate 3 and HeartMate II.[51] Candidates for this study were NYHA class III–IV patients who were receiving optimal medical therapy with a left ventricular ejection fraction <25%, were inotrope dependent or had a cardiac index <2.2 L/min/m^2 without inotropes, and were failing to respond to optimal medical therapy for 45 of the past 60 days, or had advanced heart failure for the prior 14 days with at least 7 days of IABP support. The study design is unique in that the endpoints do not distinguish between the separate indications of BTT, DT, or recovery. The primary study endpoint was a composite of survival to transplant, recovery, or a specified duration of LVAS support, free of debilitating stroke or reoperation to replace the pump.

In the short-term follow-up study, 86.2% of patients supported by the HeartMate 3 (n = 151) met the primary endpoint of survival free of disabling stroke (Modified Rankin Scale [MRS] >3) or reoperation to replace or remove the device at 6 months after implantation. The HeartMate 3 showed noninferiority to HeartMate II LVAS (n = 138), as 76.8% of the HeartMate II LVAS patients met the primary endpoint. Survival at 6 months with the HeartMate 3 was 89% and was consistent with the results of the CE mark study.[52]

The long-term follow-up study included 190 patients implanted with the HeartMate 3 and 176 with the HeartMate II. The composite primary endpoint was 2-year survival free of disabling stroke or survival free of reoperation to replace or remove a malfunctioning device.[53] The primary endpoint was reached by 151 patients (79.5%) in the HeartMate 3 group as compared with 106 (60.2%) in the HeartMate II group. Reoperation for device malfunction occurred in three (1.6%) patients with the HeartMate 3 and 30 (17%) patients with the HeartMate II (P=0.001). The rate for suspected or confirmed pump thrombosis remained very low for the HeartMate 3 (1.1%) compared to the HeartMate II (15.7%), whereas the rates for all strokes and ischemic strokes were statistically lower for the HeartMate 3 group (P=0.002 and P=0.003, respectively). The long-term follow-up analysis of this trial revealed that the HeartMate 3 was superior to the HeartMate II with regard to a composite primary endpoint of survival free of disabling stroke or reoperation to replace or remove a malfunctioning device.

Studies have demonstrated that the HeartMate 3 offers improved hemocompatibility over other devices. One small study showed that the HeartMate 3 preserves von Willebrand multimeres better than the HeartMate II does, a factor attributed to the high incidence of gastrointestinal bleeding with continuous-flow LVADs.[54] However, in the clinical studies, the incidence of gastrointestinal bleeding has not been different between the HeartMate 3 and HeartMate II. In a substudy of the MOMENTUM trial, fewer hemocompatibility-related adverse events (i.e., thrombosis and stroke) were reported with the HeartMate 3, likely contributing to better outcomes.[55]

The Food and Drug Administration (FDA) approved the premarket approval application for HeartMate 3 in 2017 to be used as a short-term hemodynamic support system, and approval for long-term support is pending.

HeartWare HVAD

The HeartWare Ventricular Assist Device (HVAD) (Medtronic, HeartWare Inc.) is a centrifugal flow pump that is implanted in the pericardial space at the apex or diaphragmatic surface of the left ventricle (Fig. 10.4). A short integral inflow cannula and the small size of

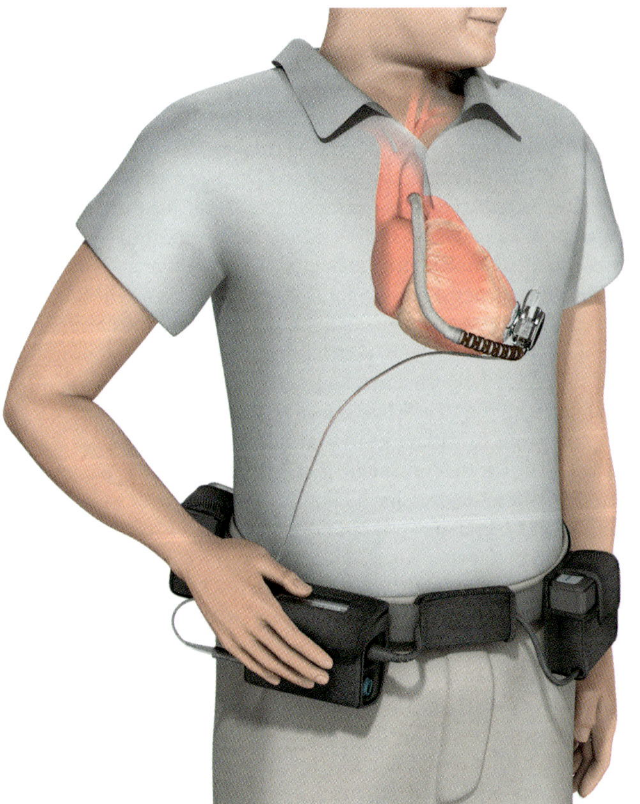

Fig. 10.4 The implanted HeartWare Ventricular Assist Device. (Reproduced with permission of Medtronic, Inc.)

the pump allow for pericardial positioning and avoidance of a pump pocket. The HVAD can generate up to 10 L/min of continuous blood flow with a pump speed operating range of 1800 to 4000 rpm. The pump contains a wide-blade impeller that is suspended by magnetic and hydrodynamic forces for frictionless rotation of the impeller.[56] The frictionless movement of the impeller minimizes heat generation and component wear. An external microprocessor-based system controller connected to the pump by a percutaneous driveline controls and monitors the implanted device. Suction detection and alternating speed modes are automatically maintained by the controller, but their use is determined by the operator. An LED display on the controller provides information on pump operating parameters and alarm conditions. A system monitor can make changes in operating parameters and collect data regarding pump function. The device can operate with AC or DC power sources. Lithium-ion batteries are used during ambulatory operation and an automobile DC adaptor allows for extended travel time.

The HVAD system was initially evaluated for BTT in a multicenter, prospective study in patients with end-stage heart failure. Patients ($n = 332$) were followed for ≥180 days following implantation or until cardiac transplantation, device removal for recovery, or death. The 180-day and 1-year survival rate was 94% and 86%, respectively.[57] Despite excellent survival rates and an adverse event profile similar to other studies, pump thrombosis was seen in 14% of patients, and the incidence of stroke was 15.3%, indicating that complications with this device exist and its use must be closely monitored. Early in the trial, the device was modified to incorporate a textured inflow conduit to help reduce device thrombosis. In addition, during the trial, the recommended anticoagulation therapy was adjusted to include an increase in aspirin dosage from 81 mg/day to 325 mg/day.[58] With the good overall survival, improved quality of life, and declining thrombotic adverse event rates, market approval for the BTT indication was gained in 2012. The Prospective, Randomized, Controlled, Unblinded, Multi-Center Clinical Trial to Evaluate the HeartWare Ventricular Assist Device System for Destination Therapy of Advanced Heart Failure (ENDURANCE DT) trial for the HVAD was conducted from 2010 to 2012 and included 446 patients who were randomized to either the HVAD or HeartMate II in a 2:1 ratio. The primary endpoint was 2-year survival free from disabling stroke (MRS ≥4). The outcome was not statistically or clinically different between HeartMate II and HVAD, 57.4% versus 55%, respectively. Importantly, more patients with the HeartMate II device required replacements due to malfunction or device failure (16.2% vs. 8.8%), while patients receiving the HVAD had a higher incidence of strokes (29.7% vs. 12.1%).[59] It was determined that careful management of anticoagulation and antiplatelet therapy with good blood pressure control was necessary to minimize neurologic adverse events during support with the HVAD device.[60,61] Results of a supplemental study that investigated the influence of blood pressure control on stroke incidence were recently published. The supplemental trial did not demonstrate noninferiority of HVAD versus control in regards to the primary endpoint of reduction of mean arterial blood pressure. However, HVAD subjects reached the composite endpoint (freedom from death, disabling stroke, and device replacement or urgent transplantation) at a higher rate than controls.[62]

Due to the small size of the HVAD pump and its intrapericardial placement, a number of variations for implantation have been evaluated. Placement of the inflow conduit through the diaphragmatic surface of the left ventricle and minimally invasive techniques may offer some advantages in reducing adverse events.[63–67] The HVAD has also been implanted for biventricular support or as part of a hybrid biventricular system.[68–75]

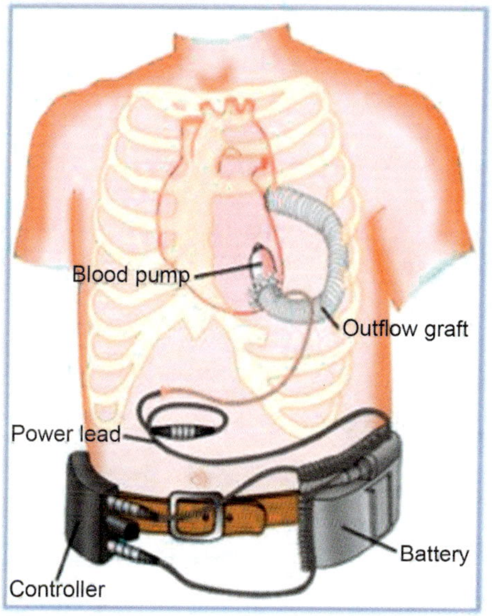

Fig. 10.5 The Jarvik 2000 left ventricular assist device (LVAD).

Jarvik 2000

The Jarvik 2000 LVAD (Jarvik Heart Inc.) is a small axial flow device in which the blood pump is uniquely positioned within the left ventricular cavity (Fig. 10.5). Outflow from the pump is through a graft that is anastomosed to either the ascending or the descending aorta. A percutaneous driveline that exits the skin in the right upper quadrant of the abdomen provides the means for power and control to the blood pump. An analog controller provides a display of alarm conditions and allows for adjustment of the pump speed from 8000 to 12,000 rpm in increments of 1000. Patients are allowed to make speed changes as their requirement for support changes. However, there is no method for monitoring the pump flow with this device. The Jarvik LVAD uses only DC battery power; AC power sources are needed to recharge batteries. There are portable lithium ion batteries for ambulatory operation and larger lead-acid batteries are for nonambulatory use.

The Jarvik 2000 has been in clinical trials for BTT approval for approximately a decade. Although the clinical trials have not been completed, numerous reports indicate that outcomes have been largely positive.[76–78] A multicenter study in Japan had 1- and 2-year survival rates of 85% and 79%, respectively.[79] Patients have been successfully supported by this device for durations greater than 7 years, with no device failures, and the mean survival time for patients supported for DT is 402 days.[80] A unique skull-pedestal power cable connector appears to allow for long-term use with a low incidence of driveline infections. An early report described an observed high incidence of gastrointestinal bleeding in patients supported by this device,[81] and this observation was later made in patients supported by the HeartMate II.[82] Detailed analysis of patients supported by axial flow devices indicates that the gastrointestinal bleeding is related to acquired von Willebrand disease.[83–85] This form of von Willebrand disease may be shear induced and may be a characteristic of continuous-flow devices. The Jarvik LVAD has also undergone a number of design enhancements and miniaturization for pediatric use.[86] Currently, the Jarvik LVAD does not have market approval in the United States, but it is used for both BTT and DT in Europe and Asia.

Berlin Heart INCOR

The INCOR LVAD (Berlin Heart GmbH) is an implantable pump that is intended for long-term support for BTT or DT (Fig. 10.6). The unique design feature of this axial flow pump is the contact-free impeller, which

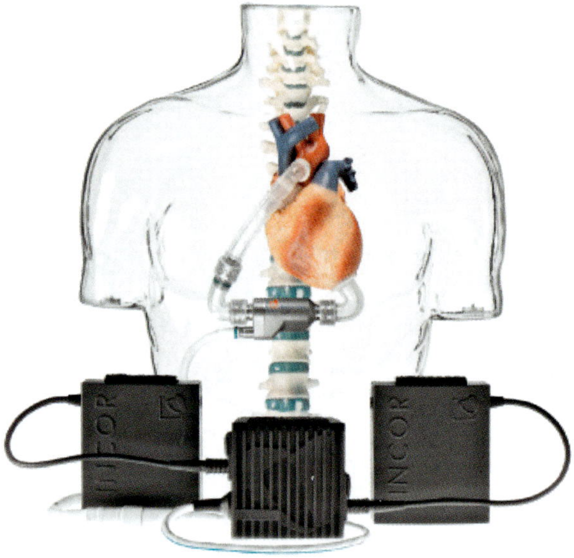

Fig. 10.6 Berlin INCOR left ventricular assist device.

is unlike other axial flow pumps that utilize blood-immersed bearings. The pump has a displacement volume of 82 mL and weighs 200 g. Active and passive magnetic force is used to suspend and rotate the impeller along the axis of the cylindrical pump housing. The operational impeller speed range is 5000 to 10,000 rpm. The pump is positioned below the left hemidiaphragm in a pump pocket with the inflow in the left ventricle and the outflow is attached to the ascending aorta. The blood contacting surfaces are coated with Carmeda to reduce thrombogenicity. A percutaneous driveline connects to an external controller that monitors and controls the function of the implanted pump. The device is powered by AC or DC sources, with small batteries for portable operation. A laptop computer interfaced with the controller sets the operating parameters.

The INCOR device was developed for long-term support and has been used for DT, BTT, and BTR.[87–89] This device has been used mainly in Europe and has not been tested in controlled trials in the United States. Clinical results indicate that hemodynamic support, incidence of adverse events, and outcomes are similar to those of other axial flow and pulsatile LVADs.[89–91] Use of the INCOR device appears to be minimal, with a very small number of reported cases in recent years.[92,93]

Berlin Heart EXCOR Pediatric Ventricular Assist Device

The Berlin Heart EXCOR Pediatric (Berlin Heart GmbH and Berlin Heart Inc., Berlin, Germany) is a small pVAD with a pneumatically powered diaphragm pump that can provide univentricular or biventricular support for weeks to months in children as small as 3 kg (Fig. 10.7).[94,95] Available blood pump sizes are 10, 15, 25, and 30 mL stroke volume for pediatric patients and larger pumps with 50, 60, and 80 mL stroke volume for larger patients. Selection of pump size is based on the patient's

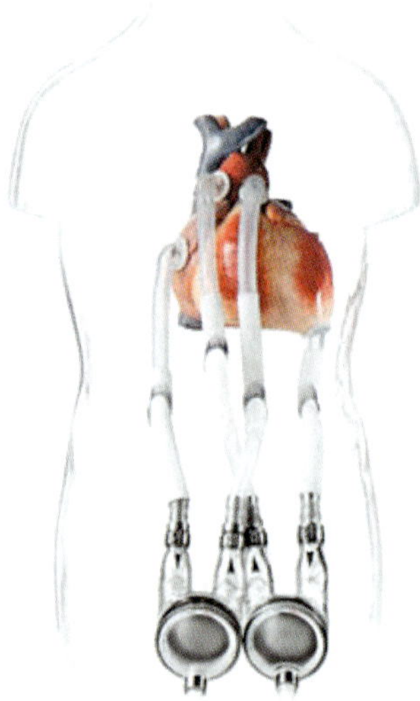

A

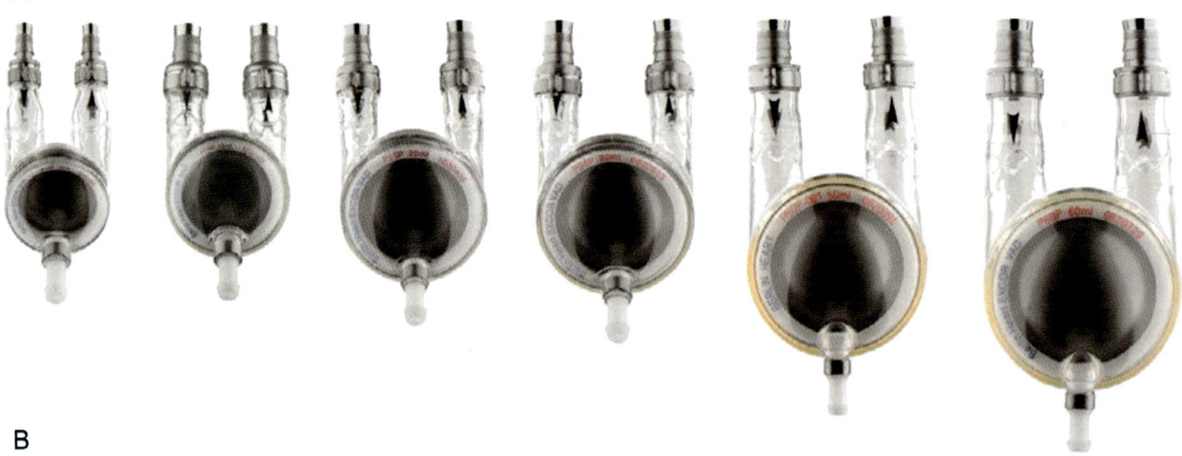

B

Fig. 10.7 Berlin Heart EXCOR. (A) Cannulation configuration for biventricular support. (B) Variety of pump sizes available.

weight: <9 kg patients have pump stroke volumes of 10 mL; 10–25 kg patients have pumps with a stroke volume of 25 or 30 mL; and patients weighing >30 kg use the adult sizes (50, 60, and 80 mL). Cannulation often depends on mediastinal anatomy, the size of the pump, and prior surgical procedures; thus, a variety of cannula sizes may be used. Direct cannulation and unloading of the ventricle are desirable, and outflow cannulas are normally placed in the main pulmonary artery and aorta. The cannula(s) are externalized through the anterior abdominal wall and connected to the extracorporeally positioned pump. Portable and stationary pneumatic drive consoles provide power and control of the pumps. Ambulation is encouraged early after implantation, and children who use the portable drive console resume an active life.

The EXCOR VAD was first implanted in an 8-year-old boy in 1990,[96] with expanded use in pediatrics after small blood pump sizes were introduced in 1992.[94] The EXCOR has been used continuously in Europe since that time and is the most widely used device for pediatric BTT. There has been a gradual increase in use in the United States. A Humanitarian Use Device Exemption was approved by the FDA in 2011, and an Investigational Device Exemption study was also initiated.[95] The US clinical trial compared the outcomes of patients implanted with the EXCOR (n = 24) for BTT to those of historical controls treated with extracorporeal membrane oxygenation (ECMO) (n = 48).[97] The primary endpoint for the VAD-treated patients was the time to death or weaning from the device with an unacceptable neurologic outcome. The most common serious adverse events were major bleeding (42% VAD; 50% ECMO), infection (63% VAD; 50% ECMO), stroke (29% for both VAD and ECMO), and hypertension (50% VAD; 33% ECMO). At 30 days, 33% of ECMO-treated patients had died, whereas in the VAD-treated group the mortality rate was 4%. Furthermore, 88% of the VAD-supported patients underwent transplantation by 6 months. On the basis of superior survival for the VAD-supported patients, market approval for the EXCOR was gained for pediatric BTT in June 2017. For pediatric patients waiting for transplantation, bridging with the EXCOR VAD is preferred to other forms of MCS.[98]

EVAHEART LVAS

The EVAHEART LVAS (Sun Medical Technologies, Corp., and Evaheart, Inc.) includes a titanium blood pump with a 40-mm diameter impeller driven by a brushless, direct current motor (Fig. 10.8). The impeller's hydrodynamically levitated bearing rotates without friction, eliminating wear and heat generation. A unique feature of this pump is the recirculating cooling system; the spinning impeller is levitated within a thin layer of water, which lubricates and cools the shaft. Blood flow through the pump is exposed to low shear stress due to the wide cross-sectional area within the pump and the relatively large diameter inflow and outflow conduits (16 mm). The inflow conduit is inserted into the left ventricle at the apex and the outflow graft is anastomosed to the ascending aorta. The pump can generate pulsatile arterial blood flow greater than 15 L/min at 1800 to 2400 rpm, with a pulse pressure of 15 to 30 mm Hg. The implanted pump is connected to an external power and control unit with a driveline externalized through the patient's abdominal wall. Rechargeable lithium-ion batteries can provide up to 12 hours of continuous support.

A prospective noncontrolled clinical trial for BTT was conducted in Japan from 2005 to 2008 in 18 patients.[99] The 6-month and 1-year survival rate was 89% and 83%, respectively. Fifteen patients were discharged from the hospital and experienced significant improvement in the quality of life. In a posttrial registry study involving 96 transplant eligible patients, the survival rate with support was 93% at 6 months, 87% at 1 year, and 87% at 2 years.[100] Serious adverse events were driveline infection (14.6%), ischemic stroke (17.7%), bleeding (13.5%), pump thrombosis (1%), and hemolysis (1%). There was a low incidence of gastrointestinal bleeding, right heart failure, pump thrombosis, and device failure.

After regulatory approval for BTT in Japan was granted, Evaheart Inc. formed a North American branch to expand the market. As of early 2018, an Investigational Device Exemption study in the United States is underway and CE mark approval in Europe is pending. The device has been slightly modified with a smaller blood pump, controller, and inflow cannula.

SynCardia Total Artificial Heart

The SynCardia temporary TAH-t (SynCardia Systems, LLC, Tucson, AZ) is the only device available that replaces the failing ventricles with intracorporeal, pneumatic, pulsatile ventricles, each with a volume of 70 cc (Fig. 10.9).[101] Implanting diagnoses have evolved over time to include failing heart transplant (acute or chronic), restrictive and infiltrative cardiomyopathy, congenital anomalies, malignant arrhythmias that do not respond to other interventions, large post-infarction ventricular septal defects, partial ventricular thrombosis, cardiac malignancies, and Chagas disease.[101–104] Rebridging with a temporary Total Artificial Heart (TAH-t) has been successful in some patients who experience LVAD/biventricular assist device failure. It is approved as a BTT therapy by the FDA and the CE Mark. There is currently

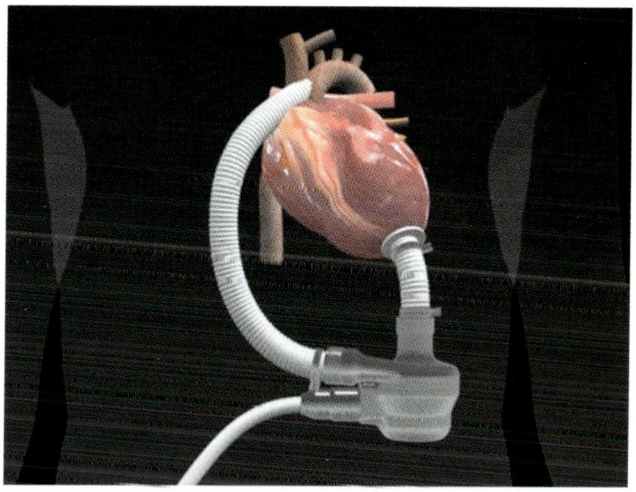

Fig. 10.8 The Evaheart Left Ventricular Assist System.

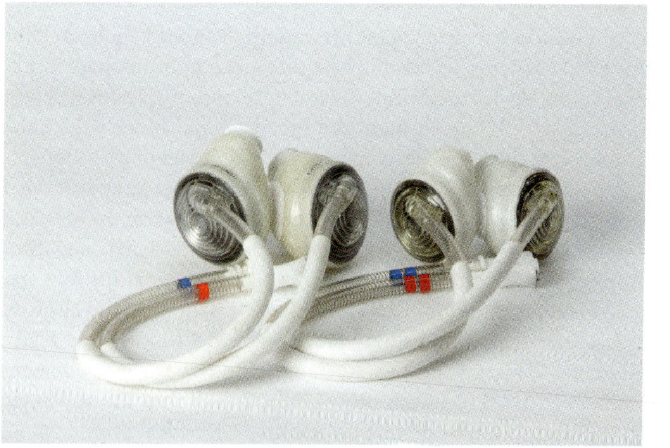

Fig. 10.9 Syncardia total artificial heart. Courtesy of Syncardia: https://urldefense.proofpoint.com/v2/url?u=http-3A__syncardia.com&d=DwIGaQ&c=o3PTkfaYAd6-No7SurnLt5qpge1aKYwPQyBFS7c8AA0&r=FBuXc-9xQ3rDss6MqtpFMM5kaX1CT38lmVaRYeJLxOg&m=CnY96lsBhF7Zb1vbbar--Vt7ZiHM8GicpevKnr4xPIE&s=_jUsLVf9PF6h7k9t8-NwDebh0zgv9gNxCBkTpfYSB88&e.

a trial for a 50cc TAH and a DT trial for the 70cc. The TAH-t allows for patients to be discharged home with the Freedom Driver.[105] A new generation of a more portable and soundless driver is forthcoming.

An INTERMACS analysis showed that patients who receive the TAH-t are generally sicker (patient profile 1 and 2) than patients who received LVADs (more frequently patient profiles 2 and 3).[106] One or more characteristics of RV failure were present in 82% of patients implanted with TAH-t. INTERMACS analysis shows that center experience with the TAH-t (particularly with >10 implants) is an essential determinant of success, with no discernible difference in the level of patient sickness at the time of implantation. The 1- and 2-year survival according to Kaplan-Meier estimates were 53.2% and 33.9%, respectively.[106] Hazard function analysis showed an early rapidly decreasing risk that merged with a constant phase at about 4 months. By competing outcomes analysis, the overall rate of transplantation was 53%, mortality was 34%, and 13% were alive on a device by 12 months. Survival outcome was highest for patients with an INTERMACS profile of 3. Among centers implanting more than 10 TAH-t during the period of study, 58% of patients received a heart transplant within 12 months, versus 43% in lower-volume centers.

The major period of risk for mortality with the TAH-t is the first 3 months. Center experience with the TAH-t (particularly with >10 implants) is an essential determinant of success, with no discernible difference in the level of patient sickness at the time of implantation.[106] The most common cause of death is multisystem organ failure (36% of deaths), followed by neurologic injury (18%) and elective withdrawal of support (12%). Successful bridging to heart-kidney transplantation has been performed with the TAH-t.

The increase in mortality with patients in cardiogenic shock (patient profile 1) has led to a decrease in the proportion of such patients receiving LVAD devices. The recent increase in the use of short-term MCS has proven to be encouraging for the severely ill patient in cardiogenic shock as a bridge to decision and durable LVAD.[107,108] However, this use is associated with an increase in early mortality, in part because of unrecognized RV failure. The encouraging survival in this patient subset with the TAH-t, particularly with sufficient center experience, provides support for consideration of the TAH as an alternative to the use of right- or left-sided VADs in patients with severe biventricular failure.

FUTURE DIRECTIONS OF MECHANICAL CIRCULATORY SUPPORT

Major advances have been made in treating advanced stage heart failure with LVAD systems, leveraging new directions in technology innovations. Future device modifications and novel system designs will target expansion of VAD application to a broader population, reduction of adverse event rates, and development of durable right heart support.

Support of children with congenital heart disease and advanced heart failure using biocompatible and safe long-term LVADs is an ongoing challenge. Recently, the National Heart, Lung, and Blood Institute, Jarvik Heart Inc., and New England Research Institute partnered to initiate the PumpKIN (Pumps for Kids, Infants, and Neonates) clinical trial that will evaluate the Jarvik 2015 for BTT or BTR in children.[109] This prospective single-arm study began enrollment in October of 2018. Preclinical studies indicate that the fully implantable Jarvik device may have a more favorable adverse event profile than the EXCOR; specifically, it may be less thrombogenic due to its valveless continuous-flow configuration and possibly have greater resistance to infection because of its intracorporeal position. Other possibilities for durable LVAD support in children, excluding infants, are the HVAD and HeartMate 3 devices, which accommodate patients with small body size.[110,111] Both Medtronic and Abbott are developing small blood pumps that could be implanted in small children for durable support.

Infectious complications have been consistent with all implantable MCS systems.[112] Infections greatly increase hospital time and increase mortality, limiting the overall effectiveness of therapy. There are two approaches in device development that may have an important impact in reducing infection complications. First, smaller pumps can be implanted less invasively, reducing surgical trauma and the likelihood of surgical wound infection. Recent studies have demonstrated that both the HVAD and HeartMate 3 can be implanted safely with less invasive approaches.[113] Second, totally implantable systems that do not have drivelines penetrating the skin are necessary to eliminate late infections that seriously add to morbidity and mortality.[114] Transcutaneous energy transmission to provide power and control to the internal pump could drastically reduce infections and the total cost of care for LVAD-supported patients.[115]

Right heart failure is also a persistent problem both early and late following LVAD implantation. Presently, there is no durable VAD for isolated right heart support that can be used either temporarily or long-term. Because of small size, the HVAD and HeartMate II devices have been applied for biventricular support with varying success.[70,116,117] In most cases, catheter-mounted or extracorporeal temporary devices are used and weaned when possible. Ideally, a VAD could be used for right heart support temporarily or with long-term LVAD support.

The Heart114Mate 3 LVAS has superior hemocompatibility, with a low incidence of thrombosis and hemolysis and better preservation of von Willebrand factor. However, stroke remains a challenge, and more research is needed in the area of hemocompatibility. Devices in the future may be miniaturized even further, but there must be a commitment to optimizing hemocompatibility. Ideally, devices in the future will be smaller, with less biomaterial-blood interaction, incorporate transcutaneous energy transfer, and utilize less invasive implantation techniques, particularly for isolated right heart support

The concept of TAH continues to evolve as more efficient drivers are developed for the SynCardia TAH-t. The CARMAT TAH has initiated a trial in Europe.[119] The BiVACOR TAH incorporates a design utilizing magnetic levitation technology that can generate continuous or pulsatile flow.[118] The quest for a long-term heart replacement continues with designs in the form of the ReinHeart TAH,[120] CCFTAH,[48] OregonHeart TAH,[121] Helical Flow TAH,[122] and a hybrid CF-TAH (50).[123]

SUMMARY

Substantial progress has been made in treating heart failure with durable VADs and TAHs, which now creates the challenge to reduce adverse events to lower morbidity. As clinical experience progresses, and as more devices become available, more heart failure patients will be treated with MCS. Increased availability in regions where the incidence of heart failure deaths is high is essential to leveraging the potential impact of MCS on the growing heart failure population.

REFERENCES

1. Holman WL, Teitel ER, Itescu S. Biologic barriers to mechanical circulatory support. In: Frazier OH, Kirklin JK, eds. *Ishlt Monograft Series*. New York: Elsevier; 2006:9–32.
2. Dennis C, Gorayeb EJ, Iticovici HN, et al. The artificial heart-lung apparatus, experimental creation and repair of interventricular septal defects. *Surg Forum*. 1956;6:185–189.
3. Gibbon JH Jr. Application of a mechanical heart and lung apparatus to cardiac surgery. *Minn Med*. 1954;37:171–185.
4. Kantrowitz A, Tjonneland S, Krakauer J, et al. Clinical experience with cardiac assistance by means of intraaortic phase-shift balloon pumping. *Trans Am Soc Artif Intern Organs*. 1968;14:344–348.

5. Liotta D, Hall CW, Henly WS, Cooley DA, Crawford ES, Debakey ME. Prolonged assisted circulation during and after cardiac or aortic surgery. Prolonged partial left ventricular bypass by means of intracorporeal circulation. *Am J Cardiol.* 1963;12:399–405.
6. DeBakey ME. Left ventricular bypass pump for cardiac assistance. Clinical experience. *Am J Cardiol.* 1971;27:3–11.
7. Cooley DA, Liotta D, Hallman GL, Bloodwell RD, Leachman RD, Milam JD. Orthotopic cardiac prosthesis for two-staged cardiac replacement. *Am J Cardiol.* 1969;24:723–730.
8. Szycher M, Clay W, Gernes D, Sherman C. Thermedics' approach to ventricular support systems. *J Biomater Appl.* 1986;1:39–105.
9. Gunby P. Utah group to implant 'Jarvik 7' heart soon. *JAMA.* 1982;248. 1944, 1946.
10. Copeland JG, Smith RG, Icenogle TB, Rhenman B, Williams R, Vasu MA. Early experience with the total artificial heart as a bridge to cardiac transplantation. *Surg Clin North Am.* 1988;68:621–634.
11. Frazier OH, Nakatani T, Duncan JM, Parnis SM, Fuqua JM. Clinical experience with the hemopump. *ASAIO Trans.* 1989;35:604–606.
12. Wiebalck AC, Wouters PF, Waldenberger FR, et al. Left ventricular assist with an axial flow pump (hemopump): clinical application. *Ann Thorac Surg.* 1993;55:1141–1146.
13. Pagani FD, Miller LW, Russell SD, Aaronson KD, et al. HeartMate II Investigators. Extended mechanical circulatory support with a continuous-flow rotary left ventricular assist device. *J Am Coll Cardiol.* 2009;54:312–321.
14. Kormos RL, Teuteberg JJ, Pagani FD, et al. Continuous flow left ventricular assist device: incidence, risk factors, and impact on outcomes. *J Thorac Cardiovasc Surg.* 2009; in press.
15. Frazier OH, Rose EA, McCarthy P, et al. Improved mortality and rehabilitation of transplant candidates treated with a long-term implantable left ventricular assist system. *Ann Surg.* 1995;222:327–336, discussion 336-328.
16. Poirier VL. The heartmate left ventricular assist system: worldwide clinical results. *Eur J Cardiothorac Surg.* 1997;11(Suppl):S39–S44.
17. Frazier OH, Rose EA, Oz MC, et al. Multicenter clinical evaluation of the HeartMate vented electric left ventricular assist system in patients awaiting heart transplantation. *J Thorac Cardiovasc Surg.* 2001;122:1186–1195.
18. Portner PM, Jansen PG, Oyer PE, Wheeldon DR, Ramasamy N. Improved outcomes with an implantable left ventricular assist system: a multicenter study. *Ann Thorac Surg.* 2001;71:205–209.
19. Rose EA, Gelijns AC, Moskowitz AJ, et al. Long-term mechanical left ventricular assistance for end-stage heart failure. *N Engl J Med.* 2001;345:1435–1443.
20. Hill JD, Farrar DJ, Hershon JJ, et al. Bridge to cardiac transplantation: successful use of prosthetic biventricular support in a patient awaiting a donor heart. *ASAIO Trans.* 1986;32:233–237.
21. Hill JD, Farrar DJ, Hershon JJ, et al. Use of a prosthetic ventricle as a bridge to cardiac transplantation for postinfarction cardiogenic shock. *N Engl J Med.* 1986;314:626–628.
22. Kirklin JK, Naftel DC, Stevenson LW, et al. INTERMACS database for durable devices for circulatory support: first annual report. *J Heart Lung Transplant.* 2008;27:1065–1072.
23. Kirklin JK, Naftel DC, Pagani FD, et al. Seventh INTERMACS annual report: 15,000 patients and counting. *J Heart Lung Transplant.* 2015;34:1495–1504.
24. Miller LW, Pagani FD, Russell SD, et al. HeartMate II Clinical Investigators. Use of a continuous-flow device in patients awaiting heart transplantation. *N Engl J Med.* 2007;357:885–896.
25. Slaughter MS, Rogers JG, Milano CA, et al. HeartMate II Clinical Investigators. Advanced heart failure treated with continuous-flow left ventricular assist device. *N Engl J Med.* 2009;361:2241–2251.
26. John R, Naka Y, Smedira NG, et al. Continuous flow left ventricular assist device outcomes in commercial use compared with the prior clinical trial. *Ann Thorac Surg.* 2011;92:1406–1413, discussion 1413.
27. Starling RC, Naka Y, Boyle AJ, et al. Results of the post-U.S. Food and Drug administration-approval study with a continuous flow left ventricular assist device as a bridge to heart transplantation: a prospective study using the INTERMACS (Interagency Registry for Mechanically Assisted Circulatory Support). *J Am Coll Cardiol.* 2011;57:1890–1898.
28. Jorde UP, Kushwaha SS, Tatooles AJ, et al. Results of the destination therapy post-Food and Drug Administration approval study with a continuous flow left ventricular assist device: a prospective study using the INTERMACS Registry (Interagency Registry for Mechanically Assisted Circulatory Support). *J Am Coll Cardiol.* 2014;63:1751–1757.
29. Kirklin JK, Naftel DC, Pagani FD, et al. Long-term mechanical circulatory support (destination therapy): on track to compete with heart transplantation? *J Thorac Cardiovasc Surg.* 2012;.
30. Allen JG, Weiss ES, Schaffer JM, et al. Quality of life and functional status in patients surviving 12 months after left ventricular assist device implantation. *J Heart Lung Transplant.* 2010;29:278–285.
31. Kiernan MS, Sundareswaran KS, Pham DT, et al. Preoperative determinants of quality of life and functional capacity response to left ventricular assist device therapy. *J Card Fail.* 2016;22:797–805.
32. Starling RC. Improved quantity and quality of life: a winning combination to treat advanced heart failure. *J Am Coll Cardiol.* 2010;55:1835–1836.
33. Kugler C, Malehsa D, Tegtbur U, et al. Health-related quality of life and exercise tolerance in recipients of heart transplants and left ventricular assist devices: a prospective, comparative study. *J Heart Lung Transplant.* 2011;30:204–210.
34. Rogers JG, Aaronson KD, Boyle AJ, et al. Continuous flow left ventricular assist device improves functional capacity and quality of life of advanced heart failure patients. *J Am Coll Cardiol.* 2010;55:1826–1834.
35. Rogers JG, Boyle AJ, O'Connell JB, et al. Risk assessment and comparative effectiveness of left ventricular assist device and medical management in ambulatory heart failure patients: design and rationale of the ROADMAP clinical trial. *Am Heart J.* 2015;169:205–210. e220.
36. Estep JD, Starling RC, Horstmanshof DA, et al. Risk assessment and comparative effectiveness of left ventricular assist device and medical management in ambulatory heart failure patients: results from the ROADMAP study. *J Am Coll Cardiol.* 2015;66:1747–1761.
37. Starling RC, Estep JD, Horstmanshof DA, et al. ROADMAP Study Investigators. Risk assessment and comparative effectiveness of left ventricular assist device and medical management in ambulatory heart failure patients: the ROADMAP study 2-year results. *JACC Heart Fail.* 2017;5:518–527.
38. Starling RC, Moazami N, Silvestry SC, et al. Unexpected abrupt increase in left ventricular assist device thrombosis. *N Engl J Med.* 2014;370:33–40.
39. Kirklin JK, Naftel DC, Pagani FD, et al. Pump thrombosis in the Thoratec HeartMate II device: an update analysis of the INTERMACS Registry. *J Heart Lung Transplant.* 2015;34(12):1515–1526.
40. Mehra MR, Stewart GC, Uber PA. The vexing problem of thrombosis in long-term mechanical circulatory support. *J Heart Lung Transplant.* 2014;33:1–11.
41. Menon AK, Gotzenich A, Sassmannshausen H, Haushofer M, Autschbach R, Spillner JW. Low stroke rate and few thrombo-embolic events after HeartMate II implantation under mild anticoagulation. *Eur J Cardiothorac Surg.* 2012;42:319–323, discussion 323.
42. Rossi M, Serraino GF, Jiritano F, Renzulli A. What is the optimal anticoagulation in patients with a left ventricular assist device? *Interact Cardiovasc Thorac Surg.* 2012;15:733–740.
43. Sponga S, Nalli C, Casonato A, Charbonneau E. Severe upper gastrointestinal bleeding in HeartMate II induced by acquired von Willebrand deficiency: anticoagulation management. *Ann Thorac Surg.* 2012;94:e41-e43.
44. Crow SS, Joyce DD. Are centrifugal ventricular assist devices the answer to reducing post-implantation gastrointestinal bleeding? *JACC Heart Fail.* 2014;2:146–147.
45. Harvey L, Holley CT, John R. Gastrointestinal bleed after left ventricular assist device implantation: incidence, management, and prevention. *Ann Cardiothorac Surg.* 2014;3:475–479.
46. Lopilato AC, Doligalski CT, Caldeira C. Incidence and risk factor analysis for gastrointestinal bleeding and pump thrombosis in left ventricular assist device recipients. *Artif Organs.* 2015;39:939–944.
47. Maltais S, Kilic A, Nathan S, et al. PREVENT Study Investigators. Prevention of HeartMate II pump thrombosis through clinical management: the PREVENT multi-center study. *J Heart Lung Transplant.* 2017;36:1–12.

48. Bourque K, Cotter C, Dague C, et al. Design rationale and preclinical evaluation of the HeartMate 3 left ventricular assist system for hemocompatibility. *ASAIO J*. 2016;62:375–383.
49. Schmitto JD, Hanke JS, Rojas SV, Avsar M, Haverich A. First implantation in man of a new magnetically levitated left ventricular assist device (HeartMate III). *J Heart Lung Transplant*. 2015;34:858–860.
50. Netuka I, Sood P, Pya Y, et al. Fully magnetically levitated left ventricular assist system for treating advanced HF: a multicenter study. *J Am Coll Cardiol*. 2015;66:2579–2589.
51. Heatley G, Sood P, Goldstein D, et al. MOMENTUM 3 Investigators. Clinical trial design and rationale of the Multicenter Study of MagLev Technology in Patients Undergoing Mechanical Circulatory Support Therapy with HeartMate 3 (MOMENTUM 3) investigational device exemption clinical study protocol. *J Heart Lung Transplant*. 2016;35:528–536.
52. Mehra MR, Naka Y, Uriel N, et al. A fully magnetically levitated circulatory pump for advanced heart failure. *N Engl J Med*. 2017;376: 440–450.
53. Mehra MR, Goldstein DJ, Uriel N, et al. MOMENTUM 3 Investigators. Two-year outcomes with a magnetically levitated cardiac pump in heart failure. *N Engl J Med*. 2018;378:1386–1395.
54. Netuka I, Kvasnicka T, Kvasnicka J, et al. Evaluation of von Willebrand factor with a fully magnetically levitated centrifugal continuous-flow left ventricular assist device in advanced heart failure. *J Heart Lung Transplant*. 2016;35:860–867.
55. Uriel N, Colombo PC, Cleveland JC, et al. Hemocompatibility-related outcomes in the momentum 3 trial at 6 months: a randomized controlled study of a fully magnetically levitated pump in advanced heart failure. *Circulation*. 2017;135:2003–2012.
56. Larose JA, Tamez D, Ashenuga M, Reyes C. Design concepts and principle of operation of the HeartWare ventricular assist system. *ASAIO J*. 2010;56:285–289.
57. Slaughter MS, Pagani FD, McGee EC, et al. HeartWare ventricular assist system for bridge to transplant: combined results of the bridge to transplant and continued access protocol trial. *J Heart Lung Transplant*. 2013;32:675–683.
58. Najjar SS, Slaughter MS, Pagani FD, et al. An analysis of pump thrombus events in patients in the HeartWare ADVANCE bridge to transplant and continued access protocol trial. *J Heart Lung Transplant*. 2014;33:23–34.
59. Rogers JG, Pagani FD, Tatooles AJ, et al. Intrapericardial left ventricular assist device for advanced heart failure. *N Engl J Med*. 2017;376:451–460.
60. Willey JZ, Boehme AK, Castagna F, et al. ADVANCE Trial Investigators. Hypertension and stroke in patients with left ventricular assist devices (LVADS). *Curr Hypertens Rep*. 2016;18:12.
61. Teuteberg JJ, Slaughter MS, Rogers JG, et al. The HVAD left ventricular assist device: risk factors for neurological events and risk mitigation strategies. *JACC Heart Fail*. 2015;3:818–828.
62. Milano CA, Rogers JG, Tatooles AJ, et al. ENDURANCE Investigators. HVAD: the ENDURANCE Supplemental Trial. *JACC: Heart Failure*. 2018;6(9):792–802. https://doi.org/10.1016/j.jchf.2018.05.012.
63. Gregoric ID, Cohn WE, Frazier OH. Diaphragmatic implantation of the HeartWare ventricular assist device. *J Heart Lung Transplant*. 2011;30:467–470.
64. Krabatsch T, Drews T, Potapov E, Weng Y, Pasic M, Hetzer R. Different surgical strategies for implantation of continuous-flow VADS-experience from Deutsches Herzzentrum Berlin. *Ann Cardiothorac Surg*. 2014;3: 472–474.
65. Maltais S, Womack S, Davis ME, et al. Surgical considerations and challenges for bilateral continuous-flow durable device implantation. *ASAIO J*. 2016;62:e18-21.
66. Ozbaran M, Yagdi T, Engin C, Nalbantgil S, Ozturk P. Left ventricular assist device implantation with left lateral thoracotomy with anastomosis to the descending aorta. *Interact Cardiovasc Thorac Surg*. 2018;.
67. Hanke JS, Rojas SV, Cvitkovic T, et al. First results of HeartWare left ventricular assist device implantation with tunnelling of the outflow graft through the transverse sinus. *Interact Cardiovasc Thorac Surg*. 2017;25:503–508.
68. Baldwin ACW, Sandoval E, Cohn WE, Mallidi HR, Morgan JA, Frazier OH. Nonidentical continuous-flow devices for biventricular support. *Tex Heart Inst J*. 2017;44:141–143.
69. Ovroutski S, Miera O, Krabatsch T, Berger F, Photiadis J, Potapov E. Two pumps for single ventricle: mechanical support for establishment of biventricular circulation. *Ann Thorac Surg*. 2017;104:e143–e145.
70. Stein ML, Yeh J, Reinhartz O, et al. HeartWare HVAD for biventricular support in children and adolescents: the Standford experience. *ASAIO J*. 2016;62:e46-51.
71. Krabatsch T, Potapov E, Stepanenko A, et al. Biventricular circulatory support with two miniaturized implantable assist devices. *Circulation*. 2011;124:S179-186.
72. Strueber M, Meyer AL, Malehsa D, Haverich A. Successful use of the HeartWare HVAD rotary blood pump for biventricular support. *J Thorac Cardiovasc Surg*. 2010;140:936–937.
73. Loforte A, Montalto A, Della Monica PL, Contento C, Musumeci F. Biventricular support with the HeartWare implantable continuous flow pump: an additional contribution. *J Heart Lung Transplant*. 2010;29:1443–1444.
74. Hetzer R, Krabatsch T, Stepanenko A, Hennig E, Potapov EV. Long-term biventricular support with the HeartWare implantable continuous flow pump. *J Heart Lung Transplant*. 2010;.
75. Arabia FA, Milano CA, Mahr C, et al. Biventricular support with intracorporeal, continuous flow, centrifugal ventricular assist devices. *Ann Thorac Surg*. 2018;105:548–555.
76. Feller ED, Sorensen EN, Haddad M, et al. Clinical outcomes are similar in pulsatile and nonpulsatile left ventricular assist device recipients. *Ann Thorac Surg*. 2007;83:1082–1088.
77. Siegenthaler MP, Frazier OH, Beyersdorf F, et al. Mechanical reliability of the Jarvik 2000 heart. *Ann Thorac Surg*. 2006;81:1752–1758, discussion 1758-1759.
78. Frazier OH, Myers TJ, Westaby S, Gregoric ID. Clinical experience with an implantable, intracardiac, continuous flow circulatory support device: physiologic implications and their relationship to patient selection. *Ann Thorac Surg*. 2004;77:133–142.
79. Kohno H, Matsumiya G, Sawa Y, et al. The Jarvik 2000 left ventricular assist device as a bridge to transplantation: Japanese Registry for Mechanically Assisted Circulatory Support. *J Heart Lung Transplant*. 2018;37:71–78.
80. Westaby S, Siegenthaler M, Beyersdorf F, et al. Destination therapy with a rotary blood pump and novel power delivery. *Eur J Cardiothorac Surg*. 2010;37:350–356.
81. Letsou GV, Shah N, Gregoric ID, Myers TJ, Delgado R, Frazier OH. Gastrointestinal bleeding from arteriovenous malformations in patients supported by the Jarvik 2000 axial-flow left ventricular assist device. *J Heart Lung Transplant*. 2005;24:105–109.
82. Stern DR, Kazam J, Edwards P, et al. Increased incidence of gastrointestinal bleeding following implantation of the HeartMate II LVAD. *J Card Surg*. 2010;25:352–356.
83. Malehsa D, Meyer AL, Bara C, Struber M. Acquired von Willebrand syndrome after exchange of the HeartMate XVE to the HeartMate II ventricular assist device. *Eur J Cardiothorac Surg*. 2009;35:1091–1093.
84. Geisen U, Heilmann C, Beyersdorf F, et al. Non-surgical bleeding in patients with ventricular assist devices could be explained by acquired von Willebrand disease. *Eur J Cardiothorac Surg*. 2008;33:679–684.
85. Yoshida K, Tobe S, Kawata M, Yamaguchi M. Acquired and reversible von Willebrand disease with high shear stress aortic valve stenosis. *Ann Thorac Surg*. 2006;81:490–494.
86. Selzman CH, Koliopoulou A, Glotzbach JP, McKellar SH. Evolutionary improvements in the Jarvik 2000 left ventricular assist device. *ASAIO J*. 2018;.
87. Komoda T, Komoda S, Dandel M, Weng Y, Hetzer R. Explantation of incor left ventricular assist device after myocardial recovery. *J Card Surg*. 2008;23:642–647.
88. Garatti A, Bruschi G, Colombo T, et al. Clinical outcome and bridge to transplant rate of left ventricular assist device recipient patients: comparison between continuous-flow and pulsatile-flow devices. *Eur J Cardiothorac Surg*. 2008;34:275–280, discussion 280.

89. Galantier J, Moreira LF, Benicio A, et al. Hemodynamic performance and inflammatory response during the use of VAD-INCOR as a bridge to transplant. *Arq Bras Cardiol.* 2008;91:327–334.
90. Schmid C, Jurmann M, Birnbaum D, et al. Influence of inflow cannula length in axial-flow pumps on neurologic adverse event rate: results from a multi-center analysis. *J Heart Lung Transplant.* 2008;27:253–260.
91. Schmid C, Tjan TD, Etz C, Schmidt C, et al. First clinical experience with the INCOR left ventricular assist device. *J Heart Lung Transplant.* 2005;24:1188–1194.
92. Camboni D, Zerdzitzki M, Hirt S, Tandler R, Weyand M, Schmid C. Reduction of INCOR driveline infection rate with silicone at the driveline exit site. *Interact Cardiovasc Thorac Surg.* 2017;24:222–228.
93. Pieri M, Muller M, Scandroglio AM, et al. Surgical treatment of mediastinitis with omentoplasty in ventricular assist device patients: report of referral center experience. *ASAIO J.* 2016;62:666–670.
94. Hetzer R, Kaufmann F, Delmo Walter EM. Paediatric mechanical circulatory support with Berlin Heart EXCOR: development and outcome of a 23-year experience. *Eur J Cardiothorac Surg.* 2016;50:203–210.
95. Almond CS, Buchholz H, Massicotte P, et al. Berlin Heart EXCOR pediatric ventricular assist device investigational device exemption study: study design and rationale. *Am Heart J.* 2011;162:425–435. e426.
96. Warnecke H, Berdjis F, Hennig E, et al. Mechanical left ventricular support as a bridge to cardiac transplantation in childhood. *Eur J Cardiothorac Surg.* 1991;5:330–333.
97. Fraser Jr CD, Jaquiss RD, Rosenthal DN, et al. Berlin Heart Study Investigators. Prospective trial of a pediatric ventricular assist device. *N Engl J Med.* 2012;367:532–541.
98. Almond CS, Morales DL, Blackstone EH, et al. Berlin Heart EXCOR pediatric ventricular assist device for bridge to heart transplantation in US children. *Circulation.* 2013;127:1702–1711.
99. Yamazaki K, Saito S, Nishinaka T, et al. Japanese clinical trial results of new generation LVAS EVAHEART. *J Card Fail.* 2009;15:S147.
100. Saito S, Yamazaki K, Nishinaka T, et al. J-MACS Research Group. Post-approval study of a highly pulsed, low-shear-rate, continuous-flow, left ventricular assist device, EVAHEART: a Japanese multicenter study using J-MACS. *J Heart Lung Transplant.* 2014;33:599–608.
101. Copeland JG, Smith RG, Arabia FA, et al. Total artificial heart bridge to transplantation: a 9-year experience with 62 patients. *J Heart Lung Transplant.* 2004;23:823–831.
102. El-Banayosy A, Arusoglu L, Morshuis M, et al. CardioWest total artificial heart: Bad Oeynhausen experience. *Ann Thorac Surg.* 2005;80:548–552.
103. Meyer A, Slaughter M. The total artificial heart. *Panminerva Med.* 2011;53:141–154.
104. Copeland JG, Copeland H, Gustafson M, et al. Experience with more than 100 total artificial heart implants. *J Thorac Cardiovasc Surg.* 2012;143:727–734.
105. Friedline K, Hassinger P. Total artificial heart freedom driver in a patient with end-stage biventricular heart failure. *AANA J.* 2012;80:105–112.
106. Arabia FA, Cantor RS, Koehl DA, et al. Interagency registry for mechanically assisted circulatory support report on the total artificial heart. *J Heart Lung Transplant.* 2018;.
107. Zeriouh M, Mohite P, Raj B, et al. Short-term ventricular assist device as a bridge to decision in cardiogenic shock: is it a justified strategy? *Int J Artif Organs.* 2016;39. 0.
108. den Uil CA, Akin S, Jewbali LS, et al. Short-term mechanical circulatory support as a bridge to durable left ventricular assist device implantation in refractory cardiogenic shock: a systematic review and meta-analysis. *Eur J Cardiothorac Surg.* 2017;.
109. Baldwin JT, Adachi I, Teal J, et al. Closing in on the pumpkin trial of the Jarvik 2015 ventricular assist device. *Semin Thorac Cardiovasc Surg Pediatr Card Surg Annu.* 2017;20:9–15.
110. Miera O, Kirk R, Buchholz H, et al. A multicenter study of the HeartWare ventricular assist device in small children. *J Heart Lung Transplant.* 2016;35:679–681.
111. Adachi I, Burki S, Zafar F, Morales DL. Pediatric ventricular assist devices. *J Thorac Dis.* 2015;7:2194–2202.
112. Goldstein DJ, Naftel D, Holman W, et al. Continuous-flow devices and percutaneous site infections: clinical outcomes. *J Heart Lung Transplant.* 2012;31:1151–1157.
113. Ricklefs M, Hanke JS, Dogan G, et al. Less invasive surgical approaches for left ventricular assist device implantation. *Semin Thorac Cardiovasc Surg.* 2018;.
114. Hernandez GA, Breton JDN, Chaparro SV. Driveline infection in ventricular assist devices and its implication in the present era of destination therapy. *Open J Cardiovasc Surg.* 2017;9:. 1179065217714216.
115. Slaughter MS, Myers TJ. Transcutaneous energy transmission for mechanical circulatory support systems: history, current status, and future prospects. *J Card Surg.* 2010;25:484–489.
116. Potapov EV, Kukucka M, Falk V, Krabatsch T. Biventricular support using 2 HeartMate 3 pumps. *J Heart Lung Transplant.* 2016;35: 1268–1270.
117. Tran HA, Pollema TL, Silva Enciso J, Greenberg BH, Barnard DD, Adler ED. Pretorius VG. Durable biventricular support using right atrial placement of the HeartWare HVAD. *ASAIO J.* 2017;.
118. Mohacsi P, Leprince P. The carmat total artificial heart. *Eur J Cardiothorac Surg.* 2014;.
119. Timms D, Fraser J, Hayne M, Dunning J, McNeil K, Pearcy M. The BiVACOR rotary biventricular assist device: concept and in vitro investigation. *Artif Organs.* 2008;32:816–819.
120. Pelletier B, Spiliopoulos S, Finocchiaro T, et al. System overview of the fully implantable destination therapy—ReinHeart-therapy artificial heart. *Eur J Cardiothorac Surg.* 2015;47:80–86.
121. Glynn J, Song H, Hull B, et al. The OregonHeart total artificial heart: design and performance on a mock circulatory loop. *Artif Organs.* 2017;41:904–910.
122. Abe Y, Isoyama T, Saito I, et al. Animal experiments of the helical flow total artificial heart. *Artif Organs.* 2015;39:670–680.
123. Fox C, Chopski S, Murad N, Allaire P, Mentzer R, Rossano J, et al. Hybrid continuous-flow total artificial heart. *Artif Organs.* 2018;42:500–509.

11

Operative Techniques and Intraoperative Management

Erin M. Schumer, Mark S. Slaughter, Walter Dembitsky

KEY POINTS

Historical Note
Principles of Device Selection
Preoperative Assessment and Preparation
Implant Operation
Intraoperative Considerations
Postoperative Care

HISTORICAL NOTE

The first left ventricular assist device (LVAD) was implanted in 1963 by Dr. DeBakey in a patient with postcardiotomy shock.[1] As the incidence of heart failure rose to epidemic proportions, the LVAD emerged as a new solution to this devastating disease, and superiority over medical treatment was demonstrated in the Randomized Evaluation of Mechanical Assistance for the Treatment of Congestive Heart Failure (REMATCH) trial.[2] The first-generation devices were pulsatile, in an attempt to replicate native cardiac physiology. When compared to medical management alone, therapy with these devices showed improved survival. However, their large size limited patient selection to mainly male patients, required large pneumatic drivers, and demonstrated limited durability.

Thus, second- and third-generation devices were developed using continuous-flow pumps. These devices were smaller, allowing implantation in a broader population including women and children. The improved technology allowed for lengthened battery life, longer support times, and overall better quality of life for patients with advanced heart failure.[3] Continuous-flow devices have continued to dominate the market since their introduction and are implanted in over 90% of patients with advanced heart failure.[4]

PRINCIPLES OF DEVICE SELECTION

Chronic support of the left ventricle (LV) requires long-term reliability and durability, portability, and adequate cardiac flow for active patients. Three devices currently on the market are widely used: the HeartMate II (HMII) LVAS (Abbott, Lake Bluff, IL, USA), the Heartware HVAD (Medtronic, Minneapolis, MN, USA), and the newly approved HeartMate 3 (HM3) LVAS (Abbott, Lake Bluff, IL, USA). All three pumps have inflow cannulas that are placed in the LV apex. The inflow cannula is connected to a pump body, which then is attached to an outflow cannula and graft that is subsequently sewn onto the ascending aorta. An electrical driveline from the pump exits the patient via a subcutaneous tunnel in the upper abdomen.

These pumps differ in several significant ways. The HMII, a second-generation device, uses an axial flow pump and, in general, requires a preperitoneal pocket for placement.[3] Both the HVAD and HM3, third-generation devices, utilize centrifugal flow in a smaller configuration allowing for intrapericardial implantation.[5] While the survival outcomes are similar for the HMII and HVAD,[6] complication rates differ. The HVAD has a higher stroke rate, while the HMII has a higher rate of driveline infection and hemolysis/thrombosis, all with significant clinical impact[7] (see also Chapter 13). The smaller size of the HVAD is more conducive to a minimally invasive approach via thoracotomy, either at the initial operation or if a redo operation is required. Additionally, biventricular configuration of the HVAD has been reported, which is not feasible with the HMII. Early results with the HM3 are promising, as this device appears to have a lower rate of hemolysis/thrombosis. However, survival and disabling stroke rates are similar when compared to the HMII.[8] Ultimately, it appears that device selection must be individualized for each patient, underscoring the importance of patient selection.[9]

PREOPERATIVE ASSESSMENT AND PREPARATION

Indication for LVAD placement varies by individual patient and continues to evolve. Historically, LVAD implantation has been indicated for patients with New York Heart Association Class IV heart failure refractory to medical treatment and may include those patients with intractable arrhythmias and/or angina, end-organ dysfunction attributed to heart failure, or postcardiotomy shock.[10] Patients are classified by therapy goals into bridge to transplantation, destination, bridge to recovery, and bridge to decision therapy.

The Interagency Registry for Mechanically Assisted Circulatory Support (INTERMACS) scoring system is useful to identify appropriate patients and timing of LVAD support.[4] Optimal patient selection is crucial for the success of chronic LVAD implantation and is achieved through an array of diagnostic studies.

Assessment is divided into cardiac and noncardiac considerations. Cardiac considerations include right ventricular (RV) function, valvular function and structure, intracardiac shunting, apical thrombus, and arrhythmias. Transesophageal echocardiography (TEE) is an essential part of the preoperative evaluation. Irreversible, advanced right heart failure is a contraindication to the placement of an isolated LVAD, and these patients may be considered for biventricular ventricular assist devices (VADs), total artificial heart placement, or heart transplantation. Noncardiac considerations include end-organ function (particularly

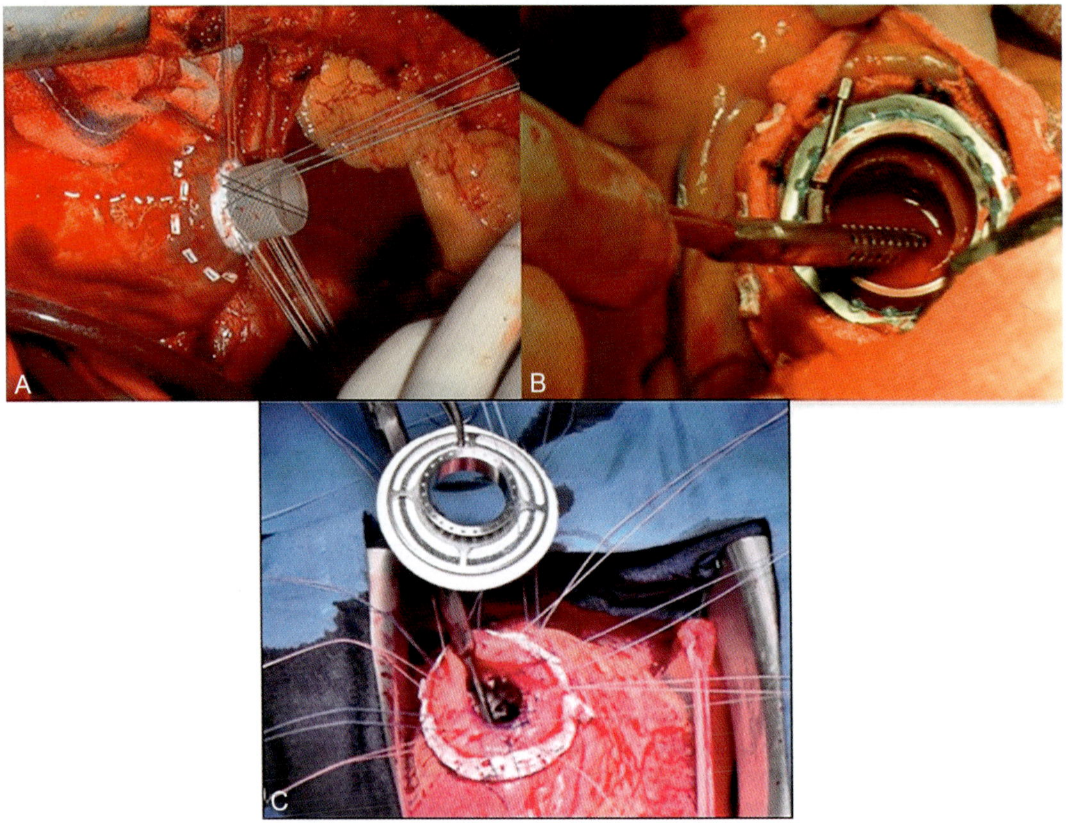

Fig. 11.1 Sutures are placed circumferentially around the left ventricular apex for the sewing ring. The sutures are passed through the sewing ring, and the ring is seated after the sutures are tied down. (A) HeartMate II. (B) HVAD. (C) HeartMate 3.

pulmonary, renal, and hepatic), nutrition, body habitus, and social and psychiatric issues. End-organ function must be optimized through the use of inotropes and potentially intra-aortic balloon pump and/or extracorporeal membrane oxygenation if shock is present.

IMPLANT OPERATION

Hemodynamic monitoring is performed using a pulmonary artery catheter, arterial line, and TEE. After induction and skin preparation, a midline sternotomy incision is performed. A preperitoneal pocket is made using sharp and blunt dissection in the case of HMII implantation. As VAD placements are frequently repeat sternotomies, accurate dissection of the LV from surrounding scar tissue is required. Following this dissection, the patient is systemically heparinized.

Aortic cannulation should be placed as high as possible, close to the arch. Single two-stage venous cannulation will suffice in the majority of cases. If more dissection of the LV is required, it is performed during cardiopulmonary bypass (CPB) with the heart beating but decompressed. The driveline is tunneled percutaneously under the rectus muscle to exit usually over the left upper quadrant of the abdomen and can be done prior to heparinization.

The heart is elevated, bringing the LV to the midline of the wound. Pledgeted braided polyester sutures are placed from the myocardium through the sewing ring around a chosen spot for the inflow cannula (Fig. 11.1), which must point toward the mitral valve and parallel to the septum (Fig. 11.2). The sutures are then placed through the sewing ring, which is then seated and tied down. In the case of HMII implantation, coring can be performed prior to placement of the sewing ring.

The patient is placed in the Trendelenburg position in preparation for coring. Strong suction is maintained on an aortic needle vent to capture any air that may be ejected from the ventricle. The heart is emptied and a cruciate incision is made at the apex. The coring tool is used to perform the left ventriculotomy (Fig. 11.3), removing a core of LV muscle. The ventricle is inspected for crossing fibers, thrombus, or obstructing muscle, which, if identified, is removed or resected. Once clear, the heart is deaired, and the inflow cannula of the pump is inserted (Fig. 11.4). Continuous surveillance for air in the ascending

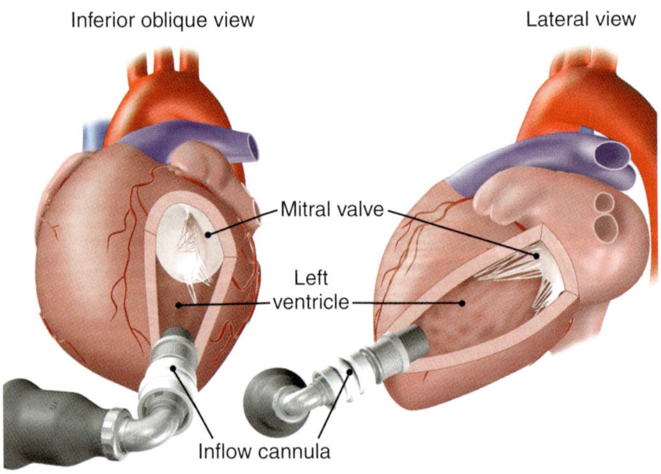

Fig. 11.2 Proper placement of the inflow cannula within the left ventricle. (Reproduced with permission from Slaughter M. Chapter 11: Surgical methods for mechanical circulatory support. In: Kormos RL, Miller LW, eds. *Mechanical Circulatory Support: A Companion to Braunwald's Heart Disease Ebook*. Elsevier Health Sciences; 2011: 141–152.)

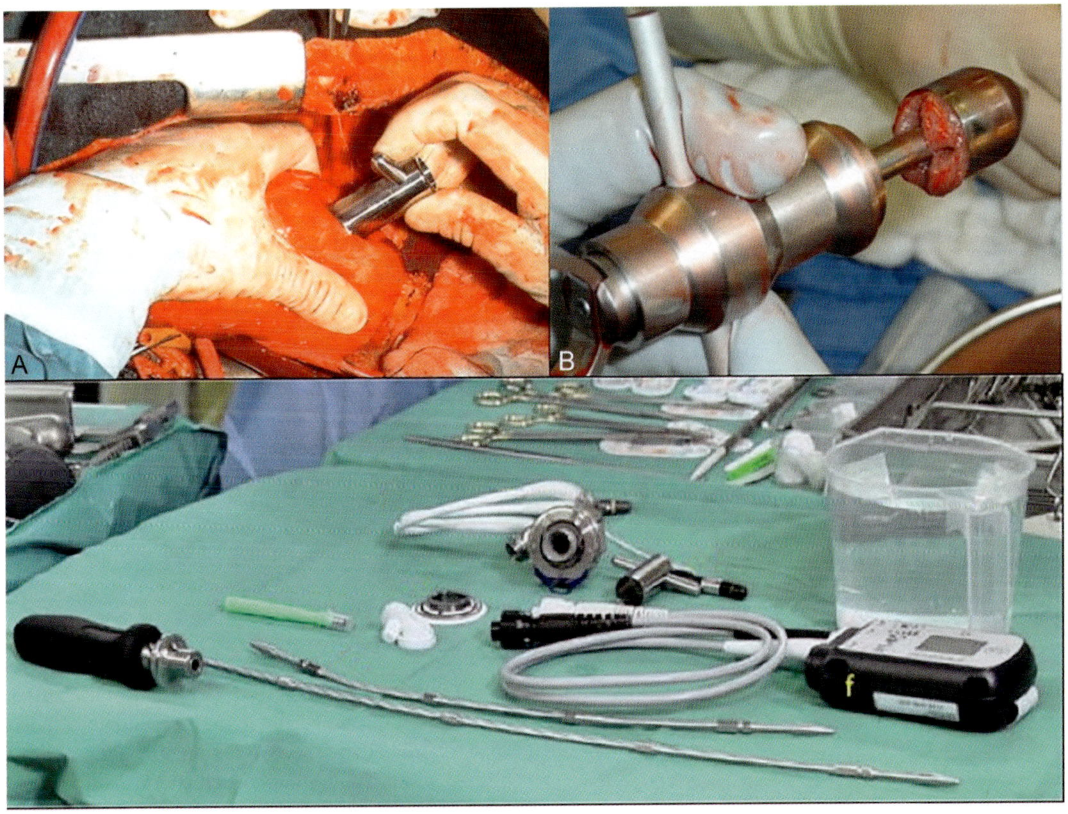

Fig. 11.3 Coring is performed using the coring tool. (A) HeartMate II. (B) HVAD. (C) HeartMate 3.

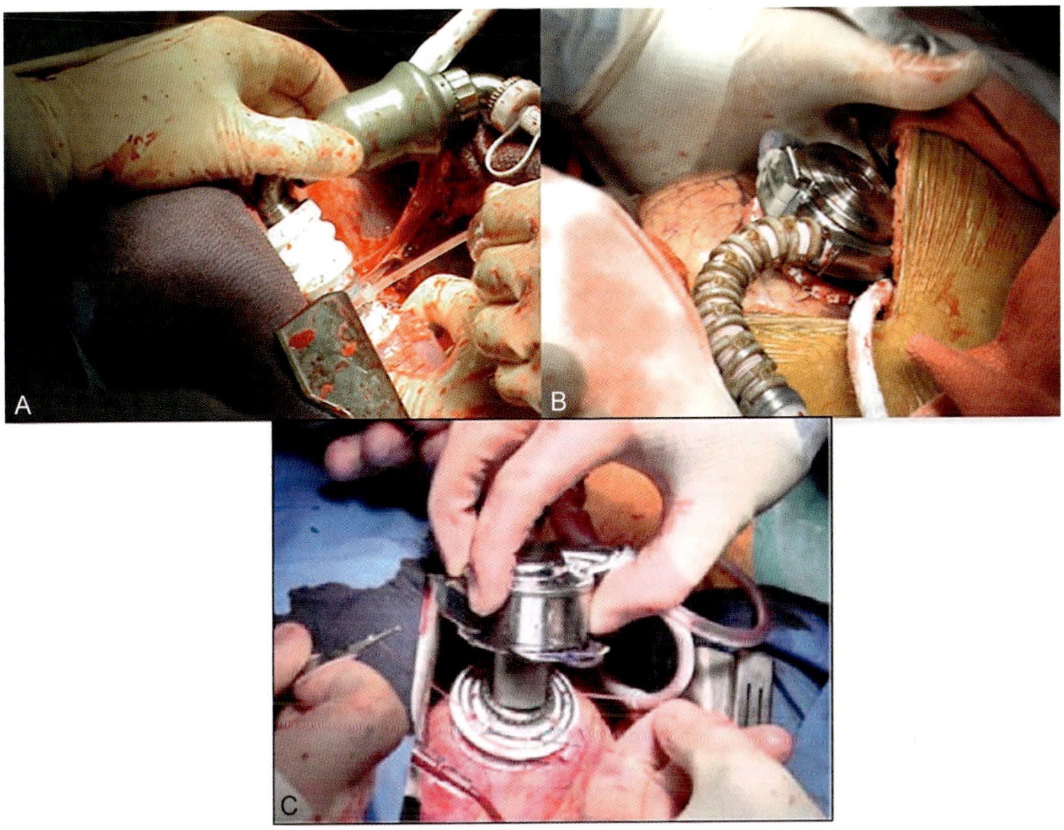

Fig. 11.4 The inflow cannula of the pump is inserted into the ventriculotomy and secured within the sewing ring. (A) HeartMate II. (B) HVAD. (C) HeartMate 3.

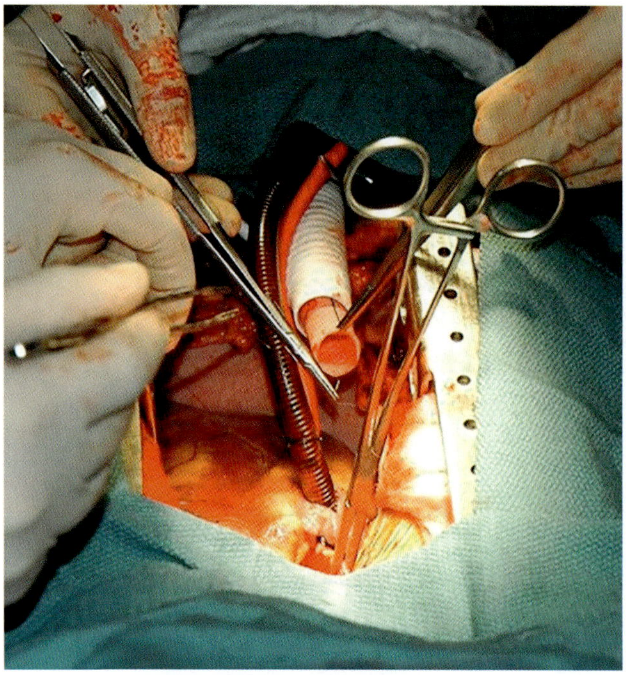

Fig. 11.5 The aortic anastomosis is performed using a running Prolene suture in an end-to-side fashion.

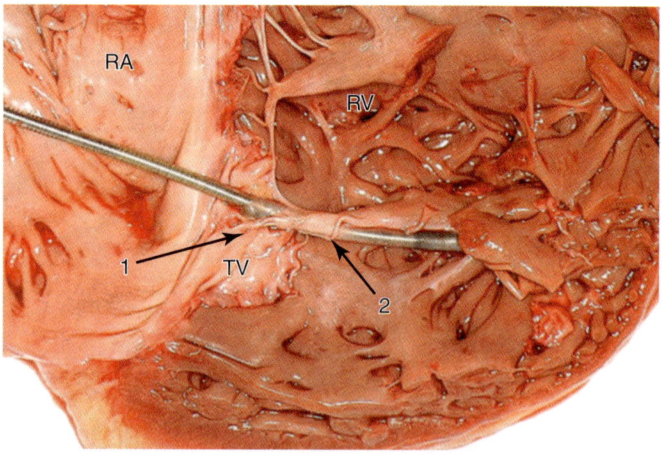

Fig. 11.6 Transvalvular pacing wires with associated destruction of the tricuspidseptal leaflet and the subvalvular mechanism (2). *RA*, Right atrium; *RV*, right ventricle (1); *TV*, tricuspid valve. (Reproduced with permission from Dembitsky W, Naka Y. Chapter 11. In: Kormos RL, Miller LW, eds. *Mechanical Circulatory Support: A Companion to Braunwald's Heart Disease Ebook*. Elsevier Health Sciences; 2011:153–164.)

aorta is maintained by the echocardiographer or anesthesiologist during this portion of the operation. The pump is secured after proper orientation is confirmed, and the heart is then placed back in normal anatomic position in the chest.

Further deairing is then performed through the outflow graft. The bend relief and outflow graft can be placed inside a 20-mm woven Dacron graft for further protection during subsequent explant for transplantation. The graft is then measured, clamped, and cut. A partial occluding clamp is placed on the greater curvature of the ascending aorta. After aortotomy, the outflow graft is anastomosed to the ascending aorta with continuous polypropylene suture (Fig. 11.5).

Normal ventilation is resumed, and inhaled nitric oxide or prostaglandin and inotropes are initiated. The driveline is passed off the field and connected to the system controller. Following rewarming to normothermia, thorough deairing of the heart and pump is again performed, and CPB is weaned while increasing the LVAD pump speed to achieve adequate flow.

After weaning from CPB, the right heart should be assessed before reversing heparin. Pulmonary hypertension by itself is not an indication for RV support unless accompanied by RV failure. Destabilizing bleeding, with ongoing transfusion requirement, will often lead to RV failure and should be corrected before weaning from bypass. Protamine infusion is administered, and the patient is decannulated. Left pleural, mediastinal, and right pleural drains are inserted. Once adequate hemostasis is achieved, the chest is closed.

INTRAOPERATIVE CONSIDERATIONS

Valvular Incompetence and Repair

The intraoperative management of native valvular incompetence during LVAD insertion remains an area of controversy. The expected duration of LVAD support and patient characteristics both influence the decision to repair insufficient native valves. However, since the duration of support can never be certain, it seems advisable to correct severe forms of aortic, mitral, and tricuspid insufficiency at the time of implantation, especially if the physiologic response to LV support appears unlikely to improve the insufficiency, and if it can be accomplished without additional mortality and morbidity.[11] During and after LVAD implantation, both the right and the left native valves are subjected to new demands that can influence their performance acutely and chronically. In general, a greater likelihood of recovery should prompt serious consideration for repair of severely insufficient atrioventricular or aortic valves. However, consensus has not been reached on the specific indications for repair.

Tricuspid Regurgitation

Correction of tricuspid regurgitation (TR) reinforces the integrity of the RV pumping complex, which comprises the RV and the pulmonary vascular resistance (PVR). Tricuspid insufficiency in LVAD recipients is multifactorial; advancing age, chronic atrial fibrillation, and pulmonary hypertension with chronic right heart pressure and volume overload can all dilate the tricuspid annulus.[12] In patients with a compliant interventricular septum, increased venous return to the right heart following LVAD insertion can be accompanied by a septal shift to the left. The increased RV volume can exacerbate existing TR. The TR in LVAD recipients is also often worsened by the adverse effects of the transvalvular lead components of automatic internal cardioverter defibrillators and pacemakers (Fig. 11.6). Both the incidence and the degree of TR increase with the number and size of the transvalvular leads.[13] These leads can develop clots within days, inflammation within weeks, and sclerosis within a year. Usually, the posterior leaflet is affected. Perforation can occur, as can entanglement of the subvalvular apparatus. Secondary TR may abate over time if the LV–LVAD complex is functioning properly and is accompanied by important reduction in pulmonary hypertension and pulmonary insufficiency.

An INTERMACS analysis reported a 40% incidence of moderate to severe TR at the time of implantation.[14] The impact of surgical treatment of TR on survival and functional outcome has not been established. The controversy is confounded by the finding that moderate–severe TR is a marker for less good survival post implantation, but in two multi-institutional studies, tricuspid valve repair did not improve short or longer term survival,[14–16] suggesting that moderate to severe

TR is a marker for greater derangement of RV function. Furthermore, moderate to severe TR usually improves with LVAD implant alone, since reactive pulmonary hypertension and RV afterload are reduced.[14] Some data suggest that leaving severe TR is associated with worsening RV function and progressive TR over time.[17,18]

In practice, the actual threshold for repairing the tricuspid valve varies among surgeons; approximately one-third of patients with severe TR at implantation undergo TV repair.[14] The threshold is lower for patients who are not expected to recover RV and/or tricuspid valve function.[13] There does appear to be growing consensus that if preimplant TR is severe and tricuspid valve annulus is >40 mm, TV repair is advisable.

Tricuspid annuloplasty can be effective in decreasing TR resulting from annular dilatation. However, if leaflet tethering is severe, annuloplasty is not usually successful.[14] In instances where annuloplasty is not possible, tricuspid valve replacement, using a bioprosthesis inserted over existing pacemaker leads without excision of the tricuspid apparatus, has produced good long-term results.[13] The disadvantage of having a bioprosthesis in the right heart is the increased possibility of incurring a prosthetic infection and potential heterograft degeneration. Because the post-LVAD RV afterload is usually reduced, transvalvar flow patterns and reduced pressures are likely to favor longer durability of bioprostheses in the tricuspid position.

Mitral Regurgitation

With continuous-flow pumps, the mitral valve may remain open throughout the entire natural cardiac cycle. This is especially noticeable in the early postoperative period when native LV function is most compromised. As the LV recovers, attenuated pulsatile flow becomes the norm. The reduced pressure reduces the work demands on the mitral valve.

The impact of severe mitral regurgitation (MR) on long-term outcome remains controversial.[19–21] It is also unknown if these abnormal pressure and flow patterns affect the native mitral valve function and whether this impacts long-term prognosis.[19] However, there are increasing data that repair of severe MR may improve overall survival.[20]

MR caused by chordal tethering is diminished during LVAD support because LV volumes are reduced and the interpapillary muscle distance is lessened by the functioning LVAD. Annular dilation and contraction may recover as LV function recovers. However, if MR is >2+, an annuloplasty ring can be placed and provides a secure remedy at a low risk. In rare cases where structural valve leaflet abnormalities exist, repair is advised using standardized techniques, including chordal replacement, edge-to-edge repair, and annuloplasty. The edge-to-edge repair, although not a perfect solution, can be performed effectively through the LV apex at the time of apical cannula insertion. In some patients, mitral valve replacement may be necessary, in which case a bioprosthetic valve should be used.

Management of mechanical mitral valve prostheses with LVAD implantation is controversial. Minimizing the potential for thrombus on the prosthesis depends on intermittent pulsatile flows to wash areas of stasis. In recipients of long-term LVAD support, the chronic bleeding consequences imposed by LVADs may necessitate temporary cessation of anticoagulation, with a potentially adverse effect on implanted mechanical valves. However, successful LVAD support in patients with mechanical mitral prosthetic valves has been reported for up to 689 days.[22]

Aortic Valve

The new functional demands on the native aortic valve during LVAD support are not physiologic. Aortic root flow conditions favoring stasis have been observed with continuous-flow VADs and are more severe as the distance from the aortic entry of the outflow graft to the aortic valve is increased. Thrombus has been observed on the noncoronary cusp[23] and in the left coronary sinus in patients with previous coronary bypass grafting and in patients with aortic root closure, presumably due to the static flow conditions. This thrombotic liability can result in systemic or coronary artery embolization.[24]

Aortic insufficiency (AI) can lead to failure of the LV to reduce in size and progressive congestive heart failure with chronically elevated left atrial pressure in VAD patients. In vitro studies have shown an increase in leaflet stress during LVAD support. Radial stress was greater than circumferential stress in a model using a continuous-flow pump in an LVAD support configuration.[25] The clinical importance of AI during LVAD support depends on its severity and the underlying native LV function (see also Chapter 13 on Adverse Events During VAD Support). As AI progresses, more blood recirculates centrally through the LV–LVAD complex and causes systemic hypoperfusion and progressive LV volume loading. Patients with progressive or significant AI may have signs of low systemic flow and high LVAD flows with increased pulmonary capillary wedge pressure (PCWP) and pulmonary congestion. The severity of this malady can be confirmed by measuring right heart output and finding that it is less than the flows calculated from the LVAD performance interpretation displayed on the VAD console.

No absolute rules currently exist to guide treatment of AI seen in the operating room. However, aortic valve repair or closure should be considered when more than moderate (and perhaps moderate) AI is noted on the pre-CPB TEE. If the heart is maintained in a beating state during implantation, important AI will also be apparent when viewed through the apical cannulation site.

An effective technique for aortic valve closure is that described by Adamson et al.[26] (Fig. 11.7). In patients with sclerotic valves where progression is unlikely, central suture closure of insufficient leaflets may suffice,[27] but central coaptation sutures in otherwise normal valves do not prevent progression of AI and its sequelae.

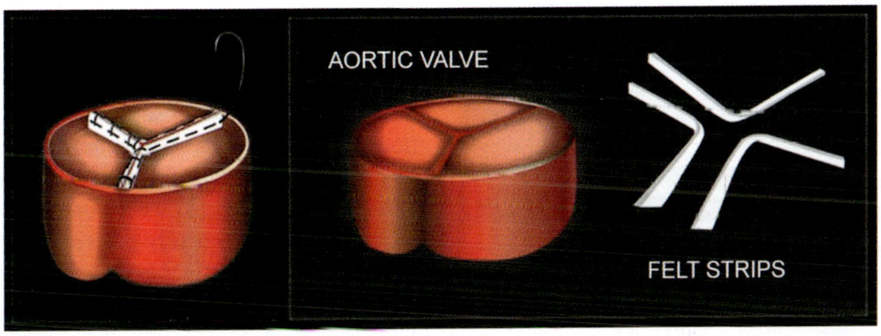

Fig. 11.7 Adamson technique for closure of the aortic valve using 4-0 prolene sutures and felt strips.

If AI is severe in the operating room *after* LVAD implantation, it can be readily detected by the intraoperative TEE. If the degree of AI cannot by effectively handled by the LVAD, the echocardiogram will show a dilated LV and shift of the atrial septum to the right. High pulmonary artery pressure and high PCWP confirm the presence of intolerable failure due to AI. In this setting, prompt repair/closure of the regurgitant aortic valve is mandatory. Since late repair may become necessary, and historically required a surgical reintervention, early valve closure is warranted in patients with existing/progressive AI following VAD implant, especially in long-term LVAD recipients with thin leaflets.[28]

Protracted low intermittent transvalvar flows cause both mechanical and bioprosthetic valves to thrombose following LVAD implantation. Patients with existing mechanical aortic prostheses are at extra risk for thromboembolism. Permanent closure of these prostheses is probably advisable since it seems to minimize systemic embolization of valve thrombus during intermittent opening. A variety of techniques have been suggested to reduce that liability, including sutures to retard the valve leaflets, patch closure over the valve, replacement of the valve with a bioprosthesis, and replacement of the valve using a patch in the aortic root.

Chronic LV outflow tract closure has been reported without adverse long-term consequences to date.[26] The incidence of thromboembolism does not appear to be increased but has not been eliminated. Reported survival is as good as in patients without outflow tract closure, and hemodynamics are excellent if the apical inflow cannula is well positioned. Patients with LV outflow tract who recover ventricular function and are able to be weaned from the device will require aortic valve replacement.

Patent Foramen Ovale

An LVAD may create a pressure gradient from the right to left atrium, which exaggerates right to left shunting through a patent foramen ovale (PFO), resulting in marked oxygen desaturation.[2] Profound hypoxia will result from a persistent PFO as the LVAD reduces the left atrial pressure and the right atrial pressure rises. The incidence of PFO is between 20% and 30%, depending on whether it is defined by physiologic testing with a left shifted septum or by direct inspection. Routine intraoperative TEE Doppler examination of the interatrial septum should be a routine part of the TEE assessment before CPB (Fig. 11.8). All PFOs should be surgically closed prior to leaving the operating room, with no demonstrated increase in surgical risk.[21,29,30]

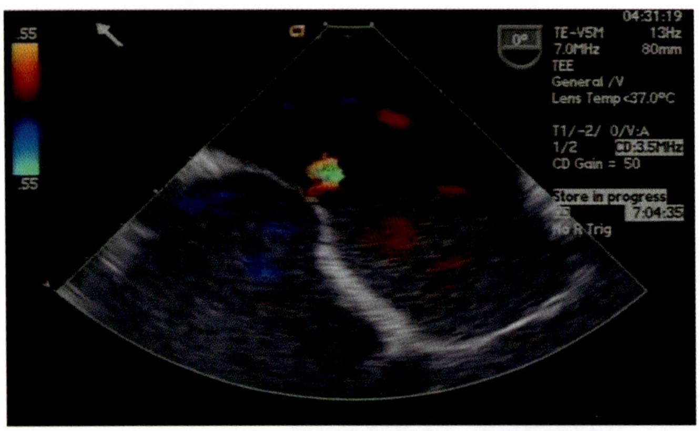

Fig. 11.8 Confirmation of the physiologic significance of right to left shunt through a patent foramen ovale using a transesophageal echocardiogram to image the interatrial septum being shifted to the left by compressing the pulmonary artery prior to the institution of cardiopulmonary bypass.

Ventricular Arrhythmias

Recipients with severe ventricular arrhythmias may require biventricular support, but such arrhythmias may improve or be better tolerated after isolated LVAD insertion. Standard ventricular arrhythmia ablation techniques can be used to eliminate or attenuate these rhythms. In the setting of recurrent ventricular tachycardia, preoperative mapping can serve as a guide to intraoperative ablation. It may also be prudent to connect the apical cannulation site to any proximate scar using cryoablation. This procedure eliminates the formation of an isthmus of myocardium between the scar and the apical cannulation site. The left atrial appendage is usually oversewn in patients with chronic atrial fibrillation.

Management of Weaning From Cardiopulmonary Bypass

When LVAD implantation is completed, pharmacologic cardiac support is initiated. After complete deairing of the device, the patient is weaned from CPB. The pump speed in revolutions per minute (rpm) is then gradually increased, allowing the LV to be filled and serve as a safe reservoir to supply the implanted LVAD. During the critical weaning interval, assiduous attention must be directed toward maintaining LV filling volume. If the ventricle is emptied, a suction event can occur in rotary blood pumps. Suction events can create transient ventricular arrhythmias or, worse, cause air to be sucked in around the apical cannula and pumped into the ascending aorta, the right coronary artery, and the cerebral circulation. In cases in which the aortic valve is closed, the LVAD is actuated and its flow is increased as CPB is weaned.

The interventricular and interatrial septa are monitored by TEE and maintained in a neutral position. Correct position of the apical cannula can be confirmed by increasing the pump rpm and observing a reduction of LV volume. The appropriate shape of the LV in TEE short axis view is a round shape; a flattened or convex septum ("D"-shaped LV) indicates excessive suction by the LVAD. In patients with a compliant septum, dynamic interventricular interaction through the ventricular septum can significantly change after LVAD initiation and compromise RV function, especially with continuous-flow devices. If the LV is overly aspirated, temporarily decreasing pump speed usually restores the shape of the LV and the hemodynamics.

Management of the Right Ventricle

Right Heart Failure

The interaction between the two ventricles is altered in the presence of an LVAD. During LVAD support, global RV performance can be impaired by excessive reduction of LV volume and chamber size in patients with a compliant septum resulting in a shift of the interventricular septum to the left and into the LV. This shift distorts the geometry of the RV and reduces its pumping ability. Myocardial efficiency and power output can often be maintained through a decrease in pulmonary artery pressure and an increase in RV filling pressure.[31,32]

Unlike heart transplantation, high pulmonary artery pressures before LVAD implantation usually indicate a RV that is at least partially conditioned to high afterload. Any diminution of RV contractile performance during LVAD support is usually neutralized by the reduction in afterload created by reducing the left atrial pressure stimulus to elevated pulmonary artery pressure. Reduction of LV end-diastolic pressure is reflected back to the pulmonary circulation, resulting in a reduced pulmonary artery pressure, decreased RV afterload, and enhanced RV function. Increased systemic blood pressure enhances right coronary blood flow. However, increasing the speed of a rotary pump LVAD increases its output, which augments systemic blood flow and secondarily increases venous return to the RV. Excessive venous return can worsen TR and compromise overall RV performance. It is the balance between these competing forces that ultimately determines the degree of RV dysfunction or failure.

Proactive and aggressive treatment of subtle signs of RV dysfunction can prevent deterioration of hemodynamics soon after CPB. The fragile nature of the RV myocardium, with its dependence on LV function and its sensitivity to RV afterload, creates vulnerability to rapid right heart failure if these conditions get out of control. A myriad of factors can elevate PVR in the operating room; their impact must be anticipated and a preventive strategy implemented. Patients with chronic vasoactive pulmonary hypertension can be treated pharmacologically with pulmonary vasodilators, including nitric oxide, milrinone, dobutamine, prostacyclin, isoproterenol, iloprost, and sildenafil. Ventilation is adjusted to reduce the end-tidal CO_2 to about 25 mm Hg, and oxygen saturation is kept high using appropriate inspired oxygen concentrations. Systemic acidosis should be corrected to optimize the pulmonary vascular response to drugs. Pulmonary effusions should be evacuated and endobronchial secretions removed, even endoscopically if necessary. Proper position of the LV inflow cannula is confirmed by TEE. LV chamber size is adjusted so that the septum is midline. Excessive suction can cause the apical cannula to impinge on the ventricular septum or free wall and generate ventricular arrhythmias.

Extreme care is taken to avoid air embolization to the right coronary artery. To minimize the impact of coronary gas embolization, the operative field is flooded with CO_2 during the entire implantation procedure. The heavy CO_2 displaces lighter atmospheric gases in the pericardium, and if it embolizes to the right coronary artery, it can be quickly absorbed from the blood without causing significant ischemic myocardial injury. Consideration should be given to addressing major occlusive disease in the coronary arterial supply of the RV using saphenous vein grafts.

The following parameters are key factors in hemodynamic assessment: preload (central venous pressure [CVP]), afterload (pulmonary systolic pressure and PVR), contractility of the RV, interventricular interaction, heart rate, rhythm, and systemic vascular resistance. Overdistention of the RV must be avoided. A CVP greater than 15 mm Hg is a sign of RV dysfunction. Increased stress of the thin RV wall can lead to worsening TR and decreased forward flow. PVR is frequently elevated after LVAD implantation. If the lung resistance is high and the cardiac output is low due to a failing RV, the pulmonary artery pressures may be normal or low.

Inotropic therapy with either milrinone (0.25 to 0.5 μg/kg/min) or dobutamine (3 to 5 μg/kg/min) is routinely administered to support RV contraction and provide pulmonary vasodilation. These two drugs may be combined with isoproterenol. All three drugs have a synergistic pulmonary vasodilatory effect when combined with nitric oxide. Inhaled nitric oxide (up to 40 parts per million) with low tidal volumes can be preemptively initiated during CPB. Epinephrine is added for further assistance without delay if subtle signs of RV dysfunction appear. Heart rate and rhythm are controlled with pacing or administration of antiarrhythmic agents, or both. Maintenance of coronary perfusion is achieved by maintaining systemic vascular resistance and adequate perfusion pressure (mean systemic blood pressure approximately 80 mm Hg). Arginine vasopressin is effective in treating vasodilatory hypotension in these patients.[33] However, excessive afterload can impair pump flow with continuous-flow devices.[34]

Decisions About Right Ventricular Support

Pulmonary hypertension prior to LVAD implant is usually secondary to chronic elevation of left atrial pressure. Conversely, high CVP and low pulmonary artery pressures (high right atrial pressure to PCWP ratio) in patients with low cardiac output indicates a failing RV that is incapable of generating a high pulmonary artery pressure. Right atrial pressure may be the best marker of RV function. In the presence of chronic sequelae of advanced right heart failure (marked peripheral edema, ascites, chronic elevation of CVP above 20 mm Hg), the need for biventricular support is likely. In the more acute state, CVP above 20 mm Hg despite medical optimization in hospital (and particularly if CVP > PCWP) indicates a high likelihood of needing biventricular support. Scoring systems using hemodynamic parameters or echocardiography have not provided great assistance in decision making.[23,24]

Usually, the decision to proceed to RV assist device (RVAD) support is made in the operating room. In general, if the patient requires progressive escalation of inotropic or vasopressor support following weaning from CPB (see previous section), an RVAD (usually a temporary device) should be promptly inserted. As a temporizing maneuver when acute RV failure develops in the operating room post-CPB, temporary support can be established using the CPB circuit. A cannula is placed in the pulmonary artery through a simple purse string. Using a "Y" connector,[35] the arterial flow from the bypass circuit can be redirected from the aorta into the pulmonary artery.[25] This allows the RV to remain decompressed while gradually elevating the systemic pressure and enhancing RV recovery. Increased cardiac output elevates the systemic venous oxygen saturation, and intrapulmonary shunting is reduced. During this period of temporary right heart support, the oxygenator gas flow is reduced and the gas exchange function of the natural lung can be assessed. The PVR is pharmacologically reduced. Gradually, the temporary pump flow is reduced from the initial flows of 4 to 5 L/min, and the CVP is allowed to rise to between 10 and 15 mm Hg. If the native RV cannot assume the burden of pulmonary flow necessary to fill the LVAD within half an hour to 1 hour, a short-term device is implanted, heparin is reversed, hemostasis is obtained, and the chest is closed.

Pump Selection for Right Heart Support

Published reports of reduced survival for RVAD recipients have incorrectly discouraged the appropriate application of RVADs. Their underuse may impair patient recovery in the early perioperative period by allowing RV pressure and CVP to remain high and LVAD outputs to be low. The resultant low mean arterial pressure and high systemic venous pressure reduce the tissue perfusion gradient below the desired minimum of 40 mm Hg. This condition and the independent adverse effect of increased CVP compromise RV, hepatic, renal, gastrointestinal, and cerebral recovery and may directly lead to worsening function.

Before selecting a pump to support the failing right circulation, the duration of support must be estimated. Most patients require only short periods of support. If more than 1 or 2 hours but less than 2 weeks of assistance is needed, widely available short-term pumps may be used. Percutaneously placed continuous-flow paracorporeal rotary pumps are well suited for brief use. If more than 2 weeks of support is anticipated, long-term support devices are usually selected. To date, long-term support devices have usually been paracorporeal pulsatile pumps, although successful biventricular support using implantable centrifugal pumps has become more common.

Intraoperative Bleeding

Intraoperative and perioperative bleeding associated with general cardiac surgery is usually easily managed. However, at least currently, the bleeding associated with LVAD insertion, particularly in a reoperative setting, is considerably more challenging. Excessive bleeding increases mortality and morbidity due to right heart failure, renal dysfunction, respiratory failure, and multiple organ dysfunction (see also Chapter 13: Adverse Events).

The hemostatic system is a dynamic balance between thrombotic and thrombolytic influences, often acting simultaneously and setting the stage for hemorrhagic or thrombotic consequences. Bleeding causes are multifocal, so hemostatic management should be guided by a systematic approach.

To reduce intraoperative bleeding and its attendant morbidity, coagulopathic drugs are discontinued prior to device implantation, and the hemodynamics are optimized. The hemodynamic strategy is directed toward normalizing visceral organ responsiveness by reducing venous congestion while maintaining cardiac output and blood pressure. Congestive hepatopathy and its clinical features, including jaundice and ascites, may respond dramatically to diuretics to reduce CVP. In addition, blood pressure, cardiac output, and venous pressure are optimized using appropriate inotropes and vasodilators in conjunction with fluid removal techniques, including diuretics, hemofiltration, peripheral ultrafiltration, and therapeutic paracentesis. Excessive diuresis should be avoided, which could impair hepatic and renal perfusion by reducing cardiac output and lowering blood pressure.

The large internal blood exposed surfaces of rotary pumps, with varying degrees of sheer stress, also influence the coagulopathy of recipient patients. The effect of foreign surfaces on coagulation and lytic interaction are precipitated by the protein adherence to foreign blood-contacting surfaces within the device. Indiscriminate attachment of proteins can favor fibrinogen, which then precipitates an intravascular coagulopathy. Certain proteins, including albumin, can passively coat surfaces and have successfully been used to minimize initiating this cascade. CPB generates its own universe of coagulopathy; insertion of VADs without CPB and via a less invasive approach may be associated with less bleeding.[36,37]

Minimizing bleeding from apical cannulation sites requires special attention to detail. A recommended technique is to use a circumferential Teflon felt bolster to attach the cannula to the apical ventriculotomy with horizontal mattress sutures. When inserting the cannula into a friable, infarcted ventricle, the emphasis is to achieve hemostasis without excessive suture tension, which can tear the weakened muscle. A large felt cone extended over the surface of the heart and attached to normal myocardium can rectify this problem. In cases where extensive ventricular apical infarction is present, effective apical cannulation sites can be reconstructed by sandwiching the myocardium between two felt patches in the affected areas. Since LV pressures during VAD support are greatly reduced, apical bleeding is usually controllable.

Sternal Reentry

Sternal reentry after VAD implantation is frequently needed, most commonly for subsequent heart transplantation, which is then complicated by dense adhesions around the heart and the device. Dissection of adhesions and mobilization of the heart for cardiectomy extend the time on CPB, possibly prolonging ischemic time of the donor heart and increasing the risk of posttransplantation bleeding.

Various materials have been tried to reduce these adhesions after VAD implantation. The most commonly used material is an expanded polytetrafluoroethylene membrane. This pericardial substitute reduces the risk of cardiac injury during sternal reentry for various types of cardiac reoperations including those after VAD implantation.[38] With advances in tissue engineering, elements of the extracellular matrix (ECM) have gained attention as important components in maintaining the characteristics of three-dimensional cardiac cell aggregates.[39] ECM is composed primarily of collagen, is found in all humans and animals, and has been studied in regenerative medicine to replace and reconstruct native tissue such as pericardium. The synthetic ECM technology is applicable to reconstructing pericardium through a commercially available product, CorMatrix (CorMatrix Cardiovascular, Inc.). The edge of the CorMatrix is placed in contact with the edge of opened pericardium with 4-0 polypropylene running suture to cover the entire heart, inflow, and outflow conduit. A drain is placed underneath the membrane and the device is left uncovered in the preperitoneal space.

POSTOPERATIVE CARE

Following implantation, hemodynamic monitoring in the cardiac intensive care unit usually includes a pulmonary artery catheter and echocardiography that guide titration of pump speed, parenteral fluids, inotropes, and vasopressor agents. Pump speed is optimized to several parameters, including maintenance of midline septal position and reduction of MR, while maintaining adequate flow to end organs. Average pump speed ranges from 8000 to 10,000 rpm, from 2200 to 2800 rpm, and from 3000 to 9000 rpm for the HMII, HVAD, and HM3, respectively. If an intraaortic balloon pump is present, it should be removed as soon as possible in the postoperative period.

Additionally, right heart function is monitored by echocardiography and filling pressures. PVR is minimized by careful ventilator adjustments in addition to judicious fluid management. Agents such as inhaled nitric oxide or intravenous prostaglandins can help lower PVR. However, if right heart failure develops and is refractory to medical management, then RVAD support may be required, usually with a temporary device.

Anticoagulation with heparin is initiated once postoperative bleeding is minimal, making meticulous intraoperative hemostasis crucial to this aspect of postoperative care. Transition to long-term anticoagulation with warfarin is not started until the patient is stable, usually 48–72 hours postimplantation. In the absence of ongoing bleeding, an international normalized ratio (INR) of 2.5–3.5 is generally targeted. Antiplatelet therapy is additionally started at this point. The most common strategy is a full aspirin once a day. Currently, there are no consistent practice recommendations for monitoring platelet activity.

Other aspects of postoperative care include the use of perioperative prophylactic antibiotics for a period of 72 hours to provide coverage of both gram-positive and gram-negative organisms (see discussion in Chapter 13). The driveline dressing changes are performed daily under sterile conditions, and the technique is taught to the patients and their caregiver. Enteral nutrition should be initiated as soon as the patient's clinical condition warrants. Finally, a multidisciplinary team is crucial to the success of the patient both as an inpatient and after discharge.

REFERENCES

1. DeBakey ME. Development of mechanical heart devices. *Ann thorac Surg.* 2005;79:S2228–S2231.
2. Rose EA, Gelijns AC, Moskowitz AJ, et al. Long-term use of a left ventricular assist device for end-stage heart failure. *New Engl J Med.* 2001;345:1435–1443.
3. Slaughter MS, Rogers JG, Milano CA, et al. Advanced heart failure treated with continuous-flow left ventricular assist device. *New Engl J Med.* 2009;361:2241–2251.
4. Kirklin JK, Naftel DC, Pagani FD, et al. Seventh INTERMACS annual report: 15,000 patients and counting. *J Heart Lung Transplant.* 2015;34:1495–1504.
5. Slaughter MS, Pagani FD, McGee EC, et al. HeartWare ventricular assist system for bridge to transplant: combined results of the bridge to transplant and continued access protocol trial. *J Heart Lung Transplant.* 2013;32:675–683.
6. Lalonde SD, Alba AC, Rigobon A, et al. Clinical differences between continuous flow ventricular assist devices: a comparison between HeartMate II and HeartWare HVAD. *J Cardiac Surg.* 2013;28:604–610.

7. Stulak JM, Davis ME, Haglund N, et al. Adverse events in contemporary continuous-flow left ventricular assist devices: a multi-institutional comparison shows significant differences. *J Thorac Cardiovasc Surg*. 2016;151:177–189.
8. Mehra MR, Goldstein DJ, Uriel N, et al. Two-year outcomes with a magnetically levitated cardiac pump in heart failure. *N Engl J Med*. 2018;378:1386–1395.
9. Shah P, Birk S, Maltais S, et al. Left ventricular assist device outcomes based on flow configuration and pre-operative left ventricular dimension: An interagency registry for mechanically assisted circulatory support analysis. *J Heart Lung Transplant*. 2017;36:(6)640–649.
10. Go AS, Mozaffarian D, Roger VL, et al. Heart disease and stroke statistics—2014 update: a report from the American Heart Association. *Circulation*. 2014;129:e28–e292.
11. Tanaka A, Kitahara H, Onsager D, et al. Impact of residual valve disease on survival after implantation of left ventricular assist devices. *Ann Thorac Surg*. 2018;106:1789–1796.
12. Nakanishi K, Homma S, Han J, et al. Prevalence, predictors, and prognostic value of residual tricuspid regurgitation in patients with left ventricular assist device. *J Am Heart Assoc*. 2018;7.
13. Mazine A, Bouchard D, Moss E, et al. Transvalvular pacemaker leads increase the recurrence of regurgitation after tricuspid valve repair. *Ann Thorac Surg*. 2013;96:816–822.
14. Song HK, Gelow JM, Mudd J, et al. Limited utility of tricuspid valve repair at the time of left ventricular assist device implantation. *Ann Thorac Surg*. 2016;101(6):2168–2174.
15. Robertson JO, Grau-Sepulveda MV, Okada S, et al. Concomitant tricuspid valve surgery during implantation of continuous-flow left ventricular assist devices: a Society of Thoracic Surgeons database analysis. *J Heart Lung Transplant*. 2014;33(6):609–617.
16. Milano C, Pagani FD, Slaughter MS, et al. Clinical outcomes after implantation of a centrifugal flow left ventricular assist device and concurrent cardiac valve procedures. *Circulation*. 2014;130(11 suppl 1):S3–S11.
17. Kwak JJ, Kim YJ, Kim MK, et al. Development of tricuspid regurgitation late after left-sided valve surgery: a single-center experience with long-term echocardiographic examination. *Am Heart J*. 2008;155:732–737.
18. Fujita T, Kobayashi J, Hata H, et al. Right heart failure and benefits of adjuvant tricuspid valve repair in patients undergoing left ventricular assist device implantation. *European Journal of Cardio-Thoracic Surgery*. 2014;46(5):802–807.
19. Maltais S, Anwer LA. The importance of mitral regurgitation in patients with left ventricular assist devices: an ongoing conundrum. *JACC Heart Fail*. 2017;5:89–91.
20. Kassis H, Cherukuri K, Agarwal R, et al. Significance of residual mitral regurgitation after continuous flow left ventricular assist device implantation. *JACC Heart Fail*. 2017;5:81–88.
21. Robertson JO, Naftel DC, Myers SL, et al. Concomitant mitral valve procedures in patients undergoing implantation of continuous-flow left ventricular assist devices: an INTERMACS database analysis. *J Heart Lung Transplant*. 2018 Jan 1;37(1):79–88.
22. ABIOMED AB5000 Circulatory Support System AB5000 ventricle instructions for use. Danvers, MA: Abiomed; 2003.
23. Dang NC, Topkara VK, Mercando M, et al. Right heart failure after left ventricular assist device implantation in patients with chronic congestive heart failure. *J Heart Lung Transplant*. 2006;25:1-6.
24. Saito T, Wassilew K, Gorodetski B, et al. Aortic valve pathology in patients supported by continuous-flow left ventricular assist device. *Circ J*. 2016;80:1371–1377.
25. Pak SW, Uriel N, Takayama H, et al. Prevalence of de novo aortic insufficiency during long-term support with left ventricular assist devices. *J Heart Lung Transplant*. 2010;29:1172–1176.
26. Adamson RM, Dembitsky WP, Baradarian S, et al. Aortic valve closure associated with HeartMate left ventricular device support: technical considerations and long-term results. *J Heart Lung Transplant*. 2011;30:576–582.
27. Park KM, Park YJ, Yang SS, Kim DI, Kim YW. Treatment of failing vein grafts in patients who underwent lower extremity arterial bypass. *J Korean Surg Soc*. 2012 Nov 1;83(5):307–315.
28. Truby LK, Garan AR, Givens RC, et al. Aortic insufficiency during contemporary left ventricular assist device support: analysis of the INTERMACS registry. *JACC Heart Fail*. 2018;6:951–960.
29. Kapur NK, Conte JV, Resar JR. Percutaneoius closure of patent foramen ovale for refractory hypoxemia after HeartMate II left ventricular assist device placement. *J Invasive Cardilo*. 2007;19:E268–E270.
30. Pal JD, Klodell CT, John R, et al. Low operative mortality with implantation of a continuous-flow left ventricular assist device and impact of concurrent cardiac procedures. *Circulation*. 2009;120(suppl 1):S215–S219.
31. Baldwin RT, Duncan JM, Frazier OH, Wilansky S. Patent foramen ovale: a cause of hypoxemia in patients on left ventricular support. *Ann Thorac Surg*. 1991;52:865–867.
32. Santamore WP, Gray Jr LA. Left ventricular contributions to right ventricular systolic function during LVAD support. *Ann Thorac Surg*. 1996;61:350–356.
33. Stewart GC, Kittleson MM, Cowger JA, et al. Who wants a left ventricular assist device for ambulatory heart failure? Early insights from the MEDAMACS screening pilot. *J Heart Lung Transplant*. 2015;34:1630–1633.
34. Dandel M, Potapov E, Krabatsch T, et al. Load dependency of right ventricular performance is a major factor to be considered in decision making before ventricular assist device implantation. *Circulation*. 2013;128:S14–S23.
35. Loebe M, Potapov E, Sodian R, Kopitz M, Noon GP. A safe and simple method of preserving right ventricular function during implantation of a left ventricular assist device. *J Thorac Cardiovasc Surg*. 2001;122:1043.
36. Gaffey AC, Chen CW, Chung JJ, et al. Improved approach with subcostal exchange of the HeartMate II left ventricular assist device: difference in on and off pump? *Ann Thorac Surg*. 2017;104:1540–1546.
37. Mohite PN, Sabashnikov A, Raj B, et al. Minimally invasive left ventricular assist device implantation: a comparative study. *Artif Organs*. 2018;.
38. Leprince P, Rahmati M, Bonnet N, et al. Expanded polytetrafluoroethylene membranes to wrap surfaces of circulatory support devices in patients undergoing bridge to heart transplantation. *Eur J Cardiothorac Surg*. 2001;19:302–306.
39. Akhyari P, Kamiya H, Haverich A, Karck M, Lichtenberg A. Myocardial tissue engineering: the extracellular matrix. *Eur J Cardiothorac Surg*. 2008;34:229–241.

12

Postoperative VAD Management: Operating Room to Discharge and Beyond

Surgical and Medical Considerations

William L. Holman, Robb D. Kociol, Sean Pinney

KEY POINTS

Perioperative Management
Considerations in the Operating Room Relevant to Subsequent ICU Care
Early Postimplantation ICU Care
Early Postimplantation Medical Management in the ICU
Pharmacologic Management in the ICU
Preparing for Home Discharge
Standard Outpatient Visit

PERIOPERATIVE MANAGEMENT

This chapter focuses on the early postoperative care of patients with ventricular assist devices (VADs). Appropriate patient selection and optimal implantation techniques greatly simplify postoperative management. Indeed, some problems created by suboptimal implantation techniques are difficult or impossible to correct, short of a return to the operating room. This chapter commences with a discussion of operative factors that influence the early intensive care unit (ICU) course of a VAD patient, reviews early postoperative challenges in the ICU and their management, and addresses the further hospital course leading up to discharge and considerations of postdischarge management once the patient first returns to the community. We start in the operating theatre.

CONSIDERATIONS IN THE OPERATING ROOM RELEVANT TO SUBSEQUENT ICU CARE

Appropriate de-airing of the pump and heart is crucial to a successful outcome. The surgeon carries out the de-airing maneuvers in conjunction with the perfusionist and the anesthesiologist while monitoring the transesophageal echocardiogram. A substantial amount of air can be removed from the patient's left ventricle (LV) and VAD before completing the final connections of the system (i.e., 1—outflow graft anastomosis to aorta *or* 2—outflow graft connection to the pump housing). If the final step is to anastomose the outflow graft to the aorta, attaching a sump sucker to the outflow graft and then filling the beating heart with blood pushes blood from the heart through the VAD and into the sump sucker. If the final step is to attach the outflow graft to the pump housing, a vent tube can be attached to the pump outlet thread protector. The surgeon and perfusionist fill the beating heart with blood to push blood and air into the vent line.

While the pump and heart are in this initial phase of de-airing, the lungs should be gently ventilated with the patient in a head-down (Trendelenburg) position with a second venting device aspirating blood from the aortic root. While this initial de-airing occurs, the surgical team can accomplish other tasks, including placement of the percutaneous driveline and positioning of the outflow graft in the desired position (e.g., along the diaphragmatic surface of the pericardium and lateral to the right atrium), with a few sutures to prevent migration.

The final de-airing takes place after the pump connections are complete. It is best for each team to develop their own protocol for de-airing; however, the general plan contains the following features. The process begins by fully reinflating the lungs and setting the ventilator to resume regular respirations. The rhythm of the heart is optimized using pacing and medications as necessary. Ideally, the patient will be in a normal sinus or paced atrial rhythm. The perfusionist then decreases venous return and begins partial cardiopulmonary bypass. When the surgeon feels that there is adequate blood in the LV, the pump is powered up and rotor rotation is started, but with a cross-clamp in place on the outflow graft. Blood and air are aspirated from the outflow graft proximal to the clamp via a venting needle. After completing the initial de-airing, the outflow graft is slowly unclamped while monitoring the LV and ascending aorta for air. The vent in the ascending aorta captures any air that escapes the outflow graft vent. Shaking the heart and forcefully ventilating the lungs dislodge smaller bubbles of air trapped along the walls of the heart and pump. After completing the de-airing sequence with the patient in a head-down position, the maneuvers are repeated with the patient in a supine (flat) position.

Air that enters the cerebral circulation may cause brain injury ranging from confusion to more severe focal and global brain injury (e.g., multiple small regions of stroke). Air entering the ascending aorta and right coronary artery (RCA) may cause—at least transiently—right ventricle (RV) dysfunction, resulting in immediate RV dilation and free wall hypokinesis. At this point, it is prudent to go back on full cardiopulmonary bypass in order to push the air through the right coronary circulation and recover RV function.

As the echocardiographer and surgeon monitor for air, they can also assess native cardiac function and the effects of the VAD on the heart. This includes determining valve function (e.g., assessments for mitral, aortic, and tricuspid valve insufficiency) and the position of the ventricular septum relative to the LV and RV cavities. Another important item to check with echocardiography is the position of the inflow cannula relative to the LV septum and free wall. Ideally, the orifice of the inflow cannula will point posteriorly, directly at the mitral valve orifice. Doppler interrogation of the LV cavity confirms nonturbulent flow directly from the mitral valve into the VAD. The inflow cannula should not be angled toward the intraventricular septum, but rather parallel to the septum to avoid septal suction, turbulent flow, and potential ventricular tachycardia.

As the LV fills and begins to eject blood through the aortic valve, the surgeon increases pump rotor speed (revolutions per minute) to a point where the VAD provides adequate systemic blood flow without pulling the ventricular septum toward the LV. Upon achieving this balance of native ventricular function and pump function, the flow of the cardiopulmonary bypass circuit is decreased and eventually discontinued. At this point, the patient's cardiac output is a combination of the native LV ejection and left VAD (LVAD) pump flow. If systemic flow is adequate and the other echocardiographic indicators of VAD function are satisfactory (e.g., inflow cannula position, septal position, and absence of air in the heart or aorta), the surgeon removes the cardiopulmonary bypass cannulas as the anesthesiologist administers protamine.

Pharmacological management of circulation early after VAD implantation focuses primarily on RV function. This includes inotropic medications (often milrinone, which simultaneously reduces RV afterload) to stimulate RV contractility, vasopressors to maintain adequate systemic blood pressure required for right coronary artery perfusion, and inhaled pulmonary vasodilators (often inhaled prostanoids as a less expensive alternative to inhaled nitric oxide) to reduce pulmonary vascular resistance without causing V/Q mismatch and resultant hypoxemia or systemic hypotension. If blood pressure is low or the patient has poor renal function, low-dose epinephrine or dobutamine may be used for inotropic support of the RV in place of milrinone. Some centers use both low-dose epinephrine and milrinone for support.

After administering protamine, the surgical team typically turns its attention to obtaining hemostasis. The surgeon must also decide whether to close the chest primarily or leave the sternum unclosed and either packed or treated with a vacuum-assisted wound management device. When the wounds are closed or sealed, the implantation team transports the patient to the ICU. If there is significant RV dysfunction, either due to a marginal RV prior to surgery or an injury to the RV intraoperatively, the surgeon may leave the chest open to assist RV function or implant a temporary right VAD (RVAD) either surgically or percutaneously for initial RV support.

EARLY POSTIMPLANTATION ICU CARE

The early postimplantation care of patients with a VAD is similar in many ways to the care of other postcardiac surgery patients who arrive from the operating room. The following section focuses on the unique aspects of caring for VAD patients.

LVAD placement among patients with end-stage heart disease has a high prevalence of postoperative bleeding,[1] although the incidence of bleeding in the first 12 months postimplantation has significantly decreased from the 2008 to 2010 era (when compared to the 2011–2013 era).[1] The causes of postimplantation bleeding include scarring and adhesions from prior cardiac operations, as well as chronic congestion of the liver that may result in liver dysfunction and resultant coagulopathy. Known cirrhosis would typically be a contraindication to durable LVAD implantation.[2] It is difficult to measure hepatic reserve in a patient with chronic congestion from heart failure. Low serum protein and albumin levels, along with an elevated international normalized ratio (INR), suggest that hepatic synthesis of clotting factors in response to incisional bleeding and cardiopulmonary bypass will be diminished and that a fibrinolytic state may be prolonged after surgery. Preoperative right upper quadrant ultrasound can be suggestive of cirrhosis, although liver biopsy is considered the gold standard. Some groups routinely use thromboelastography to monitor the rate of clot formation, clot strength, and fibrinolytic activity. However, many groups rely on prothrombin time/partial thromboplastin time (PTT)/INR and platelet count to guide blood product and blood factor therapy early after VAD implantation.

Another useful maneuver for managing postimplantation coagulopathic bleeding is packing of the mediastinum to encourage clotting and allow time for the coagulopathy to resolve. This can be accomplished by placing sponges or laparotomy pads around cannulation sites, anastomotic sites, and against cut tissue edges followed by closure of the skin. Another useful maneuver is to pack the mediastinum as described earlier and then apply a vacuum-assisted wound closure device (e.g., Wound V.A.C.; KCI, San Antonio, TX).[3] Use of delayed sternal closure minimizes the chance of tamponade by leaving the sternal halves separated and optimizing drainage of the mediastinum. Of note, the vacuum module for negative pressure wound management systems can be set to a variety of levels measured in mm Hg (typically ranging from −50 to −125 mm Hg) that exceed the maximum suction that a chest tube drainage system can provide (typical maximum suction, −40 cm water). To ensure that one system does not prevent drainage from the other, it is important to balance the vacuum-assisted wound closure and chest tube drainage systems at the bedside. The conversion factor is 1 cm H_2O = 0.736 mm Hg. Thus, the maximal suction for a typical chest drainage system (e.g., Pleur-evac; Teleflex, Morrisville, NC) is 40 cm H_2O, which equals 29.4 mm Hg. This is below the preset suction options for vacuum modules. A reasonable starting point is 75 mm Hg vacuum for the mediastinal sponge dressing. This provides 102 cm H_2O suction at the top of the wound sponge, but less in the deeper planes of the mediastinum. Typically, 75 mm Hg of vacuum still allows some of the chest drainage to exit via the chest tube drainage system. Low negative pressures (50–100 mm Hg suction) provide chest wall stability that is similar to stability at higher vacuum settings, so higher vacuum settings do not provide an advantage in this regard. Of note, high vacuum settings can cause air leaks at the edge of the dressing or organ injury.[4,5] Complications from prolonged use of negative pressure wound therapy in the setting of poststernotomy mediastinitis are uncommon (7% in one series[6]). Complications from short-term (1–3 days) use of negative pressure wound therapy include clogging of the drainage tube with clot and loss of the air-seal at the wound edges. In our experience, these problems are rare and easily remedied.

Use of packing sponges or a vacuum system requires a return trip to the operating room for removal of the dressings and packing sponges. Mediastinal reexploration provides an opportunity for removal of mediastinal thrombus. Clot removal reduces the chances of late infection, since bacteria, especially *Staphylococcus*, have an affinity for growing in blood clots. This is due to the limited number of viable phagocytes in clots and the presence of nutrients, including free hemoglobin, that support bacterial growth. Use of an irrigation system (e.g., Pulsavac; Zimmer, Inc., Warsaw, IN) is helpful is removing residual thrombus from the surfaces of the mediastinal tissues and from the external surfaces of the pump. The pulsing irrigation helps wash out fibrin, necrotic debris, and any bacteria that may have inoculated the wound. A small amount of Betadine soap (1–2 mL per liter saline irrigation) (Betadine; Purdue Pharma, LP, Stamford, CN) helps remove any bacteria that adhere to tissue surfaces and disrupts small colonies of bacteria that are in the early stages of biofilm development.[7,8]

RV failure that limits LVAD performance is a relatively common and serious problem. Placement of an RVAD before the sequelae of low cardiac output development will improve patient survival.[9] Typically, the RV performance improves as pulmonary vascular resistance diminishes and the heart recovers from acute surgery.[10,11] Early after LVAD implantation, pharmacologic measures to decrease pulmonary vascular resistance are helpful. If these do not produce the desired result within a few hours, placement of an extracorporeal centrifugal RVAD such as the Centrimag centrifugal flow extracorporeal VAD (Abbott Inc., Abbott Park, IL) or a novel percutaneously inserted RVAD should be considered before the patient is exposed to prolonged marginal circulatory support, as well as high doses of inotropes and vasopressors. One such novel percutaneous device is the Impella RP (Abiomed, Danvers, MA), shown to be feasible in a very small prospective study that included a post-LVAD, RV failure cohort.[12,13] Another such device is the TandemLife pump with Protek Duo cannula (TandemLife, Pittsburg, PA) that is inserted as a single dual-lumen cannula through the internal jugular vein, as opposed to the Impella RP,[14] which is inserted through the femoral vein, thus offering greater mobility. Some centers routinely bring their LVAD patients out of the operating room on inhaled prostanoids (or inhaled nitric oxide) and low-dose inotropes for empiric RV support and wean the support as tolerated by the individual patient. The efficacy of this strategy has not been proven. Associations between the length of inotropic support of the RV after LVAD implantation and death awaiting transplant have been demonstrated in retrospective analyses[15]; however, this may represent a population with severely compromised RV function prior to LVAD implantation.

Surgical techniques for implanting a second durable LVAD in the RV position have been described.[16] Placement of a second durable device within the chest can be challenging, since the volume of the two pumps within the chest may compromise cardiac and pulmonary function. The combined volume of two implanted devices can make sternal closure challenging, unless the patient's chest is relatively large. The flow of the two pumps must be balanced to avoid high mean pressures in the left or right atrium due to overcirculation of one pump relative to the other. Use of right and left atrial pressure monitoring catheters aid in appropriately setting the speed of the pumps in the early postoperative period. The ability of the native ventricles to balance the right and left circulation and the load-responsiveness of rotary pumps is helpful in achieving a right-left balance. Placement of the RVAD inflow cannula is difficult if the patient has a small RV or a fragile right atrium. Therefore, placement of the inflow cannula is best individualized to each patient. It is important to remember that all durable centrifugal pumps were designed for use in the systemic circulation. As such, the optimal pump speed for durable LVADs in the right heart position is unknown. Some groups use constricting sutures on the RVAD outflow graft to mimic systemic vascular resistance.[17–21] The benefit of outflow graft constricting sutures has not been proven, although outflow graft constriction may improve the long-term performance of centrifugal pumps in the pulmonary circulation by maintaining optimal rotor position in the stator housing. Importantly, in the short-term, constricting the outflow graft adds resistance such that running the pump within its optimal speed range will not result in excess cardiac output overloading the LV or over-perfusing the pulmonary circulation. The most extensive experience in using two durable LVADs for a biventricular assist device configuration comes from the implantation of dual HeartWare HVAD (Medtronic, Minneapolis, MN) devices. Over 600 such cases have been reported in the Interagency Registry for Mechanically Assisted Circulatory Support (INTERMACS). Recently, a case series of similar implantation of two pumps using the HeartMate 3 centrifugal flow pump has been published consisting of a series of 18 total patients.[17] As opposed to positioning the HVAD on the right side, where the outflow graft must often be constricted to simulate systemic vascular resistance and allow the pump to run at speeds (rpm >2400) within its required parameters to avoid touch-down events, this does not seem to be required of the HeartMate 3 device (Fig. 12.1). Because it employs full magnetic levitation (MagLev), the HeartMate 3 rotor will not have touch-down events at any speed. Regardless, patients requiring biventricular durable LVADs have a significantly increased risk of early death or death prior to transplantation.[22]

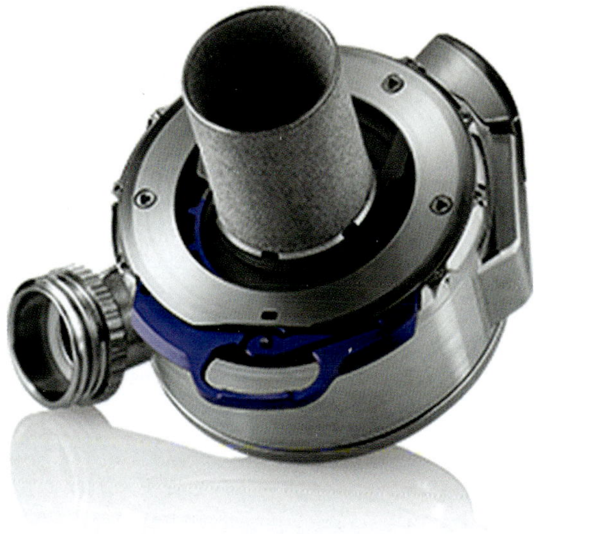

Fig. 12.1 Picture of the HeartMate 3 left ventricular assist system pump.

The role of tricuspid valve repair at the time of LVAD placement remains controversial because improved RV contractility, lower pulmonary artery pressure, and falling pulmonary vascular resistance over time may decrease tricuspid regurgitation (TR) following LVAD implantation even if tricuspid repair is not performed at the time of implantation. During the 2000–2013 timeframe, most, but not all, studies suggested a benefit for tricuspid valve repair with an undersized annuloplasty ring among those with moderate to severe TR, and this was the common practice.[4,5] More recent data suggest that even severe TR will improve over time as the patient's pulmonary pressures come down and the heart remodels. The extra time on bypass to repair the tricuspid valve may be worth the risk in those at high risk for development of right heart failure (RHF), but not necessarily in all comers.[12,23–26] Some centers are moving away from this practice in patients with mild and moderate TR, performing tricuspid valve repair or replacement only among those with tenuous RV function and severe TR. The quality of the data, both for and against tricuspid repair, is limited by the single-center design in most cases, although there were a few studies using INTERMACS data. Nonetheless, the studies' retrospective design and the possibility of selection bias potentially confound the study results. Whether the procedure is beneficial among LVAD patients with moderate to severe TR can only truly be answered by a prospective, randomized trial.

Measures during the perioperative period to prevent infection include prophylactic antibiotics and appropriate driveline dressing with aseptic technique. The 2017 International Society for Heart and Lung Transplantation (ISHLT) Consensus Document on MCS Infections recommends intravenous antibiotics to target *Staphylococcus* species administered within 1 hour of skin incision. Among those whose nares are positive for methicillin-resistant *Staphylococcus aureus* (MRSA) and in hospitals with a high prevalence of MRSA, the recommendation is vancomycin administered intravenously at least 2 hours prior to skin incision. Current recommendations do not advocate broad-spectrum

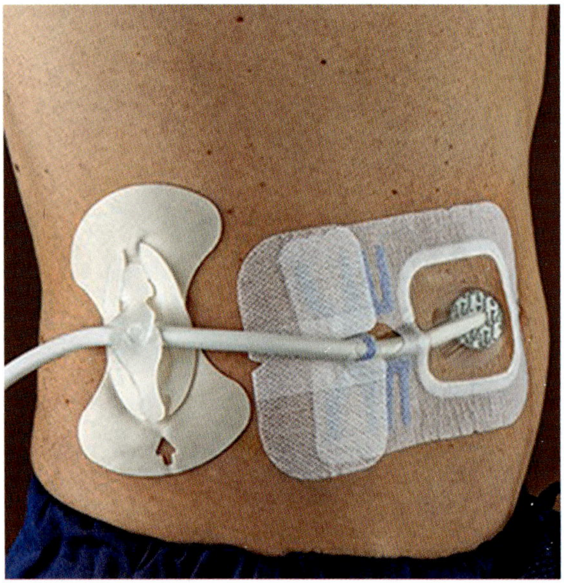

Fig. 12.2 Demonstration of a commercially available driveline dressing kit including dressing material, skin cleanser, a "biopatch," and stabilizer/tension relief. (© Medline Industries, Inc. 2019.)

gram-negative or antifungal prophylaxis; however, this depends upon the institutional microbiological data and resistance patterns.[27] Equally important is the meticulous management and care of the percutaneous driveline. Management of the driveline in the early postimplantation period primarily includes placement of a protective dressing, a stabilizer, and daily wound cleansing with a mild antiseptic until there is no longer drainage and the wound appears to have superficially epithelialized after which time chlorhexidine is utilized one to three times per week with dressing changes, under sterile conditions with driveline immobilization (Fig. 12.2).[28] Our practice at University of Alabama at Birmingham is to use two driveline fixation devices in addition to a suture at the exit site. The use of a stabilizing percutaneous exit site suture is controversial.[29] If the surgeons place an exit site suture, it is important to remove it within 2–3 weeks of implantation to prevent accumulation of detritus around the stabilizing suture, which encourages infection.

Prevention of driveline trauma begins when the patient is mobilized. It is important to assign a sufficient number of helpers to move the patient from a sitting position to a standing one and during ambulation early after surgery. Dropping the controller can pull the driveline fixation devices away from the skin and traumatize the exit site during the initial phase of healing, thereby predisposing the wound to infection. Excellent driveline care using standardized protocols for driveline implantation and management can decrease the incidence of driveline infection,[30] which remains at about 20% in the first 12 months after device implantation.[29,31,32] If a patient drops the controller or in any other way traumatizes the driveline exit site, the patient will require careful initial inspection of the driveline exit site and frequent monitoring, as trauma to the exit site is one of the leading causes of bacterial driveline infections. Directly asking the patient about any instances of driveline exit site trauma at each postdischarge clinic visit should be a routine part of the history.

The cumulative incidence of driveline infections is high and may represent the Achilles heel of pumps that require percutaneous energy delivery.[33] Several groups are working on novel transcutaneous energy transmission systems,[34] and the first generation of fully implanted pumps (i.e., pumps with no percutaneous components) has been tested.[35,36] Patients and physicians agree that fully implanted systems are highly desirable. However, there are several important design challenges. The implanted components (energy receiver, controller, and back-up battery) must be highly reliable, not result in additional infection risk, and not be prohibitively expensive to manufacture. The external energy transmitter and receiver coupling may only cause mild local warming and tissue pressure to prevent local skin damage. Replacement of individual components that fail (e.g., controller) or reach end of life (e.g., back-up battery) must have acceptable associated morbidity and hospital length of stay. A fully implantable VAD system is not currently available, although there were prior trials of a fully implanted LVAD and a fully implanted total artificial heart.

Risk factors for driveline infection include obesity,[37–39] cachexia, and malnutrition.[40] Several methods have been developed for preimplantation nutritional risk assessment.[41] However, it remains challenging to actually improve a patient's nutritional state prior to VAD implantation or in the early phase of postimplantation recovery due to hemodynamic instability, poor gastrointestinal motility, depressed appetite, and the patient's catabolic state in severe heart failure or early after surgery.[42–45] Some have advocated for the initiation of parenteral nutrition prior to implantation and continuing through the postimplantation period to provide uninterrupted protein and calorie support. This has been achieved without a concomitant increase in line-related infection.[46] It is nevertheless important to aggressively optimize the patient's nutrition before and after implantation.[47]

Inflow cannula position should be checked in the operating room with transesophageal echocardiography after the chest is closed. Typically, this is done with transthoracic echocardiography early after return to the ICU, and then as needed.

Optimal positioning of the inflow cannula relative to the LV walls and the mitral valve orifice is crucial to pump function. The anteroposterior (AP) chest radiograph (CXR) provides a reasonable initial determination of pump position for axial-flow devices (e.g., HeartMate II; Abbott Inc., Abbott Park, IL).[42,46,48] Pump position (especially the angle between the pump housing and the inflow cannula for axial flow designs) is one factor that appears to influence pump thrombosis. Moreover, suboptimal inflow cannula position will limit pump flow due to obstruction of the inflow cannula. Excessive outflow graft length or suboptimal positioning of the outflow graft anastomosis on the aorta can lead to kinking that diminishes pump flow and can cause hemolysis. With the initial HeartMate 3 experience (Abbott Laboratories), excessive outflow graft twisting or kinking resulted in a US Food and Drug Administration class I recall due to the frequency of flow interruption and thrombus formation when these events occurred.[49–51] Positioning of centrifugal LVADs (e.g., HeartWare, Medtronic, Minneapolis, MN; and HeartMate 3, Abbott, Abbott Park, IL) has not been studied as extensively as axial flow pumps. However, an AP CXR will provide an estimate of inflow cannula position relative to the mitral orifice. For both axial and centrifugal flow pumps, echocardiography and three-dimensional reconstructions of gated computed tomography (CT) images provide the most precise information to describe the position of the inflow cannula relative to the ventricular walls and the mitral orifice.[52] Echocardiography has the added advantage of flow assessment within the LV. Continuous laminar flow from the mitral orifice to the inflow cannula suggests an optimal inflow cannula position. Shifting of pump position within the body following implantation has been documented for axial flow devices.[53,54] These shifts, if sufficiently severe, are associated with increased incidence of pump thrombosis.[49] Shifts of inflow cannula position in centrifugal pumps are less of a problem than in axial flow VADs; however, in small patients and in patients with massive ventricles, the chest wall can push the inflow cannula for a centrifugal pump medially into a position near the chordae tendineae or mitral leaflets. Leaving the pericardium open or adding relaxing incisions to the right and/or left pericardial edges will allow the heart to move away from the pump.

Another important aspect of device management in the early postoperative period is modulation of pump speed (rpm). When the speed of a continuous-flow pump is changed, the results should be assessed not just by pump output but also by the effect on pulsatility (either the Pulsatility Index (PI) for the HeartMate II or 3 device or wave form amplitude on the HeartWare HVAD device). Most speed changes should be accompanied by direct visualization, with careful attention to avoid septal suction toward the left or bowing. Diminished pulsatility or loss of pulsatility suggests that the rpm is set to too high, which predisposes the pump to suction events and can worsen RV contractility. Loss of RV contractility because of septal shifting is an important concept that was developed by David Farrar, John Woodard, and Edna Chou in a canine heart failure model.[50] The ventricular septum provides an important contribution to RV contractile function (up to 20%–40%).[55,56] When an excessively high pump speed pulls the ventricular septum toward the LV, the septal contribution to RV function is lost. Combined with the resultant RV dilatation and increased wall stress, this can lead to a cycle of diminishing cardiac output (LVAD + native LV) and rising central venous pressure (CVP).

Assessment of the VAD patient's incision sites, for instance, the sternotomy incision and/or thoracotomy incision, is similar to other surgical procedures. Wounds should be periodically inspected for the development of incisional separation, erythema, or pain. Purulent discharge suggests that a superficial wound infection may be present, while sternal instability may indicate sternal dehiscence or osteomyelitis (mediastinitis). Mediastinitis is a grave complication in a patient with an implanted LVAD and should be treated aggressively following diagnosis. Diagnosis of mediastinitis is based on wound culture, blood culture, wound assessment, leukocyte count, and imaging of the sternum with plain films and CT scan.[56] Serious complications with deep wound infections were encountered early in the use of durable implanted devices. The large space required for pulsatile implanted LVADs predisposed patients to infections of the pump pocket that could involve the inflow and outflow cannulas. Success in managing these patients, at least for limited periods of time to allow transplantation, was achieved with antibiotic-eluting beads of bone cement[57] and the use of autologous tissue such as rectus flaps and omental transfers.[58] Similar methods can be used to manage infections of implanted rotary pumps and mediastinitis in patients with VADs. The collaboration of plastic-reconstruction surgeons to plan and perform these operations is extremely helpful, especially when components of the pump are exposed. Fortunately, deep infections that involve the pump or cannulas are less common with rotary pumps because they require a smaller pocket than a pulsatile LVAD does (e.g., axial flow pumps) or no pocket (e.g., centrifugal pumps attached to the LV apex).

EARLY POSTIMPLANTATION MEDICAL MANAGEMENT IN THE ICU

Postimplantation, patients will arrive intubated and sedated to the ICU with chest tubes, a mediastinal tube, a pulmonary artery catheter, an arterial line, an orogastric tube, peripheral intravenous lines, and, generally, at least one inotrope and one vasopressor running. Vasoplegic patients, or those with RV failure, may be receiving high doses of multiple inotropes and vasopressors, and they may have inhaled nitric oxide or epoprostenol connected to the ventilator. Some may have a temporary RVAD, surgical or percutaneous, in place.

Initial attention should be paid to transferring the many drips from anesthesia pumps to the ICU pumps, without interrupting the infusions (or for the shortest time possible), leveling the arterial-line and pulmonary artery catheter (PAC) transducers so the hemodynamic monitoring is accurate, and placing the patient on the ICU ventilator. Often, during this period of transition, the patient's stability may be tenuous at best and several nurses, an intensivist, respiratory therapy, and a medical assistant should be on hand to receive the patient. Fluid shifts during this period are expected, including those from bleeding and third spacing due to inflammation and capillary leak. These events may require both resuscitation with crystalloid, colloid, or blood and increased vasopressor or inotropic support for vasoplegia and RV failure, respectively. All ICU intravenous infusions should be prepared in advance, including inotropes, vasopressors, and sedatives. Crystalloid and colloid should be immediately available should the blood pressure become dangerously low. The patient's mean arterial pressure (MAP) on the arterial line should be maintained at >65 mm Hg and no higher than 80 mm Hg. The amount of blood drained into the chest/mediastinal tube containers should be marked with time and date. Finally, a trained LVAD nurse or coordinator should inspect the driveline dressing to be sure it has been placed correctly and the tension-relief stabilizer is likewise being used and appropriately positioned.

Echocardiographic and hemodynamic speed optimization is an iterative process, initiated in the operating room and performed as needed in the ICU and prior to discharge with the same basic targets in mind. The LVAD speed is initially optimized in the operating room with transesophageal echocardiogram (TEE) guidance. It should be at the lowest speed possible, which generates adequate flow (confidence interval [CI], 2.2–2.6 L/Min × M^2), does not suck the septum leftward, minimizes mitral regurgitation (MR), and allows a perfusing blood pressure (often with the support of a low-dose vasopressor infusion for improved vascular tone). The reason for minimizing the pump speed and LV output from the pump is to avoid an acute volume load on the RV since it is not accustomed to robust venous return, is often dysfunctional as well, and without the benefit of mechanical support. Rather the speed should be increased slowly over the first few hours to days and likely will need to be increased as third-spaced fluid returns to the intravascular space and the LV needs increased unloading. Evidence suggests that after this initial perioperative phase, pump speed changes among patients with an implanted LVAD are much less likely to affect the RV performance if done carefully.

If the patient arrived in the operating room with an intraaortic balloon pump (IABP) in place, the augmentation is decreased and the IABP is removed as soon as possible after arrival in the ICU. The pulsation of the IABP creates a pulsatile waveform; however, conventional wisdom has it that IABP inflation will stop the forward flow or actually reverse the flow of blood out of a rotary LVAD. On the other hand, a small study in 2015 at Barnes-Jewish Hospital in St. Louis looked at 51 flow tracings from LVAD patients with an IABP *in situ* postimplantation at inflation ratios of 1:1, 1:2, and 1:3 versus off and actually found no statistically significant difference in mean flow among groups, although there was a statistically significant reduction in minimum flow rates and increase in maximal flow rates, thus widening the pulsatility.[59–62] However, since the IABP is often on a 1:2 or 1:3 setting postimplantation, there is a risk of thrombus formation and thromboembolism from the balloon pump. As long as the activated clotting time (ACT) has dropped sufficiently, the balloon pump should be pulled, and appropriate hemostasis achieved.

The initial hours in the ICU are critical to establishing stability and recognizing potential problems that, if untreated, may lead to increased morbidity, mortality, and prolonged ICU length of stay. These include bleeding, progressive right heart dysfunction, vasoplegia, and pericardial tamponade. Close attention to vital signs, invasive hemodynamics, mixed venous oxygen saturation, and serum lactate values will often hint at potential problems ahead. One must also be attuned to changes in VAD parameters, urine output, and chest tube output.

The development of a low pump output is a frequent clinical challenge in the early postoperative period. Clinicians must pay particular attention to trends in the CVP levels as well as the hourly chest tube output and LVAD parameters such as pump flow and pulsatility. The postoperative events that lead to low pump output include bleeding, hypovolemia, pericardial tamponade, and acute RHF (Fig. 12.3). Differentiating one from the other can be accomplished by using invasive hemodynamics and clinical acumen. For example, in the case of tamponade, an elevation of CVP and the sudden cessation of mediastinal tube drainage or an insidious fall in pump output should prompt echocardiographic confirmation and early chest exploration.[63] Other typical signs, such as muffled heart sounds and paradoxical pulse, are unreliable in the setting of a continuous-flow blood pump and a recent sternotomy. Acute RHF can be identified by a sudden drop in flow, a dampening of wave forms on a centrifugal-flow device with a waveform display, and/or a sudden drop in the mixed venous oxygen saturation combined with a rising CVP and serum lactate level. A transesophageal echocardiogram can help rapidly make the diagnosis and the surgeon may intervene in time (by placing a temporary RVAD) to prevent damage to end-organs from low cardiac output (Fig. 12.4).

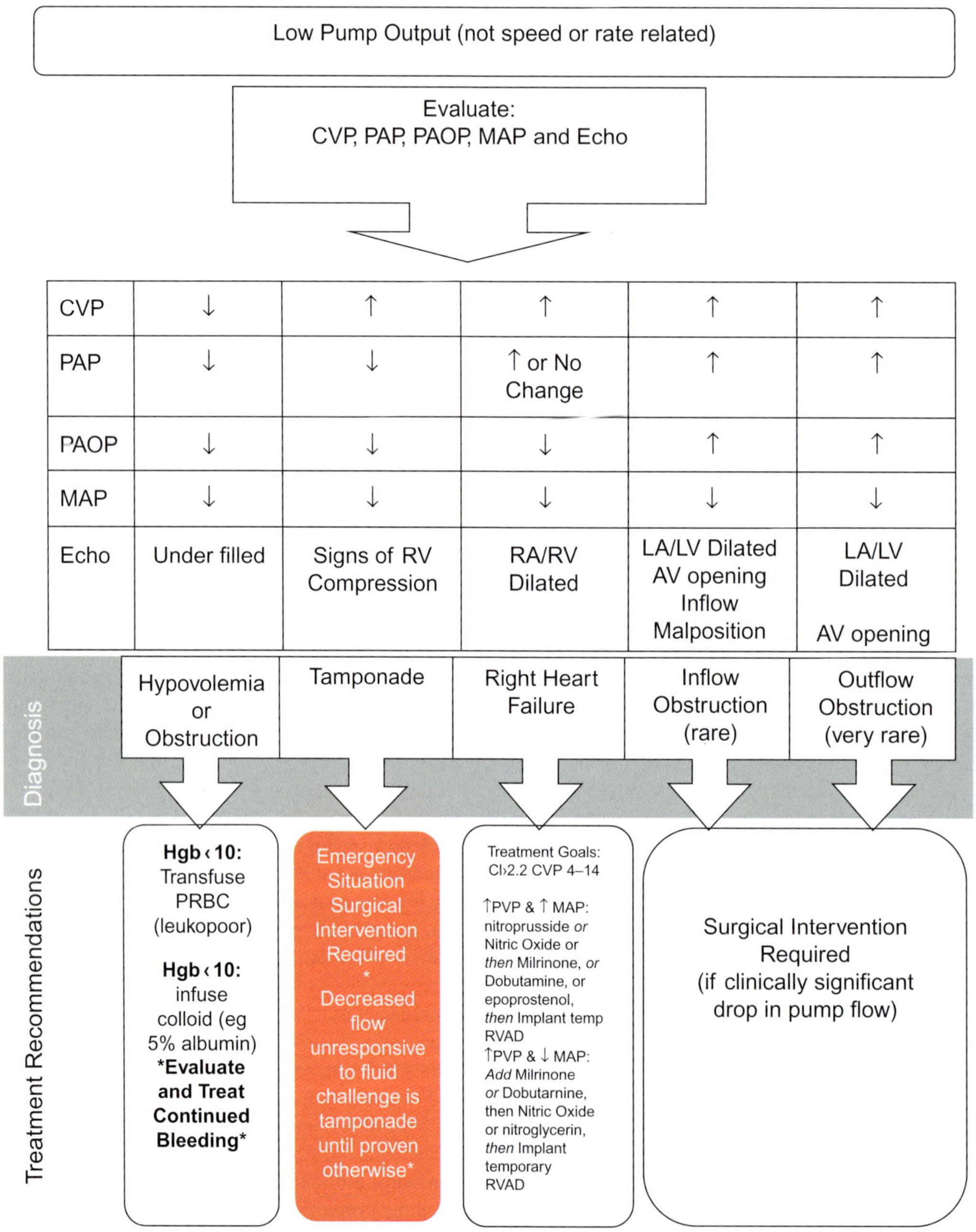

Fig. 12.3 Algorithm for rapid evaluation of new or worsening low pump output postoperatively. Note that the CVP is the first point of decision-making, since a low CVP will almost always reflect hypovolemia due to bleeding or third-spacing while an elevated CVP is seen in most other conditions and requires further evaluation. *AV*, aortic valve; *CVP*, central venous pressure; *LA*, left atrium; *LV*, left ventricle; *MAP*, mean arterial pressure; *PAOP*, pulmonary artery occlusive pressure; *PAP*, pulmonary artery pressure; *PRBC*, packed red blood cells; *PVR*, pulmonary vascular resistance; *RA*, right atrium; *RV*, right ventricle; *RVAD*, right ventricular assist device.

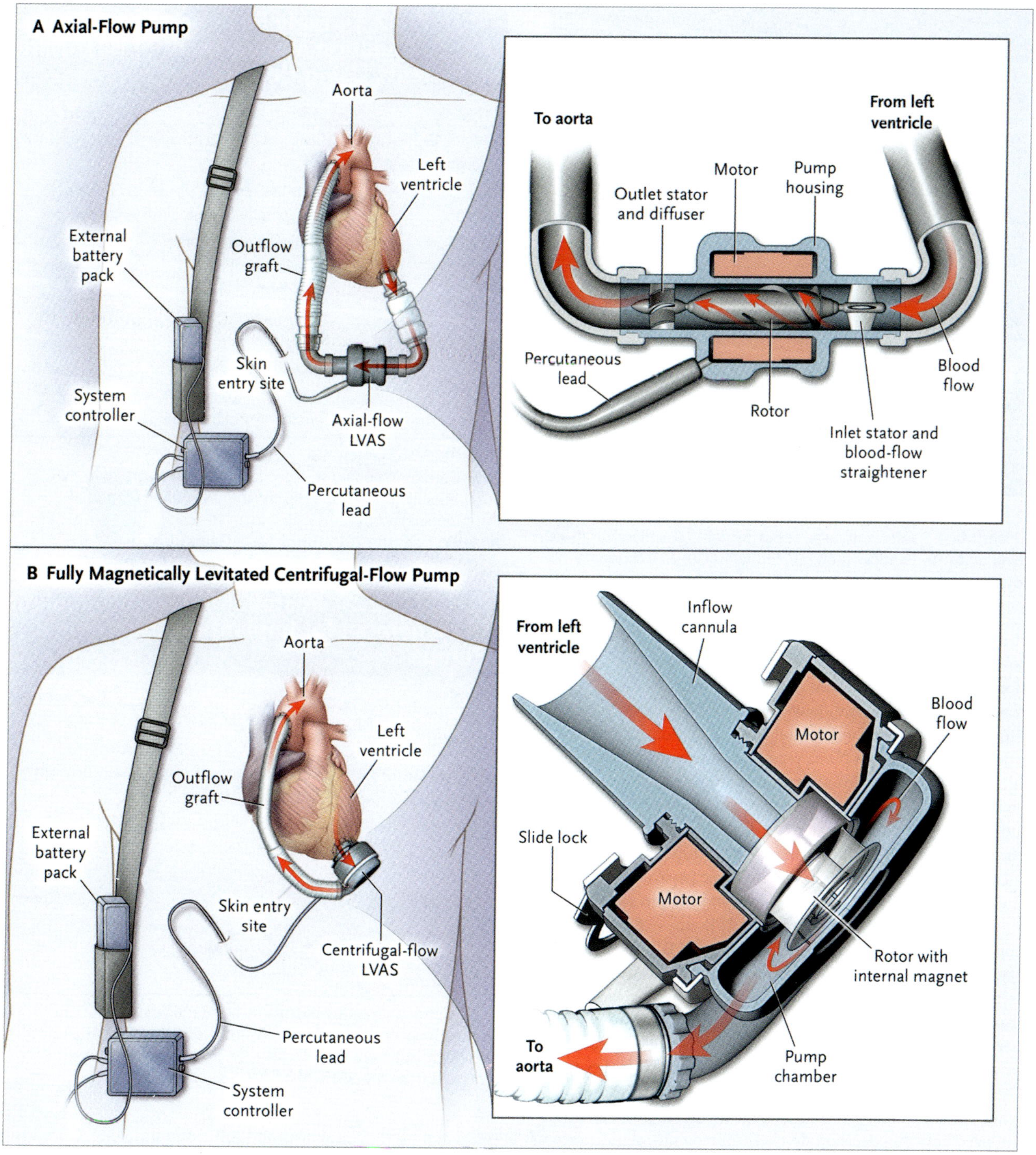

Fig. 12.4 Illustration of the (A) axial-flow design of the HeartMate 2 left ventricular assist system *(LVAS)* and (B) centrifugal-flow, MagLev design of the HeartMate 3 LVAS. (From Abbott Inc., Abbott Park, IL.)

PHARMACOLOGIC MANAGEMENT IN THE ICU

Generally, epinephrine and other vasopressors should be weaned first, as long as the patient can maintain an adequate, perfusing MAP. Next, any inhaled pulmonary vasodilators should be weaned off, again slowly and as tolerated. Generally, the weaning of inhaled epoprostenol is protocolized in most institutions. As epoprostenol or inhaled nitric oxide (iNO) is weaned, some centers will start oral sildenafil or low-dose digoxin for RV support. The evidence for these practices is slim and mostly anecdotal and requires further validation in high-quality clinical trials. Many centers continue to infuse low doses of a positive inotrope, such as milrinone, to patients with impaired RV function until such time as the RA and RV filling pressures have been optimized to the point where they are no longer impacting RV function.

Early extubation should be the goal with all postimplantation patients along with early mobilization. Of course, this varies widely based upon the intraoperative and early postoperative course. Often, patients remain intubated postoperative day (POD) 0 to POD 1 in order to gain stability and begin the process of diuresing third-spaced volume that has since been mobilized into the intravascular space. Some centers may prefer an initial bolus of furosemide, followed by a low-dose drip

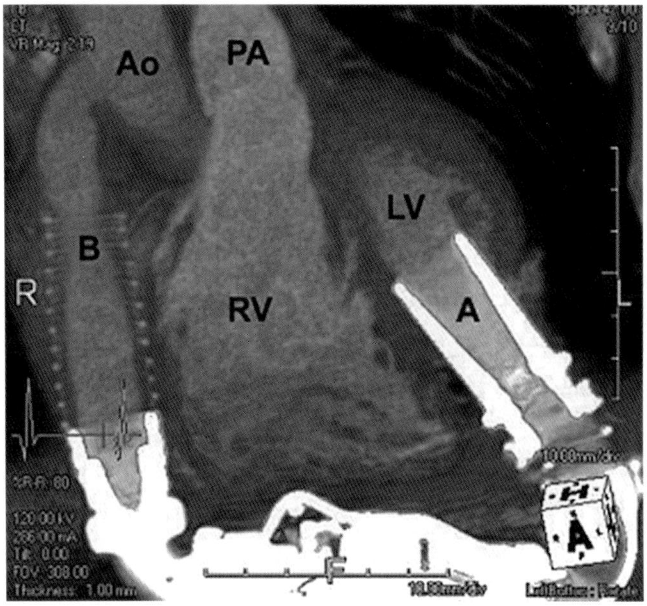

Fig. 12.5 Gated CTA of the chest demonstrating proper placement of the HeartMate 2 left ventricular assist system. *A*, inflow graft; *Ao*, Ascending aorta; *B*, Outflow graft; *LV*, left ventricle; *R*, (on original film to denote the right side of the body); *RV*, right ventricle.

TABLE 12.1 Early Postoperative Anticoagulation Management of HeartMate II[a] Patients Using Heparin

Timing	Action	Target
After CPB—leaving operating room	Complete reversal of heparin	Not applicable
ICU admission—24 hours	No action required, consider acetylsalicylic acid	Not applicable
Postoperative day 1–2	IV heparin or alternative anticoagulation, if no evidence of bleeding	PTT (40–60 seconds)
Postoperative day 2–3	Continue heparin	PTT (60–80 seconds)
	Start warfarin and aspirin (81–325 mg daily) after removal of chest tubes	INR (2.0–3.0)

[a]Thoratec, Pleasanton, CA.
CPB, Cardiopulmonary bypass; *ICU*, intensive care unit; *INR*, international normalized ratio; *IV*, intravenous; *PTT*, partial thromboplastin time.
Adapted from the 2013 ISHLT MCS Guidelines.

TABLE 12.2 Postoperative Anticoagulation Management for Implantable Centrifugal Pumps

Timing	Action	Target
After CPB—leaving operating room	Complete reversal of heparin	Not applicable
ICU admission—24 hours	No action required, consider acetylsalicylic acid	Not applicable
Postoperative Day 1–2	IV heparin or alternative anticoagulation, if no evidence of bleeding	PTT (40–60 seconds)
Postoperative Day 2–3	Continue heparin	PTT (60–80 seconds)
	Start warfarin and aspirin (81–325 mg daily) after removal of chest tubes	INR (2.0–3.0)

CPB, Cardiopulmonary bypass; *ICU*, intensive care unit; *INR*, international normalized ratio; *IV*, intravenous; *PTT*, partial thromboplastin time.
Adapted from the 2013 ISHLT MCS Guidelines.

to start a gentle diuresis with a goal of maintaining a CVP <16 mm Hg, above which renal and hepatic congestion can develop, causing a reduction in glomerular filtration rate and protracted coagulopathy. If increasing doses of furosemide with or without a thiazide diuretic added for synergy do not provide for an adequate diuresis to maintain or decrease the patient's filling pressures, continuous veno-venous hemofiltration (CVVH) or ultrafiltration should be employed early to manage intravascular volume and pressure until the patient can mobilize fluid with the assistance of pharmacologic diuretics alone.

Anticoagulation should be started early postoperatively with the introduction of aspirin on POD 1 and low-dose heparin drip without a bolus and an initial goal PTT of 40–60 seconds within 48 hours and ideally a goal PTT of 60–80 seconds within 72 hours. Guidance for the initiation of anticoagulation can be found in the ISHLT and American Association for Thoracic Surgery Guidelines in addition to the manufacturer's instructions for use. These guidelines were developed in the era of the HeartMate 2 and HVAD pumps (Fig. 12.5). It remains to be seen if anticoagulation can be delayed further and the intensity reduced among those with the newer generation of fully MagLev (magnetically levitated) centrifugal pumps. Of course, centers have evolved significant variation in the timing of beginning anticoagulation and often, in part, base this decision on chest tube output, significance of bleeding in the operating room, and prior personal experience. The ISHLT guidelines are summarized in Tables 12.1 and 12.2. The caveat, of course, is that anticoagulation is withheld as long as there is significant bleeding ongoing.

As alluded to previously, early mobility is also a primary goal among patients with a fresh LVAD implant in order to prevent further deconditioning, muscle atrophy, and myopathy. In an ideal situation, patients who have been removed from mechanical ventilation will be able to sit upright in a chair for a few hours daily in the early postoperative period. The ability of intubated patients to tolerate enough lightening of sedation to be able to safely sit in a chair varies widely but is not tolerated by most. Even if the patient remains intubated, trained physical therapists can work with the patient who is arousable to perform either active extremity movement or passive range of motion exercises to prevent muscle contractures and soft tissue stiffening. Once extubated, the patient should be treated for pain with appropriate narcotic medication such that they can deeply inspire (especially while chest tubes are in place) and stand at the bedside with minimal discomfort while not being so heavily medicated that they lack the ability to participate in their rehabilitation.

Lines and tubes are barriers to patient ambulation and are a source of infection risk and should be removed as soon as possible. Chest tubes are often a significant source of pain, irritating and inflaming the pleura with every motion. Guidelines recommend timeframes for removal of lines and tubes. Generally, chest tubes should come out when the output is less than 100 mL over 6 hours despite repositioning and within the 48 hours it takes to start heparin. The pocket drain should be removed within 72 hours and when output is <100 mL over 6 hours. The pulmonary artery catheter should be pulled within 48–72 hours as long as the patient is not exhibiting severe RHF requiring high-dose inotropes, where hemodynamics need to be monitored more closely. The arterial line should stay in until all vasoactive medications are discontinued. Some centers may choose to place a peripherally inserted central catheter (PICC), as opposed to a central venous catheter. This not only allows infusion access for medications such as furosemide, heparin, or inotropes but also provides facilitated access for blood draws and the sampling of central venous oxygenation saturation. Such PICC use may be associated with a lower risk of central-line-associated blood stream infection.

Once patients are able to stand, they should be encouraged to ambulate three times daily regardless of the distance walked or the assistance required. The patient should also be out of their bed and sitting in a chair for meals each day. As the patient's conditioning improves, longer walks with physical therapy and nursing staff are encouraged. Ideally, the patient's stay in the ICU postoperatively should be limited to 3–5 days until he/she moves to a skilled step-down floor, with nurses well trained in VAD management and who can reinforce teaching started by the VAD coordinator preoperatively and in the ICU. Of course, there are outliers in both directions—patients with a complicated postoperative course who remain intubated for an extended period and develop myopathy or ICU delirium and those needing a higher level of care than a step-down unit can provide. Also, there are patients who do extraordinarily well, are extubated on POD 0, and are off all drips, with tubes and lines out within 48 hours, ready to move to step-down. While chance complications can certainly play a role in a patient's immediate postoperative course, the elective placement of a durable LVAD in a patient who is INTERMACS class 3 and has been admitted prior to surgery for careful hemodynamic optimization is likely to have a smoother postoperative course than one who is INTERMACS class 2 (sliding despite inotropes) and rushed into the operating room just before multiorgan system failure was to develop.

In addition to mobilization, once on the step-down floor, attention is turned to teaching and reinforcing teaching regarding the independent management of the LVAD. The patient should become the device expert. Patients must demonstrate the ability to perform battery exchanges, switching effortlessly from the power module to batteries and back again. The caregiver also needs to learn these skills should the patient be incapacitated. A caregiver must be selected who can perform driveline dressing changes and be taught aseptic technique, learn how to examine the driveline dressing site for signs of infection or drainage, and can take pictures of it, if in doubt, to send to the VAD coordinator.

Patients are taught diet management with respect to coumadin, to avoid foods that contain high levels of vitamin K, and, most importantly, to follow a consistent diet. The importance of attending clinic visits in a consistent fashion (Table 12.3) is underscored by the need for frequent INR checks when levels are labile. Similarly, patients with LVADs are encouraged to call the clinic or use the LVAD hotline should any concerns arise, day or night. Concerning events include weight gain, new-onset shortness of breath (SOB), fever, and change in the appearance of the driveline exit site such as erythema, purulent drainage, and increased serous drainage especially if accompanied by warmth, tenderness, or fluctuance. This is all part of the teaching process that patients and their caregivers must go through and be "signed off" on by the VAD coordinators or designated nursing staff.

Perhaps the most important thing a patient and their caregiver need to learn prior to discharge is how to change out the system controller in case of malfunction. This is especially true among patients whose aortic valves have been sutured closed during the implantation due to aortic insufficiency (AI). However, even with a functional aortic valve, many patients would lose consciousness should they lose pump function for a sustained period of time. Therefore, changing out the system controller must be second nature and is taught over and over again during the index hospitalization, using demonstration equipment. They are taught to change out the system controller in a very controlled, yet expeditious and systematic, manner. Patients are taught to always carry with them a back-up controller with the same settings as their live system controller. Some centers, as a "final exam," have the patients change out their own live system controller to their back-up controller while supervised to be sure they can do it correctly under that type of pressure. However, many centers have moved away from that type of teaching, given the small, but nonzero, risk that if there is a small thrombus in the impeller, the result of abruptly stopping the pump and then starting back up again might lead to its dislodgement, embolization, and stroke. Providers rely on adequate demonstration utilizing the teaching equipment that the patient has learned the skill and can do it smoothly, without hesitation, and in a systematic, efficient fashion.

The final optimization step prior to discharge is the so-called echo optimization study. This is done once the patient is perceived to be euvolemic and optimized on his/her discharge medication regimen. Each center has their own style of performing the echo optimization study, but it is typically intended to find the optimal speed that, in decreasing priority, optimizes septal position, decreases MR, allows for at least intermittent aortic valve opening, maximizes flow, and does not compromise a perfusing mean arterial blood pressure. This is often performed by stepwise increases in speed in fixed increments until the aortic valve no longer opens, taking measurements of LV end-diastolic dimension (LVEDD), degree of MR, degree of AI, frequency and degree of aortic valve opening (i.e., opens partially every other beat), appearance of septum in multiple planes (midline, flattened, and bowed leftward) along with the speed (rpm), flow, and pulsatility. We recommend pausing at each new speed for at least 2 minutes to allow for reequilibration prior to taking measurements. Once this has been done across a wide range of speeds, the optimal speed is determined by the LVAD physician and coordinator. If this speed is different from the current speed, then the back-up controller must be reprogrammed for the new speed as well.

These echocardiography-guided ramp studies worked well with axial flow devices, but it seems that reduction in LV volume with axial flow devices is more pronounced in the short axis and results in larger degrees of changes in the measurement of LVEDD than a relatively similar change performed on a centrifugal flow pump, which results in a more circumferential change in LV size.[64] Some have advocated for LVAD optimization using not only echocardiography but also hemodynamic measurements with a pulmonary artery catheter to directly measure the right- and left-sided filling pressures and changes in the Fick cardiac output. Among those with centrifugal flow pumps, the combination of echocardiography and simultaneous hemodynamic measurements, while time-intensive, has been shown to improve filling pressures and cardiac output.[65]

PREPARING FOR HOME DISCHARGE

The successful transition from hospital to home begins with achieving clinical stability. In theory, this means achieving a sufficient cardiac and pump output to sustain organ perfusion coupled with an ability to ambulate and care for oneself. In practical terms, this means several things. First, the circulation should be sustained without the need for inotropic or pressor support. There should be resolution of, or at least significant improvement from, organ injury that occurred either as a result of surgery or the heart failure state that preceded it. Chest and mediastinal tubes should have been removed along with temporary pacing wires, and pleural effusions have been drained. Wounds should be granulating and covered and not actively bleeding. Additionally, patients should be able to feed themselves and consume a sufficient quantity of protein and calories to facilitate wound healing and organ recovery.

TABLE 12.3 Schedule of Visits

	Week 1	Week 2	Week 4	Week 6	Month 2	Month 3	Month 4	Month 5	Month 6	Month 7	Month 8	Month 9	Month 10	Month 11	Month 12
AHF clinic	X	X	X	X	X	X	X	X	X	X	X	X	X	X	X
Surgeon visit		X		X											
PT/INR/LDH	X	X	X	X	X	X	X	X	X	X	X	X	X	X	X
Echocardiogram						X			X			X			X
Right heart cath.						X			X			X			X
6-minute walk test/ CPET						X									X
Chest CT					X								X		
PRA			X			X			X			X			X

RHC need not be performed at months 6 and 9 in the absence of pulmonary hypertension.
A positive HIT screen should be confirmed with a serotonin release assay (SRA).
HIT screening need not be performed at months 6 and 9 in the absence of a positive screen at month 3 or subsequent heparin exposure.
PRA should be repeated 2–4 weeks after a sensitizing event (blood transfusion, pregnancy, etc.).
AHF, Advanced heart failure; *Chest CT*, chest computerized tomography; *CPET*, cardiopulmonary exercise test; *HIT*, heparin induced antibody; *PT/INR/PFH*, prothrombin time/international normalized ratio/plasma free hemoglobin; *PRA*, panel reactive antibodies; *Right heart cath.*, right heart catheterization.

Preparing for home discharge includes a physical therapy assessment. Challenges that may be encountered at home, such as the need to climb stairs, should be addressed prior to discharge. A physical therapy assessment including an ability to walk unassisted and climb a minimum number of steps can be very useful in providing assurances that patients can safely handle their home environment. Patients should demonstrate an ability to carry out their activities of daily living including grooming, dressing, and feeding themselves. Some programs may choose to have patients shower in hospital prior to discharge, but this need should be balanced with the potential for infection and is not an absolute prerequisite for discharge.

Sufficient time should be set aside to teach patients and their caregivers about living with an LVAD. This includes understanding and troubleshooting various device alarms, demonstrating proper technique for battery exchanges, and performance of driveline wound care while maintaining sterile technique. These tasks are considered to be the most challenging for patients and caregivers to handle so one should not expect full mastery and retention after a single education session.[64]

Rather, one should plan for multiple sessions over time while employing teach-back methodology to ensure that patients and caregivers have achieved working knowledge and comfort with these tasks. This is an appropriate time to ensure that a home safety survey has been completed, making sure that there are grounded power outlets. Patients must have an emergency plan to follow in the case of a power outage or environmental emergency to ensure uninterrupted access to alternating current to power the power module and charge batteries.

Nothing can fully prepare patients for the adjustments in lifestyle required to live well with an LVAD, but some strategies to ease this transition can be helpful. Meeting another LVAD patient prior to discharge can provide insights and reduce anxieties over the challenges ahead. Participation in LVAD support groups and meeting with social work or palliative care specialists can help prepare one to address the emotional challenges that may arise at home. Simply being made aware that disruptions to normal living, such as difficulty dressing, bathing, and sleeping, may occur can often facilitate adjustment and acceptance of this new way of living. Honest discussions about the potential for sexual dysfunction and ways to restore intimacy are often important to patients even though they may find it difficult to express these concerns in the open.[66]

All patients should be provided a schedule of outpatient appointments prior to being discharged. A typical schedule (see Table 12.2) includes an early follow-up visit, followed by outpatient visits at regular intervals such as every 2–4 weeks. Most programs find it helpful to repeat an outpatient echocardiogram within the first 3 months to ensure proper LV unloading and identification of any significant valvular insufficiency or RV dysfunction. Follow-up right heart catheterizations, particularly for those awaiting heart transplant, can be useful to document reductions in pulmonary arterial pressures and may facilitate the optimization of pump speed programming.[67]

STANDARD OUTPATIENT VISIT

There are several objectives that must be addressed during a standard outpatient visit. The first is to ensure the safe operation of the LVAD and patient well-being. The second is to identify whether patients are encountering any potential adverse events. The third is to assess for health-related quality of life (HRQoL) and to screen for depression. Each encounter should start with a thorough examination of the patient's recent history inquiring about such things as their daily activities, quality and quantity of sleep, the presence of any exertional dyspnea or fatigue, the occurrence of any abnormal bleeding, any drainage from the driveline exit site, and any change in the color or quantity of their urine. Patients should be asked whether they have encountered any device alarms and should report how long they are being supported on battery before needing to change them.

A thorough physical assessment should not only include a complete cardiopulmonary examination but should also hone in on those aspects that are unique to the LVAD itself. This begins with proper blood pressure measurement. The reduced pulse pressure produced by continuous-flow LVADs makes it challenging to auscultate a blood pressure or to palpate a peripheral pulse. This reduces the accuracy of automated oscillatory blood pressure cuffs to properly estimate systolic, diastolic, and MAP. This limitation can be overcome through the use of a manual sphygmomanometer combined with a Doppler ultrasound to detect the opening pressure. Due to dampened arterial pulsatility, the opening Doppler blood pressure is often considered equivalent to the

MAP, although this may be less true in those patients with preserved pulsatility and a widened pulse pressure. Other measurement techniques that employ a slow cuff-deflation system (Terumo, Elemano) more closely approximate the measurements obtained from an arterial line and may be more accurate than Doppler blood pressure.[64] Some uncertainty exists regarding blood pressure monitoring in those patients supported with newer CF-LVADs that include pulsatility algorithms, such as the HeartMate 3, as these patients may have an intermittently palpable pulse. In these individuals, it may be appropriate to record blood pressures taken with both an automated blood pressure cuff and with a Doppler ultrasound.

The proper examination of an LVAD patient continues with additional aspects unique to the LVAD itself. Pump speed, power, and flow should be recorded along with some mention of the flow pulse or pulsatility index. A review of recent alarms should look for any low flow events or power disruptions that may have arisen either through improper disconnection or exhausted batteries. Although it may be challenging to auscultate heart sounds in LVAD patients, clinicians should document whether it is possible to hear the continuous hum of the pump itself. The driveline exit wound should be examined at each visit, looking for signs of infection that may include erythema, bleeding, or drainage from the site. The integrity of the driveline itself should also be inspected for the presence of any tears or disruptions from mechanical trauma. Minor tears can usually be repaired with the use of specialized tape provided from the manufacturer. More extensive tears or those associated with low flow alarms should be examined radiographically for evidence of disruptions to the wires themselves. The proper anchoring technique should be reviewed with patients and caregivers to ensure that the driveline is immobilized and the wound is being properly cleaned and dressed.

Most visits will include laboratory studies that are reflective of device-patient hemocompatibility.[68] Perhaps the singular, most important goal is to ensure a proper level of anticoagulation through the use of INR monitoring. Current guidelines support maintaining a patient's INR between 2 and 3, although reduced targets may ultimately be appropriate in some patients with newer MagLev technologies.[69] An elevated level of lactate dehydrogenase may be indicative of hemolysis arising from pump thrombosis and should be regularly assessed along with a complete blood count to screen for anemia. Elevations in white blood cell count may be a sign of infection in the right clinical context. For those patients being bridged to transplantation, the measurement of alloantibodies at frequent intervals (every 1–3 months) may be helpful in screening for sensitization and planning a cross-match at the time of organ offer.

Cardiac rhythm disturbances are common after LVAD implantation.[70] Both atrial and ventricular tachyarrhythmia may arise without loss of consciousness. Clues to their presence may include an unexpected drop in pump output, orthostasis, or exertional symptoms. For these reasons, all patients should have an electrocardiogram performed with every visit. This is all the more imperative for patients who have not received an implantable cardioverter defibrillator (ICD) or whose ICD shock therapies are disabled.

A routine CXR need not be performed every visit but should be obtained at baseline and with any change in symptoms. Not only can a CXR be helpful in diagnosing pleural effusion or pulmonary edema, but it may also aid in understanding the reasons behind pump malfunction. The identification of an enlarging cardiac silhouette or a "boot-shaped" heart could suggest the presence of a pericardial effusion leading to cardiac tamponade. Improper alignment of the inflow cannula either at the time of placement or from device movement over time may lead to acute angulation, cannula deflection away from the mitral valve, and partial obstruction to flow. The resulting turbulent flow may produce hemolysis and could possibly contribute to low flow and the development of pump thrombosis.[71]

Perhaps no single test is as useful as a transthoracic echocardiogram in the overall management of an LVAD patient.[50] Surveillance two-dimensional echocardiography with Doppler flow assessment should be performed at regular intervals to monitor both pump and native heart function. Such studies should be performed with the pump set at its baseline speed setting and include both LVAD-specific views in addition to all the elements of a standard exam. The frequency of these protocol studies may vary between institutions, but a baseline study just prior to hospital discharge may be followed by additional studies at 1, 3, 6, and 12 months postimplantation and every 6–12 months thereafter. Key elements of these exams include measuring biventricular size and function, examining the interventricular septal position, documenting the frequency of aortic valve opening, and assessing native heart valve integrity. Additionally, echocardiography should be employed in the evaluation of pump malfunction or the emergence of clinical heart failure. Echocardiography can be readily used to assess for pericardial tamponade, RHF, AI, inflow or outflow cannula obstruction, and excessive LV unloading leading to suck-down events. Echocardiographic ramp studies that employ changing pump speeds can be helpful both to optimize pump speed setting and to evaluate for suspected pump thrombosis.[72] One additional function of echocardiography is to screen for recovery of native heart function. Although many patients experience some improvement in LV function with durable LVAD support, it remains the small minority of patients who enjoy enough recovery to allow safe device removal.

One final objective of the routine outpatient visit is to assess HRQoL and screen for depression. Although LVADs improve survival and HRQoL for most patients, fully one-third of patients will either die or continue to experience poor quality of life during the first year after implantation.[64] Patients who are more likely to experience poor HRQoL are those who had more advanced heart failure symptoms and poorer functional status prior to implantation, as well as those with device-related complications. Several validated tools, such as the Euroqol 5-Dimensions and Kansas City Cardiomyopathy Questionnaire, have been used as research tools in outcome studies but can be challenging to employ in routine clinical practice. In contrast, the Patient Health Questionnaire-9 is a self-administered depression screening tool that patients can complete during outpatient visits. Patients with more than mild symptoms of depression should be considered for referred to a mental health or palliative care specialist. Finally, functional status as measured by the standardized 6-minute walk test is required by INTERMACS and allows for an objective measure of both cardiopulmonary progress and regression. Many centers protocolize the frequency of this test to coincide with INTERMACS requirements.

REFERENCES

1. Kirklin JK, Pagani FD, Kormos RL, et al. Eighth annual INTERMACS report: special focus on framing the impact of adverse events. *J Heart Lung Transplant*. 2017;36:1080–1086.
2. Kirklin JK, Naftel DC, Pagani FD, et al. Sixth INTERMACS annual report: a 10,000-patient database. *J Heart Lung Transplant*. 2014;33:555–564.
3. Feldman D, Pamboukian SV, Teutcberg JJ, et al. The 2013 International Society for Heart and Lung Transplantation Guidelines for mechanical circulatory support: executive summary. *J Heart Lung Transplant*. 2013;32:157–187.
4. Fleck T, Kickinger B, Moidl R, et al. Management of open chest and delayed sternal closure with the vacuum assisted closure system: preliminary experience. *Interact Cardiovasc Thorac Surg*. 2008;7:801–804.

5. Obdeijn MC, de Lange MY, Lichtendahl DH, de Boer WJ. Vacuum-assisted closure in the treatment of poststernotomy mediastinitis. *Ann Thorac Surg*. 1999;68:2358–2360.
6. Mokhtari A, Petzina R, Gustafsson L, Sjogren J, Malmsjo M, Ingemansson R. Sternal stability at different negative pressures during vacuum-assisted closure therapy. *Ann Thorac Surg*. 2006;82:1063–1067.
7. Petzina R, Malmsjo M, Stamm C, Hetzer R. Major complications during negative pressure wound therapy in poststernotomy mediastinitis after cardiac surgery. *J Thorac Cardiovasc Surg*. 2010;140:1133–1136.
8. Anglen J, Apostoles PS, Christensen G, Gainor B, Lane J. Removal of surface bacteria by irrigation. *J Orthop Res*. 1996;14:251–254.
9. Kormos RL, Teuteberg JJ, Pagani FD, et al. Right ventricular failure in patients with the HeartMate II continuous-flow left ventricular assist device: incidence, risk factors, and effect on outcomes. *J Thorac Cardiovasc Surg*. 2010;139:1316–1324.
10. Aissaoui N, Morshuis M, Paluszkiewicz L, Lauenroth V, Borgermann J, Gummert J. Comparison of biventricular and left ventricular assist devices for the management of severe right ventricular dysfunction in patients with end-stage heart failure. *ASAIO J*. 2014;60:400–406.
11. Cleveland Jr JC, Naftel DC, Reece TB, et al. Survival after biventricular assist device implantation: an analysis of the Interagency Registry for Mechanically Assisted Circulatory Support database. *J Heart Lung Transplant*. 2011;30:862–869.
12. Atluri P, Fairman AS, MacArthur JW, et al. Continuous flow left ventricular assist device implant significantly improves pulmonary hypertension, right ventricular contractility, and tricuspid valve competence. *J Card Surg*. 2013;28:770–775.
13. Lazar JF, Swartz MF, Schiralli MP, et al. Survival after left ventricular assist device with and without temporary right ventricular support. *Ann Thorac Surg*. 2013;96:2155–2159.
14. Anderson MB, Goldstein J, Milano C, et al. Benefits of a novel percutaneous ventricular assist device for right heart failure: The prospective RECOVER RIGHT study of the Impella RP device. *J Heart Lung Transplant*. 2015;34:1549–1560.
15. Ravichandran AK, Baran DA, Stelling K, Cowger JA, Salerno CT. Outcomes with the Tandem Protek Duo Dual-Lumen Percutaneous Right Ventricular Assist Device. *ASAIO J*. 2018;64:570–572.
16. Schenk S, McCarthy PM, Blackstone EH, et al. Duration of inotropic support after left ventricular assist device implantation: risk factors and impact on outcome. *J Thorac Cardiovasc Surg*. 2006;131:447–454.
17. Hetzer R, Krabatsch T, Stepanenko A, Hennig E, Potapov EV. Long-term biventricular support with the Heartware implantable continuous flow pump. *J Heart Lung Transplant*. 2010;29:822–824.
18. Krabatsch T, Potapov E, Stepanenko A, et al. Biventricular circulatory support with two miniaturized implantable assist devices. *Circulation*. 2011;124:S179–S186.
19. Krabatsch T, Stepanenko A, Schweiger M, et al. Alternative technique for implantation of biventricular support with HeartWare implantable continuous flow pump. *ASAIO J*. 2011;57:333–335.
20. Song HK, Tibayan FA, Mudd J, Gelow J, Slater MS. Right ventricular outflow tract cannulation for right ventricular assist device implantation. *Ann Thorac Surg*. 2013;96:333–335.
21. Strueber M, Schmitto JD, Kutschka I, Haverich A. Placement of 2 implantable centrifugal pumps to serve as a total artificial heart after cardiectomy. *J Thorac Cardiovasc Surg*. 2012;143:507–509.
22. Lavee J, Mulzer J, Krabatsch T, et al. An international multicenter experience of biventricular support with HeartMate 3 ventricular assist systems. *J Heart Lung Transplant*. 2018;37:1399–1402.
23. Fujita T, Kobayashi J, Hata H, et al. Right heart failure and benefits of adjuvant tricuspid valve repair in patients undergoing left ventricular assist device implantation. *Eur J Cardiothorac Surg*. 2014;46:802–807.
24. Maeder MT, Leet A, Ross A, Esmore D, Kaye DM. Changes in right ventricular function during continuous-flow left ventricular assist device support [corrected]. *J Heart Lung Transplant*. 2009;28:360–366.
25. Miyawaki F, Murata M, Mukai F, Tsuji T. Split-circulation assist device facilitates heart failure management and increases effects of intra-aortic balloon pumping. *ASAIO J*. 1998;44:M628–M633.
26. Piacentino V 3rd , Troupes CD, Ganapathi AM, et al. Clinical impact of concomitant tricuspid valve procedures during left ventricular assist device implantation. *Ann Thorac Surg*. 2011;92:1414–1418, discussion 1418–9.
27. Song HK, Gelow JM, Mudd J, et al. Limited Utility of Tricuspid Valve Repair at the Time of Left Ventricular Assist Device Implantation. *Ann Thorac Surg*. 2016;101:2168–2174.
28. Kusne S, Mooney M, Danziger-Isakov L, et al. An ISHLT consensus document for prevention and management strategies for mechanical circulatory support infection. *J Heart Lung Transplant*. 2017;36:1137–1153.
29. Stahovich M, Sundareswaran KS, Fox S, et al. Reduce driveline trauma through stabilization and exit site management: 30 days feasibility results from the multicenter RESIST study. *ASAIO J*. 2016;62:240–245.
30. Fudim M, Brown CL, Davis ME, et al. Driveline infection risk with utilization of a temporary external anchoring suture after implantation of a left ventricular assist device. *ASAIO J*. 2016;62:291–296.
31. Holman WL, Pamboukian SV, McGiffin DC, Tallaj JA, Cadeiras M, Kirklin JK. Device related infections: are we making progress? *J Card Surg*. 2010;25:478–483.
32. McCandless SP, Ledford ID, Mason NO, et al. Comparing velour versus silicone interfaces at the driveline exit site of HeartMate II devices: infection rates, histopathology, and ultrastructural aspects. *Cardiovasc Pathol*. 2015;24:71–75.
33. Goldstein DJ, Naftel D, Holman W, et al. Continuous-flow devices and percutaneous site infections: clinical outcomes. *J Heart Lung Transplant*. 2012;31:1151–1157.
34. Zierer A, Melby SJ, Voeller RK, et al. Late-onset driveline infections: the Achilles' heel of prolonged left ventricular assist device support. *Ann Thorac Surg*. 2007;84:515–520.
35. Wang JX, Smith JR, Bonde P. Energy transmission and power sources for mechanical circulatory support devices to achieve total implantability. *Ann Thorac Surg*. 2014;97:1467–1474.
36. Waters BH, Smith JR, Bonde P. Innovative Free-range Resonant Electrical Energy Delivery system (FREE-D System) for a ventricular assist device using wireless power. *ASAIO J*. 2014;60:31–37.
37. Boehmer JPe-B A, Korfer R, Arusoglu L, Hetzer R, Weng Y, et al. Destination therapy with a totally implantable left ventricular assist device system: results of the LionHeart CUBS Trial. *Circulation*. 2003;108. IV-364-IV-365.
38. Dowling RD, Gray Jr LA, Etoch SW, et al. Initial experience with the AbioCor implantable replacement heart system. *J Thorac Cardiovasc Surg*. 2004;127:131–141.
39. Pae WE, Connell JM, Adelowo A, et al. Does total implantability reduce infection with the use of a left ventricular assist device? The LionHeart experience in Europe. *J Heart Lung Transplant*. 2007;26:219–229.
40. Raymond AL, Kfoury AG, Bishop CJ, et al. Obesity and left ventricular assist device driveline exit site infection. *ASAIO J*. 2010;56:57–60.
41. Imamura T, Kinugawa K, Nitta D, et al. Readmission due to driveline infection can be predicted by new score by using serum albumin and body mass index during long-term left ventricular assist device support. *J Artif Organs*. 2015;18:120–127.
42. Holdy K, Dembitsky W, Eaton LL, et al. Nutrition assessment and management of left ventricular assist device patients. *J Heart Lung Transplant*. 2005;24:1690–1696.
43. Yost G, Gregory M, Bhat G. Short-form nutrition assessment in patients with advanced heart failure evaluated for ventricular assist device placement or cardiac transplantation. *Nutr Clin Pract*. 2014;29:686–691.
44. Yost G, Gregory M, Bhat G. Nutrition assessment with indirect calorimetry in patients evaluated for left ventricular assist device implantation. *Nutr Clin Pract*. 2015;30:690–697.
45. Yost G, Tatooles A, Bhat G. Preoperative nutritional assessment with the prognostic nutrition index in patients undergoing left ventricular assist device implantation. *ASAIO J*. 2018;64:52–55.
46. Montgomery TD, Cohen AE, Garnick J, Spadafore J, Boldea E. Nutrition assessment, care, and considerations of ventricular assist device patients. *Nutr Clin Pract*. 2012;27:352–362.
47. Scurlock C, Pinney SP, Lin HM, et al. Safety of parenteral nutrition in patients receiving a ventricular assist device. *ASAIO J*. 2014;60:376–380.
48. Kugler C, Malehsa D, Schrader E, et al. A multi-modal intervention in management of left ventricular assist device outpatients: dietary

counselling, controlled exercise and psychosocial support. *Eur J Cardiothorac Surg.* 2012;42:1026–1032.
49. Adamson RM, Mangi AA, Kormos RL, Farrar DJ, Dembitsky WP. Principles of HeartMate II implantation to avoid pump malposition and migration. *J Card Surg.* 2015;30:296–299.
50. Kazui T, Zhang A, Greenberg J, et al. Left ventricular assist device inflow angle and pump positional change over time adverse impact on left ventricular assist device function. *Ann Thorac Surg.* 2016;102:1933–1940.
51. Taghavi S, Ward C, Jayarajan SN, Gaughan J, Wilson LM, Mangi AA. Surgical technique influences HeartMate II left ventricular assist device thrombosis. *Ann Thorac Surg.* 2013;96:1259–1265.
52. Administration USFD. *Abbott Recalls the HeartMate 3™ Left Ventricular Assist System Due to Potential Malfunction that may Lead to Graft Occlusion.* 2018.
53. Acharya D, Hashim T, Kirklin JK, et al. Use of retrospectively gated CT angiography to diagnose systolic LVAD inflow obstruction. *ASAIO J.* 2013;59:542–546.
54. Acharya D, Singh S, Tallaj JA, et al. Use of gated cardiac computed tomography angiography in the assessment of left ventricular assist device dysfunction. *ASAIO J.* 2011;57:32–37.
55. Chow E, Farrar DJ. Right heart function during prosthetic left ventricular assistance in a porcine model of congestive heart failure. *J Thorac Cardiovasc Surg.* 1992;104:569–578.
56. Woodard JC, Chow E, Farrar DJ. Isolated ventricular systolic interaction during transient reductions in left ventricular pressure. *Circ Res.* 1992;70:944–951.
57. Hannan MM, Husain S, Mattner F, et al. Working formulation for the standardization of definitions of infections in patients using ventricular assist devices. *J Heart Lung Transplant.* 2011;30:375–384.
58. McKellar SH, Allred BD, Marks JD, et al. Treatment of infected left ventricular assist device using antibiotic-impregnated beads. *Ann Thorac Surg.* 1999;67:554–555.
59. Arabia FA, Copeland JG, Smith RG, et al. Infections with the CardioWest total artificial heart. *ASAIO J.* 1998;44:M336–M339.
60. Hutchinson OZ, Oz MC, Ascherman JA. The use of muscle flaps to treat left ventricular assist device infections. *Plast Reconstr Surg.* 2001;107:364–373.
61. Milano CA, Georgiade G, Muhlbaier LH, Smith PK, Wolfe WG. Comparison of omental and pectoralis flaps for poststernotomy mediastinitis. *Ann Thorac Surg.* 1999;67:377–380, discussion 380–1.
62. Turowski GA, Orgill DP, Pribaz JJ, Eriksson E, Couper GS. Salvage of externally exposed ventricular assist devices. *Plast Reconstr Surg.* 1998;102:2425–2430.
63. Swinney C, Itoh A, Keith A, Balsara K, Joseph S, Silvestry S. Defining the impact of intraaortic balloon pump setting on ventricular assist device flow. *J Heart Lung Transplant.* 2015;34:993–995.
64. Uriel N, Sayer G, Addetia K, et al. Hemodynamic ramp tests in patients with left ventricular assist devices. *JACC Heart Fail.* 2016;4:208–217.
65. Uriel N, Levin AP, Sayer GT, et al. Left ventricular decompression during speed optimization ramps in patients supported by continuous flow left ventricular assist devices: device-specific performance characteristics and impact on diagnostic algorithms. *J Card Fail.* 2015;21:785–791.
66. Widmar SB, Dietrich MS, Minnick AF. How self-care education in ventricular assist device programs is organized and provided: a national study. *Heart Lung.* 2014;43:25–31.
67. Eckman PM, Dhungel V, Mandras S, et al. Sexual function after left ventricular assist device. *J Am Coll Cardiol.* 2013;61:2021–2022.
68. Lanier GM, Orlanes K, Hayashi Y, et al. Validity and reliability of a novel slow cuff-deflation system for noninvasive blood pressure monitoring in patients with continuous-flow left ventricular assist device. *Circ Heart Fail.* 2013;6:1005–1012.
69. Mehra MR. The burden of haemocompatibility with left ventricular assist systems: a complex weave. *Eur Heart J.* 2017;40(8):673–677.
70. Netuka I, Ivak P, Tucanova Z, et al. Evaluation of low-intensity anti-coagulation with a fully magnetically levitated centrifugal-flow circulatory pump—the MAGENTUM 1 study. *J Heart Lung Transplant.* 2018;37:579–586.
71. Enriquez AD, Calenda B, Gandhi PU, Nair AP, Anyanwu AC, Pinney SP. Clinical impact of atrial fibrillation in patients with the HeartMate II left ventricular assist device. *J Am Coll Cardiol.* 2014;64:1883–1890.
72. Stainback RF, Estep JD, Agler DA, et al. Echocardiography in the management of patients with left ventricular assist devices: recommendations from the American Society of Echocardiography. *J Am Soc Echocardiogr.* 2015;28:853–909.

13

Adverse Events and Mitigation Strategies

J. Eduardo Rame, James K. Kirklin, William L. Holman, Garrick C. Stewart

KEY POINTS

Introduction
Definitions
Time-Related Occurrence, Contributing Factors, and Causation
Adverse Event Burden and Era Effect
Adverse Events Contributing to Death
Perioperative Bleeding
Surgical Wound Infections
Pump-Related Infection
Gastrointestinal Bleeding
Neurologic Dysfunction
Renal Failure
Device Failure
Pump Thrombosis
Other Thromboembolic Events
Right Heart Failure
Aortic Insufficiency
Arrhythmias

INTRODUCTION

The evolution of ventricular assist devices (VAD) since the year 2000 has allowed patients with end-stage heart failure to survive with increased functional capacity and quality of life (QOL).[1] Since the beginning of randomized clinical trials in the field, survival, QOL, and resource requirements have been limited by adverse events. In the case of the Randomized Evaluation of Mechanical Assistance for the Treatment of Congestive Heart Failure (REMATCH) trial,[2] pump malfunction due to nondurable components requiring a surgical exchange and stroke caused significant morbidity and mortality. As engineering in the field of mechanical circulatory support (MCS) has applied novel solutions to increase durability and to miniaturize the pumps for more facile implantation, the incidence and manifestations of certain adverse events have been altered or amplified, such as gastrointestinal (GI) bleeding and neurologic dysfunction, with a more complex pathogenesis in association with continuous-flow (CF) device support. As pump technology evolves over time, we should expect that newer devices designed to improve upon previous platforms will be associated with adverse events that require rigorous investigation and novel proposals to eliminate or mitigate their occurrence.

MCS with current-generation CF devices has provided a major improvement in duration of survival on device compared to prior pulsatile pumps.[3] With current documented survival exceeding 80% at 1 year and 70% at 2 years, extension of this therapy into the ambulatory advanced heart failure population (Interagency Registry for Mechanically Assisted Circulatory Support [INTERMACS] levels 4–6) has been extensively discussed and implemented to a limited degree.[4] However, the success of this therapy is a function not only of survival but also of QOL among survivors. A major determinant of QOL with CF pumps is the frequency, severity, and sequelae of major adverse events. Grady and colleagues demonstrated the major deleterious effect on QOL of certain adverse events at 6 months postimplantation.[5] The Randomized Evaluation of VAD Intervention Before Inotropic Therapy (REVIVE-IT) trial was designed to test the hypothesis that device therapy was superior to optimal medical therapy for such patients.[6] However, the presence of a higher-than-expected incidence of pump thrombosis in the HeartMate II (HMII) device during the era of the planned study[7] caused the investigators to terminate the study prior to performing the first implantation.[7] With increased awareness of the frequency and impact of major adverse events during CF MCS support, the application of these devices in patients with ambulatory class IV advanced heart failure has declined during recent years. The proportion of patients in INTERMACS levels 4–7 at implantation represented 18% from 2012 to 2014 and decreased to 13% in 2015–2016.[4] With the exception of right heart failure, other adverse events are equally as likely in ambulatory heart failure patients as in patients more critically ill (Figs. 13.1–13.3).[1] Thus, understanding the frequency, severity, and impact of major adverse events is of critical importance; both for truly informed decision making by patient, family, and caregiver and to inform decisions about future pump design and patient management. Moreover, increased device durability and dramatically lower adverse events (AE) rates must be achieved before a substantial increase in mechanical circulatory support device (MCSD) usage occurs in less ill populations (e.g., INTERMACS levels 4–7).

DEFINITIONS

Accurate identification of adverse events and reliable calculation of incidence requires clear definitions. Throughout the history of MCS trials, differing applications and definitions have been applied. When INTERMACS was created in 2006 as the national database for US durable MCS devices approved by the Food and Drug Administration, extensive deliberations among expert clinicians, industry, governmental personnel, and engineers focused on adverse event definitions. These were incorporated into the national INTERMACS database. More recently, the Academic Research Consortium has participated in attempts to harmonize definitions of adverse events

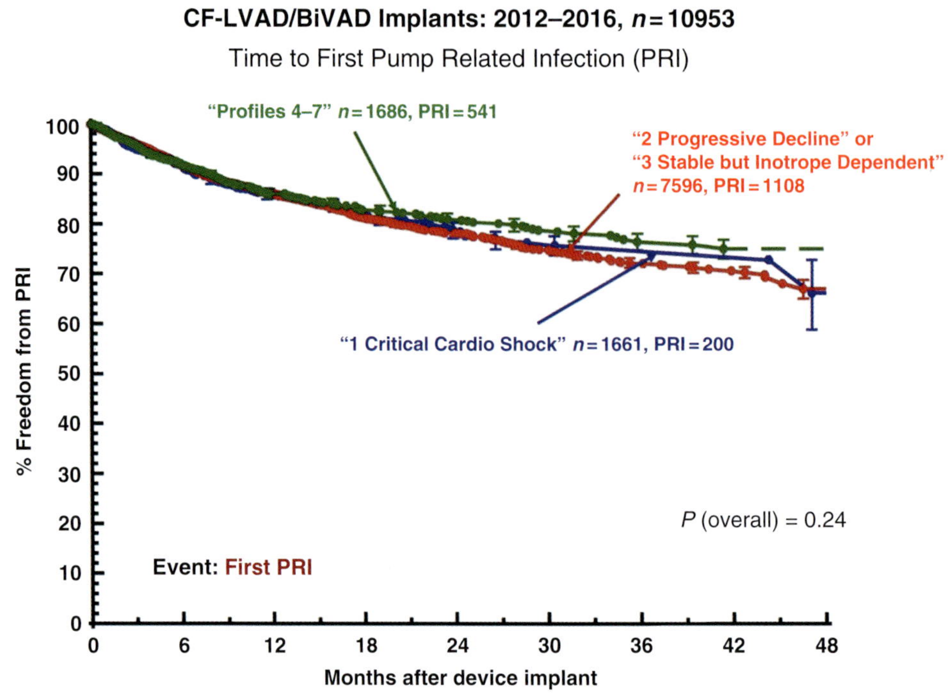

Fig. 13.1 Kaplan-Meier freedom from pump-related infection *(PRI)*, stratified by Interagency Registry for Mechanically Assisted Circulatory Support profile. *BiVAD*, Biventricular assist device; *CF-LVAD*, continuous-flow left ventricular assist device. (Modified with permission from Kirklin JK, Pagani FD, Kormos RL, et al. Eighth annual INTERMACS report: special focus on framing the impact of adverse events. *J Heart Lung Transplant* 2017;36(10):1080–1086.)

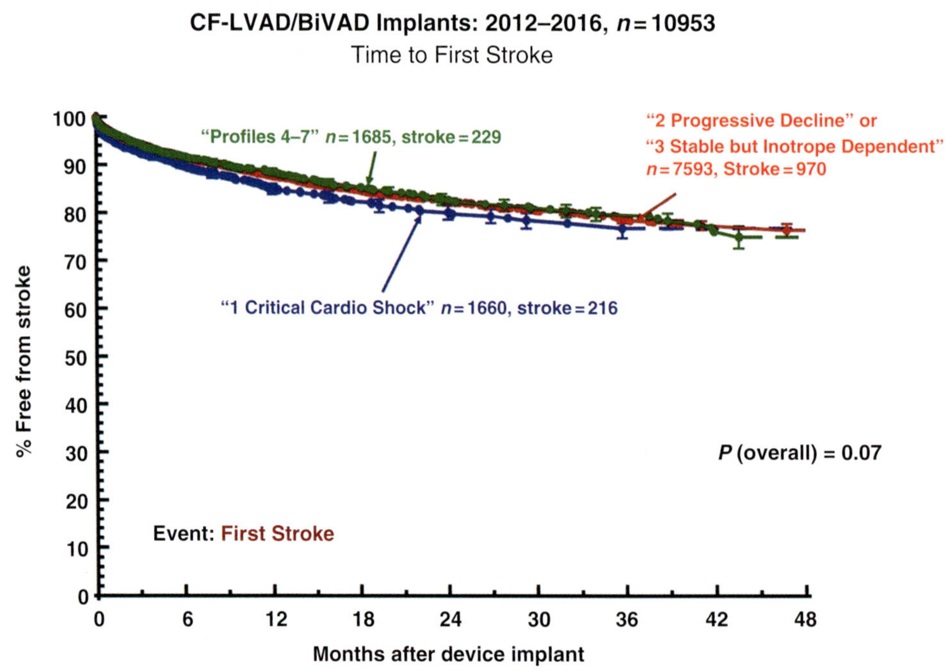

Fig. 13.2 Freedom from first stroke, stratified by Interagency Registry for Mechanically Assisted Circulatory Support profile. *BiVAD*, Biventricular assist device; *CF-LVAD*, continuous-flow left ventricular assist device. (Modified with permission from Kirklin JK, Pagani FD, Kormos RL, et al. Eighth annual INTERMACS report: special focus on framing the impact of adverse events. *J Heart Lung Transplant* 2017;36(10):1080–1086.)

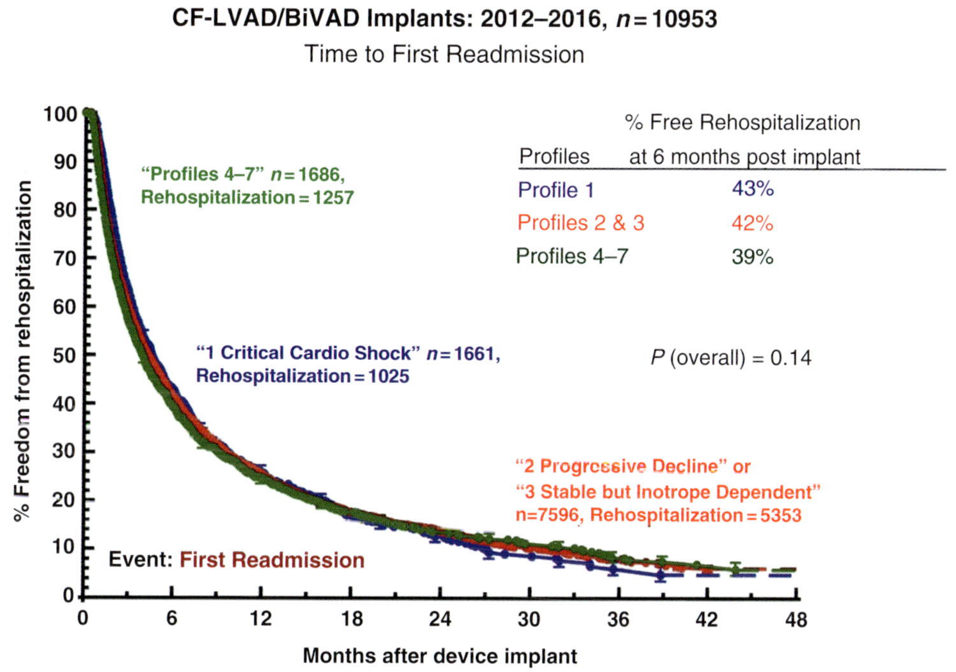

Fig. 13.3 Freedom from first readmission, stratified by Interagency Registry for Mechanically Assisted Circulatory Support profile. *BiVAD*, Biventricular assist device; *CF-LVAD*, continuous-flow left ventricular assist device. (Modified with permission from Kirklin JK, Pagani FD, Kormos RL, et al. Eighth annual INTERMACS report: special focus on framing the impact of adverse events. *J Heart Lung Transplant* 2017;36(10):1080–1806.)

among countries. The definitions used by INTERMACS in the collection of postimplantation data on more than 20,000 patients are included in the Appendix.

TIME-RELATED OCCURRENCE, CONTRIBUTING FACTORS, AND CAUSATION

Adverse events occurring early after implantation are often ascribed to the preoperative condition of the patient and often reflect the risks associated with preoperative morbidity—major cardiac surgery is being performed in patients with advanced heart failure, often decompensated and with altered metabolic status and end-organ injury. In contrast, the more chronically occurring events generally result from device design issues or management strategies.

From an analytic perspective, both the time to occurrence of a given adverse event and its repetitive nature (incidence) help characterize its impact. Although the exact "cutoff" is rather arbitrary, multiple analyses have identified different adverse events and frequencies that are more prominent early or later after implantation (Table 13.1). Additional challenges are highlighted by the following examples. A single stroke can have relatively minor or devastating effects on the patient's QOL. Strokes are discrete events in many cases, although extension of a stroke by hemorrhagic conversion may occur. By contrast, infections and especially device-related infections have slow onset so that the date of an infection AE often describes the date of diagnosis rather than the date of onset. Moreover, the date for resolution for an infection may reflect the cessation of antimicrobial therapy rather than a bona-fide eradication of infection. For example, driveline percutaneous exit site infections are typically treated for weeks with antibiotics and then the antibiotics are stopped. If erythema and purulent drainage at the site worsen, the patient will presumably be placed back on antibiotic therapy. Should this be counted as a de novo infection or persistence of a prior infection? If a driveline percutaneous exit site infection occurs, should all other episodes of driveline infection be considered recurrences of the initial event or only if the infecting organism changes? If the patient is placed on chronic suppressive antibiotic therapy, should the initial episode of driveline infection be considered as resolved or ongoing? Thus, considerable analytic challenges exist as we seek "truths" about the potential life-threatening complications of this therapy.

Risk Factors

The need for *biventricular support* because of severe left and right heart failure increases the risk of many adverse events, including respiratory failure, neurologic events, renal dysfunction, and cardiac arrhythmias. Obesity is a risk factor for adverse events in general, with greatest impact on infection incidence.[8,9]

ADVERSE EVENT BURDEN AND ERA EFFECT

The overall impact of adverse events can be discussed under the descriptive category of "adverse event burden." While nonquantitative, depictions such as freedom from any of a group of adverse events are a first step in such a description (Fig. 13.4). As experience has accumulated in the care of patients with CF devices, the incidence of many adverse events has gradually decreased (Table 13.2).[4] This era effect is also in part accounted for by cumulative experience with these devices over time. For example, evaluation of multiple adverse events, along with survival (event-free survival), was an integral part of clinical trials with the HeartMate 3 (HM3) magnetically levitated centrifugal flow pump with wide pathways engineered to minimize friction during propulsion and avoid stasis with an intrinsic pulse design.[10] The primary endpoint of the Multicenter Study of MagLev Technology in Patients Undergoing Mechanical Circulatory Support Therapy with HeartMate 3 (MOMENTUM 3)

TABLE 13.1 **Baseline Risk Factors by Multivariate Model of Mortality**

	EARLY		CONSTANT	
Variable	**Hazard Ratio**	***P* Value**	**Hazard Ratio**	***P* Value**
Demographics				
Age (by 10-year increase)	1.5	<0.0001	1.23	<0.0001
Female	1.37	0.0001		
BMI (increase by 5 units)	1.11	0.0008	1.05	0.0053
Not blood type O			1.15	0.0007
Europe	2.3	<0.0001		
Americas			1.71	<0.0001
Active smoking			1.21	0.017
Peripheral vascular disease			1.28	0.002
Ischemic etiology			1.15	0.0011
Concomitant surgery	1.39	<0.0001		
Clinical Status				
Ventilator support	1.42	0.0003		
ECMO	1.83	<0.0001		
IABP			1.18	0.0002
Dialysis	2.27	<0.0001		
INTERMACS 1–3			1.17	0.0026
Destination therapy	1.29	0.0009	1.14	0.0032
Laboratory Values				
Creatinine (per 1-mg/dL increase)	3.67	0.0034	1.13	0.0009
BUN (per 25-mg/dL increase)			1.16	<0.0001
AST (per 10-μL increase)	1.08	<0.0001		
Sodium (per 10-mEq/L increase)	0.77	0.0002		
White blood cell count (per 100-μL increase)	1.32	<0.0001		
Total bilirubin (per 1-mg/dL increase)	3.27	<0.0001		
Hemodynamics				
Central venous pressure (per 10-mm Hg increase)	1.59	<0.0001		
Pulmonary diastolic pressure (per 10-mm Hg increase)	0.82	<0.0001		
Echocardiographic Parameters				
Tricuspid regurgitation moderate/severe	1.41	<0.0001		

AST, Aspartate aminotransferase; *BMI*, body mass index; *BUN*, blood urea nitrogen; *ECMO*, extracorporeal membrane oxygenation; *IABP*, intraaortic balloon pump; *INTERMACS*, Interagency Registry for Mechanically Assisted Circulatory Support.

trial was survival free of disabling stroke and pump exchange. This combined endpoint showed superiority in the HM3 versus the HMII at 6 months and 2 years,[11] largely related to a major reduction in pump exchange for thrombosis. The primary endpoint of comparing the CE Mark trial for the HM3 device to a recent report of "real-world" experience in Germany demonstrated improvement in the incidence of multiple adverse events during the first year in the postclinical trial experience: GI bleeding (12%–7%), right heart failure (10%–7.4%), stroke (18%–0%), and all bleeding (44%–30%).[12,13]

ADVERSE EVENTS CONTRIBUTING TO DEATH

The risk of death caused by various adverse events changes over time (Fig. 13.5).[14] The risk of death from right heart failure is greatest early postimplantation, whereas infection death has an early peak and then gradually increases again after about 2 years. The risk of neurologic death decreases rapidly during the first 6 months and then remains relatively constant.[1] When viewed over a 6-year period, neurologic events account for the greatest cumulative risk of death, followed by infection adverse events (Fig. 13.6).[4] The dramatic impact of adverse events on subsequent mortality is underscored in an analysis from INTERMACS, which demonstrates the strong predictive value of multiple adverse events during the first 3 months on subsequent survival (Table 13.3, Fig. 13.7).[4]

PERIOPERATIVE BLEEDING

Perioperative bleeding, with the associated transfusion requirement, increases the risk of infection, allosensitization, and acute lung injury. In the presence of lung injury and destabilizing bleeding, right ventricular failure may lead to reduced left VAD (LVAD) output, end-organ ischemia, and reduced survival.[15,16] The potential need for reoperation to evacuate clot, particularly if tamponade is present, further exacerbates the spiral of hemodynamic instability and the potential for mediastinal infection. Nearly one-third of patients require reoperation for bleeding post VAD implantation. Several factors increase the risk of an increased bleeding diathesis following VAD implantation. A chronic coagulopathy often accompanies chronic right heart failure.[15,17] The

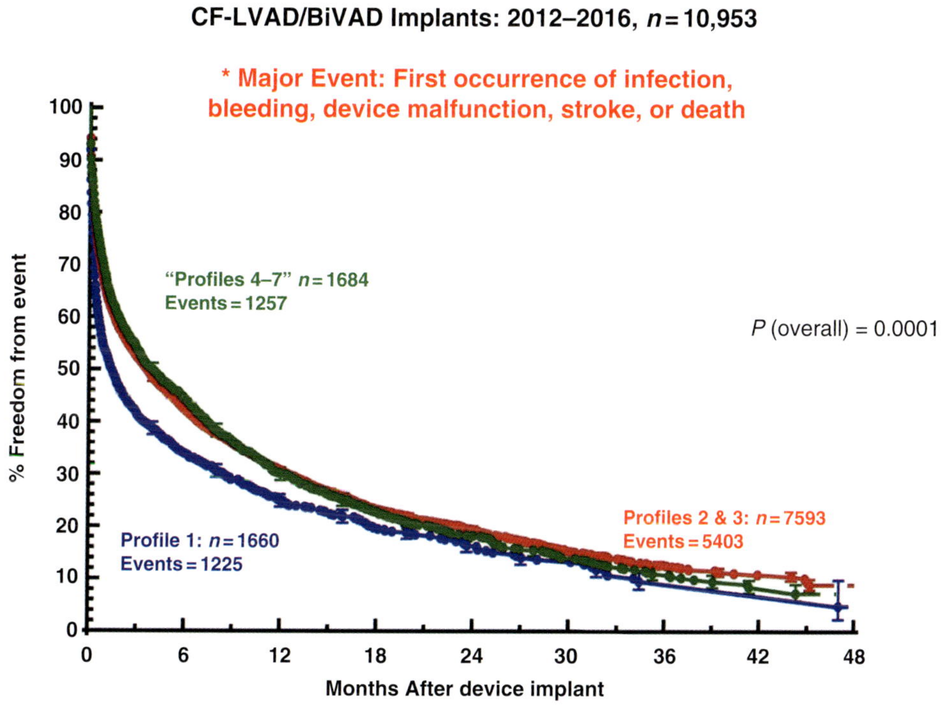

Fig. 13.4 Freedom from the combined major event of first infection, bleeding, device malfunction, stroke, or death. *BiVAD*, Biventricular assist device; *CF-LVAD*, continuous-flow left ventricular assist device. (Modified with permission from Kirklin JK, Pagani FD, Kormos RL, et al. Eighth annual INTERMACS report: special focus on framing the impact of adverse events. *J Heart Lung Transplant* 2017;36(10):1080–1086.)

TABLE 13.2 Adverse Event Rates (Events/100 Patient Months) in the First 12 Months Postimplantation by Era for CF-LVADs/BiVADs (n = 12,030)

	ERA 1 (n = 4744) CONTINUOUS 2008–2011		ERA 2 (n = 7286): CONTINUOUS 2012–2014		ERA 1 vs. ERA 2 2008–2011/2012–2014	
Adverse Event	**Events**	**Rate**	**Events**	**Rate**	**Ratio**	***P* Value**
Bleeding	3,932	9.41	4,420	7.79	1.21	<0.0001
Cardiac/vascular						
Right heart failure	238	0.57	276	0.49	1.17	0.07
Myocardial infarction	29	0.07	34	0.06	1.16	0.55
Cardiac arrhythmia	2,007	4.80	2,303	4.06	1.18	<0.0001
Pericardial drainage	271	0.65	305	0.54	1.21	0.02
Hypertension	182	0.44	115	0.20	2.15	<0.0001
Arterial non-CNS thrombosis	70	0.17	94	0.17	1.01	0.93
Venous thrombotic event	304	0.73	286	0.50	1.44	<0.0001
Hemolysis	200	0.48	314	0.55	0.87	0.11
Infection	3,435	8.22	4,132	7.28	1.13	<0.0001
Stroke	487	1.17	916	1.61	0.72	<0.0001
Renal dysfunction	601	1.44	876	1.54	0.93	0.19
Hepatic dysfunction	246	0.59	326	0.57	1.02	0.76
Respiratory failure	1,104	2.64	1,551	2.73	0.97	0.39
Wound dehiscence	81	0.19	96	0.17	1.15	0.36
Psychiatric episode	486	1.16	525	0.93	1.26	0.0003
Total burden	13,673	32.72	16,569	29.20	1.12	<0.0001

BiVAD, Biventricular assist device; *CF*, continuous flow; *CNS*, central nervous system; *LVAD*, left ventricular assist device.

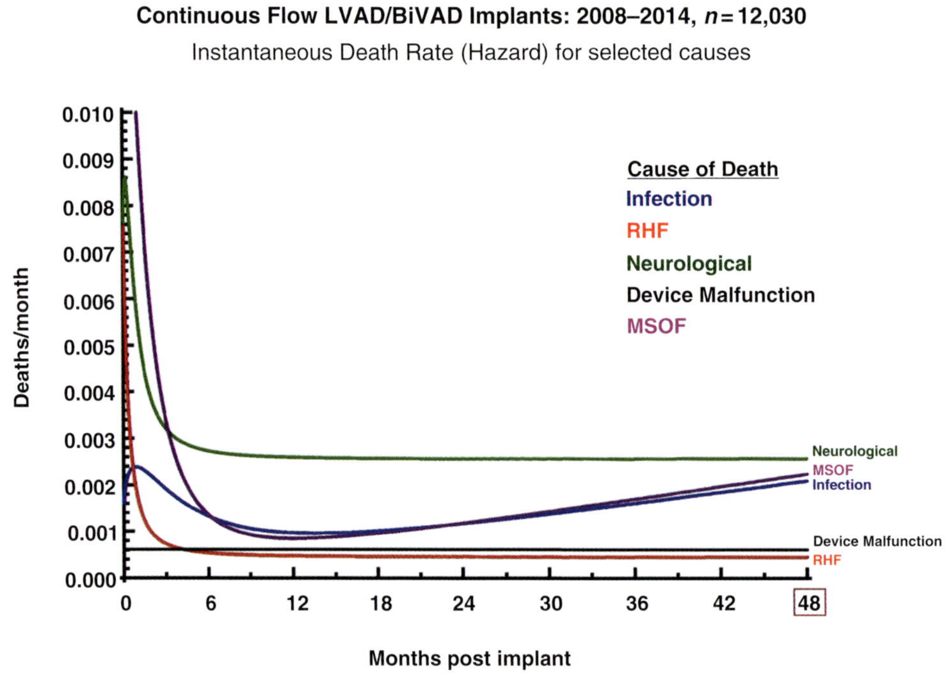

Fig. 13.5 Hazard function curves indicating the instantaneous risk of death over time for the major causes/modes of death. *BiVAD*, Biventricular assist device; *LVAD*, left ventricular assist device; *MSOF*, multisystem organ failure; *RHF*, right heart failure. (Modified with permission from Kirklin JK, Naftel DC, Pagani FD, et al. Seventh INTERMACS annual report: 15,000 patients and counting. *J Heart Lung Transplant* 2015;34(12):1495–1504.)

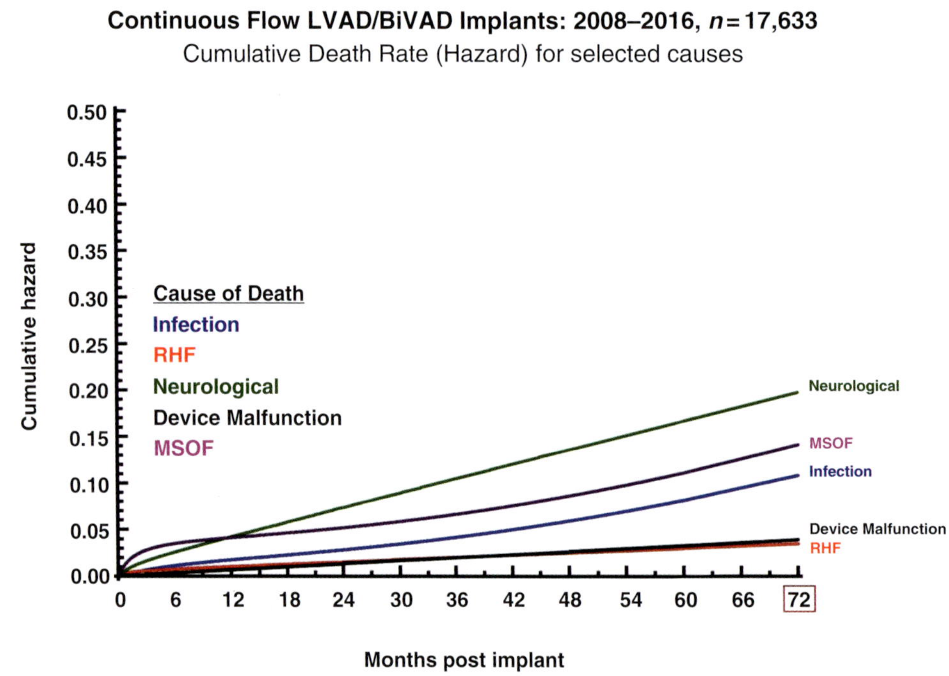

Fig. 13.6 Cumulative hazard function for major causes/modes of death. *BiVAD*, Biventricular assist device; *LVAD*, left ventricular assist device; *MSOF*, multiple system organ failure; *RHF*, right heart failure. (Modified with permission from Kirklin JK, Naftel DC, Pagani FD, et al. Seventh INTERMACS annual report: 15,000 patients and counting. *J Heart Lung Transplant* 2015;34(12):1495–1504.)

preoperative Model for End-Stage Liver Disease (MELD) score, which is a weighted sum of serum creatinine, bilirubin, and international normalized ratio (INR), is correlated with the risk of bleeding and death after LVAD implantation.[18] Chronic administration of platelet inhibitors and warfarin add to the coagulopathic state, particularly in the presence of prior cardiac operations. Therefore, an elevated INR should be normalized before implantation. Patients more critically ill at the time of implantation (INTERMACS level 1) are also poised for greater coagulopathy.

TABLE 13.3 Continuous-Flow LVAD/BiVAD Implantations: 2008–2016 (n = 17,633)

	CONSTANT PHASE OF HAZARD	
Risk Factors	**HR**	***P* Value**
Preimplantation		
Age (older)[a]	1.09	<0.0001
Race: white	1.32	<0.0001
Device strategy: destination therapy	1.18	0.0003
ICD prior to implant	1.22	0.0005
Clinical Events During 3 Months		
Number of strokes	1.47	<0.0001
Number of respiratory failures	1.16	0.0003
Number of infections	1.16	<0.0001
Number of device malfunctions	1.30	<0.0001
Days in acute care	1.01	<0.0001
Clinical Condition at 3 Months		
BUN (higher)	1.01	<0.0001
Creatinine (higher)	1.12	<0.0001
Albumin (lower)	0.97	<0.0001
LDH (higher)	1.00	<0.0001
Ascites	1.73	0.003
Peripheral edema	1.30	0.0008
Inotropes	1.70	<0.0001
Warfarin (nonuse)	0.74	<0.0001
Quality of Life/Neurocognitive		
Visual analog scale (lower)[b]	0.93	<0.0001
Mobility problems	1.31	<0.0001
Trail-making test (higher)[c]	1.07	<0.0001

[a] Comparing age 60–50.
[b] HR is for a 10-unit decrease.
[c] HR is for a 60-second increase.
Risk factors for death in patients who were alive at 3 months postimplantation (n = 14,887).
Event: Death after 3 months postimplantation and before 24 months (deaths = 2372).
Risk factors: Preimplantation, during the first 3 months after implant and at the 3 month follow-up evaluation.
BUN, Blood urea nitrogen; *HR*, hazard ratio; *ICD*, implantable cardioverter defibrillator; *LDH*, lactate dehydrogenase.

Accurate dissection, meticulous hemostasis, reversal of coagulopathy, and careful inspection of suture lines are the key elements of prevention of postoperative bleeding.[19] In the event of a severe ongoing coagulopathy after reversal of protamine following cardiopulmonary bypass, initial placement of a wound vacu-system, followed by secondary sternal closure, is safe and common practice.[20,21] An irrigation system (e.g., Pulsavac, Zimmer Biomet, Warsaw, IN) used with sterile saline, possibly with 3–5 mL Betadine soap (Purdue Pharma LP, Stamford, CT) added per liter, can be used to clean the mediastinal surfaces after removal of the packing sponges. Care must be taken not to stimulate arrhythmias or excessively cool the heart during the irrigation. The goal is to minimize the residual clot and fibrin deposits in the wound prior to final closure.

SURGICAL WOUND INFECTIONS

In the presence of the large foreign body (i.e., the LVAD), infection of the mediastinum is particularly dangerous. True mediastinitis may require debridement, followed by coverage with rectus or omental flaps, wound vac systems, or, in the worst instance, device exchange or removal. Surgical management of the infected mediastinum in a patient with an implanted MCSD may be challenging. Collaboration with an experienced plastic and reconstructive surgeon often provides useful ideas for tissue coverage, including which tissue substitutes are best suited for covering the pump and thoracic organs when there is insufficient autologous tissue (e.g., omentum or myocutaneous rotational flaps) available.

The presence of simple wound dehiscence may reveal chronic infections that may promote colonization of the wound or pump pocket. These complications and a prolonged inflammatory state are more likely in the presence of malnutrition, particularly when associated with a prealbumin <15 mg/dL within the first 2 weeks after VAD implantation.[21,22]

PUMP-RELATED INFECTION

During the 1990s, individual center experiences and multicenter trials confirmed that infection was a relatively common adverse event and mode of death,[23] with a prevalence ranging from 20% to 70% of implants.[23] By 2000, investigators recognized the importance of reporting the incidence rather than the prevalence of infection because of the steadily increasing duration of MCS as a bridge to cardiac transplantation, the advent of destination therapy, and the need to identify time points during implantation with the greatest risk for infection (e.g., the first 30 days after implantation).

INTERMACS defined infection adverse events for durable MCS devices (INTERMACS 2010). Infections can be categorized as device related, device specific, and non-device related.[23] Analysis of INTERMACS infection data has identified the following risk factors for cumulative number of infections: greater severity of preimplantation illness (i.e., INTERMACS level 1), use of biventricular support, older patient age, and higher blood urea nitrogen at implantation.[23] Pneumonia is the most commonly reported infection, occurring in 23% of patients, followed by bacteremia (20%) and driveline infection (20%).[24] Bloodstream infections occur in about 10% of patients, the majority of which are non-VAD-related and occur in the first 3 months after device implantation.[25] Non-device-related infections have the highest incidence in the first 3 months, with pneumonia, bloodstream infection, urinary tract infection, and GI infection being most common.[26]

Infection-related mortality is a function of causative organism and location, as well as other risk factors. Fungal infections carry the highest mortality but are relatively uncommon, documented in <8% of patients.[27] Most commonly, fungal infections are non–VAD-related pneumonia, line-sepsis, or urinary tract infections. VAD-related fungal infections tend to occur early, with an associated mortality of 20% at 1 month and 50% by 6 months.

Consideration of the microbiology of device infection is important to understand infection etiology, prevention, and management. The concepts of inoculation of pump surfaces, microbial adhesion, colony proliferation, and biofilm formation are fundamental to this understanding.[28] Bacteria and fungi that exist in biofilms have several characteristics that make their eradication challenging.[29] First, some

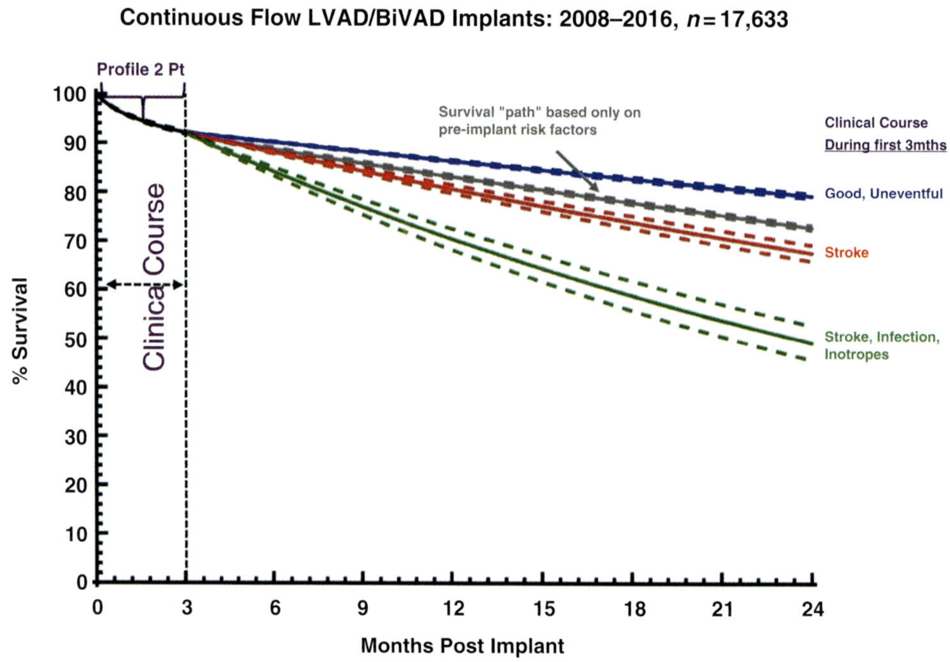

Fig. 13.7 Solution to the multivariable equation for risk of death after 3 months, conditional on 3-month survival. The dashed lines indicate the 70% confidence limits. *BiVAD*, Biventricular assist device; *LVAD*, left ventricular assist device. (Modified with permission from Kirklin JK, Naftel DC, Pagani FD, et al. Seventh INTERMACS annual report: 15,000 patients and counting. *J Heart Lung Transplant* 2015;34(12):1495–1504.)

members of the colony may switch on genes for substances that cleave or otherwise inactivate antimicrobial drugs. Second, organisms that live in relatively nutrient-poor and oxygen-poor regions of the biofilm slow their metabolism and develop higher tolerance to antimicrobial drugs that depend on actively metabolizing cells for their microbicidal activity. A third mechanism for survival has been described that represents an extreme form of slowed metabolism. This is the "persister state," whereby an individual organism becomes essentially metabolically inert and is highly tolerant to environmental stresses, including antimicrobial drugs.[30,31] The state of persistence seems to be a spontaneously occurring phenotype that is present in a small percentage of organisms within a biofilm and that can be responsible for the resurgence of a colony after eradication of the actively metabolizing organisms.

Based on the robust properties of microbes for attaching to prosthetic surfaces, thriving on the surface, and surviving efforts at eradication, it is not surprising that device-related infection has emerged as a major challenge to the survival and QOL for recipients of MCS devices. Prevention of infection is based on minimizing the inoculation of the wound and pump surfaces at the time of surgery and meticulous care of the percutaneous driveline exit site. Management of established device infection is based on removal of the biofilm by any means possible and extended therapy with antimicrobial drugs, disinfectants, or host defenses (e.g., omental coverage of infected pump pocket) to suppress or eradicate any resurgence of infection.

Preoperative cleansing of the patient's skin with antimicrobial substances (e.g., disinfectants such as chlorhexidine) and detergents in conjunction with clipping of body hair rather than shaving decreases the microbial burden at the cutaneous incision site. However, viable bacteria remain in the epidermis and deep in hair follicles that can inoculate the wound at the time of implantation. There is evidence that pathogenic bacteria (e.g., methicillin-resistant *Staphylococcus aureus* [MRSA]) from sites such as the nose or perineum are additional risk factors for postimplantation infection. Some centers use rapid screening for nasal or perineal MRSA based on polymerase chain reaction assays to identify patients colonized with MRSA, and reported a lower sternal infection rate after application of topical antimicrobials to eradicate MRSA.[32] Despite all of these measures, some inoculation of bacteria into the surgical wound and onto the exterior surface of the implanted pump components is inevitable. Thus, routine prophylactic antibiotics are utilized. The most common prophylactic regimens include vancomycin, cefazolin, and fluconazole for 24 hours.[33] Bacteria that exist in retained clot, pump interstices, or in a pump pocket may survive prophylactic antibiotics. As they multiply, some organisms contact and adhere to the surface of implanted MCS device components. The individual microbes that initially colonize the surface are able to detect the presence of other microbes in the immediate vicinity through a process termed "quorum sensing,"[34] which is the mechanism for triggering alterations in microbial gene expression that result in biofilm formation. The colony encases itself in a slime layer or biofilm, defined as "a structured community of bacterial cells enclosed in a self-produced polymeric matrix."[35] The biofilm stabilizes the microbial colony on the prosthetic surface and markedly increases the resistance of the individual organisms to antimicrobial drugs or host immune attack.[34,36]

Percutaneous Driveline Infection

The incidence of driveline infection peaks at about 6 months, but the risk continues throughout the period of VAD support, with 20% of patients affected by 1 year and 25% by 2 years.[24] Among adults, younger age is a strong risk factor for driveline infection, likely related to greater activity level and higher risk of accidents and mechanical damage.

Prevention of driveline infection begins with careful intraoperative management. Minimizing movement across the percutaneous exit site is important to prevent migration of bacteria off the skin edge and into the fabric that is ultimately left in a subcutaneous position. Some groups routinely soak the driveline fabric in antimicrobial solutions.[37] Others use a plastic sheath from a pulmonary artery catheter insertion kit to cover the driveline, and the driveline is soaked in a solution of vancomycin and gentamicin. As a final step in the implantation procedure, the plastic sheath is pulled out of the driveline tunnel, and the driveline is stabilized by skin stitches and an external appliance (Horizontal Drain/Tube Attachment Device; Hollister, Inc., Libertyville, IL). Consistent stabilization of the driveline and educational reinforcement to the patient to minimize or avoid any pulling or twisting of the driveline is essential in preventing late infections of the percutaneous driveline site. The optimal management for the percutaneous site has not yet been defined but probably involves periodic cleaning to remove shed epithelial cells and kill microbes followed by a dry dressing to minimize contamination.

The optimal driveline design to prevent infection is controversial. There is general agreement that the percutaneous driveline should be covered in a fabric that encourages ingrowth by fibroblasts to create a stable and infection-resistant collagen bond to the fabric. However, the exact fabric material, the diameter and flexibility of the driveline, and whether or not the fabric crosses the dermis are debated. A fabric that has adequate durability against degradation and physical stresses (e.g., pulling, repetitive flexion, and torque) is required. The driveline should be supple so that bending forces are not transmitted to the healed edge of the skin-driveline junction, but there must be resistance to overbending that jeopardizes the integrity of the electrical wires within the driveline. Smaller driveline circumference minimizes the area at risk for infection, but after a certain point, the circumferential length of healed tissue has insufficient strength to resist pulling or torque.

The question of whether to bring the fabric (velour) across the skin or leave it a few millimeters below the dermal layer has been studied for many years. Most of this research focused on the design of catheters for long-term peritoneal dialysis (e.g., Tenckhoff and related catheters)[38] or for intravenous access. Designs for peritoneal dialysis catheters typically employ a fibrous cuff at the level of the fascia to discourage leakage of the dialysate and a second fibrous cuff in the subcutaneous tissue 10–15 mm below the dermis. In humans, an epithelial-lined sinus forms from the dermis down to the fibrous cuff. The edge of the fibrous cuff is covered with a small rim of granulation tissue.[39] Makers of the C-Pulse counterpulsation MCS device have chosen this approach for their pneumatic percutaneous driveline (Sunshine Heart, Inc., Tustin, CA), whereas makers of other implanted and paracorporeal MCS devices design the velour-covered percutaneous driveline or cannulas to cross the dermal junction. There are no trials that compared MCS device driveline design in humans, and long-term animal models are unlikely to provide useful information to answer this question.

Even if initial driveline healing is adequate, infection can still occur. Cumulative driveline infection rates approach 100% in some studies.[39] The mechanism for late infection is probably a tear in the dermal-fabric healing because of abrupt pulling or twisting. This problem is a testimony to, and a consequence of, the marked increase in mobility and activity reported by many patients after LVAD implantation. This opening can allow a nidus of infection to begin that produces further loosening of the collagen that has grown into the driveline velour. Exuberant and moist granulation tissue forms as the infection progresses. This moist tissue encourages further bacterial growth and tunneling along the driveline. A surface adhesion molecule of *Staphylococcus epidermidis* that has affinity for collagen and the polyester velour has been identified in fully healed drivelines explanted from humans.[40] Experimental murine models support a postulated mechanism that organisms that are adherent to tissue and material in the vicinity of a tear will invade a breach in the barrier and tunnel along the collagen-fiber interface over the subcutaneous portion of the driveline.[41]

The management of a driveline infection begins with proper patient and caregiver education emphasizing the importance of early reporting (often with uploaded photos) of local purulent drainage, increasing local pain, and/or advancing erythema at the exit site. Topical disinfectants such as chlorhexidine can be added to the regimen for driveline care, and if appropriate, antibiotics that cover *Staphylococcus* may be added. If moist granulation tissue has formed, cauterization with silver nitrate promotes regression of granulations. If the infection begins to tunnel along the driveline, debridement of the infected tissue should be considered. Some groups have used vacuum-assisted healing devices (Vacuum Assisted Closure; Kinetic Concepts, Inc., San Antonio, TX) to accelerate the healing of the resulting wound,[42,43] but there is a high recurrence rate of tunnel infection. Local disinfectants such as hydrogen peroxide are useful, and wound cultures guide antimicrobial therapy. Comparing devices, the larger driveline in the HMII device has a higher incidence of driveline infection than the HVAD.[44]

Pump Pocket Infections

Patients with infected pump pockets may present with sepsis syndrome, fevers without other symptoms, or minimal signs and symptoms (e.g., low-grade fever and mild leukocytosis). Infection of the pocket should be suspected when the patient has positive blood cultures (often *Staphylococcus* species) and mild to severe pain over the device. The diagnosis can be confirmed by either computed tomography scan or ultrasound evidence of fluid around the implanted pump. Patients with other reasons for positive blood cultures, such as long-term indwelling intravenous lines, pose a diagnostic challenge because an ultrasound scan of the pump pocket may show fluid that is uninfected and occupying the potential space around the device. In the presence of bacteremia and no other identifiable source, consideration should be given to local exploration of a symptomatic pump pocket.

Management of an infected pump pocket begins with initial exploration and drainage. Cultures for bacteria and fungi are obtained, and the tissue and pump surfaces are thoroughly cleaned. A dilute solution of povidone-iodine soap (Betadine; Purdue Pharma L.P., Stamford, CT) consisting of 5–10 mL of Betadine soap per liter of sterile saline and a pulsating irrigation device (Pulseavac Irrigation System; Zimmer, Inc., Warsaw, IN) is useful for cleaning and debriding the pocket. The detergent action of the soap disrupts biofilms. After irrigation, beads of bone cement can be fabricated with heat-stabile antibiotic powder and left in the wound.[45,46] These beads elute antibiotics at bactericidal levels for about 6–8 weeks after placement, depending on the size of the beads and the number that are placed. Initially, the regional concentration of antibiotics is high, and absorption of the antibiotics is detectable in peripheral blood samples. The levels are typically well below toxic levels; however, if the patient is receiving the same antibiotic intravenously (e.g., vancomycin), the treating physician may wish to obtain one or two serum levels to ensure safety. Many patients require more than one round of therapy with pump pocket irrigation and antibiotic beads. With multiple rounds of therapy, patients can live as outpatients with their infection, and in some instances, the infection appears to be eradicated. Appropriate systemic antibiotics are given long-term and stopped only with careful monitoring (e.g., temperature, leukocyte count, and surveillance blood cultures).

Infections of Blood Contacting Pump Components (Pump Endocarditis)

Pump endocarditis is rare but can involve inflow or outflow cannulas and the pump interior, with or without vegetations. Differentiating bloodstream infection from pump endocarditis is challenging. Obtaining blood cultures from the left ventricle and outflow graft and nuclear tagged leukocyte scans[47] can help, but the diagnosis may ultimately rest with exclusion of other potential sources. The options for treating pump endocarditis are limited and entail substantial risk.

If the infection is low grade, device removal with transplantation is an option.[48] Other options include replacing an infected component of the pump[47] or complete device replacement.[49]

GASTROINTESTINAL BLEEDING

A major disadvantage of CF pumps compared to previous pulsatile technology is the higher incidence of GI bleeding. An analysis by Crow and colleagues[50] reported a 10-fold higher incidence of GI bleeding with CF pumps compared to pulsatile devices (46.5 vs. 4.7 events/100 patient-years). Over 95% of patients on pulsatile flow devices were free from GI bleeding at 1 year versus 66% of patients on CF pumps. The most common finding on endoscopy is angiodysplasia—often multiple and typically in the stomach or early portions of the small bowel. This pattern of multiple small arteriovenous malformations (AVMs) is believed to be associated with a low pulse pressure in CF pump patients similar to patients with aortic stenosis (Heyde's syndrome).[51–53] Patibandla and colleagues have provided experimental evidence suggesting that the degree of pulsatility within the CF system may influence the likelihood of submucosal AVM formation.[52]

Another major associated factor appears to be a deficiency in high-molecular-weight multimers of von Willebrand factor (vWF) in patients supported on CF devices.[52] One study showed a near-total depletion of levels of vWF at the time of GI bleed.[54] Possible differences among axial flow and centrifugal flow devices in the depletion of vWF remain unresolved. Elderly patients (>age 60 years) appear more susceptible to GI bleeding.

NEUROLOGIC DYSFUNCTION

Although many types of neurologic events have been observed during CF pump support, the most devastating complication is stroke, either embolic (ischemic) or hemorrhagic, which among all adverse events is associated with the highest morbidity and mortality, longest hospital stay, and greatest cost.[55] Predisposing factors associated with ischemic strokes are areas of flow stagnation within the device, thrombogenic surfaces, hypercoagulable states, ineffective anticoagulation, and intracavitary left atrial or ventricular thrombus.

The predisposing factors for hemorrhagic strokes are more enigmatic. Recent studies have identified relative hypertension as an important factor associated with hemorrhagic strokes.[56] The association between intestinal AVMs and GI bleeding is well established (see section on Gastrointestinal Bleeding), but such a relationship in central nervous system bleeding has not been established.

The incidence of stroke in the HMII bridge to transplant and destination therapy trials[57,58] was 19% and 17%, respectively. In these series, the incidence of hemorrhagic and ischemic strokes was 2% and 6% for the bridge-to-transplant patients and 11% and 8% for the destination-therapy patients, respectively.

Between 2012 and 2015, the INTERMACS database reported that 11% of patients suffered at least one stroke, with an incidence of 0.12 strokes per patient-year and nearly equal distribution between hemorrhagic and ischemic.[59] Stroke occurred at similar rates in young and old LVAD recipients and did not differ by device implantation strategy. Among patients with a first stroke, 13% suffered a subsequent stroke. Among all patients, 9% suffered one stroke, 1% suffered two strokes, and <0.2% suffered a third or fourth stroke. Preimplantation risk factors for postimplantation stroke included female gender, higher preimplantation systolic blood pressure, history of heparin-induced thrombocytopenia, and preoperative intraaortic balloon pump. The unique environment conferred by CF pumps that disposes to neurologic events is supported by the finding that a history of stoke does not increase the susceptibility to a postimplantation stroke (P=0.17).[59] The risk of stroke persists throughout follow-up, with >80% of strokes occurring after the first 2 weeks. The cumulative risk for stroke was 15% at 3 years (8% for hemorrhagic and 7% for ischemic). Diabetes and malnutrition increase the risk of later stroke.

Survival after stroke on a CF durable device is generally poor (Fig. 13.8).[59] Survival at 1 and 6 months after an ischemic stroke is 81% and 66%, and after hemorrhagic stroke is 45% and 35%, respectively.[59] Among patients awaiting heart transplantation on device, the occurrence of a stroke reduced the chances of transplantation by 50%.

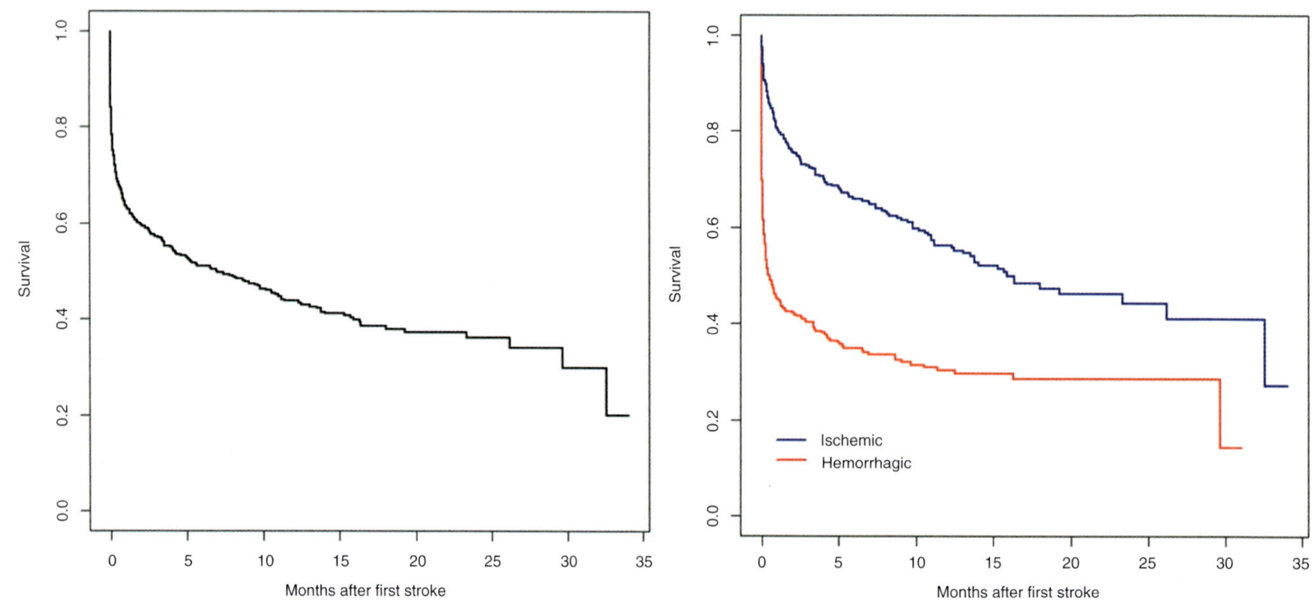

Fig. 13.8 Kaplan-Meier curves of patient survival following stroke: overall (left) and by stroke type (right). (Modified with permission from Acharya D, Loyaga-Rendon R, Morgan CJ, et al. INTERMACS analysis of stroke during support with continuous-flow left ventricular assist devices: risk factors and outcomes. *JACC: Heart Fail* 2017;5(10):703–711.)

Comparing the stroke rates among devices, the HVAD had a higher incidence of stroke compared to the HMII in the HeartWare ADVANCE-HVAD (Advanced Heart Failure Bridge to Transplant) trial, with an equivalent proportion of ischemic and hemorrhagic strokes.[58,60] In the MOMENTUM 3 trial, the short-term cohort showed no difference in the overall freedom from disabling stroke between the HM3 and the HMII.[10,61] However, in the long-term cohort, the 2-year stroke rate was twice as high in the HMII (19%) as the HM3 (10%).[62] The reduced stroke rate was evenly divided between hemorrhagic and ischemic etiologies.

A rare neurologic adverse event associated with VAD therapy is cerebral hyperperfusion syndrome,[63] a life-threatening syndrome in which a chronically hypoperfused cerebral vasculature suddenly experiences normal cerebral blood flow following VAD implantation. The mechanism is not clear but may relate to overwhelming cerebral autoregulation, leading to brain edema and, in severe cases, hemorrhage. The clinical picture is one of confusion and encephalopathy.[64]

An important association has been established between bloodstream or device infection and subsequent stroke. One study reported that 40% of stokes occurred in the setting of active infection.[65] In addition to infection, stroke rate is increased after GI bleeding,[59] possibly related to alterations in anticoagulation.

Strict blood pressure control and frequent anticoagulation monitoring are known to reduce the risk of hemorrhagic stroke.[56] The use of clot extraction techniques for patients with acute embolic strokes involving the accessible intracranial arteries is warranted in selected cases.[59,66]

RENAL FAILURE

Chronic renal insufficiency may be part of the chronic heart failure state (cardiorenal syndrome), as a sequelae of prolonged elevation of filling pressures, marginal cardiac output, and an abnormal neurohormonal milieu.[67–70] The frequent coexistence of diabetes and hypertension adds other direct causes of renal damage to the mix. Acute renal failure postimplantation is more likely in the presence of preexisting renal insufficiency,[71] and especially if circulatory performance is suboptimal early postimplantation. Proteinuria is a preimplantation risk factor for postimplantation renal failure; 30% of such patients developed renal failure in one study.[72]

Preimplantation renal dysfunction is also a risk factor for subsequent mortality, especially when renal failure occurs postimplantation.[68,73,74] Although at least one single-center study failed to identify at least moderate renal dysfunction as a risk for mortality,[75] a large INTERMACS analysis of the US CF device experience (2006–2012) showed a significant correlation between worse preimplantation renal dysfunction and postimplantation mortality, with the major effect occurring in the first 3 months (Fig. 13.9).[3] By multivariable analysis, several studies have identified increasing renal dysfunction as a major risk factor for early mortality and a minor risk factor in the longer-term.[3,76,77] Early mortality was especially high among patients in shock and requiring renal replacement therapy at the time of implantation (Fig. 13.10).[3] Among patients with severe renal dysfunction at implantation, right ventricular failure, infection, and multisystem failure were the most common causes of death. These analyses support the importance of proceeding with VAD therapy before the onset of advanced cardiorenal syndrome.

Despite the increased risk associated with greater degrees of preimplantation renal dysfunction, most patients with abnormal renal function experience improvement within the first few weeks of LVAD support (Fig. 13.11).[3]

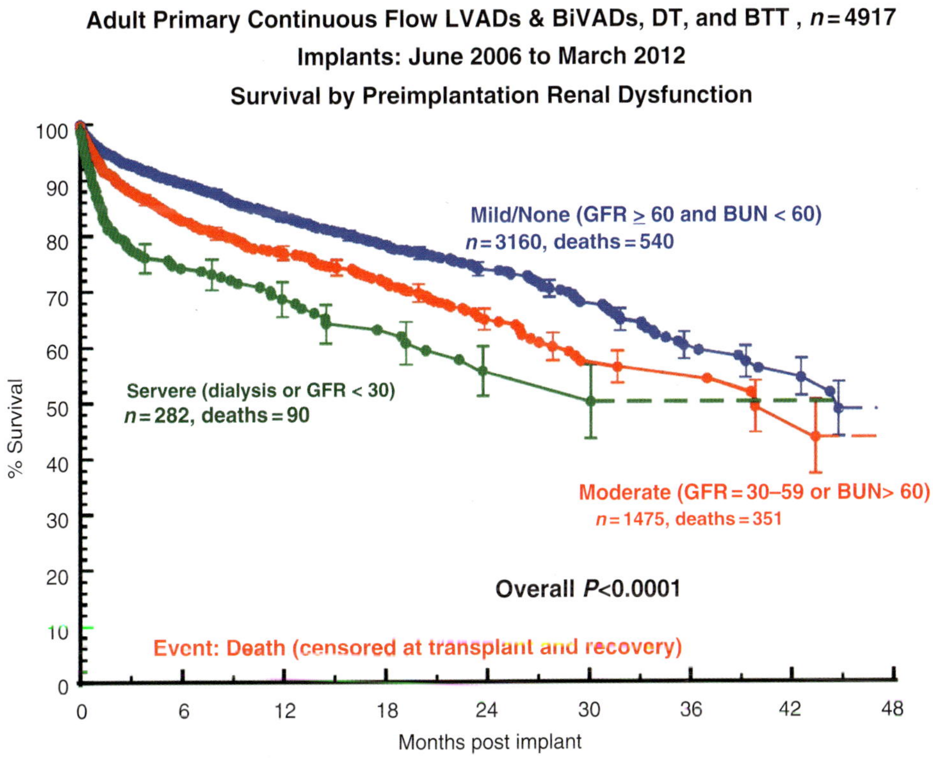

Fig. 13.9 Actuarial curves show survival stratified by severity of preimplantation renal dysfunction. The error bars indicate ± 1 standard error. *BiVAD*, Biventricular assist device; *BTT*, bridge to transplant; *BUN*, blood urea nitrogen; *DT*, destination therapy; *GFR*, glomerular filtration rate; *LVAD*, left ventricular assist device. (Modified with permission from Kirklin JK, Naftel DC, Kormos R, et al. Quantifying the effect the effect of cardiorenal syndrome on mortality after left ventricular implant. *J Heart Lung Transplant* 2013;32(12)1205–1213.)

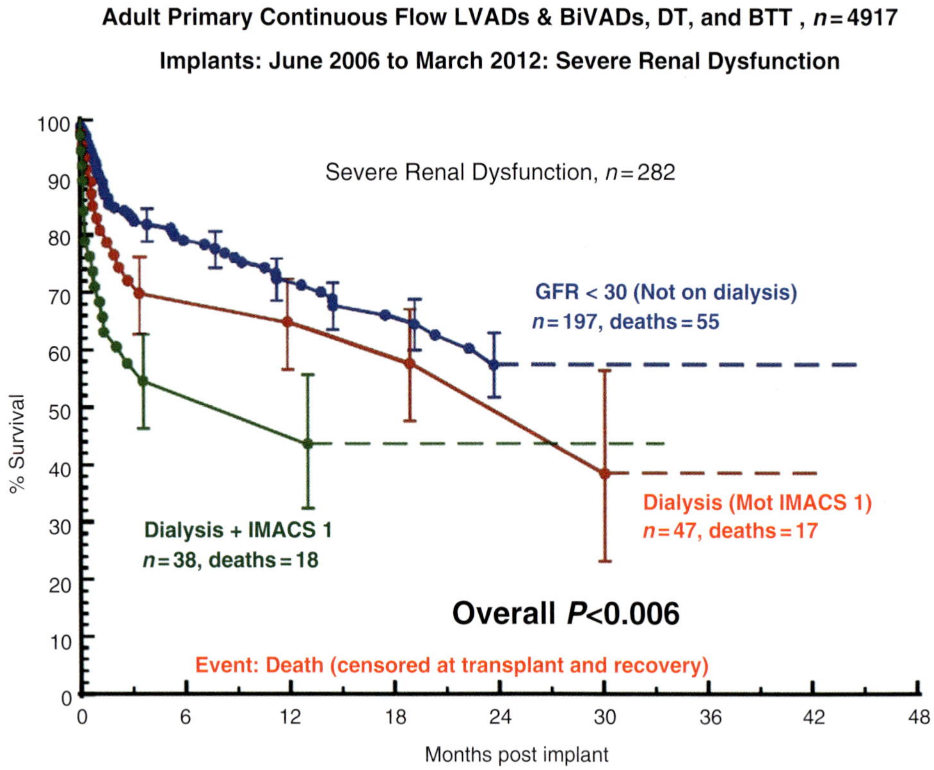

Fig. 13.10 Actuarial survival postimplantation, stratified by combinations of risk factors. The error bars indicate ± 1 standard error. *BiVAD*, Biventricular assist device; *BTT*, bridge to transplant; *DT*, destination therapy; *IMACS 1*, INTERMACS level 1; *LVAD*, left ventricular assist device. (Modified with permission from Kirklin JK, Naftel DC, Kormos R, et al. Quantifying the effect the effect of cardiorenal syndrome on mortality after left ventricular implant. *J Heart Lung Transplant* 2013;32(12)1205–1213.)

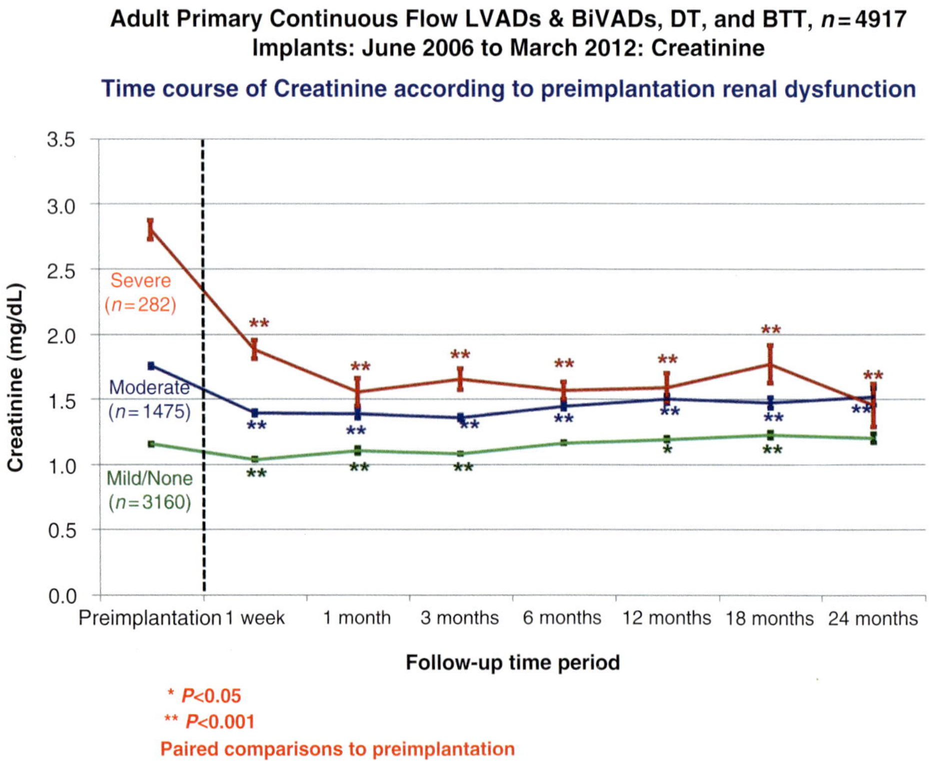

Fig. 13.11 Time course of average serum creatinine among surviving patients at designated follow-up points, stratified by severity of preimplantation renal dysfunction. The error bars indicate ± 1 standard error. *BiVAD*, Biventricular assist device; *BTT*, bridge to transplant; *DT*, destination therapy; *LVAD*, left ventricular assist device. (Modified with permission from Kirklin JK, Naftel DC, Kormos R, et al. Quantifying the effect the effect of cardiorenal syndrome on mortality after left ventricular implant. *J Heart Lung Transplant* 2013;32(12)1205–1213.)

DEVICE FAILURE

An engineering definition for device failure is "the nonperformance or inability of a component or system to perform its intended function for a specified time under specified environmental conditions."[78] For MCS devices, failures include hardware and software failures. *Hardware* failures are usually caused by degradation of components or unrecognized defects in fabrication, which can be minimized by specifying appropriately low tolerance limits for variation in components, excellent quality control in the assembly process, and adequate prepackaging testing of the assembled MCS device. *Software failures* usually equate with controller failure and can often be resolved by installing a new version of the software on existing hardware. *Human factors* are defined as "the application of the scientific knowledge of human capabilities and limitations to the design of systems and equipment to produce products with the most efficient, safe, effective, and reliable operation."[79] Engineers are assigned to develop the human-device interface during initial MCS device design. The human-device interface takes into account numerous factors, including the need to change energy sources (e.g., battery power to power base unit and vice versa), appropriate recognition and response to various alarm conditions, and environmental factors (e.g., exposure to water, extreme heat, or repetitive bending of the driveline).

The most commonly cited major human error is when the patient or caregiver mistakenly disconnects all power from a rotary (CF) pump while changing batteries or while changing from battery power to a power base unit. Removing all power from a rotary pump can be catastrophic because these pumps have no valves, and retrograde flow occurs immediately after cessation of forward pumping. The capacity for retrograde flow depends on the pressure differential between the aorta and the left ventricle and is not quantified for the various rotary pumps currently available. Based on anecdotal reports, some patients seem to tolerate retrograde flow from a stopped rotor quite well, whereas other patients develop acute heart failure and cardiogenic shock within minutes, depending on the ability of the native heart to generate forward flow. If the patient is alone at this time, an acute decrease in blood pressure can cause syncope, which is followed by death. The number of deaths that occurred in elderly patients suggests that the mistake was not recognized and successfully resolved by the patient before he or she lost consciousness. The need for a caregiver within hearing range of the device alarms is increased for patients with limited cognitive abilities.

Failure modes for rotary pumps have not been fully developed, and all such devices have the potential for rapid decompensation and death owing to pump. The tradeoff for this disadvantage is the superior durability of rotary pumps compared to existing pulsatile devices. However, repetitive strain secondary to bending of the driveline can cause wire fractures and interruption of power to the motor. Design modification to increase the strength of the driveline and patient education to avoid sudden entrapment have decreased catastrophic driveline-associated failures. The ultimate solution is elimination of drivelines with the use transcutaneous energy transmission systems.

PUMP THROMBOSIS

Pump thrombosis is a major complication of VAD support with most current CF VADs. Related to considerable variability in axial and centrifugal flow pump design, there is considerable variability among current generation pumps regarding the propensity for pump thrombosis.

The interactions of a mechanical pump with human blood are complex. They depend first on microlevel interactions of blood with the biomaterials chosen for the blood path within the pump. The interactions secondarily depend on macrolevel aspects of pump design, for instance, strategic placement of smooth and rough surfaces along the flow path and the patterns of flow created by movement of blood within the pump. In addition, the propensity for clot formation within a pump changes according to pharmacologic modifications of the coagulation system with drugs like heparin, coumadin, or aspirin.

The ideal biocompatible surface for blood would be normally functioning endothelium. Unfortunately, it is not possible to fabricate or grow a confluent endothelial layer over biomaterials at the current time. The means to minimize unwanted thrombus formation are limited to avoiding highly thrombogenic biomaterials, developing optimal pump designs using the methods described below, and pharmacologic inhibition of clotting. Platelet activation and the formation of platelet aggregates (i.e., white thrombus) within a blood pump result from a complex interaction of the biomaterial surface, shear forces generated within the pump, and the duration of exposure of platelets to these influences. The prediction of platelet adhesion, activation, and aggregation using computer simulations of flow within a pump is feasible but complex.[80]

The intrinsic clotting system is responsible for clot (i.e., red thrombus) formation on biomaterial surfaces. This cascade is initiated when the foreign surface, particularly a negatively charged surface, encounters a group of plasma proteins including factor XII (Hageman factor), prekallikrein, factor XI, and high molecular weight kininogen.[81–83] If the active forms of the proteins are allowed to dwell in vicinity to one another before they are washed away and diluted, the clotting reaction is amplified and a clinically apparent thrombus will form. This typically occurs at defects in the blood flow path (e.g., a small gap between the pump housing and the housing of a prosthetic valve, or at the connection to an inflow or outflow cannula), in zones of stagnation, or within stable vortices where shear rates and washout are low. Pump designers use computational flow dynamics (CFD) analysis to identify thrombosis-prone regions within the blood flow paths and eliminate them from pump designs. Prefabrication CFD analysis can help define the hemolytic and platelet damaging potential of a pump by quantitatively defining shear forces within the flow paths,[84–86] as well as vortices and other regions of potential stagnation.

Iterations of prototypes eliminate these areas as the pump design is optimized in computer-based renderings (i.e., in-silico studies). Physical models of the pump, typically using transparent plastic components, allow particle imaging within mock circulation loops to validate the CFD design.[87,88] Optimizing pump design prior to animal testing saves considerable time and money in pump development.[89,90]

Every pump design has regions within the flow paths that are vulnerable to thrombus formation. In pulsatile devices, regions in the vicinity of the valves are prone to stasis during pump diastole. Rotary pumps with shafts that attach the rotor to the drive mechanism (e.g., Evaheart left VAD; Houston, TX) require constant irrigation of the shafted impeller. Rotary pumps with bearings (e.g., HMII; Abbott, Chicago, IL) rely on washing of the bearing by plasma flowing across the surfaces of the bearing to prevent the buildup of fibrin. Deposits of fibrin in the rear (aft) bearing of the HMII left VAD can create substantial hemolysis, even with sustained pump flow. Without treatment such as a pump exchange, turbulent flow results in high levels of plasma-free hemoglobin that will injure the kidneys. Importantly, ring thrombus on the aft bearing can propagate into the cylindrical (axial) rotor that is rotating at high rpm (about 9000 rpm) with impeller blades that are very close to the pump housing. Propagation of ring thrombus into the rotor increases the magnitude of hemolysis and can even cause acute pump stoppage. Problems with thrombus formation within HMII left VADs stimulated renew interest in CFD analysis of this device, including the effects of pulsatility from the native heart on flow within an axial flow pump (i.e., HMII) and novel CFD models for defining thrombotic risk.[80,91–93]

Levitated rotors have no attachment to their electromagnetic drive mechanism, so there are no shafts or physical bearings. Levitated rotors have a primary flow path through which the majority of blood passes before exiting the pump. Secondary flow paths around the rotor are smaller; they rely on washing to remain free of fibrin and thrombus.[94]

The secondary flow paths of hydrodynamically levitated rotors have relatively small clearances from surrounding pump structures. Small pieces of thrombus that wash into a pump with hydrodynamic bearings (e.g., Heartware VAD; Medtronic, Minneapolis, MN) or buildup of a fibrin layer over the pump housing can lead to increased turbulence of the blood near the rotor. This results in lysis of blood elements, most notably red blood cells, with consequent release of free hemoglobin and other intracellular contents such as lactate dehydrogenase (LDH).

The HM3 LVAD (Abbott, Chicago, IL) uses magnetic forces (MAGLEV) to center the shrouded impeller (a.k.a. rotor). The MAGLEV positioning system allows larger secondary flow paths that may result lower potential for thrombus formation.[94] A randomized prospective trial of the HM3 with an axial flow left VAD (HMII) showed significantly fewer reoperations for pump malfunction of the HM3 within 2 years of implantation.[11] The reason for replacement of the axial flow pump was most often pump thrombosis or severe hemolysis.

All current CF pumps are susceptible to hemolysis, which can be affected by abnormal blood-surface interactions and alterations in blood flow dynamics, which can increase sheer stress, contribute to red cell fragmentation, and induce hemolysis.[95,96] The precise relationship between hemolysis and subsequent pump thrombosis remains under investigation.[95,96] Using a definition for hemolysis of plasma-free hemoglobin >40 mg/dL, Katz and colleagues found that patients with documented hemolysis had a 20% chance of requiring pump exchange within 6 months.[95] Mortality (Fig. 13.12)[6] after pump exchange is considerable (and gets worse with subsequent exchanges) (Fig. 13.13),[97a] and the incidence of subsequent infection and strokes is increased.[6] In an important analysis that described the clinical presentation of pump thrombosis, Birati and colleagues found a broad spectrum of clinical syndromes—from asymptomatic patients to stroke and cardiogenic shock—which afflicted the cases of pump thrombosis from a single-center study.[97b]

The HMII device has received the most detailed analysis for pump thrombosis. In the pivotal premarket approval study conducted between 2005 and 2008, the likelihood of pump thrombosis at 6 months was about 2% and at 1 year was about 3%.[7] After an initial clinical experience suggesting a low incidence of pump thrombosis, isolated reports of an increased frequency of pump thrombosis with the HMII surfaced in 2012. A subsequent INTERMACS analysis documented a five- to six-fold increase in pump thrombosis between 2010 and 2012, with the greatest risk occurring in the first 3 months.[6] Multivariable analysis identified later implantation year, younger adult age, female gender, history of noncompliance, larger body mass index, history of severe right heart failure, and evidence of greater hemolysis (higher LDH level) at 1 month (especially when greater than 600 ml/dl) (Fig. 13.14)[1] as risk factors for pump thrombosis in the HMII.[1,6] With tightening of anticoagulation protocols and increased focus on optimal pump positioning and operative technique, the event rate had improved some (Fig. 13.15).[1] These registry data enabled clinicians to provide better informed consent and patient education about risk of pump thrombosis and recurrent thrombosis, including the importance of vigilant adherence to anticoagulation protocols. The recent International Society for Heart and Lung Transplantation guidelines for anticoagulation targets are device specific, usually a target INR of 2.0–3.0 or 2.5–3.5.[98,99]

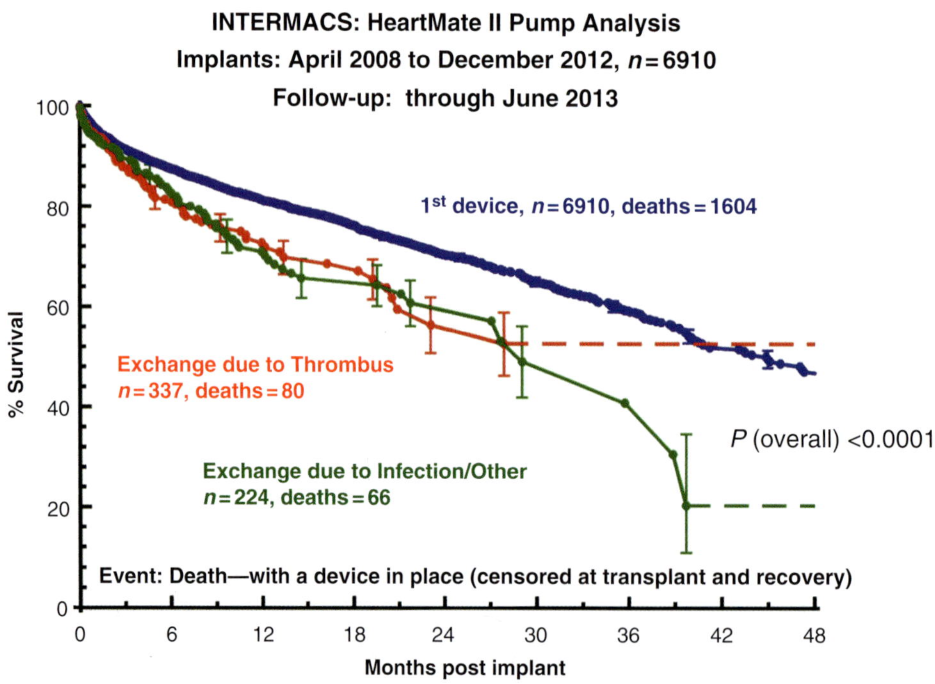

Fig. 13.12 Actuarial survival after initial or subsequent pump exchange. The error bars represent ± 1 standard error. *INTERMACS*, Interagency Registry for Mechanically Assisted Circulatory Support. (Modified with permission from Kirklin JK, Naftel DC, Kormos RL, et al. Interagency Registry for Mechanically Assisted Circulatory Support (INTERMACS) analysis of pump thrombosis in the HeartMate II left ventricular assist device. *J Heart Lung Transplant* 2014;33(1):12–22.)

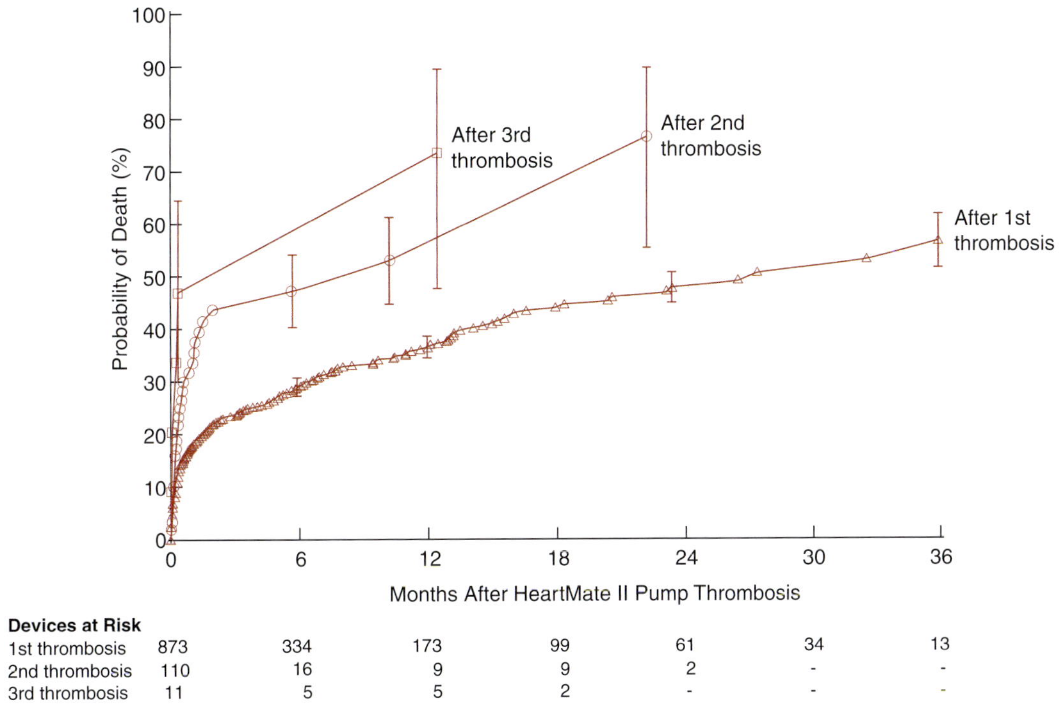

Fig. 13.13 Probability of death after HeartMate II pump thrombosis while remaining on mechanical circulatory support, according to whether a subsequent thrombosis occurred. This is from a nested nonparametric analysis with pump thrombosis as time zero. Symbols are nonparametric estimates and vertical bars are the 68% confidence limits equivalent to 1 standard error. (Modified with permission from Smedira NG, Blackstone EH, Ehrlinger J, et al. Current risks of HeartMate II pump thrombosis: non-parametric analysis of Interagency Registry for Mechanically Assisted Circulatory Support data. *J Heart Lung Transplant* 2015;34(12):1527–1534.)

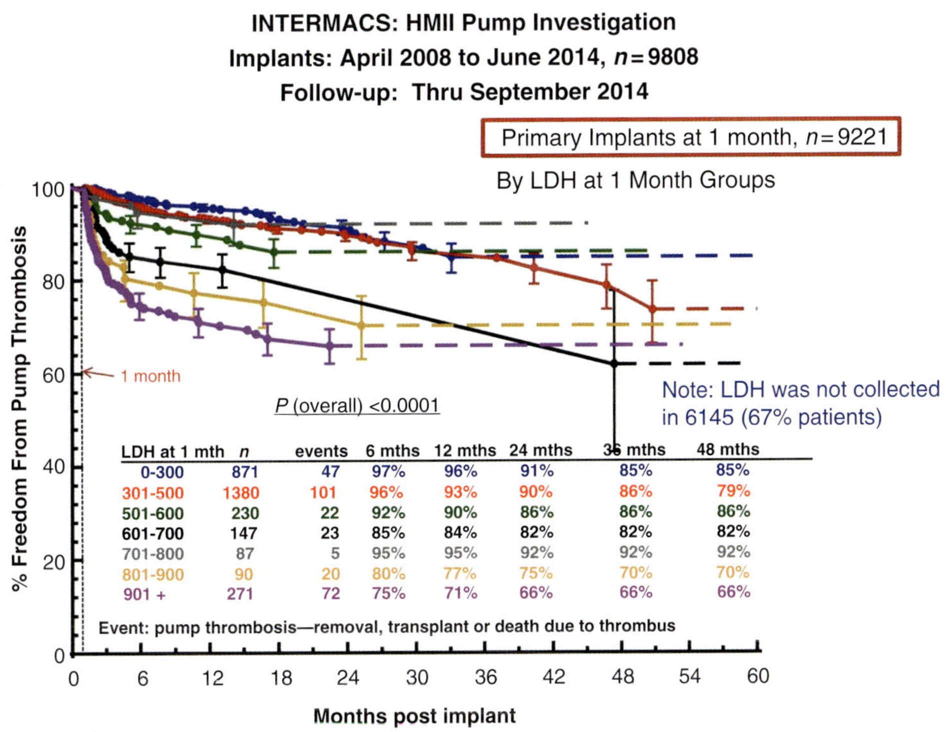

Fig. 13.14 Actuarial freedom from HMII pump thrombosis, stratified by maximum LDH at 1 month (±2 weeks) postimplantation. Note that time 0 in this depiction is 1 month postimplantation. *HMII*, HeartMate II device; *INTERMACS*, Interagency Registry for Mechanically Assisted Circulatory Support; *LDH*, lactate dehydrogenase. (Modified with permission from Kirklin JK, Naftel DC, Pagani FD, et al. Pump thrombosis in the Thoratec HeartMate II device: an update analysis of the INTERMACS Registry. *J Heart Lung Transplant* 2015;34(12):1515–1526.)

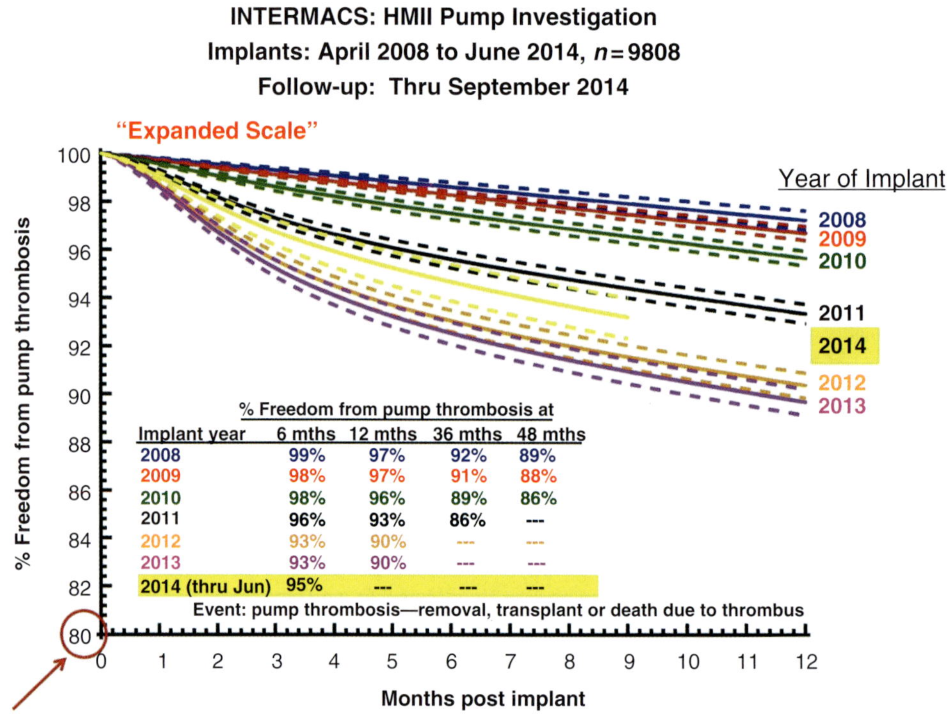

Fig. 13.15 Parametric solution of the hazard model for the effect of implant year on freedom from HMII pump thrombosis. The dashed lines indicate the 70% confidence limits. The table contains the parametric point estimates. Note that the *y*-axis scale goes from 80 to 100. *HMII*, HeartMate II device; *INTERMACS*, Interagency Registry for Mechanically Assisted Circulatory Support. (Modified with permission from Kirklin JK, Naftel DC, Pagani FD, et al. Pump thrombosis in the Thoratec HeartMate II device: an update analysis of the INTERMACS Registry. *J Heart Lung Transplant* 2015;34(12):1515–1526.)

OTHER THROMBOEMBOLIC EVENTS

Other (nonneurologic) thromboembolic events during VAD support are more common than strokes during the first month postimplantation, but they are relatively uncommon after that.[98] Preoperative atrial fibrillation does not appear to increase the risk of postimplantation thromboembolic events.

RIGHT HEART FAILURE

Right heart failure before and after VAD implantation is covered in Chapter 14. Management of intraoperative right heart failure is discussed in Chapter 11.

AORTIC INSUFFICIENCY

The development of aortic insufficiency (AI) during the period of long-term support on CF-LVAD has been well documented, affecting approximately one in four patients who will develop mild or greater AI after 1 year of MCS.[100–103] Mechanisms proposed for the cause of worsening AI during CF-LVAD use include leaflet deterioration, commissural fusion, aortic sinus dilation, and increased transvalvular gradients, all of which may have implications for device function, thromboembolism, and myocardial recovery.[104,105] Patients with preimplantation underlying aortic valve pathology with moderate or greater degree of insufficiency undergo surgical addressment at the time of implantation per the current guidelines (Class I, LOE C, reference) with oversewing the atrioventricular (AV) structure, partially closing the aortic valve with pledgeted sutures through the midpoint of each leaflet, closure of the ventriculoaortic junction with a surgical patch, or valve replacement using a bioprosthesis.[106,107]

It is well accepted that progression of AI takes place over time on long-term CF device support, with periodic echocardiograms performed routinely (every 6 months) to assess the frequency of aortic valve opening, the aortic valve structure, and the severity of AI. The degree of AI which develops on CF-LVAD support may be more difficult to measure with routine, standard echocardiography. Whereas in a native heart, AI occurs in diastole; in an LVAD-implanted heart, AI is pancyclic, occurring throughout systole and diastole in response to the constant positive and reversed transaortic pressure gradient. Traditional echocardiographic indices of AI severity such as vena contracta do not take into consideration the pancyclic nature of AI jets in patients with LVADs and one study that measured the regurgitant fraction across the aortic valve found a weak correlation with traditional echo parameters of AI and proposed two novel parameters unique to LVAD physiology—the diastolic flow acceleration and the systolic-to-diastolic peak velocity (S/D) ratio of the LVAD outflow cannula.[108]

Strategies have been developed to promote aortic valve opening in an effort to prevent the development and progression of AI.[106] With limited sample size, single-center studies have not demonstrated the significant impact on morbidity and mortality after the development of clinically significant AI. Using INTERMACS, a recent study has demonstrated the progressive nature of de novo AI on LVAD support, with over 50% of patients developing mild AI and 15% of patients developing moderate to severe AI at 2 years of support.[106] This progressive hemodynamic load of continuous, pancyclic AI leads to adverse ventricular remodeling and increased mitral regurgitation, which has further impact on left ventricular load and remodeling. Furthermore, the study identified the risk factors of older age, small body surface area, female gender, and the presence of mild AI at the time of implantation as determinants of progression to moderate and severe AI with ongoing mechanical assist device support—consistent with prior single-center reports. In terms of clinical impact, this INTERMACS analysis identified increased rehospitalization and decreased survival after 1 year of CF-LVAD support.[106]

Strategies to overcome the hemodynamic effects of AI that can improve clinical outcomes have not been well studied to date. One study demonstrated improved hemodynamics when patients with mild or greater AI were optimized with a full ramp optimization of pump speed, but at the cost of worsening AI in 80% of patients who were optimized.[109] The effects of medical management with therapies that target afterload reduction—which may or may not improve the transvalvular gradients depending on the impact on left ventricular preload have not been studied. Single-center studies have demonstrated early success in the addressment of AI with transcatheter aortic valve implantation (TAVI), but the safety and long-term efficacy in a multicenter study have not been demonstrated. In an INTERMACS analysis of AI, aortic valve closure at LVAD implantation led to less frequent development of moderate to severe AI, but adjusted analysis suggested closure was associated with a significant increased risk of mortality (hazard ratio, 1.87; 95% confidence interval, 1.39–2.53).[110] Efforts are currently underway to design clinical trials that will identify the safety and clinical impact of correcting AI with surgical approaches such as TAVI, and these studies will be very important in further elucidating the natural history of this complication of long-term CF-LVAD support.

Arrhythmias

Cardiac arrhythmias on devices are classified as one of two types: (1) sustained ventricular arrhythmias requiring defibrillation or cardioversion or (2) sustained supraventricular arrhythmias requiring drug treatment or cardioversion. Supraventricular arrhythmias that lead to AV dys-synchrony can affect right ventricular output. Control of supraventricular arrhythmias using standard medical therapy optimizes LVAD function. In patients with chronic atrial fibrillation and slow ventricular response, ensuring an adequate ventricular rate with the use of temporary pacing wires may be beneficial in the immediate postoperative period.

Sustained ventricular tachycardia usually results in diminished LVAD output, whereas ventricular fibrillation diminishes LVAD flow further. Since right ventricular contraction will not contribute to pulmonary blood flow during ventricular fibrillation, the effectiveness of an isolated LVAD in that setting depends on pulmonary vascular resistance and other factors.

If a patient being considered for LVAD support has a history of medically refractory arrhythmias and biventricular support is feasible, this is a preferred mode of therapy over single ventricle support. If it is available, the total artificial heart is the best solution for the management of refractory ventricular arrhythmias.

When patients with an LVAD have sustained ventricular arrhythmias and as a consequence experience a decrease in flow, they can be treated with cardioversion or defibrillation. The patient should be adequately sedated before receiving external electrical shocks if flow remains adequate for consciousness. MCS devices are designed to withstand internal and external electrical shocks for cardioversion and defibrillation, but the instructions for use should be consulted before employing external shocks. Detaching the driveline from the controller or other measures may be required. Implantable cardioverter defibrillators (ICDs) use sufficiently low energy levels that their potential for affecting pump components is substantially less. The ICD should be checked after VAD implantation to ensure that the pacing and sensing thresholds have not changed and that the device is functioning properly. In some instances, the radiofrequency energy emitted by the implanted pump (e.g., HMII) interferes with radiofrequency signals sent transcutaneously to the ICD. In such cases, the power to the pump must be temporarily interrupted to allow communication with the ICD. The patient should be comfortable and in a supine position if interruption of pump power is necessary. If the patient develops syncope or presyncope, power is immediately restored to the pump. The most recent versions of ICDs have successfully resolved the problem with radiofrequency interference by using another frequency.

REFERENCES

1. Kirklin JK, Naftel DC, Pagani FD, et al. Seventh INTERMACS annual report: 15,000 patients and counting. *J Heart Lung Transplant.* 2015;34(12):1495–1504.
2. Rose EA, Gelijns AC, Moskowitz AJ, et al. Long-term use of a left ventricular assist device for end-stage heart failure. *New Engl J Med.* 2001;345(20):1435–1443.
3. Kirklin JK, Naftel DC, Kormos RL, et al. Fifth INTERMACS annual report: risk factor analysis from more than 6,000 mechanical circulatory support patients. *J Heart Lung Transplant.* 2013;32(2):141–156.
4. Kirklin JK, Pagani FD, Kormos RL, et al. Eighth annual INTERMACS report: special focus on framing the impact of adverse events. *J Heart Lung Transplant.* 2017;36(10):1080–1086.
5. Grady KL, Wissman S, Naftel DC, et al. Age and gender differences and factors related to change in health-related quality of life from before to 6 months after left ventricular assist device implantation: findings from Interagency Registry for Mechanically Assisted Circulatory Support. *J Heart Lung Transplant.* 2016;35(6):777–788.
6. Pagani FD, Aaronson KD, Kormos R, et al. The NHLBI REVIVE-IT study: understanding its discontinuation in the context of current left ventricular assist device therapy. *J Heart Lung Transplant.* 2016;35(11):1277–1283.
7. Kirklin JK, Naftel DC, Pagani FD, et al. Sixth INTERMACS annual report: a 10,000-patient database. *J Heart Lung Transplant.* 2014;33(6):555–564.
8. Forest SJ, Xie R, Kirklin JK, et al. Impact of body mass index on adverse events following implantation of left ventricular assist devices: an IMACS registry analysis. *J Heart Lung Transplant.* 2018; 37(10): 1207–1217.
9. Kiernan MS, Grandin EW, Brinkley M Jr, et al. Early right ventricular assist device use in patients undergoing continuous-flow left ventricular assist device implantation: incidence and risk factors from the interagency registry for mechanically assisted circulatory support. *Circ Heart Fail.* 2017;10(10):e003863.
10. Cleveland JC, Goldstein DJ. The HeartMate 3 pump: Overcoming the hemocompatibilty gap. *The Journal of Thoracic and Cardiovascular Surgery.* 2018 Dec 01;156(6):2140–2142.
11. Mehra MR, Goldstein DJ, Uriel N, et al. Two-year outcomes with a magnetically levitated cardiac pump in heart failuree. *N Engl J Med.* 2018;378(15):1386–1395.
12. Goldstein DJ. HeartMate 3: bridging from clinical trial experience to real-world use. *The Journal of thoracic and cardiovascular surgery.* 2018;156(2): 660–661.
13. Hanke JS, Dogan G, Zoch A, et al. One-year outcomes with the HeartMate 3 left ventricular assist device. *The Journal of thoracic and cardiovascular surgery.* 2018.
14. Kirklin JK, Naftel DC, Pagani FD, et al. Pump thrombosis in the Thoratec HeartMate II device: an update analysis of the INTERMACS Registry. *J Heart Lung Transplant.* 2015;34(12):1515–1526.
15. McKenna Jr DH, Eastlund T, Segal M, et al. HLA alloimmuization in patients requiring ventricular assist device support. *J Heart Lung Transplant.* 2002;21:1218–1224.
16. Sihler KC, Napolitano LM. Complications of massive transfusions. *Chest.* 2010;137:209–220.

17. Gaudino M, Luciani N, Giungi S, et al. Different profiles of patients who require dialysis after cardiac surgery. *Ann Thorac Surg*. 2005;79:825–829.
18. Oz MC, Cosgrove DM III , Badduke BR, et al. Controlled clinical trial of a novel hemostatic agent in cardiac surgery. *Ann Thorac Surg*. 2000;69:1376–1382.
19. Schumer EM, Slaughter M, Dembitsky W. Intraoperative Operative Technique. In Braunwald's companion guide, 2nd Ed. Kirklin JK, Rogers JG, ed.
20. Stulak JM, Romans T, Cowger J, et al. Delayed sternal closure does not increase late infection risk in patients undergoing left ventricular assist device implantation. *JHLT*. 2012;31(10):1115–1119.
21. Schulman AR, Martens TP, Russo MJ, et al. Effect of left ventricular assist device infection on post-transplant outcomes. *J Heart Lung Transplant*. 2009;28:237–242.
22. Asadollahi K, Beeching NJ, Gill GV. Leukocytosis as a predictor for non-infective mortality and morbidity. *QJM*. 2010;103:285–292.
23. Holman WL, Kirklin JK, Naftel DC, et al. Infection after implantation of pulsatile mechanical circulatory support devices. *J Thorac Cardiovasc Surg*. 2010;139:1632–1636.
24. Goldstein DJ, Naftel D, Holman W, et al. Continuous-flow devices and percutaneous site infections: clinical outcomes. *J Heart Lung Transplant*. 2012;31:1151–1157.
25. Aslam S, Xie R, Chu V, et al. Epidemiology of bloodstream infections in MCSD recipients in the IMACS Registry. *J Heart Lung Transplant*. 2017;36(4):S26–S27.
26. Hannan MM, Xie R, Kusne S, et al. Huprikar S. Antimicrobial Surgical Prophylaxis in MCS Implant Surgery and Surgical Site Infection, IMACS January 2013 to December 2015. *J Heart Lung Transplant*. 2017;36(4):S40.
27. Morrissey O, Xie R, Schaenman J, et al. Epidemiology of fungal infections (FI) in mechanical circulatory support device (MCSD) recipients: analysis of IMACS registry 2013–2015. *J Heart Lung Transplant*. 2017;36(4):S27.
28. Holman WL. Microbiology of infection in mechanical circulatory support. *Int J Artif Organs*. 2007;30:764–770.
29. Fux CA, Costerton JW, Ps Stewart, et al. Survival strategies of infectious biofilms. *Trends Microbiol*. 2005;13:34–40.
30. Kussell E, Kishony R, Balaban NQ, et al. Bacterial persistence: a model of survival in changing environments. *Genetics*. 2005;169:1807–1814.
31. Balaban NQ, Merrin J, Chait R, et al. Bacterial persistence as a phenotypic switch. *Scieance*. 2004;305:1622–1625.
32. Cimochowski GE, Harostock MD, Brown R, et al. Intranasal mupirocin reduces sternal would infection after open heart surgery diabetics and nondiabetics. *Ann Thorac Surg*. 2001;71:1572–1578.
33. Hannan MM, Xie R, Kusne S, et al. Huprikar S. Antimicrobial surgical prophylaxis in mcs implant surgery and surgical site infection, IMACS January 2013 to December 2015. *J Heart Lung Transplant*. 2017;36(4):S40.
34. Fux CA, Costerton JW, Stewart PS, Stoodley P. Survival strategies of infectious biofilms. *Trends in microbiology*. 2005;13(1):34–40.
35. Rani SA, Pitts B, Stewart PS. Rapid diffusion of flurescent tracers into *Staphylococcus epidermidis* biofilms visualized by time lapse microscopy. *Antimicrob Agents Chemother*. 2005;4:728–732.
36. Hall-Stoodley L, Costerton JW, Stoodley P. Bacterial biofilms: from the natural environment to infectious disease. *Nature*. 2004;2:95–108.
37. Hernandez MD, Mansouri MD, Aslam S, et al. Efficacy of combination of N-acetylcysteine, gentamicin, and amphotericin B for prevention of microbial colonization of ventricular assist device. *Infect Control Hosp Epidemiol*. 2009;30:190–192.
38. Twardowski ZJ. History and development of the access for peritoneal dialysis. *Contrib Nephrol*. 2004;142:387–401.
39. Twardowski ZJ, Dobbie JW, Moore HL, et al. Morphology of peritoneal dialysis catheter tunnel: macroscopy and light microscopy. *Perit Dial Int*. 1991;11:237–251.
40. Zierer A, Melby SJ, Voeller RK, et al. Late-onset driveline infections: the Achilles' heel of prolonged left ventricular assist device support. *Ann Thorac Surg*. 2007;84:515–520.
41. Arrecubieta C, Toba FA, von Bayern MP, et al. SdrF, a *Staphylococcus epidermidis* surface protein, contributes to the initiation of ventricular assist device driveline infections. *PLoS Pathog*. 2009;5:1–13.
42. Yuh DD, Albaugh M, Ullrich S, et al. Treament of ventricular assist driveline infection with vacuum-assisted closure system. *Ann Thorac Surg*. 2005;80:1493–1495.
43. Baradarian S, Stahovich M, Krause S, et al. Case series clinical management of persistent mechanical assist device driveline drainage using vacuum-assisted closure therapy. *ASAIO J*. 2006;52:354–356.
44. Stulak JM, Davis ME, Haglund N, et al. Adverse events in contemporary continuous-flow left ventricular assist devices: a multi-institutional comparison shows significant differences. *J Thorac Cardiovasc Surg*. 2016;151(1):177–189(1).
45. McKellar SH, Allred BD, Marks JD, et al. LVAD pocket infection controlled with antibiotic-impregnated polymethylmethacrylate beads. *Ann Thorac Surg*. 1999;67:554–555.
46. Holman WL, Fix RJ, Foley BA, et al. Management of wound and left ventricular assist device pocket infection. *Ann Thorac Surg*. 1999;68:1080–1082.
47. de Jonge KC, Laube HR, Dohmen PM, Ivancevic V, Konertz WF. Diagnosis and management of left ventricular assist device valve-endocarditis: LVAD valve replacement. *Ann Thorac Surg*. 2000;70(4):1404–1405.
48. Poston RS, Husain S, Sorce D, et al. LVAD bloodstream infections: therapeutic rationale for transplantation after LVAD infection. *J Heart Lung Transplant*. 2003;22:914–921.
49. Nurozler F, Argenziano M, OZ MC, et al. Fungal left ventricular assist device endocarditis. *Ann Thorac Surg*. 2001;71:614–618.
50. Crow S, John R, Boyle A, et al. Gastrointestinal bleeding rates in recipients of non-pulsatile and pulsatile left ventricular assist devices. *J Thorac Cardiovasc Surg*. 2009;137:208–215.
51. Huang RJ, Wong RJ, Draper KV, Winter TA. De novo arteriovenous malformations following implantation of the heartmate ii left ventricular assist device. *Endoscopy*. 2012;44. (suppl 2 UCTN):E441.
52. Patibandla PK, Rajasekaran NS, Shelar SB, Giridharan GA, Litovsky SH, Sethu P. Evaluation of the effect of diminished pulsatility as seen in continuous flow ventricular assist devices on arterial endothelial cell phenotype and function. *J Heart Lung Transplant*. 2016;35:930–932.
53. Letsou GV, Shah N, Gregoric ID, et al. Gastrointestinal bleeding from arteriovenous malformation in patients supported by the Jarvi 2000 axial-flow left ventricular assist device. *J Heart Lung Transplant*. 2005;24:105–109.
54. Uriel N, Pak SW, Jorde UP, et al. Acquired von Willebrand syndrome after continuous flow mechanical device support contributes to a high prevalence of bleeding during long-term support and a t the time of heart transplantation. *J Am Coll Cardiol*. 2010;56:1207–1213.
55. Lazar RM, Shapiro PA, Jaski BE, et al. Neurological events during long-term mechanical circulatory support for heart failure: the Randomized Evaluation of Mechanical Assistance for the Treatment of Congestive Heart Failure (REMATCH) experience. *Circualtion*. 2004;109:2423–2427.
56. Teuteberg JJ, Slaughter MS, Rogers JG, et al. The HVAD left ventricular assist device. *Risk factors for neurological events and risk mitigation strategies*. *J Am Coll Cardiol: Heart Failure*. 2015;3(10):818–828.
57. Miller LW, Pagani FD, Russell SD, et al. Use of a continuous-flow device inpatients awaiting heart transplantation. *N Engl J Med*. 2007;357:885–896.
58. Slaughter MS, Rogers JG, Milano CA, et al. Advanced heart failure treated with continuous-flow left ventricular assist device: analysis of outpatient anti-coagulation. *J Heart Lung Transplant*. 2009;28:881–887.
59. Acharya D, Loyaga-Rendon R, Morgan CJ, et al. INTERMACS analysis of stroke during support with continuous-flow left ventricular assist devices: risk factors and outcomes. *JACC: Heart Failure*. 2017 Oct 1;5(10):703–711.
60. Aaronson KD, Slaughter MS, Miller LW, et al. Use of an intrapericardial, continuous flow, centrifugal pump in patients awaiting heart transplantation. *Circulation*. 2012;125:3191–3200.
61. Mehra MR, Goldstein DJ, Uriel N, et al. Two-year outcomes with a magnetically levitated cardiac pump in heart failure. N Engl J Med 2018; 378(15):1386-1395.
62. Uriel N, Colombo PC, Cleveland JC, et al. Hemocompatibility-related outcomes in the MOMENTUM 3 trial at 6 months: a randomized controlled study of a fully magnetically levitated pump in advanced heart failure. *Circulation*. 2017 May 23;135(21):2003–2012.

63. Lietz K, Brown K, Ali SS, et al. The role of cerebral hyperperfusion in postoperative neurologic dysfunction after left ventricular assist device implantation for end-stage heart failure. *J Thorac Cardiovasc Surg.* 2009;137:1012–1019.
64. Boyle AJ, Park SJ, Colvin-Adams MM, et al. Cerebral hyperperfusion syndrome following LVAD implantation (abstract). *J Heart Lung Transplant.* 2003;22(suppl):S203.
65. Tsukui H, Abla A, Teuteberg JJ, et al. Cerebrovascular accidents in patients with a ventricular assist device. *J Thorac Cardiovasc Surg.* 2007;134:114–123.
66. Al-Mufti F, Bauerschmidt A, Claassen J, Meyers PM, Colombo PC, Willey JZ. Neuroendovascular interventions for acute ischemic strokes in patients supported with left ventricular assist devices: a single-center case series and review of the literature. *World Neurosurgery.* 2016;88:199–204.
67. Russell SD, Rogers JG, Milano CA, et al. Renal and hepatic function improve in advanced heart failure patients during continuous-flow support with the HeartMate II left ventricular assist device. *Circulation.* 2009;120:2352–2357.
68. Sandner SE, Zimpfer D, Zrunke P, et al. Renal function and outcome after continuous flow left ventricular assist device implantation. *Ann Thorac Surg.* 2009;87:1072–1078.
69. Radovancevic B, Vrtovec B, de Kort E, et al. End-organ function in patients on long term circulatory support with continuous-or pulsatile-flow assist devices. *J Heart Lung Transplant.* 2007;26:815–818.
70. James KB, McCarthy PM, Jaalouk S, et al. Plasma volume and its regulatory factors in congestive heart failure after implantation of long-term left ventricular assist devices. *Circulation.* 1996;93(8):1515–1519.
71. Gaudino M, Luciani N, Giungi S, et al. Different profiles of patients who require dialysis after cardiac surgery. *Ann Thorac Surg.* 2005;79:825–829.
72. Muslem R, Caliskan K, Akin S, et al. Proteinuria in patients receiving left ventricular assist devices is highly associated with renal failure and mortality. *Journal of the American College of Cardiology.* 2017;69(11 suppl):699.
73. Kanter KR, Swart MT, Pennington DG, et al. Renal failure inpatients with ventricular assist devices. *ASAIO Trans.* 1987;33:426–428.
74. Kaltenmaier B, Pommer W, Kaufmann F, et al. Outcome of patients with ventricular assist devices and acute renal failure requiring renal replacement therapy. *ASAIO J.* 2000;46:330–333.
75. Kilic A, Chen CW, Gaffey AC, Wald JW, Acker MA, Atluri P. Preoperative renal dysfunction does not affect outcomes of left ventricular assist device implantation. *The Journal of thoracic and cardiovascular surgery.* 2018;156(3):1093–1101.
76. Cowger J, Sundareswaran K, Rogers JG, et al. Predicting survival in patients receiving continuous flow left ventricular assist devices: the HeartMate II risk score. *Journal of the American College of Cardiology.* 2013;61(3):313–321.
77. Pagani FD. Left ventricular assist device outcomes and preoperative kidney dysfunction: the truth be told. *The Journal of thoracic and cardiovascular surgery.* 2018.
78. Fries RC. Human factors. In: *Reliable Design of Medical Devices.* New York: Marcel Dekker; 1997:11–21.
79. Fries RC. The concept of failure. In: *Reliable Design of Medical Devices.* New York: Marcel Dekker;1997:313-355.
80. Wu WT, Yang F, Wu J, Aubry N, Massoudi M, Antaki JF. High fidelity computational simulation of thrombus formation in Thoratec HeartMate II continuous flow ventricular assist device. *Sci Rep.* 2016;6:38025. https://doi.org/10.1038/srep38025.:38025.
81. Zhuo R, Miller R, Bussard KM, Siedlecki CA, Vogler EA. Procoagulant stimulus processing by the intrinsic pathway of blood plasma coagulation. *Biomaterials.* 2005;26(16):2965–2973.
82. Vogler EA, Graper JC, Harper GR, Sugg HW, Lander LM, Brittain WJ. Contact activation of the plasma coagulation cascade. I. Procoagulant surface chemistry and energy. *J Biomed Mater Res.* 1995;29(8):1005–1016.
83. Colman RW, Scott CF, Schmaier AH, Wachtfogel YT, Pixley RA, Edmunds Jr LH. Initiation of blood coagulation at artificial surfaces. *Annals of the New York Academy of Sciences.* 1987 Dec;516(1):253–267.
84. Song X, Throckmorton AL, Wood HG, Antaki JF, Olsen DB. Computational fluid dynamics prediction of blood damage in a centrifugal pump. *Artif Organs.* 2003;27:938–941.
85. Song X, Wood HG, Olsen D. Computational Fluid Dynamic (CFD) study of the 4th generation prototype of a continuous flow Ventricular Assist Device (VAD). *J Biomech Eng.* 2004;126:180–187.
86. Hochareon P, Manning KB, Fontaine AA, Tarbell JM, Deutsch S. Wall shear-rate estimation within the 50 cc Penn State artificial heart using particle image velocimetry. *J Biomech Eng.* 2004;126:430–437.
87. Day SW, McDaniel JC, Wood HG, Allaire PE, Landrot N, Curtas A. Particle image velocimetry measurements of blood velocity in a continuous flow ventricular assist device. *ASAIO J.* 2001;47:406–411.
88. Bachmann C, Hugo G, Rosenberg G, Deutsch S, Fontaine A, Tarbell JM. Fluid dynamics of a pediatric ventricular assist device. *Artif Organs.* 2000;24:362–372.
89. Burgreen GW, Antaki JF, Wu ZJ, Holmes AJ. Computational fluid dynamics as a development tool for rotary blood pumps. *Artif Organs.* 2001;25:336–340.
90. Chung MKH, Zhang N, Tansley GD, Qian Y. Experimental determination of dynamic characteristics of the VentrAssist implantable rotary blood pump. *Artif Organs.* 2004;28:1089–1094.
91. Meyer AL, Kuehn C, Weidemann J, et al. Thrombus formation in a HeartMate II left ventricular assist device. *The Journal of thoracic and cardiovascular surgery* 2008;135(1):203–204.
92. Chiu WC, Slepian MJ, Bluestein D. Thrombus formation patterns in the HeartMate II ventricular assist device: clinical observations can be predicted by numerical simulations. *ASAIO J.* 2014;60(2):237–240.
93. Yang F, Kormos RL, Antaki JF. High-speed visualization of disturbed pathlines in axial flow ventricular assist device under pulsatile conditions. *J Thorac Cardiovasc Surg.* 2015;150(4):938–944.
94. Bourque K, Cotter C, Dague C, et al. Design rationale and preclinical evaluation of the HeartMate 3 left ventricular assist system for hemocompatibility. *ASAIO J.* 2016;62(4):375–383.
95. Katz JN, Jensen BC, Chang PP, Myers SL, Pagani FD, Kirklin JK. A multicenter analysis of clinical hemolysis in patients supported with durable, long-term left ventricular assist device therapy. *J Heart Lung Transplant.* 2015;34(5):701–709.
96. Shah P, Mehta VM, Cowger JA, Aaronson KD, Pagani FD. Diagnosis of hemolysis and device thrombosis with lactate dehydrogenase during left ventricular assist device support. *J Heart Lung Transplant.* 2014;33(1):102–104.
97a. Smedira NG, Blackstone EH, Ehrlinger J, et al. Current risks of HeartMate II pump thrombosis: non-parametric analysis of Interagency Registry for Mechanically Assisted Circulatory Support data. *J Heart Lung Transplant.* 2015;34(12):1527–1534.
97b. Birati EY, Quiaoit Y, Wald J, et al. Ventricular assist device thrombosis: A wide spectrum of clinical presentation. *The Journal of Heart and Lung Transplantation.* 2015 Apr 1;34(4):613–615.
98. Xia Y, Stern D, Friedmann P, Goldstein D. Preoperative atrial fibrillation may not increase thromboembolic events in left ventricular assist device recipients on midterm follow-up. *J Heart Lung Transplant.* 2016;35(7):906–912.
99. Feldman D, Pamboukian SV, Teuteberg JJ, et al. The 2013 International Society for Heart and Lung Transplantation Guidelines for mechanical circulatory support: executive summary. *J Heart Lung Transplant.* 2013;32(2):157–187.
100. Jorde U, Uriel N, Nahumi N, et al. Prevalence, significance, and management of aortic insufficiency in continuous flow left ventricular assist device recipients. *Circ Heart Fail.* 2014;7(2):310–319.
101. Pak S, Uriel N, Takayama H, et al. Prevalence of de novo aortic insufficiency during long-term support with left ventricular assist devices. *J Heart Lung Transplant.* 2010;29(10):1172–1176.
102. Truby L, Garan A, Givens R. Aortic Insufficiency During Contemporary Left Ventricular Assist Device Support. *Analysis of the INTERMACS Registry JACC.* 2018;6(11):951–960.
103. Cowger J, Pagani F, Haft J, Romano M, Aaronson K, Kolias T. The development of aortic insufficiency in left ventricular assist device-supported patients. *Circ Heart Fail.* 2010;3(6):668–674.
104. Mudd J, Cuda J, Halushka M, Soderlund K, Conte J, Russell S. Fusion of aortic valve commissures in patients supported by a continuous axial flow left ventricular assist device. *J Heart Lung Transplant.* 2008;27(12):1269–1274.
105. John R, Mantz K, Eckman P, Rose A, May-Newman K. Aortic valve pathophysiology during left ventricular assist device support. *J Heart Lung Transplant.* 2010;29(12):1321–1329

106. Cowger J, Rao V, Massey T, et al. Comprehensive review and suggested strategies for the detection and management of aortic insufficiency in patients with a continuous-flow left ventricular assist device. *J Heart Lung Transplant*. 2014;34(2):149–157.
107. Park S, Liao K, Segurola R, Madhu K, Miller L. Management of aortic insufficiency in patients with left ventricular assist devices: a simple coaptation stitch method (Park's stitch). *Journal of Thoracic and Cardiovascular Surgery*. 2004;127(1):264–266.
108. Grinstein J, Kruse E, Sayer G, et al. Accurate quantification methods for aortic insufficiency severity in patients with LVAD. Role of diastolic flow acceleration and systolic-to-diastolic peak velocity ratio of outflow cannula. *JACC: Cardiovasc Imaging*. 2016;9(6):641–651.
109. Sayer G, Sarswat N, Kim G, et al. The hemodynamic effects of aortic insufficiency in patients supported with continuous-flow left ventricular assist devices. *Journal of Cardiac Failure*. 2017;23(7):545–551.
110. Robertson JO, Naftel DC, Myers SL, et al. Concomitant aortic valve procedures in patients undergoing implantation of continuous-flow left ventricular assist devices: an INTERMACS database analysis. *J Heart Lung Transplant*. 2015;34:797–805.

APPENDIX INTERMACS Definitions of Clinically Significant Acute Adverse Events After Ventricular Assist Device Implantation

Event Type	Definition
Cardiac/Vascular	
Arrhythmia (ventricular or atrial)	Any documented ventricular or atrial arrhythmia that results in a clinical compromise (e.g., diminished VAD outflow, oliguria, presyncope, or syncope) that requires hospitalization or occurs during the hospital stay.
	Ventricular arrhythmia: Sustained ventricular arrhythmia requiring defibrillation or cardioversion.
	Atrial arrhythmia: Sustained supraventricular arrhythmia requiring drug treatment or cardioversion.
Right heart failure	Symptoms and signs of persistent right ventricular dysfunction (central venous pressure >18 mm Hg with cardiac index <2.0 L/min/m^2 in the absence of elevated left atrial or pulmonary capillary wedge pressure [>18 mm Hg], tamponade, ventricular arrhythmias, or pneumothorax) requiring RVAD implantation or inotropic therapy, ≥14 days after LVAD implantation.
Hypertension	New-onset blood pressure elevation ≥140 mm Hg systolic or 90 mm Hg diastolic (pulsatile pump) or 110 mm Hg mean pressure (rotary pump).
Thromboembolism (arterial or venous)	*Arterial thromboembolism:* Acute systemic arterial perfusion deficit in any noncerebrovascular organ system confirmed by clinical and laboratory findings, operative, or autopsy.
	Venous thromboembolism: Evidence of deep vein thrombosis or other venous thrombotic event.
Hemolysis	Plasma free hemoglobin >40 mg/dL in association with clinical signs of hemolysis (e.g., anemia, low hematocrit, and hyperbilirubinemia) occurring within the first 72 hours after implantation. Hemolysis related to documented non–device-related causes (e.g., transfusion or drug) is excluded from this definition.
MI	Two categories of MI:
	Perioperative MI: Clinical suspicion of MI together with CK-MB or troponin >10 times the local hospital upper limits of normal, found within 7 days after VAD implantation together with ECG findings consistent with acute MI. This definition uses the higher suggested limit for serum markers because of apical coring at the time of VAD placement and does not use wall motion changes because the apical sewing ring inherently creates new wall motion abnormalities.
	Nonperioperative MI: The presence of two of the following three criteria at >7 days after implantation: 1. Chest pain that is characteristic of myocardial ischemia 2. ECG with a pattern or changes consistent with MI 3. Troponin or CK (measured by standard clinical pathology or laboratory medicine methods) greater than the normal range for the local hospital with positive MB fraction (≥3% total CK). This should be accompanied by a new regional left ventricular or right ventricular wall motion abnormality on a myocardial imaging study.
Other Organ Systems	
Respiratory (tracheostomy or reintubation)	Impairment of respiratory function requiring reintubation, tracheostomy, or (for patients >5 years old) the inability to discontinue ventilator support within 6 days (144 hours) after VAD implantation. This excludes intubation for reoperation or temporary intubation for diagnostic or therapeutic procedures.
Neurologic (infarct or hemorrhagic CVA or TIA)	Any new, temporary or permanent, focal or global neurologic deficit ascertained by standard neurologic examination (administered by a neurologist or other qualified physician and documented with appropriate diagnostic tests and consultation note). The examining physician distinguishes between TIA, which is fully reversible within 24 hours (and without evidence of infarction), and stroke, which lasts >24 hours (or <24 hours if there is evidence of infarction). The NIH Stroke Scale (for patients >5 years old) must be readministered at 30 days and 60 days after the event to document the presence and severity of neurologic deficits. Each neurologic event must be subcategorized as follows: 1. TIA (acute event that resolves completely within 24 hours with no evidence of infarction) 2. Ischemic or hemorrhagic CVA (event that persists >24 hours or <24 hours and associated with infarction on an imaging study) In addition, for patients <6 months old, any of the following: 3. New abnormality on head ultrasound 4. EEG positive for seizure activity with or without clinical seizure.

APPENDIX INTERMACS Definitions of Clinically Significant Acute Adverse Events After Ventricular Assist Device Implantation—cont'd

Event Type	Definition
Renal	Acute renal dysfunction (abnormal kidney function requiring dialysis in patients who did not require this procedure before implantation or increase in serum creatinine >3 times normal baseline or >5 mg/dL) and chronic renal dysfunction (increase in serum creatinine of ≥2 mg/dL above baseline or requirement of hemodialysis for at least 90 days).
Hepatic	Increase in any two hepatic laboratory values (total bilirubin, AST, or ALT) to a level >3 times the upper limit of normal 14 days after implantation (or if hepatic dysfunction is the primary cause of death).
Gastrointestinal	Cholecystitis, Crohn disease, diverticulitis, esophagitis, gastroesophageal reflux disease, hiatal hernia, ischemic bowel requiring surgical exploration, pancreatitis with abnormal amylase or lipase requiring nasogastric suction therapy, polyps, or ulcer.
Bleeding (coagulopathy, mediastinum or pocket, thorax, gastrointestinal)	Episode of internal or external bleeding in the mediastinum, pocket, thorax, or gastrointestinal system that results in death or the need for reoperation or hospitalization, or necessitates transfusions of red blood cells (≥4 U packed red blood cells within any 24-hour period in the first 7 days after implantation or ≥2 U packed red blood cells within any 24 hour period after 7 days after implantation).
Infection (driveline, bloodstream, pulmonary, mediastinum, or pocket)	Driveline, bloodstream, or pulmonary infection accompanied by pain, fever, drainage, or leukocytosis that is treated by antimicrobial agents (nonprophylactic).
	Driveline infection: Positive culture from the skin, tissue, or both surrounding the driveline or from the tissue surrounding the external housing of a pump, with the need for treatment, when there is clinical evidence of infection (pain, fever, drainage, leukocytosis). A positive culture from the infected site or organ should be present unless strong clinical evidence indicates the need for treatment despite negative cultures. The general categories of infection are:
	Localized nondevice infection: Infection localized to any organ system or region (e.g., mediastinitis) without evidence of systemic involvement (see sepsis definition), ascertained by standard clinical methods and either associated with evidence of bacterial, viral, fungal, or protozoal infection or requiring empirical treatment.
	Percutaneous site or pocket infection: Positive culture from the skin or tissue surrounding the driveline or from the tissue surrounding the external housing of a pump implanted within the body, coupled with the need to treat with antimicrobial therapy, when there is clinical evidence of infection, such as pain, fever, drainage, or leukocytosis.
	Internal pump component, inflow or outflow tract infection: Infection of blood-contacting surfaces of LVAD documented by positive site culture. There should be a separate data field for paracorporeal pump that describes infection at the percutaneous cannula site (e.g., Thoratec PVAD).
	Sepsis: Evidence of systemic involvement by infection, manifested by positive blood cultures or hypotension, or both.
Reoperation (bleeding, infection, wound dehiscence, wound debridement)	Return operation secondary to bleeding, infection, or disruption of the apposed surfaces of a surgical incision requiring surgical repair.
Pericardial fluid collection	Accumulation of fluid or clot in the pericardial space that requires surgical intervention or percutaneous catheter drainage.
	This event is subdivided into events with clinical signs of tamponade (e.g., increased central venous pressure and decreased cardiac or VAD output) and events without signs of tamponade.
Device malfunction	Device malfunction denotes a failure of one or more of the components of the MCS device system, which either directly causes or could potentially induce a state of inadequate circulatory support (low cardiac output state) or death. The manufacturer must confirm device failure. A failure that was iatrogenic or recipient induced would be classified as an iatrogenic/recipient-induced failure.
	Device failure should be classified according to which components fail: 1. Pump failure (blood-contacting components of pump and any motor or other pump-actuating mechanism that is housed with the blood-contacting components). In the special situation of pump thrombosis, thrombus is documented to be present within the device or its conduits that results in or could potentially induce circulatory failure 2. Nonpump failure (e.g., external pneumatic drive unit, electric power supply unit, batteries, controller, interconnect cable, compliance chamber).
Psychiatric episode	Disturbance in thinking, emotion, or behavior that causes substantial impairment in functioning or marked subjective distress requiring intervention. Intervention is the addition of new psychiatric medication, hospitalization, or referral to a mental health professional for treatment. Suicide is included in this definition.

ALT, Alanine aminotransferase; *AST*, aspartate aminotransferase; *CK-MB*, creatine kinase muscle-band; *CVA*, cerebrovascular accident; *ECG*, electrocardiogram; *EEG*, electroencephalogram; *INTERMACS*, Interagency Registry for Mechanically Assisted Circulatory Support; *LVAD*, left ventricular assist device; *MCS*, mechanical circulatory support; *MI*, myocardial infarction; *NIH*, National Institutes of Health; *PVAD*, paracorporeal ventricular assist device; *RVAD*, right ventricular assist device; *TIA*, transient ischemic attack; *VAD*, ventricular assist device.

14

Right Heart Failure in Patients With Mechanical Circulatory Support

Nader Moazami, Pavan Atluri, J. Eduardo Rame

KEY POINTS

INTRODUCTION

For end-stage heart failure (HF), heart transplantation or implantation of a left ventricular assist device (LVAD) is lifesaving and provides a significant improvement in quality of life.[1,2] Despite the therapeutic success of LVADs,[3] concomitant right ventricular failure (RVF) and the lack of appropriate long-term, right ventricular (RV) support devices has limited the full potential that mechanical circulatory support (MCS) can offer to patients with biventricular failure.[4–7]

Despite the relatively low rate of temporary RV assist device (RVAD) support in the United States, a significant number of patients who have been successfully discharged after receiving an LVAD remain symptomatic from RVF and undergo recurrent readmissions for the management of HF. In addition, delayed RVF is being increasingly recognized in a subset of patients on chronic LVAD support.[8] In this chapter, we will discuss the pathophysiology of RVF, which can be potentially exacerbated after LVAD implantation, and the nonsurgical and surgical management strategies to address this extremely important issue.

PHYSIOLOGY AND ANATOMY OF THE RIGHT VENTRICLE

The RV is a complex three-dimensional structure that appears triangular in sagittal section, unlike the cone-shaped left ventricle (LV) chamber (Fig. 14.1).[9–13] Both the RV and LV are linked with a common meshwork of fibers that encircle the ventricles (Fig. 14.2). The muscle mass of the RV is approximately one-sixth that of the LV and, under normal conditions, it functions in a low-pressured working environment.

Another uniqueness of RV structure is its high level of "reinforcement" with interweaving strands of muscle (trabeculae carneae) and a coarse endocardial inner surface.[14] The pattern of RV trabeculae carneae in the ventricle is an efficient means of gaining power without excessively thickening the wall of the chamber (normally 3–5 mm in thickness). In patients with increased RV pressure, the trabeculae are more likely to be coarser, which may result in substantial alterations of RV volume, mass, and ejection fraction.[15,16]

In addition, the shared interventricular septum (IVS) plays an important role in RV output. It has been suggested that a substantial portion of RV systolic pressure and stroke volume results from LV contraction, much of which is contributed through the IVS. As the IVS contracts, it adds to the contraction effort of the RV free wall and may in fact contribute as much as 40% to the output of the RV. In addition, the contracting free wall of the RV pushes against the IVS as its supporting structure. This ventricular interdependence of RV output on the IVS and on LV contractility has been demonstrated in animal models.[17–19] As discussed later in the chapter, this has particular importance once an LVAD is implanted because it can significantly alter the loading conditions of both the RV and LV and their respective geometric relationship to each other.

Under normal baseline conditions, the unique anatomy, myocardial ultrastructure, and coronary blood flow physiology of the RV reflect the characteristics of a high-volume/low-pressure pump. Because of low pulmonary vascular resistance (PVR), the RV pumps the same stroke volume as the LV does, but with ~25% of the stroke work. Contraction of the extremely compliant, thin-walled RV (by virtue of the Laplace relationship) is a process starting at the inlet, then free wall, and subsequently ending at the infundibulum. Of note, unlike the LV, in which coronary perfusion is predominately during diastole, the low-pressured RV is perfused throughout the cardiac cycle. Hence, significant elevations in the RV end-diastolic pressure, without a concomitant increase in mean arterial pressure, may be accompanied by ischemia in a relatively hypertrophied RV.[19] In chronic HF, the RV pressure-volume loop shifts from a normal trapezoidal shape, reflecting its high efficiency/low impedance, to a rectangular shape, which becomes indistinguishable from a normal LV pressure-volume loop, suggesting an ongoing RV adaptation to increased volume overload (Fig. 14.3).[11]

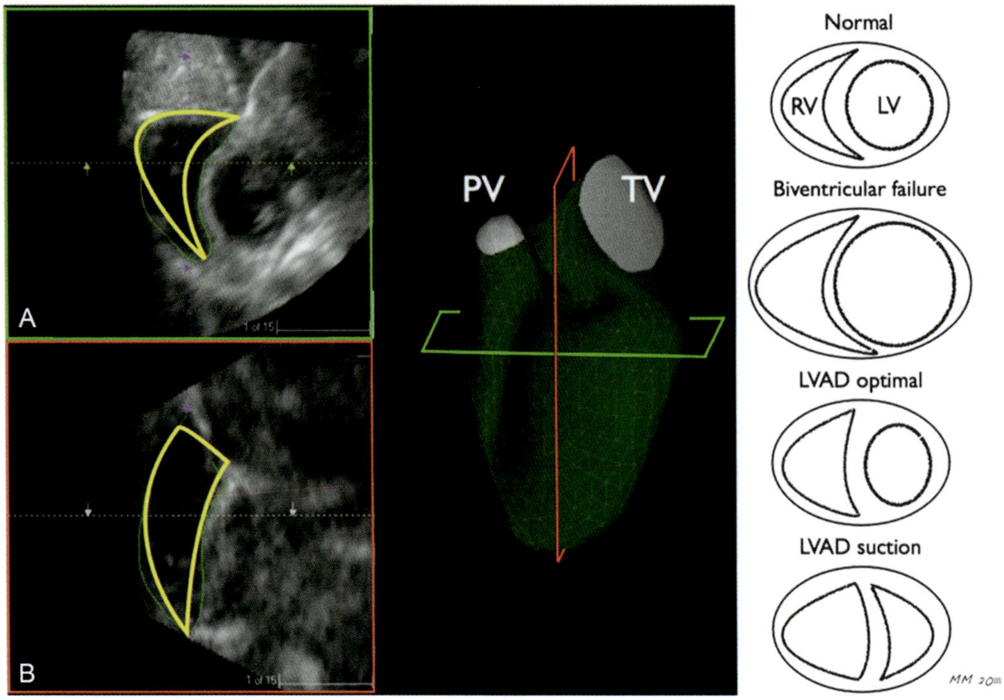

Fig. 14.1 Ventricular interdependence. Three-dimensional transesophageal echocardiographic reconstruction of the right ventricle *(RV)* from the pulmonary *(PV)* to the tricuspid *(TV)* valve. (A) Cross-section showing the crescent shape of the RV. (B) Sagittal section showing the triangular shape of the RV. Ventricular interdependence between the left ventricle *(LV)* and RV during systole relies on the position of the interventricular septum, as shown in cross-section within different clinical scenarios. (From Meineri M, Van Rensburg AE, Vegas A. Right ventricular failure after LVAD implantation: prevention and treatment. *Best Pract Res Clin Anaesthesiol* 2012;26(2):217–229.)

RIGHT VENTRICULAR FAILURE IN PATIENTS WITH CHRONIC HEART FAILURE AFTER LVAD

Definition of Right Ventricular Failure

The common working definition of RVF according to the Interagency Registry for Mechanically Assisted Circulatory Support (INTERMACS) is a persistence of signs and symptoms of RV dysfunction evident by central venous pressure (CVP) >18 mm Hg with a cardiac index <2.0 L/min/m^2 and in the absence of increased pulmonary capillary wedge pressure (PCWP) >18 mm Hg, cardiac tamponade, ventricular arrhythmias, or pneumothorax. Alternatively, placement of an RVAD or the use of intravenous inotropes or inhaled nitric oxide for >14 days post-LVAD implantation fits into this definition. The development of RVF that requires RVAD support in LVAD recipients is associated with high mortality irrespective of the timing of device insertion[8] Patients who require RVAD support have higher in-hospital mortality (48% vs. 9.5%) and worse 1-year survival rates (40% vs. 82%) compared to those who received LVAD only.

Pathophysiology of Right Ventricular Failure After LVAD Placement

The pathophysiologic mechanisms that lead to manifestations of RVF are multifactorial, with some related to preexisting conditions and others to the hemodynamic changes brought on by the device. First, in patients with generic "dilated" cardiomyopathies (whether genetic predisposition, chemotherapy induced, or other mechanisms), it is expected that the same cardiomyopathic processes that affect the LV will also involve the RV. To a large extent, the decrement in RV systolic and diastolic function and RV dilation is likely determined by this pathologic process and is further exacerbated by the afterload imposed by chronic pulmonary hypertension. Similarly, in patients with ischemic cardiomyopathy, coronary artery perfusion may be compromised by atherosclerotic disease in the distribution of the right coronary artery. The malperfusion can also be further exacerbated by decreased perfusion pressure related to high CVP and low systemic blood pressure, which are the defining characteristics of patients in end-stage HF.

Cardiopulmonary bypass during the surgery can also exacerbate RVF by causing an acute increase in PVR, likely due to inflammatory mediators. There is also a decrease in vasodilating mediators, such as nitric oxide and prostacyclin, with an increase in vasoconstricting mediators such as thromboxane A2 and endothelin.[20] Blood transfusion and protamine administration have been shown to cause pulmonary vasoconstriction and exacerbate RV dysfunction as well. Many pulmonary vasodilators have been utilized to treat acute increases in PVR, including inhaled nitric oxide, prostaglandin E1 and prostacyclin, phosphodiesterase 5 inhibitors, and endothelin receptor antagonists.[21] While these causes of postoperative pulmonary vasoconstriction have been well studied in the general cardiac surgery patient, there is a dearth of evidence analyzing the relative importance of these mechanisms specifically in the MCS population.

During the perioperative phase, the altered physiology created by the LVAD may also exacerbate RVF by several mechanisms. The effect of ventricular interdependence is most prominent in the setting of loading changes after LVAD implantation. Excessive LV unloading results in leftward shift of the IVS, thus jeopardizing efficient RV contraction and output.[22] In addition, augmentation of cardiac output and systemic blood flow by the LVAD increases the amount of venous return to the failing RV. In the absence of a significant and immediate reduction in RV afterload, RV function may become compromised.

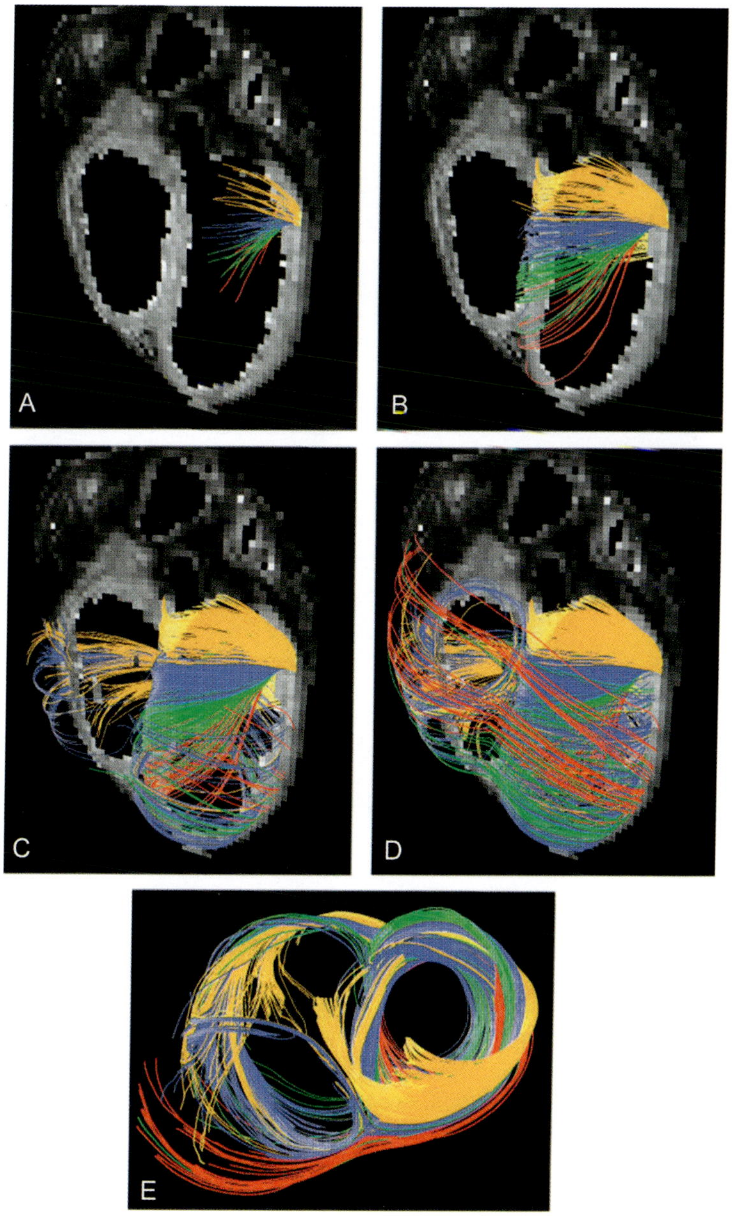

Fig. 14.2 Right ventricular architecture. This series of magnetic resonance images shows the right ventricle architecture composed of tracks originating from the parietal walls of the left ventricle. Pathways intrude from epicardium to endocardium by means of a right-hand helix movement about a transverse circular axis. (From Smerup M, Nielsen E, Agger P, et al. The three-dimensional arrangement of the myocytes aggregated together within the mammalian ventricular myocardium. *Anat Rec (Hoboken)* 2009;292(1):1–11.)

RIGHT VENTICULAR AFTERLOAD SENSITIVITY AND ADAPTATION

LVAD placement causes dramatic changes in hemodynamic markers of RV load and function. One study examined hemodynamic changes in three phases: pre-LVAD, early post-LVAD (within 6 months of implantation), and prolonged LVAD therapy (19–36 months after implantation).[23] In the early post-LVAD period, there were significant decreases in PCWP (25–10 mm Hg), effective arterial elastance (Ea; 1.04–0.43 mm Hg/mL), and PVR (2.22–1.50 Wood units), while pulmonary vascular compliance (PCA, 2.00–4.03 mL/mm Hg) increased significantly, confirming that LVAD placement reduces both resistive and pulsatile components of RV load. However, CVP did not decrease, and the CVP:PCWP ratio, an independent predictor of RVF post-LVAD, increased significantly (0.47–0.85). The data from this study suggest that despite the favorable impact of LVADs on reducing RV afterload in the early perioperative period, RV contractile dysfunction is the dominant determinant of RVF and is likely exacerbated by increased venous return. Hence, perioperative intervention continues to rely on the use of inotropes for contractile augmentation of the RV.

With prolonged LVAD therapy, PCWP and Ea remained significantly decreased (12 and 0.38 mm Hg/mL, respectively) from pre-LVAD values but were unchanged from the early post-LVAD values. In contrast, PVR further decreased between the early post-LVAD and prolonged LVAD treatment periods (1.50–1.17 Wood units). While CVP remained unchanged over both periods, CVP:PCWP decreased significantly from the early post-LVAD values (0.85–0.56) returning to

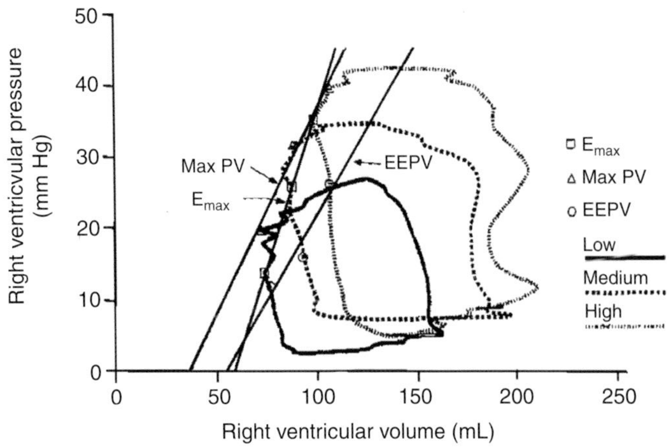

Fig. 14.3 Right ventricular pressure-volume loops at low, medium, and high loading conditions. The slopes of maximum time vary in elastance *(E_{max})*, maximum pressure/volume ratio *(max PV)*, and end ejection pressure/volume *(EEPV)* are displayed by the lines of best fit passing through three points of each pressure-volume loop. (From Dell'Italia LJ. Anatomy and physiology of the right ventricle. *Cardiol Clin* 2012;30(2):167–187.)

baseline pre-LVAD values. These results suggest that continued LVAD support beyond the perioperative period decreases RV afterload and is coupled to improved RV contractile performance.

PREOPERATIVE EVALUATION AND PREDICTIVE RISK SCORES

The importance of RVF predictors in the setting of LVAD implantation was recognized early, as evidenced by the numerous attempts to identify independent risk factors and develop RVF predictive scores. Since there are limited options for managing RVF, the purpose of these risk scores was to improve patient selection and outcomes by recognizing the need for biventricular assist devices (BIVADs) at the time of LVAD implantation. Existing risk prediction models incorporate a combination of demographics, markers of end-organ dysfunction, inotrope dependency, prior open chest procedures, and/or hemodynamic parameters.[24–27] However, certain common limitations have hindered the clinical usefulness of these risk scores: poor consistency in the definition of RVF, heterogeneity of patient populations, and variability in the types of LVADs included in each study.

One recent report investigated the use of a Bayesian statistical model to provide more accurate predictions of acute, early, and late RVF based on preoperative variables. The accuracies of all three Bayesian models were 91%–97%, with a sensitivity of 90% and specificity of 98%–99%, significantly outperforming previously published risk scores.[28] Bayesian models differ from standard multivariate analyses in that they consider the interrelationships and conditional probabilities among independent variables, making them particularly suited for combining a large sets of risk factors (each of the three independent models in this report consisted of 33–34 preoperative variables). These algorithms better reflect human logic in prioritizing dynamic clinical information but also benefit from the plethora of evidence provided by the INTERMACS.

Imaging techniques may also aid in preoperative risk assessment. Echocardiography in particular has shown promise in evaluating parameters of RV dysfunction. Tricuspid annular plane systolic excursion (TAPSE) <7.5 mm was 91% specific and 46% sensitive in predicting post-LVAD RVF.[29] Low TAPSE has not been established as a predictor of RV longitudinal function, likely because TAPSE is only a regional marker of RV function and assumes the motion of the RV free wall base represents the function of other segments. An RV:LV diameter ratio greater than 0.75 can be used as a surrogate for disproportionate RV remodeling and demonstrated an independent association with RVF.[30] Some studies have shown that RVF after LVAD implantation is associated with decreased peak systolic longitudinal strain of the basal RV free wall (−20.7% vs. −14.9%) and RV global longitudinal strain below −13%, while others found no association.[31,32] The inconsistent results between different studies evaluating echocardiographic parameters may be partly explained by user variability.

One recent study evaluated noninvasively measured preoperative liver stiffness (LS) using transient elastography, which demonstrated that LS is a predictor of post-LVAD RVF and may also be used for optimization of RV function in the perioperative period.[33] Chemokine receptor regulation patterns may also play a major role in prognostication, with one report showing that pre-LVAD chemokine receptor downregulation is associated with RVF and increased mortality after implantation.[34]

PULMONARY ARTERY PULSATILITY INDEX

The pulmonary artery pulsatility index (PAPi), defined as [(systolic pulmonary artery pressure – diastolic pulmonary artery pressure)/CVP], is a hemodynamic index originally used to predict RVF in inferior wall acute myocardial infarctions. Recently, PAPi has also been shown to be an independent predictor of postoperative RVF in continuous-flow LVAD recipients.[35,36] PAPi is unique among the risk stratification tools in that it identifies not only patients with any degree of RV dysfunction but also those who will require RVAD support. Optimal sensitivity and specificity were achieved using a cut-off value of <2.0.

PAPi further differentiates itself from other previously described hemodynamic indices, such as the CVP:PCWP ratio, in that it is purely a right-sided heart measurement. PAPi is more hemodynamically removed from the influence of left heart function and is particularly more predictive in patients on inotropic support.[36] The association between RVF and CVP:PCWP ratio, by contrast, diminished dramatically when measurements were taken on inotropes. Interestingly, the time from right heart catheterization to LVAD implantation had no effect on the effectiveness of PAPi to predict the need for RVAD therapy. It has also been suggested that recovery of PAPi values may serve as an indication of RV recovery after continuous-flow LVAD implantation. Other hemodynamic indices such as pulmonary artery compliance and elasticity have not been shown to correlate with RVF after continuous-flow LVAD implantation.

The authors use a combination of hemodynamic values (PAPi and CVP:PCWP) and echocardiographic data (RV:LV diameter, severity of tricuspid valve regurgitation (TR), objective assessment of RV free wall contractile function, and TAPSE) to predict the severity of RVF. In the absence of any standardized approach, we acknowledge that this has largely been subjective and experienced based. Hence, the most important part of our practice has focused on optimization of the procedure in all phases. This includes aggressive diuresis, inotropic support (to optimize peripheral perfusion while decongesting the liver), minimization of large transfusion requirements during implantation, use of inhaled pulmonary vasodilators, and maintenance of mean systemic blood pressure above 70 mm Hg to optimize RV performance.

PERIOPERATIVE MANAGEMENT OF RIGHT VENTRICULAR FUNCTION

Perioperative management of RV function can be critical to the hemodynamic success of LVAD placement. Management strategies for the RV include optimization of volume status, inotropic support, and use of pulmonary vasodilators to reduce RV afterload. Prerequisite to this is the assumption that the RV is not severely dysfunctional and manifests recruitable function sufficient to support the preload for an LVAD.

It is our recommendation that volume status is optimized with aggressive diuresis. This often requires preoperative admission for intravenous diuretics, potentially requiring placement of an invasive pulmonary artery catheter for determining the need for preoperative inotropes. Additional volume optimization is available while on cardiopulmonary bypass with an in-line hemoconcentrator within the cardiopulmonary bypass circuit. Target volume status should include optimal CVP and CVP:PCWP ratios as discussed earlier.

Often, RV function following LVAD placement will require intravenous inotropic support (i.e., epinephrine, milrinone, dopamine, and dobutamine) in the immediate perioperative period. While short-term use is not immediately indicative of RVF, longer-term dependence (>48 hours) can indicate postoperative RVF. High-dose inotropic support can be detrimental to systemic end-organ function and should prompt consideration for temporary mechanical support of the RV, as described later.

Great interest has been devoted to the utilization of pulmonary vasodilators as a means of reducing RV afterload and improving RV function and flow. There is significant controversy on the role of both short-acting inhaled (nitric oxide and prostaglandin) and longer-acting oral vasodilators (sildenafil and macitentan) in both reversing pulmonary vasodilation and improving RV function. The Clinical Study to Assess the Efficacy and Safety of Macitentan in Patients with Pulmonary Hypertension after Left Ventricular Assist Device Implantation (SOPRANO) trial is one such randomized prospective multiinstitutional trial (NCT02554903), which is aimed at addressing this question.

MECHANICAL CIRCULATORY SUPPORT FOR RIGHT VENTRICULAR DYSFUNCTION

Mechanical support for RV dysfunction is largely limited to temporary strategies. Off-label uses of third-generation centrifugal devices (implanted in the right atrium or ventricle) have been described.[37,38] Services approved by the US Food and Drug Administration (FDA) include the Thoratec PVAD platform and the Syncardia Total Artificial Heart for those with severe BIVAD failure. Given advances in technology the PVAD device is no longer manufactured and remains of historical interest. This device was highly effective in either RVAD or BIVAD configurations to support right HF. Currently, the Syncardia Total Artificial Heart Device remains the lone remaining FDA-approved device for long-term support of the RV, although adaptation of this technology has been limited relative to VAD technology given concerns of renal dysfunction and ability to successfully discharge a patient. This device is currently approved as a bridge to transplantation.

Most often, RVF is manifest in the immediate intraoperative or perioperative period. There are currently various options for temporarily supporting the RV immediately following implantation of an LVAD. The simplest and most cost-effective option is the surgically placed temporary VAD utilizing direct drainage of the right atrium with either a standard surgical cannula placed directly into the right atrium or peripheral placed cannula from the femoral vein with outflow most often to the pulmonary artery. Various options for outflow cannulation of the pulmonary artery have been described from the placement of a cannula using the Seldinger technique or the sewing of a dacron or polytetrafluoroethylene (PTFE) graft onto the pulmonary artery. In this configuration, a centrifugal pump head is used to support the circulation. The Centrimag device (Abbott Inc.) is one such option that has been approved for 14 days of support, although reports of much longer use are present.[39–41]

Alternatively, more recently approved options, albeit at a significantly increased cost, include the Abiomed Impella RP and Tandem Heart Protek Duo platforms (LivaNova, Inc.). The Abiomed Impella RP is a 22-Fr microaxial pump placed on an 11-Fr catheter that is inserted transfemorally via the femoral vein into the main pulmonary artery using the Seldinger technique. It is capable of 4 L/min of flow at 33,000 rpm. A randomized clinical trial of 30 patients with acute implant of the Impella RP either during postcardiotomy cardiogenic shock, postmyocardial infarction, or post-LVAD RVF conducted with comparison to a benchmark reference has demonstrated superior results (73% overall survival), thereby facilitating FDA approval for short-term use (<14 days).[42] This platform allows percutaneous placement of the VAD with ease of removal without reopening a patient's chest.

The Tandem Heart Protek Duo Platform has similarly been approved for short-term use up to 6 days. The dual lumen cannula allows for percutaneous placement via the right internal jugular vein with inflow lumen in the right atrium and outflow lumen in the pulmonary artery.[43] Placement is via a modified Seldinger technique with fluoroscopic guidance. Two cannula size options are available: 29 Fr with 16 Fr outflow and larger 31 Fr with 18 Fr outflow. The inflow and outflow cannula are connected to a centrifugal pump capable of 1.8–5.0 liters per minute (Lpm) flow. Similar to the Impella RP, the Protek Duo allows removal without reentry into the chest. Additionally, it is possible for ambulatory patients to be supported on this device given internal jugular placement.

Data strongly suggest an advantage to placement of a RVAD early following the identification of RVF for optimal outcomes.[44,45] Often, the RV can be recovered adequately to support LVAD function and to provide a patient with excellent hemodynamic support, although the long-term outlook of these dysfunctional RVs remains to be determined.

DELAYED RIGHT VENTRICULAR FAILURE

Late right HF is increasingly recognized as an important cause of morbidity and mortality in patients who have been supported long-term with LVAD therapy. Although a uniform definition for delayed RVF has not been adopted, early studies have established that right HF after the recovery from the early phase after LVAD implantation may occur at any time in the late phase of long-term MCS. The original published descriptions in continuous-flow device support defined late RHF as the appearance of persistent symptoms and signs of peripheral vascular congestion (elevated CVP, hepatomegaly or congestion-related pain of the right upper quadrant, peripheral edema, ascites, and increase in beta natriuretic peptide (BNP) values) necessitating the significant up-titration of diuretics dose or use of positive inotropic agents.[46,47] In the study from Athens, authors looked for these signs and symptoms in patients who had survived and remained on continuous-flow support beyond 1 year and identified 9 out of 20 patients who presented with right HF at a median time of 2 years post-LVAD implantation. In these patients who had a two-fold increase in the measured CVP and a significantly higher degree of neurohormonal activation (BNP greater than three-fold elevated), a significant increase in the diuretic regimen was required for initial stabilization. Despite this, four patients went on to require continuous intravenous inotropic support with an ensuing mortality due to cardiogenic shock and multiorgan system failure. In this limited single-center analysis, the authors could not identify any significant risk factor at baseline (except for a strong trend of increasing serum creatinine) that could identify the patients who would develop late RVF. In a study from Columbia University Medical Center, investigators defined delayed RVF as right HF requiring medical intervention 4 weeks after LVAD implantation and limited their analysis only to patients who were bridge to transplantation at their center.[47] Of the 141 patients who underwent cardiac transplantation with isolated LVAD, 21 (15%) developed late right HF, and 11 of these patients were bridged to cardiac transplantation with inotropic agents. The posttransplantation outcomes in patients who developed late right HF while on LVAD support were significantly worse (26% vs. 87% 5-year survival). The 15% who developed late right HF on LVAD support had increased serum creatinine, increased total bilirubin, and lower albumin at the time of heart transplantation, but no clear-cut risk factor could identify patients who would develop post-LVAD delayed RV dysfunction.

The first published multicenter analysis of delayed RVF was derived from the HMII Destination Therapy study and defined these patients on the basis of requiring inotropic support for late right HF at least 30 days *after discharge* from the index LVAD implant hospitalization.[48] Late right HF occurred in 8% (41 of 537 patients) at a median time of 1.3 years (range, 2 months to 5 years) and was associated with a very poor 1- and 2-year survival of 38% and 22%, respectively. The investigators plotted a hazard function that, 6 months after LVAD implantation, remained relatively constant, implying that a continuous risk of developing delayed RVF exists in patients on LVAD support. Consistent with the previous studies, the multicenter analysis from the HMII DT Trial could not identify any significant risk factors that could predict at baseline implantation the development of this late and clinically important syndrome. Events that occur in the post-LVAD period, such as the development of aortic insufficiency or LVAD malfunction, may present as late right HF due to recurrent left-sided failure, but this does not account for a vast majority of cases presenting with delayed RVF. In total, these studies raise the real possibility that cardiomyopathic disease progression may adversely affect RV function over time and unless we understand the mechanisms behind this phenomenon (RV-LV dys-synchrony, increased metabolic demand in the setting of altered RV mechanics, etc.) patients who are destined for long-term LVAD support will continue to face this clinically important and established adverse event.

In conclusion, RVF continues to be a major limitation in providing a stable platform for chronic mechanical LV support. Efforts at predicting which patients require RVAD support have failed to reach a consensus among experts and continue to be center specific. Furthermore, even in those who may need RVAD support, a stable reliable RVAD that can offer long-term support in one unit does not exist. In these cases, heart transplantation remains the best option. For those who are not candidates for transplantation, options are limited. These factors are even more concerning with the development of delayed RV dysfunction. The future must focus on defining better predictive tools for assessing risk of RVF after LVAD placement and developing newer MCS platforms for BIVAD support. These newer devices should ideally be supported by one common controller that is reliable and would make the patient's life outside the hospital easier to manage.

REFERENCES

1. Garbade J, Bittner HB, Barten MJ, Mohr FW. Current trends in implantable left ventricular assist devices. *Cardiol Res Pract.* 2011;2011:290561.
2. Wever-Pinzon O, Drakos SG, Kfoury AG, et al. Morbidity and mortality in heart transplant candidates supported with mechanical circulatory support: is reappraisal of the current United network for organ sharing thoracic organ allocation policy justified? *Circulation.* 2013;127(4):452–462.
3. Moazami N, Hoercher KJ, Fukamachi K, et al. Mechanical circulatory support for heart failure: past, present and a look at the future. *Expert Rev Med Devices.* 2013;10(1):55–71.
4. Fukamachi K, McCarthy PM, Smedira NG, Vargo RL, Starling RC, Young JB. Preoperative risk factors for right ventricular failure after implantable left ventricular assist device insertion. *Ann Thorac Surg.* 1999;68(6):2181–2184.
5. Kukucka M, Stepanenko A, Potapov E, et al. Right-to-left ventricular end-diastolic diameter ratio and prediction of right ventricular failure with continuous-flow left ventricular assist devices. *J Heart Lung Transplant.* 2011;30(1):64–69.
6. Simon MA. Assessment and treatment of right ventricular failure. *Nat Rev Cardiol.* 2013;10(4):204–218.
7. Steffen RJ, Halbreiner MS, Zhang L, et al. Mechanical circulatory support for the right ventricle in the setting of a left ventricular assist device. *Expert Rev Med Devices.* 2014;14:1–7. Jul.
8. Takeda K, Naka Y, Yang JA, et al. Timing of temporary right ventricular assist device insertion for severe right heart failure after left ventricular assist device implantation. *ASAIO J.* 2013;59(6):564–569.
9. Ryan JJ, Archer SL. The right ventricle in pulmonary arterial hypertension: disorders of metabolism, angiogenesis and adrenergic signaling in right ventricular failure. *Circ Res.* 2014;115(1):176–188.
10. Meineri M, Van Rensburg AE, Vegas A. Right ventricular failure after LVAD implantation: prevention and treatment. *Best Pract Res Clin Anaesthesiol.* 2012;26(2):217–229.
11. Friedberg MK, Redington AN. Right versus left ventricular failure: differences, similarities, and interactions. *Circulation.* 2014 Mar 4;129(9):1033–1044.
12. Smerup M, Nielsen E, Agger P, et al. The three-dimensional arrangement of the myocytes aggregated together within the mammalian ventricular myocardium. *Anat Rec (Hoboken).* 2009;292(1):1–11.
13. Voelkel NF, Quaife RA, Leinwand LA, et al. Right ventricular function and failure: report of a National Heart, Lung, and Blood Institute working group on cellular and molecular mechanisms of right heart failure. *Circulation.* 2006;114(17):1883–1891.
14. Whitaker RH. Anatomy of the heart. *Medicine.* 2014; 42(8):406–408.
15. Driessen MM, Baggen VJ, Freling HG, et al. Pressure overloaded right ventricles: a multicenter study on the importance of trabeculae in RV function measured by CMR. *Int J Cardiovasc Imaging.* 2014;30(3): 599–608.
16. Dell'Italia LJ. Anatomy and physiology of the right ventricle. *Cardiol Clin.* 2012;30(2):167–187.
17. Hoffman D, Sisto D, Frater RW, Nikolic SD. Left-to-right ventricular interaction with a noncontracting right ventricle. *J Thorac Cardiovasc Surg.* 1994;107(6):1496–1502.
18. Li KS, Santamore WP. Contribution of each wall to biventricular function. *Cardiovasc Res.* 1993;27(5):792–800.
19. Goldstein JA, Tweddell JS, Barzilai B, Yagi Y, Jaffe AS, Cox JL. Importance of left ventricular function and systolic ventricular interaction to right ventricular performance during acute right heart ischemia. *J Am Coll Cardiol.* 1992;19(3):704–711.
20. Winterhalter M, Antoniou T, Loukanov T. Management of adult patients with perioperative pulmonary hypertension: technical aspects and therapeutic options. *Cardiology.* 2010;116(1):3–9.
21. Itagaki S, Hosseinian L, Varghese R. Right ventricular failure after cardiac surgery: management strategies. *Semin Thorac Cardiovasc Surg.* 2012;24(3):188–194.
22. Haddad F, Hunt SA, Rosenthal DN, Murphy DJ. Right ventricular function in cardiovascular disease, part I: Anatomy, physiology, aging, and functional assessment of the right ventricle. *Circulation.* 2008;117(11):1436–1448.
23. Houston BA, Kalathiya RJ, Hsu S, et al. Right ventricular afterload sensitivity dramatically increases after left ventricular assist device implantation: a multi-center hemodynamic analysis. *J Heart Lung Transplant.* 2016;35(7):868–876.
24. Wang Y, Simon MA, Bonde P, et al. Decision tree for adjuvant right ventricular support in patients receiving a left ventricular assist device. *J Heart Lung Transplant.* 2012;31(2):140–149.
25. Cowger J, Sundareswaran K, Rogers JG, et al. Predicting survival in patients receiving continuous flow left ventricular assist devices. *The HeartMate II risk score J Am Coll Cardiol.* 2013;61(3):313–321.

26. Atluri P, Goldstone AB, Fairman AS, et al. Predicting right ventricular failure in the modern, continuous flow left ventricular assist device era. *Ann Thorac Surg*. 2013;96(3):857–863, discussion 863–854.
27. Kormos RL, Teuteberg JJ, Pagani FD, et al. Right ventricular failure in patients with the HeartMate II continuous-flow left ventricular assist device: incidence, risk factors, and effect on outcomes. *J Thorac Cardiovasc Surg*. 2010;139(5):1316–1324.
28. Loghmanpour NA, Kormos RL, Kanwar MK, Teuteberg JJ, Murali S, Antaki JF. A Bayesian model to predict right ventricular failure following left ventricular assist device therapy. *JACC Heart Fail*. 2016;4(9):711–721.
29. Puwanant S, Hamilton KK, Klodell CT, et al. Tricuspid annular motion as a predictor of severe right ventricular failure after left ventricular assist device implantation. *J Heart Lung Transplant*. 2008;27(10):1102–1107.
30 Vivo RP, Cordero-Reyes AM, Qamar U, et al. Increased right-to-left ventricle diameter ratio is a strong predictor of right ventricular failure after left ventricular assist device. *J Heart Lung Transplant*. 2013;32(8):792–799.
31. Boegershausen N, Zayat R, Aljalloud A, et al. Risk factors for the development of right ventricular failure after left ventricular assist device implantation-a single-centre retrospective with focus on deformation imaging. *Eur J Cardiothorac Surg*. 2017;52(6):1069–1076.
32. Beck DR, Foley L, Rowe JR, et al. Right ventricular longitudinal strain in left ventricular assist device surgery—a retrospective cohort study. *J Cardiothorac Vasc Anesth*. 2017;31(6):2096–2102.
33. Kashiyama N, Toda K, Nakamura T, et al. Evaluation of right ventricular function using liver stiffness in patients with left ventricular assist device. *Eur J Cardiothorac Surg*. 2017;51(4):715–721.
34. Nayak A, Neill C, Kormos RL, et al. Chemokine receptor patterns and right heart failure in mechanical circulatory support. *J Heart Lung Transplant*. 2017;36(6):657–665.
35. Kang G, Ha R, Banerjee D. Pulmonary artery pulsatility index predicts right ventricular failure after left ventricular assist device implantation. *J Heart Lung Transplant*. 2016;35(1):67–73.
36. Morine KJ, Kiernan MS, Pham DT, Paruchuri V, Denofrio D, Kapur NK. Pulmonary artery pulsatility index is associated with right ventricular failure after left ventricular assist device surgery. *J Card Fail*. 2016;22(2):110–116.
37. Krabatsch Y, Potapov E, Stepanenko A, et al. Biventricular circulatory support with two miniaturized implantable assist devices. *Circ*. 2011;124:S179–S186.
38. Tran HA, Pollema TL, Silva Enciso J, et al. Durable biventricular support using right atrial placement of the heartware HVAD. *ASAIO J*. 2018;64(3):323–327.
39. Bhama JK, Kormos RL, Toyoda Y, Teuteberg JJ, McCurry KR, Siegenthaler MP. Clinical experience using the levitronix centrimag system for temporary right ventricular mechanical circulatory support. *J Heart Lung Trans*. 2009;28:971–976.
40. Loforte A, Montalto A, Lilla Della MO. Musumeci F. Simultaneous temporary CentriMag right ventricular assist device placement in HeartMate II left ventricular assist system recipients at high risk of right ventricular failure. *Ineract Cardiovasc Thorac Surg*. 2010;10:847–850. 3.
41. Lazar JF, Swartz MF, Schiralli MP, et al. Survival after left ventricular assist device with and without temporary right ventricular support. *Ann Thor Surg*. 2013;96:2155–2159.
42. Anderson MB, Goldstein J, Milano C, et al. Benefits of a novel percutaneous ventricular assist device for right heart failure: the prospective RECOVER RIGHT study of the Impella RP device. *J Heart Lung Trans*. 2015;34:1549–1560.
43. Ravichandran AK, Baran DA, Stelling K, Cowger JA, Salerno CT. Outcomes with the tandem protek duo dual-lumen percutaneous right ventricular assist device. *ASAIO J*. 2017.
44. Lazar JF, Swartz MF, Schiralli MP, et al. Survival after left ventricular assist device with and without temporary right ventricular support. *Ann Thor Surg*. 2013;96:2155–2159.
45. Fitzpatrick JR, Frederick JR, Hiesinger W, et al. Early planned institution of a biventricular mechanical circulatory support results in improved outcomes compared with delayed conversion of a left ventricular assist device to a biventricular assist device. *J Thorac Cardiovasc Surg*. 2009;137:971–977.
46. Kapelios CJ, Charitos C, Kaldara E, et al. Late-onset right ventricular dysfunction after mechanical support by a continuous-flow left ventricular assist device. *J Heart Lung Transplant*. 2015;34: 1604–1610.
47. Takeda K, Takayama H, Colombo PC, et al. Late right heart failure during support with continuous-flow left ventricular assist devices adversely affects post-transplant outcome. *J Heart Lung Transplant*. 2015;34:667–674.
48. Rich JM, Gosev I, Patel CB, et al. The incidence, risk factors, and outcomes associated with late right-sided heart failure inpatients supported with an axial-flow left ventricular assist device. *J Heart Lung Transplant*. 2016;36:50–58.

15

Clinical Trial Results in Mechanical Circulatory Support

Stuart D. Russell, Jeffrey Teuteberg

KEY POINTS

- Disclosure
- Overview of Clinical Trials of Mechanical Circulatory Support Devices
- Pulsatile Flow
- Continuous Flow—Axial
- Continuous Flow—Centrifugal
- Quality of Life, Functional Status, and Adverse Events
- Total Artificial Hearts

DISCLOSURE

Dr. Russell is a consultant for Medtronic and serves on the Data and Safety Monitoring Board for the HeartMate 3 trial sponsored by Abbott. Dr. Teuteberg has industry relationships with Medtronic (advisory board, speaking), Abiomed (advisory board), CareDx (advisory board, speaking), Abbott (HeartMate 3 Clinical Events Committee), and EcoR1 (consulting).

OVERVIEW OF CLINICAL TRIALS OF MECHANICAL CIRCULATORY SUPPORT DEVICES

Clinical trials of mechanical circulatory support devices evolved from simple studies evaluating the efficacy of the device in a few patients to large-scale clinical trials with composite endpoints including quality of life, improvements in functional capacity, and freedom from major complications in addition to mortality. Mechanical circulatory support devices were first used clinically in 1963 when Dr. Michael DeBakey placed a device in the left thorax, connected to the left atrium and the descending thoracic aorta, and used for a patient who had a cardiac arrest 18 hours after an aortic valve replacement. The patient had clinical improvement in pulmonary edema and neurologic function, but unfortunately, he remained anuric and died 4 days later despite the continued function of the ventricular system device.[1] In 1975, based on case reports of similar patients, two short-term trials were initiated for patients who could not be weaned from cardiopulmonary bypass.[2] The trials were performed with a pneumatically powered single-chamber pump that could be placed either intraabdominally or extracorporeally. One of these case series included a 21-year-old man who successfully underwent heart transplantation after 6 days of support, which encouraged the field to move forward.[3]

In 1976, the US Congress passed the Medical Device Amendments Act, which gave the US Food and Drug Administration (FDA) the authority to preapprove the use of medical devices in the United States. The FDA's influence on clinical testing of these devices began to shape the early patient populations studied in clinical trials and the endpoints being evaluated. In 1977, the National Heart, Lung, and Blood Institute requested grant applications for the development of mechanical, electrically powered blood pumps. A second application request was issued in 1980 for long-term (2 years) left ventricular assist devices (LVADs). This support resulted in the development of the Novacor LVAD and the Thoratec LVAD, which eventually became the HeartMate XVE. Because of FDA concerns about the durability of these devices, initial clinical trials could enroll only patients who were eligible for cardiac transplantation. As devices demonstrated the ability to provide long-term support, the patient populations studied expanded to include non–transplant eligible patients. These early clinical trial populations were the source of the current indications for mechanical support: bridge to recovery, bridge to transplantation (BTT), and destination therapy (DT).

Since the mid-1980s, there have been changes in pump design from paracorporeal pumps to intracorporeal configurations and from pulsatile to continuous-flow designs. In this chapter, we review the major clinical trials that have been performed that have propelled the field forward for both BTT and DT.

PULSATILE FLOW

The first successful use of an LVAD as a BTT was reported by Hill in 1986 describing the use of the pneumatically actuated Thoratec Pierce-Donachy paracorporeal ventricular assist device (PVAD) (Fig. 15.1) in a patient after a large myocardial infarction with cardiogenic shock.[4] This was soon followed by a large series of patients successfully bridged to cardiac transplant in 1988.[5] Twenty-nine patients underwent placement of either left or left and right (14 patients) ventricular assist devices in a paracorporeal position. Twenty-one of the patients survived to transplantation after a median of 3 days of support. For those who did not survive to transplantation, the two most common causes of death were multiorgan failure and bleeding. It should be emphasized that all 29 patients had severe cardiogenic shock preoperatively, requiring multiple vasopressors, an intraaortic balloon pump ($n = 25$), and mechanical ventilation ($n = 21$). Based on these early reports, LVADs were approved for BTT in 1995.

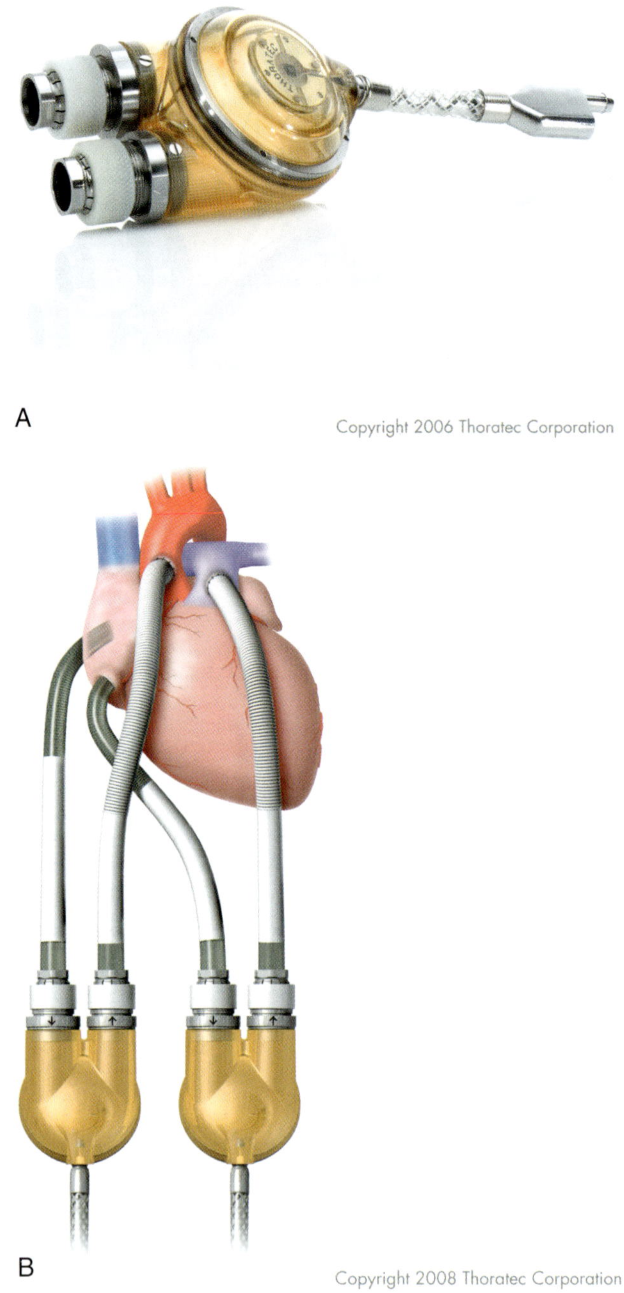

Fig. 15.1 (A) Thoratec paracorporeal ventricular assist device (PVAD) is a paracorporeal, pneumatically actuated ventricular assist device designed for right-sided, left-sided, or biventricular support. (B) Thoratec PVAD in left ventricular assist *(left)* and biventricular assist configuration *(right)*. (Courtesy of Abbott.)

Some of the drawbacks of the PVAD were its large size, need for the patient to remain hospitalized while supported, two large percutaneous cannulas, external pumping chamber, and patient discomfort. Given these limitations, an implantable version of the device was developed (Thoratec Implantable Ventricular Assist Device; Fig. 15.2). Between 2001 and 2004, 39 patients underwent implantation of this device as either BTT or for postcardiotomy failure.[6] Twenty-four of the patients had the device as left ventricular support and 15 as biventricular support, for a mean duration of 101 days. Eighteen patients were discharged from the hospital with ongoing support for a mean duration of 96 days. No survival difference was observed between the BTT and the postcardiotomy groups, and 69% of the patients were either transplanted or weaned from the device. The adverse effects of the device were quite similar to the PVAD and included infection in 22 patients, bleeding in 18 patients, and neurologic events in 14 patients. The incidence of ischemic or hemorrhagic stroke was 7.7%, which was somewhat lower than the 12.0% in the PVAD population.

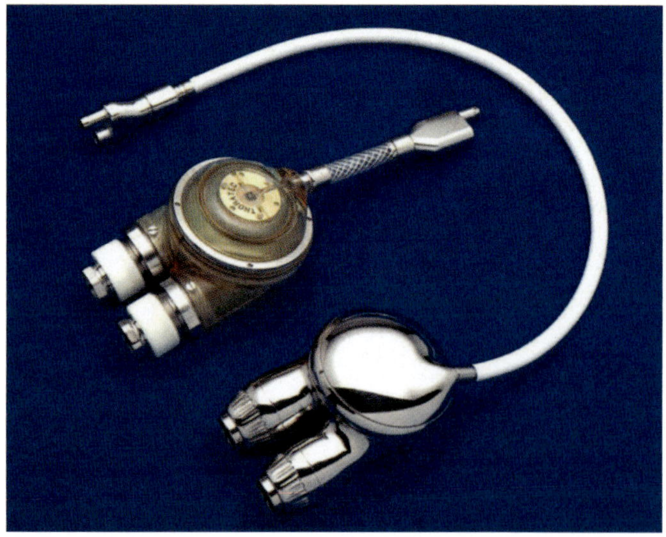

Fig. 15.2 Thoratec intracorporeal ventricular assist device (IVAD) *(lower right)* beside a Thoratec paracorporeal ventricular assist device (PVAD). The Thoratec IVAD is an implantable version of the Thoratec PVAD.

With these early successes, pump design moved to the development of long-term, left ventricular only support with intracorporeal devices. The pumps that came to clinical trial included the HeartMate IP1000 (Thoratec Corporation), HeartMate VE/XVE (Thoratec Corporation), and Novacor LVAD (World Heart Corporation).

HeartMate IP1000

In 1992, Frazier reported on 34 patients who received the HeartMate IP1000 (Fig. 15.3) as BTT and compared them to six control patients who met the enrollment criteria but did not receive the device.[7] Sixty-five percent of the patients receiving the device went on to transplantation, with a posttransplantation survival of 80%. This compared to a 50% survival to transplantation in the control arm, with no patients surviving posttransplantation. Complications of the device included bleeding in 39%, infection in 25%, and right heart failure in 21%. No thromboembolic events were reported, with the maximum time of support being 324 days. A larger study of 75 patients compared to 33 control patients was reported in 1994.[8] The survival rate to transplantation with the device was 71% compared to 36% in the controls. The adverse event profile was similar to the prior trial, with the exception of three patients having a thromboembolic complication: two with strokes and one with an embolus to the subclavian artery, which was successfully removed. This trial required a preimplantation pulmonary capillary wedge pressure >20 mm Hg with either a cardiac index <2.0 L/min/m^2 or a systolic blood pressure <80 mm Hg. In spite of these promising early results, this pump was short lived due to the development of the HeartMate VE and XVE, which had a similar pump housing but were driven by a mechanical rotor rather than pneumatically. This development allowed patients to be discharged from the hospital and have greater mobility because the pump could be powered by two smaller wearable external batteries rather than a large pneumatic console.

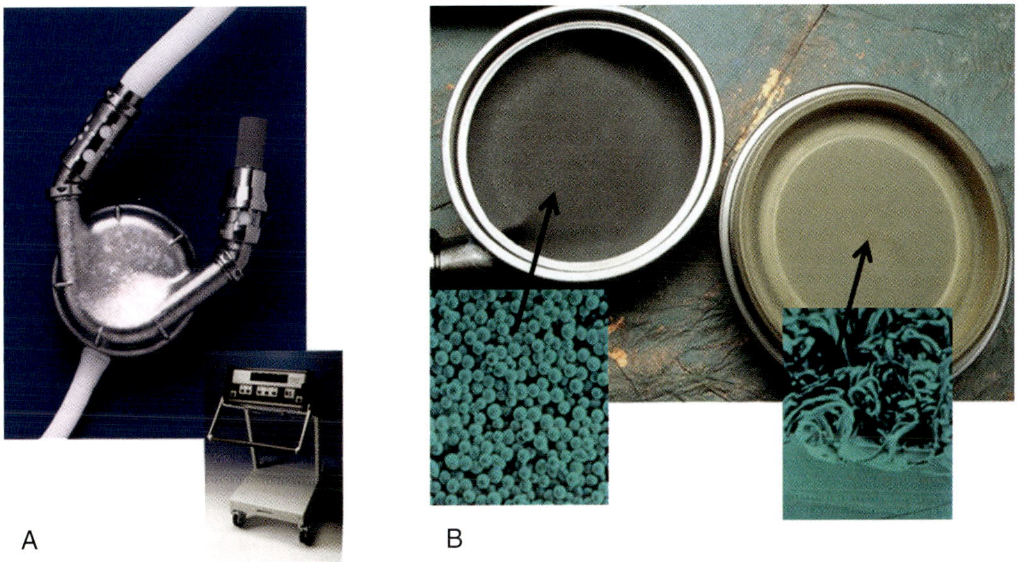

A B

Fig. 15.3 (A) The Thoratec HeartMate IP1000 is an implantable, pulsatile left ventricular assist device requiring a mobile but large drive console for pneumatic actuation of the pump's internal pusher plate. (B) The internal surfaces of the pump are coated with sintered titanium microspheres on the pump housing and integrally textured polyurethane on the flexible diaphragm covering the pusher plate. These surfaces create a pseudoendothelium that is resistant to thrombus formation.

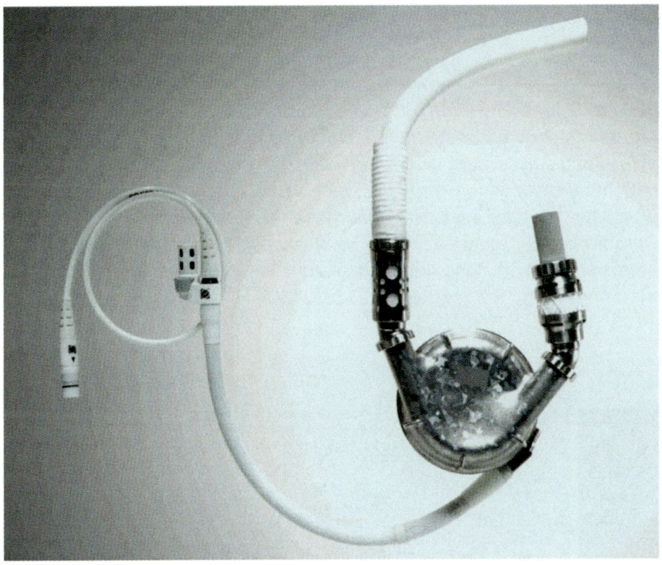

Fig. 15.4 Thoratec HeartMate XVE is an implantable, pulsatile, electrically actuated left ventricular assist device.

HeartMate VE/XVE

The HeartMate VE/XVE (Fig. 15.4) was studied in a prospective, multicenter trial of 280 transplant candidates who had poor hemodynamics despite being inotrope dependent.[9] Forty-nine percent of the patients also required a balloon pump and had a mean pulmonary capillary wedge pressure of 27 mm Hg with a systolic blood pressure of 76 mm Hg and a cardiac index of 1.67 L/min/m^2. The outcomes were compared to a control group of 48 patients who had higher blood pressure and cardiac index. The average pump support was 112 days, with 54 patients supported for over 180 days. Adverse events included bleeding in 11%, infection in 40%, neurologic dysfunction in 5%, and thromboembolic events in 6%. Only 29% of the device-supported patients died before transplantation, compared to 67% of the controls. The other highlight of this trial was that 115 of the patients were discharged from the hospital after a median of 82 days, and 86% of those patients received a transplant. This was the first major study that demonstrated that patients could be supported and successfully discharged home to await cardiac transplantation and introduced the possibility of long-term mechanical support for patients who were not eligible for cardiac transplantation, so-called destination therapy (DT).

The first trial of DT was the Randomized Evaluation of Mechanical Assistance for the Treatment of Congestive Heart Failure (REMATCH) study, which used the Thoratec VE pump.[10] This study was supported by the National Institutes of Health and was performed at 20 experienced transplant centers. Enrollment criteria included the presence of New York Heart Association (NYHA) functional class IV symptoms for at least 90 days despite optimal medical therapy, an ejection fraction (EF) <25%, and a peak oxygen consumption of <12 mL/kg/min or the need for continuous intravenous inotropic therapy due to symptomatic hypotension, decreasing renal function, or worsening pulmonary congestion. Due to slow enrollment, the criteria were later eased to include patients with 60 days of NYHA class IV symptoms and a peak oxygen consumption <14 mL/kg/min or patients who were class III/IV for 28 days plus either 14 days of either intraaortic balloon or inotropic support with at least 2 failed weaning attempts. A total of 129 patients were enrolled and randomized to either placement of an LVAD or continued medical therapy. A statistically significant improvement in survival was noted with LVAD therapy at both 1 year (52% (vs.) 25%) and 2 years (23% (vs.) 8%) (Fig. 15.5), and median survival was longer in the LVAD group, 408 days (vs.) 150 days with medical therapy. The LVAD group also had significant improvements in NYHA class and scored better on the physical-function and emotional-role subscales of the 36-item Medical Outcomes Study Short-Form General Health Survey (SF-36) and the Beck Depression Inventory. The Minnesota Living With Heart Failure score improved in the LVAD arm but not significantly ($P = 0.11$). As expected, patients in the LVAD arm had more complications, including sepsis, LVAD failure, and neurologic complications. However, the tradeoff was less mortality due to heart failure and an increase in days spent out of the hospital. This trial resulted in FDA approval of the HeartMate XVE for DT.

Improved surgical technique and enhancement of the pump design resulted in improved outcomes. Long et al. reported on 42 patients who were supported for a mean of 232 days, with a 1-year survival rate of 61% and with lower rates of adverse events and death due to sepsis.[11] Despite this, there was not widespread clinical adoption of DT for a variety of reasons, including a lack of long-term durability, requiring device replacement in over 50% of the patients by 2 years (Fig. 15.6).[12]

Novacor

The other durable pulsatile pump that was developed and studied was the Novacor left ventricular assist system (Fig. 15.7). Similar to the Thoratec device, it was initially used as bridge to transplant (BTT) in 1984 and was optimized over the years for improved outcomes. In contrast to the Thoratec device, it did not have a textured blood-contacting surface and instead used a smooth-surfaced polyurethane sac that required anticoagulation with warfarin. Registry data were published describing the outcomes in over 100 patients in a variety of US and

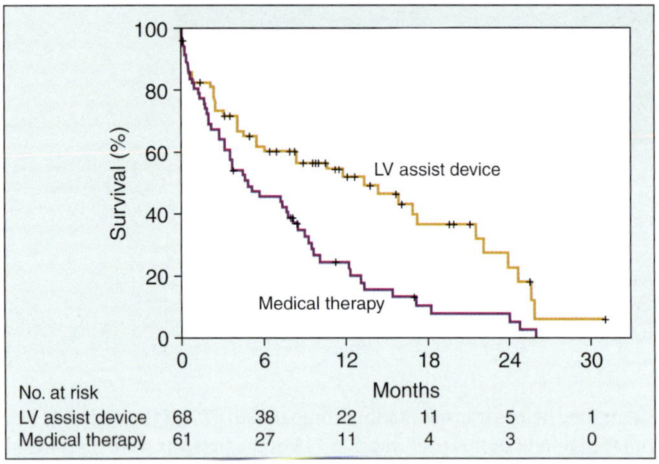

Fig. 15.5 Kaplan-Meier analysis of survival in the group that received left ventricular *(LV)* assist devices and the group that received optimal medical therapy in the REMATCH trial. *Crosses* depict censored patients. Enrollment in the trial was terminated after 92 patients had died; 95 deaths had occurred by the time of the final analysis. (From Rose EA, Gelijns AC, Moskowitz AJ, et al; Randomized Evaluation of Mechanical Assistance for the Treatment of Congestive Heart Failure [REMATCH] Study Group. Long-term mechanical left ventricular assistance for end-stage heart failure. *N Engl J Med.* 2001;345:1435–1443.)

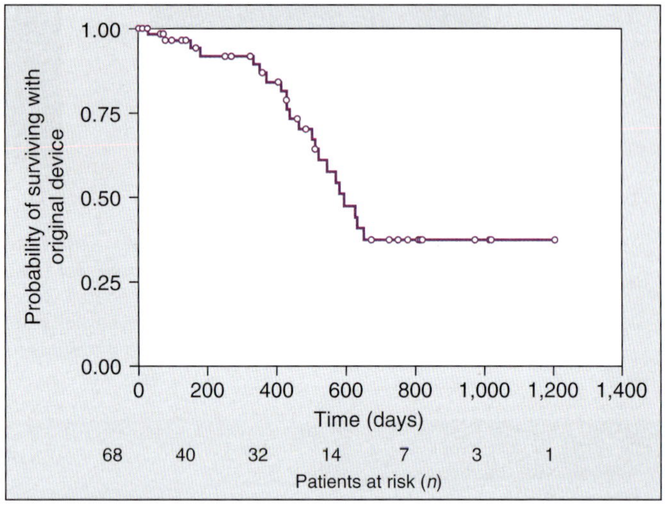

Fig. 15.6 Freedom from left ventricular assist device replacement. A product-limit estimate curve plotting the probability of being free of device replacement (vs.) time (days) on the HeartMate VE device. Patients were censored *(circles)* when they died or if, at the last date of follow-up, they had not undergone a device replacement. (From Dembitsky WP, Tector AJ, Park S, et al. Left ventricular assist device performance with long term circulatory lessons from the REMATCH trial. *Ann Thorac Surg.* 2004;78:2123–2130.)

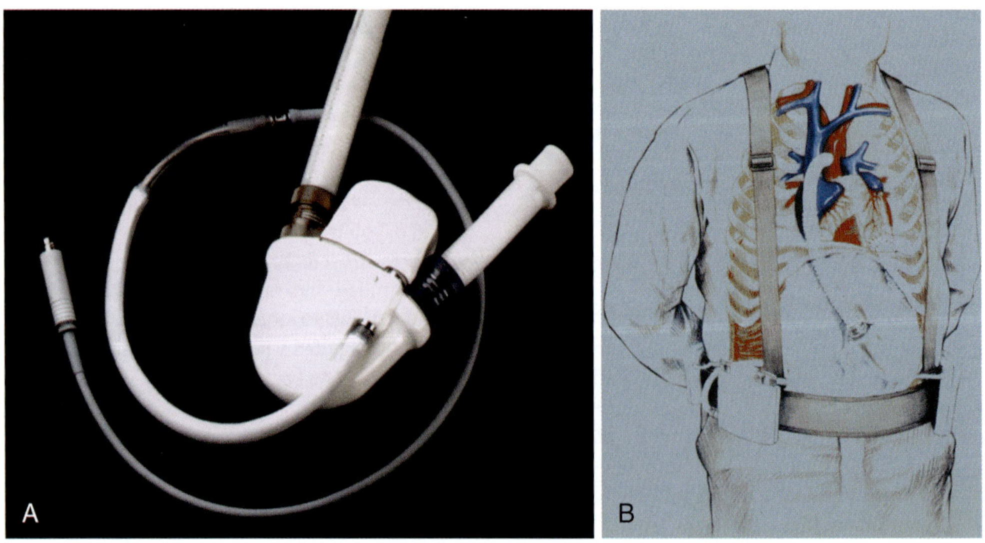

Fig. 15.7 (A) World Heart Novacor left ventricular assist device (LVAD). The Novacor LVAD is an implantable, electrically actuated pulsatile pump designed for long-term support. (B) Novacor LVAD implanted in its preperitoneal position below the diaphragm and showing the percutaneous line and external wearable components, including batteries and controller.

European studies.[13] For BTT patients, 77% of the patients were transplanted, with a mean of 80 days of support compared to 37% of the control patients. However, the stroke rate with the Novacor was higher than seen in the HeartMate XVE experience, although the device was more durable. During the 76-year cumulative support period, there were no pump failures, which set the scene for a DT trial.

The Investigation of Nontransplant-Eligible Patients who are Inotrope Dependent (INTrEPID) trial enrolled 55 patients to either the Novacor LVAD or medical therapy.[14] All patients had to meet similar eligibility criteria to the HeartMate for enrollment, and the control group consisted of patients who chose not to undergo LVAD implantation, had a mechanical aortic valve, or did not have the financial resources to cover the cost of the device or follow-up. Enrollment criteria included inotrope-dependent patients with an EF <25% and NYHA functional class IV symptoms for at least the last 3 months who were not candidates for transplant. Additionally, all patients had to have two unsuccessful weaning attempts from inotropes. The LVAD patients had improved survival at both 6 (46% (vs.) 22%) and 12 (27% (vs.) 11%) months. Unfortunately, 62% of the LVAD patients experienced a stroke or transient ischemic attack (TIA) compared to 11% of the medically managed patients.

There has been one randomized trial of the Novacor LVAD (vs.) HeartMate XVE.[15] Forty BTT patients were randomized, and there were no significant differences in survival to transplantation. The mean duration of support was 235 ± 210 days for Novacor and 175 ± 175 days for the XVE. More neurologic complications occurred with the Novacor pump, and more infections and pump durability issues with the XVE. Survival to transplantation was 65% for Novacor and 60% for the XVE. Based on the high stroke rate with the Novacor device, further development was halted in 2007.[16]

CONTINUOUS FLOW—AXIAL

With the demonstration of safety and improved survival compared to medical therapy, pulsatile pumps became the mainstay of VAD therapy worldwide through the 1990s into the early 2000s. However, major limitations related to pump design, including poor durability, pump size which did not allow implantation into shorter and smaller patients, and a large percutaneous lead required to vent air resulted in the use of these pumps being mostly restricted to short-term BTT use. The introduction of continuous-flow designs which were smaller, more durable (due to fewer moving parts), and noiseless was a significant improvement in pump design and has resulted in an increase in the use of LVADs for both BTT and DT indications.

HeartMate II

The first continuous-flow pump approved by the FDA was the HeartMate II (Thoratec) (Fig. 15.8). This axial flow rotary pump produces continuous flow to the patient at a pump speed of 8000–12,000 rpms. The first trial included 133 patients awaiting heart transplantation with no control group.[17] The primary outcome was patient survival at 180 days with either continued support, cardiac recovery, or transplantation. At 24 hours after implantation, the cardiac index increased from 2.0 ± 0.6 to 2.8 ± 0.7 L/min/m^2, with a decrease in pulmonary capillary wedge pressure from 36 ± 10 to 26 ± 7 mm Hg, showing that the pump was hemodynamically effective. Of the 133 patients, 100 (75%) reached the endpoint at 180 days, with 56 being transplanted, 43 on continued support, and 1 with recovery of function and device explantation. Thirty-three patients had an unsuccessful outcome, with 25 deaths, 5 patients removed from the transplant list due to irreversible complications, and 3 who underwent change to a different LVAD due to complications and were removed from the study. One hundred patients were discharged from the hospital, with a median of 60 days out of the hospital. Similar to the pulsatile pumps, the most common adverse events included bleeding in 31%, infection in 28%, and stroke in 8%. Causes of death included sepsis, ischemic stroke, multisystem organ failure, hemorrhagic stroke, anoxic brain injury, and right heart failure. Importantly, there was improvement in 6-minute walk distance and quality of life measured by both the Minnesota Living With Heart Failure and Kansas City Cardiomyopathy questionnaires. This study resulted in FDA approval of the device for BTT. A follow-up study was performed to evaluate longer-term outcomes with this device.[18] A total of 469 patients were enrolled and 281 patients who completed study endpoints or had 18 months of follow-up were evaluated. At 18 months, 79% of the patients were either transplanted (55.8%), had ongoing LVAD support (20.6%), died (19.9%), or had device removal (3.5%) for either recovery or exchange to another pump. Survival for patients who remained on pump support was 73% at 1 year, which was a significant improvement in survival compared to pulsatile pumps.

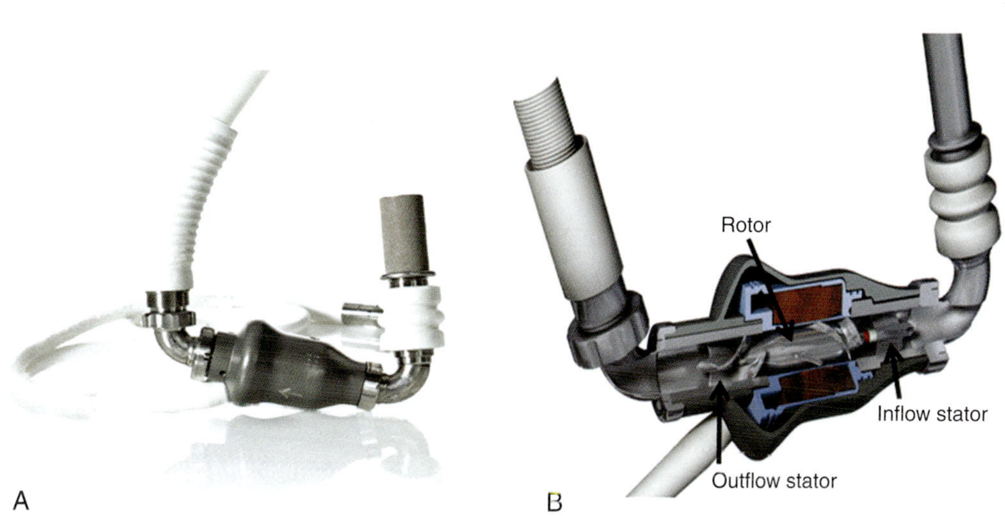

Fig. 15.8 (A) Thoratec HeartMate II is a continuous-flow rotary pump with axial design representative of the second generation of left ventricular assist device technology in clinical use in the United States. (B) Diagram showing the internal rotor suspended on bearings within the inflow and outflow stators. The internal rotor is the only moving part in the HeartMate II.

This study demonstrated the improved durability of continuous-flow pumps, resulting in improved survival with no obvious signals of untoward effects from the lack of pulsatility.

Similar to the pulsatile clinical trial experience, after approval for BTT, the HeartMate II was studied in a DT population. In contrast to a previous trial where the control arm was medical therapy, the landmark DT study randomized patients to either HeartMate II or the Thoratec XVE device in a 2:1 design.[19] Patients ineligible for transplant, usually because of advanced age, were randomized with a primary endpoint of survival free from disabling stroke and reoperation to repair or replaced the device at 2 years. Two hundred patients were randomized with a mean age of 64 and a mean EF of 17% and almost 80% were on inotropic therapy. At 2 years, the survival with HeartMate II was 58% compared to 24% with the pulsatile device. Additionally, both groups showed an improvement in NYHA class, 6-minute walk distance, and quality of life questionnaires from baseline to 24 months. Compared to the pulsatile pump, there were significant reductions in the adverse event rate, with the exception of stroke, which was similar between the two pump groups (17% (vs.) 13%). The pump replacement rate was also much lower at 9% (vs.) 34% with the HeartMate XVE. Unfortunately, despite the improvement in most side effect profiles and quality of life, the HeartMate II did not result in a reduction in hospitalizations, with 94% of the patients compared to 96% of the patients rehospitalized during the study.

The impact of clinical experience being associated with improved outcomes was also demonstrated with the HeartMate II. Park and colleagues[20] compared 281 patients who received the HeartMate II for DT to the initial 133 patients. There was a nonsignificant improvement in survival (73% (vs.) 68%, $P = 0.21$) at 1 year and a reduction in bleeding, sepsis, device-related infections, and hemorrhagic stroke.

To evaluate if the results of this study could be replicated in a nonclinical trial setting, the Interagency Registry for Mechanically Assisted Circulatory Support (INTERMACS) registry was used to assess outcomes in DT patients receiving the HeartMate II after FDA approval for DT. The first 247 patients who were enrolled in the registry were followed for 2 years and the outcomes were compared to those of the patients enrolled in the pivotal DT trial.[21] This study demonstrated the benefits of improvement in clinical care with experience. Survival at 2 years increased to 62% from 58%, with a decrease in device related infections, postoperative bleeding, and length of stay. They also demonstrated that survival varied based on the status of the patient preoperatively, with non–inotrope-dependent patients having an 82% survival at 1 year and 69% survival at year 2.

Jarvik 2000

Other axial flow LVADs have been evaluated that are not currently approved in the United States. The Jarvik 2000 (Jarvik Heart) (Fig. 15.9) pump has a pumping chamber located inside of the left ventricle, as opposed to a preperitoneal space with the HeartMate II, but the outflow graft is anastomosed to the descending thoracic aorta, in contrast to most LVADs. Frazier et al. reported the results of their first 10 implants in patients awaiting heart transplant.[22] The device was implanted through a left thoracotomy during partial cardiopulmonary bypass. The mean support period was 84 days, and seven of the patients survived to transplantation. There was a significant improvement in hemodynamics, with an improvement in cardiac index from 1.77 to 3.45 L/min/m^2 and a reduction in pulmonary capillary wedge pressure from 21.7 to 10.3 mm Hg by 48 hours. The authors did not report on adverse events in this small trial.

A report on 83 BTT patients from the Japanese Registry for Mechanically Assisted Circulatory Support was published in 2018.[23] The median support duration was 191 days, with a maximum of 758 days. Survival at 1 and 2 years was 85.0% and 79.3%, respectively. Most side effects were similar to other pumps, including a 27.7% incidence of major bleeding and 31.3% new infection. The stroke rate was high at 20.5%, with 18 hemorrhagic and 6 ischemic events. One patient developed pump thrombosis and required device exchange, and in another patient, thrombus was found at autopsy following a fatal stroke.

A clinical trial evaluating the efficacy of this pump in 150 patients has been completed, but no results have been published yet (NCT00591799). This company has also developed a driveline that is placed in a postauricular position, rather than in the upper abdomen, which they believe may reduce the incidence of serious driveline infections.

MicroMed DeBakey/HeartAssist 5

Another axial flow pump that has not yet been approved is the MicroMed DeBakey ventricular assist device, which currently is called the HeartAssist 5 (Reliant Heart) (Fig. 15.10). This device requires a small preperitoneal pocket, and the outflow graft is attached to the ascending aorta. Some unique aspects of this pump are that it is small, weighing 84 g, and it has an ultrasound flow probe attached to the outflow graft to directly measure pump flow. Goldstein reported the outcomes of the first 150 patients who underwent placement of this pump as BTT between 1998 and 2002.[24] The mean support time was 75 ± 81 days, and 55% of the patients were either bridged to transplantation, had successful explantation, or were on continued support at the end of the study. Unfortunately, 45% of the patients died, although the causes of death were not described. Major adverse events included reoperation

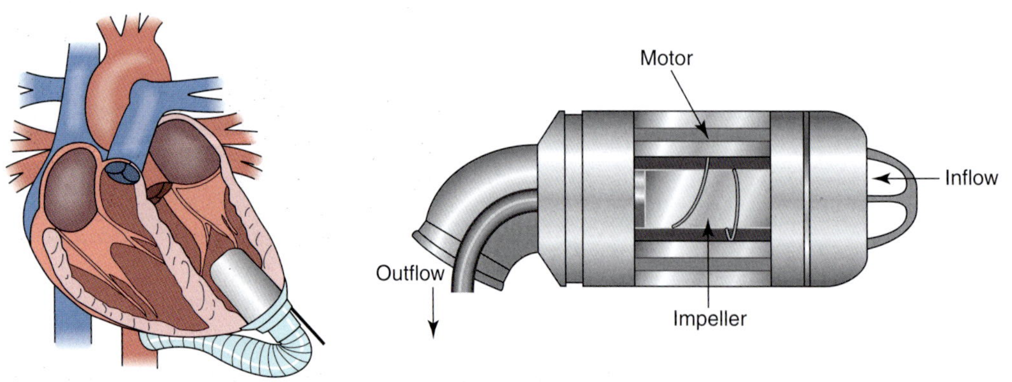

Fig. 15.9 Jarvik 2000 is a continuous-flow rotary pump with axial design and the unique feature of having the pumping chamber located within the left ventricle. (From Thunberg CA, Gaitan B, Arabia FA, et al. Ventricular assist devices today and tomorrow. *J Cardiothorac Vasc Anesth.* 2010;24:656–680.)

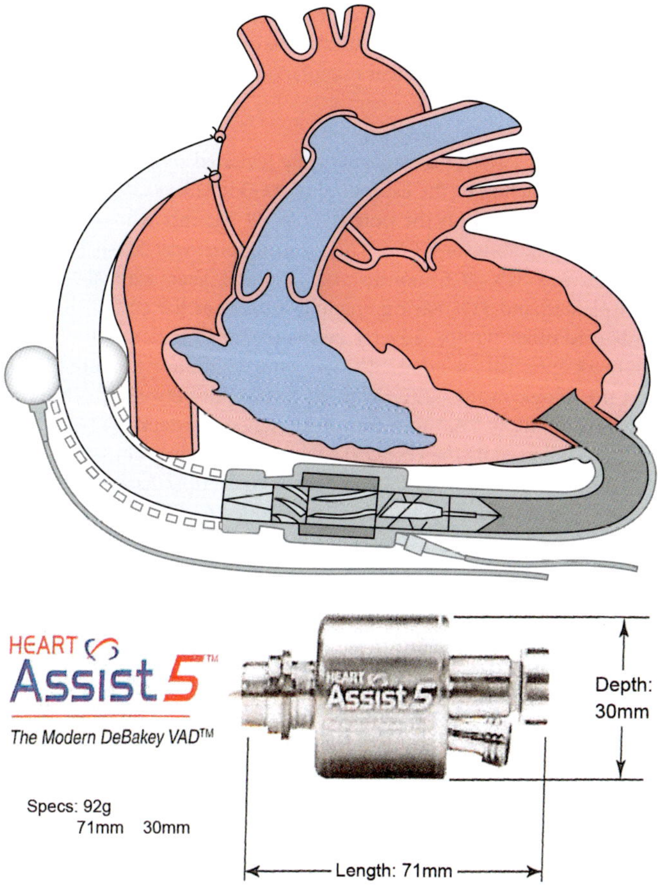

Fig. 15.10 Micromed DeBakey Heart Assist 5 is a continuous-flow rotary-pump with axial design. (Courtesy of Reliant.)

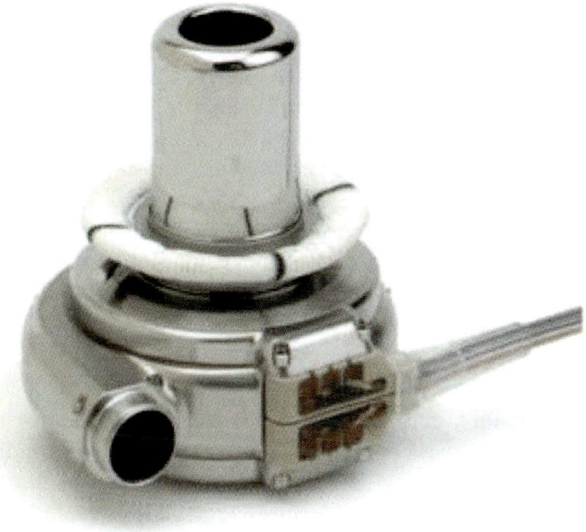

Fig. 15.11 HeartWare HVAD left ventricular assist device is a small, continuous-flow rotary pump with centrifugal and noncontact bearing design. The unique feature of the HVAD is its small size. It has a displacement volume of 45 mL and weighs 145 g but has a flow capacity of up to 10 L/min. The impeller of the HVAD is suspended in place by a combination of passive magnetic and hydrodynamic bearing systems. The impeller suspension system uses a passive magnetic bearing for radial stiffness. Axial magnetic preload and hydrodynamic bearings on top of each impeller blade provide axial constraint. The magnetic bearing consists of a stack of rare earth ring magnets near the inside diameter of the impeller that repel the magnetic force of a similar stack of magnets inside the center post. The axial alignment of the center-post magnet stack is set to provide an axial force that pushes the impeller toward the forward housing (the assembly with the inflow cannula). Physical contact between the housing and the impeller is prevented by a thin blood film generated by the hydrodynamic bearings.

for bleeding in 32%, hemolysis in 12%, thromboembolic events in 10.7%, and pump thrombus in 11.3%. This pump is currently approved for both BTT and DT in Europe. A clinical trial in the United States (NCT02205411) was terminated after the enrollment of 17 patients.

CONTINUOUS FLOW—CENTRIFUGAL

The introduction of continuous-flow axial devices has resulted in the obsolescence of prior pulsatile technology and led to a substantial increase in the number of devices being placed due to the excellent outcomes, improved adverse event profiles, smaller size, and superior durability. Despite their durability, axial-flow technology still uses mechanical bearings, and there is still a significant amount of thrombus formation on the device rotor and bearing interface, which may be part of the reason for the high incidence of pump thrombosis and embolic events, particularly strokes. Based on these risks, research proceeded on a third generation of pumps that use an impeller or rotor magnetically suspended using a non–contact-bearing design. These pumps usually have a centrifugal blood flow path and are suspended using either magnetic or hydrodynamic principles. The pumps utilizing this technology with clinical trial results include the HVAD (Medtronic), VentrAssist (Ventracor Corporation), DuraHeart (Terumo Heart Corporation), and HeartMate 3 (Abbott).

HVAD

The HVAD pump (Fig. 15.11) uses an impeller that is magnetically levitated and spun and also uses hydrodynamic thrust bearing, essentially suspending the impeller from the pump housing with a thin layer of plasma, so that there are no areas of mechanical contact or wear. The pump itself is implanted in the pericardial space. It has been the most-studied centrifugal flow pump and is approved for both BTT and DT in the United States. The initial study included 23 patients in Europe with a primary endpoint of survival to 180 days or transplantation.[25] At 180 days, 2 patients were transplanted, 2 died, and 19 had continued support for a survival of 91%, which was sustained at 86% at 1 year. This trial was followed by a larger trial of 50 patients in both Europe and the United States.[26] The primary endpoint was similar except that patients were followed-up for 2 years. Forty percent of the patients received a transplant, 8% had the pump explanted, and 34% had continued support at 2 years. The actual survival was 90% at 6 months, 84% at 1 year, and 79% at 2 years. Based on that initial success, a large 140-patient trial was conducted in BTT patients.[27] This was a nonrandomized trial that used a contemporaneous control group of patients implanted with an FDA-approved device that were enrolled in the INTERMACS registry with an implant indication of BTT. This was the first use of the INTERMACS registry as a control population. The primary endpoint was defined as survival to 180 days on the HVAD or transplantation or HVAD explantation for ventricular recovery. A total of 140 patients received an HVAD, and they were compared to 499 patients who received a control pump. There was no difference in the primary endpoint between the two groups at 180 days. Overall Kaplan-Meier survival was excellent for both groups at 180 days (94% HVAD, 90% control) and 1 year (86% HVAD, 85% control). The adverse events were collected only for the HVAD arm and included gastrointestinal bleeding in 10.7%, infection in 23.5%, right heart failure requiring inotropic support in 16.1%, and ischemic (7.1%) and hemorrhagic (5.7%)

stroke. The incidence of confirmed pump thrombosis was low at 2.1%. Similar to the results with HeartMate II, significant improvement was seen in 6-minute walk distance and the Kansas City Cardiomyopathy questionnaire quality of life score. Finally, the ReVOLVE postmarket approval study in Europe was reported in 2014.[28] This was a report of 254 patients who were implanted with an aim to show outcomes with continued use. The duration of support extended to 1057 days, with a mean support of 363 ± 280 days. At 3 years, the Kaplan-Meier survival was 73%. There was a low incidence of gastrointestinal bleeding (5%) and driveline infections (6%), with similar rates of stroke, sepsis, and right heart failure.

The HVAD pump was studied for DT patients in the ENDURANCE trial.[29] A multicenter, randomized trial of 446 patients was performed with a 2:1 randomization between the HVAD and the HeartMate II devices. The primary endpoint was survival at 2 years free from disabling stroke or device removal for malfunction or failure. A total of 297 patients received the HVAD compared to 148 patients receiving control in an intention-to-treat analysis. No difference was observed in the primary endpoint in a noninferiority analysis between the two groups. Additionally, at 2 years, survival was similar between the groups. There were significant differences in two areas, with more device replacements in the control group (16.2% (vs.) 8.8%) and more strokes in the HVAD group (29.7% (vs.) 12.1%). Functional status improved in both groups for the first 3 months and was sustained after that. A post hoc analysis of the HVAD patients showed that patients with a mean arterial blood pressure below 90 mm Hg had a lower frequency of strokes, and a follow-up study was designed to evaluate that in more detail.[30]

VentrAssist

The VentrAssist LVAD is a continuous-flow pump with a hydrodynamic bearing design (Fig. 15.12). It was first studied in 33 patients who were BTT, with the primary endpoint being survival until transplantation or transplant eligibility.[31] At the trial endpoint of 154 days, 39.4% of the patients were transplanted and 42.4% were transplant eligible, for a success rate of 82%. Five patients died during the trial. An updated report of 87 patients enrolled in all of the clinical trials (pilot trial, *n* = 9; Conformité Européene [CE] mark trial, *n* = 33; DT trial, *n* = 12; Better Results and Cost Effectiveness [BRACE] trial, *n* = 9; US BTT, *n* = 12) reported that 27 patients had ongoing support, 33 were transplanted, 1 was explanted, and 26 died on the device.[32] The maximum implant duration was 2.7 years, and the mean support duration was 103 days. In the combined experience, there have only been two documented cases of fibrin clot formation on the pump. Despite these findings, the pump is no longer manufactured.

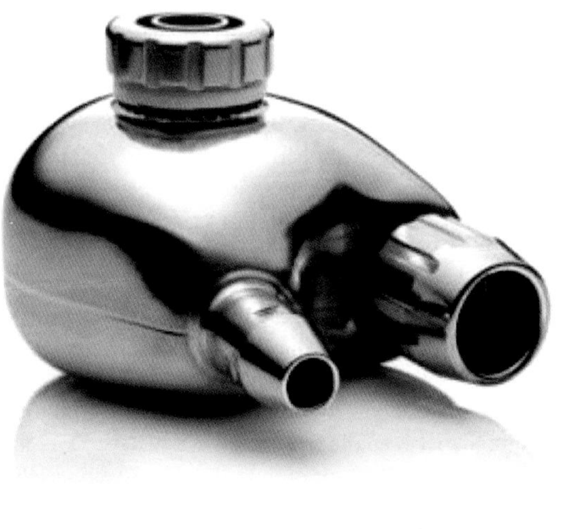

Fig. 15.12 Ventracor VentrAssist left ventricular assist device is a continuous-flow rotary pump with non–contact-bearing design. Impeller levitation inside the pump is achieved using hydrodynamic bearings.

DuraHeart

The DuraHeart LVAD is a magnetically levitated pump with an outflow graft attached to the ascending aorta (Fig. 15.13). Morshuis and colleagues reported on the outcomes of 68 patients who underwent pump implantation for BTT.[33] The mean support was 242 ± 243 days. Survival was 81% at 6 months and 77% at 1 year, with 26% being transplanted and 51% having ongoing support at the end of the trial. Similar to other pumps, adverse events in the 33 patients studied for CE mark approval included infection (58%), right heart failure (27%), and neurologic events (27%) with an equal split between cerebrovascular accidents (CVAs) and transitent ischemic attacks (TIAs). This trial was followed by the US SUSTAIN trial (A Study evaluAting Safety and effectiveness of the DuraHeart Left VenTriculAr AssIst System iN Bridge-to-Transplant patients), which enrolled 63 BTT patients in the United States.[34] Patients were followed for at least 6 months and 73% of the patients reach the primary end point of survival to transplantation, alive on device at 180 days, or explant for recovery. There were no reports of hemolysis or pump thrombosis. Unfortunately, 10% of the pumps had failure of the magnetic levitation system due to cable wire fracture but were stable in backup hydrodynamic mode. Also, the incidence of ischemic (0.17 events/patient-year) and hemorrhagic (0.09 events/patient-year) stokes remained high.

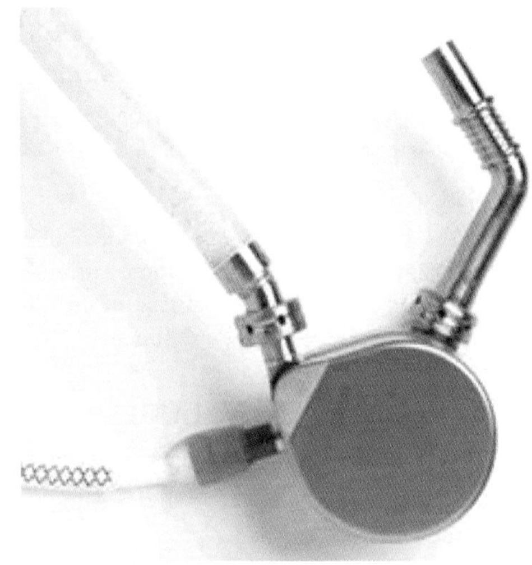

Fig. 15.13 DuraHeart left ventricular assist device is a continuous-flow rotary pump with centrifugal and noncontact bearing design. The device has a displacement volume of 180 cm^3 and a weight of 540 g. Its external dimensions are 72 mm in width and 45 mm in height. The pumping unit consists of an upper housing with the levitation system, the impeller, and a bottom housing containing the external drive motor. The device is designed with active magnetic levitation of the impeller along with hydrodynamic bearings to support impeller levitation in case the magnetic levitation system fails. The impeller is rotated through magnetic coupling between permanent magnets embedded on the motor side of the impeller and an external drive motor that uses a bearing design. Three electromagnets and three position sensors are mounted in the upper housing. Tilting and axial displacements of the impeller are monitored and controlled using a three-degrees-of-freedom controller. The ferromagnetic ring on the opposite side of the impeller is levitated by the electromagnet, and position sensors control the impeller so that it is always positioned at the center of the blood chamber. Radial impeller movement is passively suspended with a bias flux through the electromagnetic rotor and drive magnet rotor.

HeartMate 3

The newest centrifugal flow pump to be studied is the HeartMate 3 (Fig. 15.14), which is a magnetically levitated pump like the HVAD but is also suspended magnetically, which allows for larger blood flow passages than the hydrodynamic bearings of the HVAD. Additionally, it is programmed to decrease speed every 2 seconds in an attempt to provide better washing of the pump and the impeller and hopefully decrease the incidence of pump thrombosis and embolic events.

The HeartMate 3 was studied in the Multicenter Study of MagLev Technology in Patients Undergoing Mechanical Circulatory Support Therapy With HeartMate 3 (MOMENTUM 3) study, which was a non-blinded randomized trial comparing HeartMate 3 to HeartMate II.[35] A total of 294 patients were randomized in a 1:1 ratio in block randomization by trial center. The primary end point was a composite of survival free of disabling stroke or reoperation to replace or remove the device at 6 months. Secondary endpoints included survival, frequency of adverse events, functional status by both 6-minute walk and NYHA functional class, and quality of life changes. The trial was inclusive of patients with the indication of BTT, bridge to decision, and DT.

The baseline characteristics of the patients were similar between the two groups except for slightly higher systolic and mean blood pressure in the HeartMate 3 arm and more patients on diuretics in the HeartMate II arm (95.8% (vs.) 88.2%). Over a 1-year period, 151 patients were implanted with HeartMate 3 and 138 with HeartMate II. The implant hospitalization survival rate was 92.7% in the HeartMate 3 (vs.) 91.3% in the HeartMate II, with a median length of stay of 19.5 (vs.) 17.5 days, respectively. There was a significant difference in the primary endpoint (86.2% (vs.) 76.8%, $P = 0.04$ for superiority) of the HeartMate 3 driven by a decreased rate of reoperation for pump malfunction. Only one patient required reoperation (vs.) 11 patients with the HeartMate II. No significant differences existed in the rates of death or disabling stroke. Both groups had similar improvements in functional status and quality of life. Of note, no patients in the HeartMate 3 group had suspected or confirmed pump thrombosis compared with 14 patients (10.1%) in the HeartMate II arm. No differences were noted in other important adverse events, including bleeding, infection, right heart failure, or cardiac arrhythmias, between the groups.

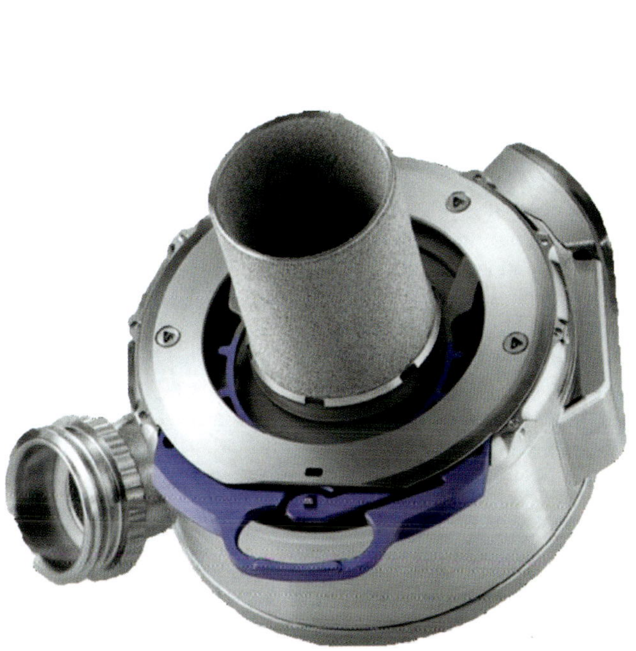

Fig. 15.14 HeartMate 3.

This trial was recently updated with 2-year outcomes.[36] The primary endpoint was survival at 2 years free of disabling strokes or reoperation to remove or replace a malfunctioning device. Additional patients were included in this trial, for a total of 366 patients (189 HeartMate 3, 172 HeartMate II, 5 randomized but not implanted). No difference was detected in initial survival to hospital discharge (93.7% (vs.) 93.0%), length of stay (20 (vs.) 18 days), or number of rehospitalization days (11 (vs.) 17) between the two groups. Similar to the 6-month data, at 2 years, there was superiority in the primary endpoint with the HeartMate 3 again driven by the reoperation or device removal endpoint (1.6% (vs.) 17.0%). The indications for pump change were driveline communication fault (1), driveline infection (1), and persistent low pump flow due to obstructive outflow-graft twist (1). The vast majority of the patients requiring pump change for the HeartMate II group were for pump thrombosis or severe hemolysis. There were no differences in mortality or rates of disabling stroke. Of note, the incidence of all strokes was reduced in the HeartMate 3 group (10.1% (vs.) 19.2%). The rates of other adverse events, including mortality, bleeding, infection, and right heart failure, were not different between the two groups.

The excellent survival and low pump thrombosis rate has been confirmed in the European trials of the HeartMate 3 as well.[37–40] The results of the pivotal CE mark trial of 50 patients who were both BTT and DT were reported in 2017.[38] This was a single-arm, prospective, nonrandomized trial with a primary endpoint of survival at 6 months compared to INTERMACS. At 1 year, 74% of the patients had ongoing support and three patients (6%) had undergone transplantation. Nine deaths were reported, two related to strokes. Adverse events were similar to other trials, with bleeding in 44%, infection in 36%, and stroke in 12% in the first 6 months and 6% in the second 6 months. Similar to the US experience, there were no incidences of hemolysis, pump thrombosis, or pump malfunction. The 2-year outcomes remained favorable, with a Kaplan-Meier survival rate of 74% ± 6%.[39] Unfortunately, gastrointestinal bleeding (11%), infection (14%), driveline infections (14%), and ischemic stroke (8%) continued to be prevalent adverse events from year 1 to 2. By the end of year 2, the overall stroke incidence was 24%, split between ischemic (16%) and hemorrhagic (8%). The rate of persistent neurologic dysfunction was lower at 10%. There were still no reports of pump thrombosis or malfunction, but one patient experienced outflow graft thrombosis.

A postregistry report of 6-month outcomes in 482 patients was recently published for both BTT and DT patients.[40] Similar to the trial data, the 6-month survival rate was 82% ± 2%. There was no pump thrombosis and other adverse events were unchanged with bleeding at 25%, infection in 35%, and stroke at 5%. Functional capacity measured by 6-minute walk and quality of life also showed significant improvements in these patients.

At this point, it appears that either the pump design or intermittent change in pump speed or both is important and has resulted in a markedly reduced incidence of pump thrombosis compared to prior pumps. The low rate of pump thrombus formation is a significant improvement in clinical outcomes for patients even if it does not result in improved survival.

QUALITY OF LIFE, FUNCTIONAL STATUS, AND ADVERSE EVENTS

Continuous-flow devices have been in use for almost 15 years. Initially, there was concern that the long-term lack of pulsatility could be detrimental to patients. This resulted in a number of analyses being performed in the HeartMate II patients to better understand the effects on other organs. Rogers et al.[41] evaluated functional capacity and quality of life in both BTT and DT populations (Figs. 15.15 and 15.16). For

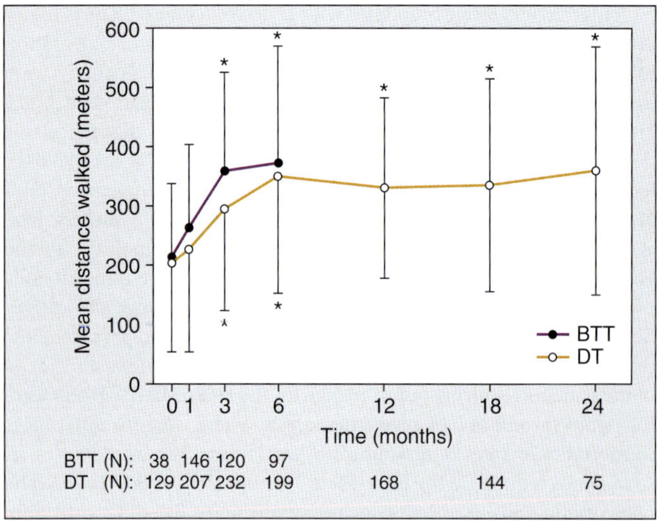

Fig. 15.15 Submaximal exercise performance after HeartMate II implantation. Mean 6-minute walk distances in the bridge to transplantation *(BTT)* and destination therapy *(DT)* trials are shown over time. Ascertainment of baseline 6-minute walk distance was limited to patients able to ambulate. The number of observations *(N)* at each time point is shown at the bottom of the figure. $*P < 0.05$ compared with baseline. (From Rogers JG, Aaronson KD, Boyle AJ, et al; HeartMate II Investigators. Continuous-flow left ventricular assist device improves functional capacity and quality of life of advanced heart failure patients. *J Am Coll Cardiol.* 2010;55:1826–1834.)

LVAD patients who had values recorded both before and at various points after implantation, there were improvements in NYHA functional class, 6-minute walk distance, and quality of life. Most of these scores improved early and continued to improve until about month 6 after implantation. Neurocognitive testing was performed in both BTT and DT patients at 1, 3, and 6 months postimplantation.[42,43] For the BTT group, 93 patients were studied and 28 patients had serial studies. There were limited improvements in visual memory, executive function, visual spatial perception, and processing speed, with no declines over these time periods. In the older DT population, there were stable or slight improvements in all domains, and importantly, even at 24 months, there was no decline in any of the domains, although fewer patients had data that far out. In the BTT population, early liver and renal function was shown to improve at 6 months.[44] The only signal of an adverse effect of continuous flow was a single center report from the University of Minnesota.[45] Crow and colleagues reported on 101 patients (55 continuous flow) and found a higher incidence of gastrointestinal bleeding, defined as guaiac-positive stool with a hemoglobin drop requiring transfusion of at least two units of packed red blood cells. The event rate was 46.5 events/100 patients-years, compared to 4.7 events/100 patient-years with pulsatile pumps. Further reports have shown that bleeding occurs in 15%–30% of these patients at a rate of 0.45 events/patient-year.[46,47] This increased rate of gastrointestinal bleeding has been a recurring issue with these devices and felt to be due to a combination of factors including therapeutic anticoagulation, development of acquired von Willebrand disease with loss of high molecular weight multimers of von Willebrand factor due to increased proteolytic cleavage of unfolded multimers from high shear stress, and the development of arteriovenous malformations throughout the gastrointestinal tract.[48] Clearly, there is a need for ongoing improvements with the continuous-flow devices to reduce the adverse events associated with them.

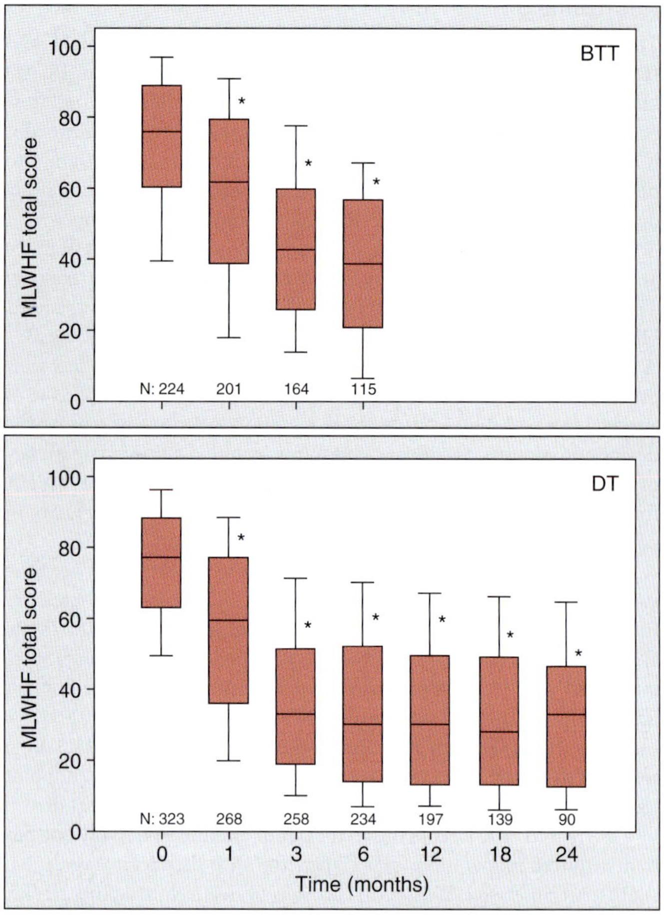

Fig. 15.16 Changes in quality of life: Minnesota Living With Heart Failure *(MLWHF)* questionnaire results in the HeartMate II bridge to transplantation *(BTT)* and destination therapy *(DT)* clinical trials. Changes in quality of life assessed with the MLWHF questionnaire are shown. Lower values signify improved quality of life. Bars indicate 25th, 50th, and 75th percentiles, whereas whiskers indicate 5th and 95th percentiles. $*P < 0.05$ compared with baseline. (From Rogers JG, Aaronson KD, Boyle AJ, et al; HeartMate II Investigators. Continuous-flow left ventricular assist device improves functional capacity and quality of life of advanced heart failure patients. *J Am Coll Cardiol.* 2010;55:1826–1834.)

The Prevention of HeartMate II pump thrombosis through clinical management (PREVENT) study was the first study to prospectively apply best practices in an attempt to reduce the adverse events associated with implantation of LVADs, in this specific case reduce the incidence of pump thrombosis.[49] Based on an observed increase in the incidence of pump thrombosis with the HeartMate II, a group of investigators tried to identify "best practices" that would hopefully result in a reduction in adverse events.[50] The trial design compared the PREVENT sites who agreed to abide by the identified surgical and medical recommendations to non-PREVENT sites who were also implanting the HeartMate II over the same period of time. The recommendations included surgical issues such as creating an adequately sized pump pocket, where to place the inflow cannula and outflow graft, pump positioning, and fixing the pump to either the diaphragm or chest wall. Anticoagulation and antiplatelet recommendations included bridging patients with unfractionated heparin or low-molecular-weight heparin within 48 hours of device implantation in nonbleeding patients with a PTT goal of 40–45 seconds and then 50–60 seconds. Warfarin was to be started within 48 hours with a goal international normalized ratio (INR) for prothrombin time of 2.0–2.5 by day 5–7 and the initiation of aspirin therapy (81–325 mg) when there was no evidence of bleeding. The goal INR throughout was 2.0–2.5. Long-term management included running with pump speeds above 9000 rpms and to only adjust the pump speed to achieve intermittent aortic valve opening if the above pump speed goals could be maintained. Finally, in all patients, the target blood pressure was a mean arterial pressure <90 mm Hg. A total of 300 patients were enrolled at 23 centers. At 6 months, 20 suspected pump thrombus events were reported, of which 15 were confirmed (5.0% of patients). Overall survival at 6 months was 89%, and survival free of pump thrombus was 84%. The adverse events in the trial included a bleeding rate of 45% at 6 months, with 21% of the patients experiencing a gastrointestinal bleed. Of interest, the hemorrhagic (2.7%) and ischemic (4%) stroke rate was much lower than in the initial clinical trials with the HeartMate II, perhaps from tight blood pressure control and a low incidence of pump thrombosis. The authors also analyzed the incidence of complications based on adherence to the surgical and medical recommendations of the trial. There was a trend to an increased incidence of pump thrombosis when the outflow graft avoided the right ventricle (15% (vs.) 5%, $P = 0.13$), and patients with a pump speed <9000 rpms at 30 days had a higher incidence of pump thrombosis at 6 months (14% (vs.) 3%, $P < 0.01$). Of note, there was no difference in mean arterial blood pressure between patients with and patients without pump thrombosis, although both groups of patients were maintained below 90 mm Hg.

The HVAD investigators also evaluated the risk factors for neurologic events.[51] Using a 382-patient BTT population, multivariable analysis predictors for ischemic events included aspirin <81 mg and atrial fibrillation. Conversely, predictors for hemorrhagic stroke included mean arterial pressure >90 mm Hg, aspirin <81 mg, and an INR >3.0. Partly through the study, the company instituted a pump design change with texturing of a segment of the inflow cannula and reinforced an INR goal of 2.0–3.0 and using aspirin at 325 mg a day. These changes resulted in a nonsignificant reduction in the prevalence of ischemic strokes from 6.3% to 2.7% ($P = 0.21$) and hemorrhagic strokes (7.4% to 6.4%, $P = 0.69$).

An analysis of pump thrombosis was also performed in patients receiving the HVAD. In 382 patients receiving the HVAD after the initial clinical trial, 8.1% of the patients experienced a pump thrombus event.[52] A multivariable analysis of possible risk factors revealed that a mean arterial pressure >90 mm Hg, aspirin dose <81 mg, an INR <2, and an INTERMACS profile of >3 at implantation were all risk factors for pump thrombosis. This was followed with the prospective trial evaluating the importance of tight blood pressure control in patients receiving the HVAD. A total of 465 patients who were ineligible for transplant were randomized 2:1 to HVAD (vs.) HeartMate II.[30] The primary endpoint was the 12-month incidence of TIA or stroke with residual deficit at 24 weeks after the event. Patients were taught to take their blood pressure twice a day for the first 3 months. If an automated blood pressure cuff was used, the goal mean arterial pressure was <85 mm Hg, and if a Doppler was used, the goal was <90 mm Hg. Only subjects receiving the HVAD were in the strict blood pressure control protocol but perhaps reflecting the overall emphasis on blood pressure control at 3 and 6 months, and there was a reduction in blood pressure in the HVAD group at each time point. When compared to the control HeartMate II, there was no difference in the primary endpoint. When compared to the HVAD group in the original DT trial, there was a 24.2% reduction in the incidence of stroke, with a 50.5% reduction in the incidence of hemorrhagic stroke. This trial demonstrates the importance of blood pressure control and also emphasizes that different pumps with different flow characteristics need to be managed differently.

Elective LVAD Therapy

Most of the trials evaluating the efficacy of LVAD therapy have been in advanced heart failure patients, most of whom were inotrope dependent with many that required intraaortic balloon pumps prior to implantation. As expected, the INTERMACS registry has reported that patients with more advanced heart failure do worse than patients with less severe heart failure, arguing that earlier implantation of an LVAD may result in better outcomes. The high adverse event rate has slowed the adoption of LVAD therapy in these patients; however, those rates are from the more advanced patients in the clinical trials. The Risk Assessment and Comparative Effectiveness of Left Ventricular Assist Device and Medical Management study was designed to evaluate the outcomes in a less advanced, ambulatory population of heart failure patients.[53] Patients with class IIIb/IV heart failure symptoms who were not inotrope dependent but otherwise met the indication for LVAD (EF <25% and on guideline-based medical therapy for 45 of the past 60 days or intolerant), who had either one heart failure hospitalization or two unscheduled emergency department/infusion clinic visits in the previous year, and a 6-minute walk distance <300 m were enrolled. Patients who met the enrollment criteria could elect to either undergo implantation of a HeartMate II LVAD or continue on medical therapy. A total of 200 patients were enrolled in the trial and 97 chose LVAD therapy. The primary endpoint was a composite of survival and improvement of ≥75 m in the 6-minute walk distance at 12 months and was achieved in 39% of the LVAD patients compared to 21% of the medical therapy patients. This endpoint was confounded by a number of the medical therapy patients asking for LVAD therapy as they became sicker. The intention to treat survival was similar at 12 months (82% LVAD (vs.) 81% medical management) but the "as treated" survival was significantly great for LVAD patients (80% (vs.) 63%). LVAD patients also experienced greater improvements in quality of life, 6-minute walk distance, and depression. As expected, the LVAD group had more frequent adverse events, with more frequent bleeding (predominantly gastrointestinal), infections, pump thrombus, arrhythmias, and borderline for stroke (eight LVAD (vs.) two medical management; $P = 0.08$). Additionally, there were more rehospitalizations in the LVAD group at 79.8% (vs.) 64%. Recently, a 2-year follow-up study was presented with similar results.[54] Survival as treated was 70% with LVAD (vs.) 41% with medical therapy, and by this time, 22% of the patients in the original medical management arm had received an LVAD. There were sustained improvements in NYHA functional class, 6-minute walk distance, and quality of life, with a tradeoff of more hospitalizations and adverse events. Additionally, patients initially in the optimal medical therapy arm who crossed over did just as well, arguing that a delayed implant strategy while being monitored closely is safe but results in a delayed improvement in quality of life parameters. A strategy of closely following patients until they are ready to proceed with LVAD implantation as long as they are not inotrope dependent seems appropriate at this time.

The INTERMACS registry was first developed as a public-private partnership between the National Institutes of Health, hospitals, and industry, with a mandate that all patients who underwent placement of FDA approved devices would be enrolled in a registry.[55] At the time of the most recent report 18,987 primary LVAD patients have been enrolled,[56] over 80% of whom have continuous-flow devices. During 2015–2016, about half of the patients in INTERMACS received an LVAD as DT, and the other half were evenly divided between those who were listed for transplant at implant and those not listed, but for whom the intent was transplant. For the most recent era, the overall 1- and 2-year survival is 82% and 73%, respectively, and BTT patients continue to have improved survival compared to DT patients because they are typically younger with fewer comorbidities. Other risk factors for mortality include more critically ill patients, older age, chronic pulmonary disease, peripheral vascular disease, and renal dysfunction. The need for a right ventricular assist device continues to be the biggest risk factor for early mortality, followed by preimplantation dialysis. Adverse events, although improved since the introduction of current devices, still continue to be a limitation of the technology and a focus of ongoing research. Unfortunately, early events, specifically the need for continuous inotropic support and strokes within the first 3 months, increase the risk of subsequent mortality. The INTERMACS registry continues to be helpful for understanding the outcomes of non–clinical trial patients and as a comparator for outcomes with new devices.

TOTAL ARTIFICIAL HEARTS

The SynCardia CardioWest total artificial heart is a pneumatic pump and replaces all four cardiac valves and both ventricles (Fig. 15.17). It currently has been used as a BTT, but with the introduction of a portable driver, it could potentially have a role for DT. The total artificial heart was studied in 81 patients and compared to 35 control patients in five centers.[57] Seventy-nine percent of the patients were successfully bridged to transplantation at an average time of 79 days compared to 46% of the control patients. Over the course of 7515 days of patient experience with the device, there was one significant device malfunction of a perforation of one of the four layers of the left ventricular diaphragm. There were also complications of fitting the device in five patients, requiring repositioning in three, and resulting in death in two others. Neurologic events including stroke (10 patients) and TIAs (four events) did occur. A more recent report of a cohort of patients who survived for at least a year with the SynCardia heart was published in 2014.[58] A total of 47 patients were included, and 72% of the patients were successfully transplanted and 24% died while on support. Major complications included device failure (10%), systemic infection (53%), driveline infections (27%), thromboembolic events (19%), and hemorrhagic events (14%).

More recently, an electro-hydraulically actuated total artificial heart was developed by Carmat. This pump was designed with bio-prosthetic blood contacting surfaces in hopes of reducing the incidence of thrombosis.[59] A four-patient experience has been reported showing implant times of 74, 270, 254, and 20 days. There was no evidence of hemolysis, clinical neurologic events, pump thrombus, or device-related infections.[60] Two of the patients were actually discharged home for a total duration of 7 months. There is an ongoing trial evaluating the safety and performance of this heart with a planned 2-year postimplantation follow-up that is estimated to be completed in 2020 (European Clinical Evaluation of the Carmat Total Artificial Heart–ADVANCE HF study: NCT02962973).

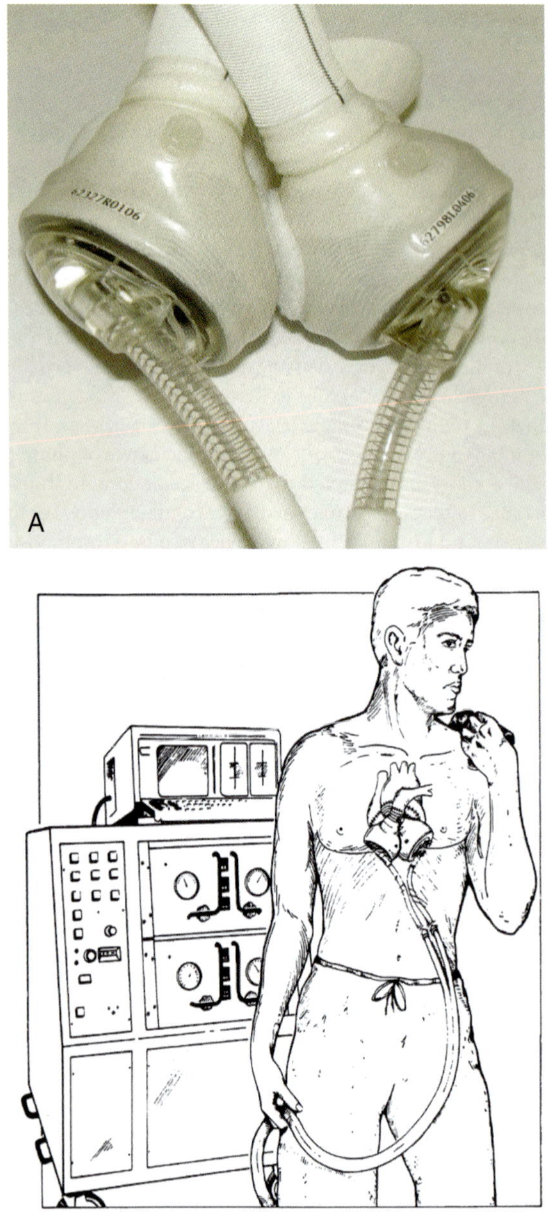

B

Fig. 15.17 (A) The Syncardia CardioWest total artificial heart is a pneumatically actuated pump designed for orthotopic replacement of the native cardiac ventricles and valves. The pump weighs 160 g, has a maximal stroke volume of 70 mL, and is capable of delivering an output of 9 L/min. (B) The standard driver for the Syncardia device allowed patients to be ambulatory but was typically limited to hospital use. A newer pneumatic driver that is smaller and enables hospital discharge is under investigation.

CONCLUSION

LVAD therapy has progressed from an early, short-term, life-sustaining therapy to an established, long-term, and viable treatment option for patients with advanced systolic heart failure, for those needing support until transplantation as well as permanent therapy for those in whom transplant is not an option. The recent studies with the currently approved centrifugal flow devices show sustained improvements in survival, with early signals of a reduction in some of the common complications associated with these devices. Further studies to understand best the techniques for the implantation and long-term care of these patients as well as design enhancements should continue to pay dividends with improved outcomes and reduced side effects.

REFERENCES

1. Hall CW, Liotta D, Henly WS, Crawford ES, DeBakey ME. Development of artificial intrathoracic circulatory pumps. *Am J Surg*. 1964;108:685–692.
2. Frazier OH. Prologue: ventricular assist devices and total artificial heart. A historical perspective. *Cardiol Clin*. 2003;21:1–13.

3. Norman JC, Duncan JM, Frazier OH, et al. Intracorporeal (abdominal) left ventricular assist devices or partial artificial hearts: a five-year clinical experience. *Arch Surg.* 1981;116:1441–1445.
4. Hill JD, Farrar DJ, Hershon JJ, et al. Use of a prosthetic ventricle as a bridge to cardiac transplantation for postinfarction cardiogenic shock. *N Engl J Med.* 1986;314:626–628.
5. Farrar DJ, Hill JD, Gray LA, et al. Heterotropic prosthetic ventricles as a bridge to cardiac transplant. A multicenter study in 29 patients. *N Engl J Med.* 1988;318:333–340.
6. Slaughter MS, Tsui SS, El-Banayosy A, et al. Results of a multicenter clinical trial with the Thoratec implantable ventricular assist device. *J Thorac Cardiovasc Surg.* 2007;133:1573–1580.
7. Frazier OH, Rose EA, Macmanus Q, et al. Multicenter clinical evaluation of the HeartMate 1000 IP left ventricular assist device. *Ann Thorac Surg.* 1992;53:1080–1090.
8. Frazier OH, Rose EA, McCarthy P, et al. Improved mortality and rehabilitation of transplant candidates treated with a long-term implantable left ventricular assist system. *Ann Surg.* 1995;222:327–338.
9. Frazier OH, Rose EA, Oz MC, et al. Multicenter clinical evaluation of the HeartMate vented electric left ventricular assist system in patients awaiting heart transplantation. *J Thorac Cardiovasc Surg.* 2001;122:1186–1195.
10. Rose EA, Gelijns AC, Moskowitz AJ, et al. Long-term use of a left ventricular assist device for end-stage heart failure. *N Engl J Med.* 2001;345:1435–1443.
11. Long JW, Kfoury AG, Slaughter MS, et al. Long-term destination therapy with the HeartMate XVE left ventricular assist device: improved outcomes since the REMATCH study. *Congest Heart Fail.* 2005;11:133–138.
12. Dembitsky WP, Tector AJ, Park S, et al. Left ventricular assist device performance with long-term circulatory support: lesson from the REMATCH trial. *Ann Thorac Surg.* 2004;78:2123–2129.
13. Dagenais F, Portner PM, Robbins RC, Oyer PE. The Novacor left ventricular assist system: clinical experience form the Novacor Registry. *J Card Surg.* 2001;16:267–271.
14. Rogers JG, Butler J, Lansman SL, et al. Chronic mechanical circulatory support for inotrope-dependent heart failure patients who are not transplant candidates: results of the INTrEPID Trial. *J Am Coll Cardiol.* 2007;50:741–747.
15. El-Banayosy A, Arusoglu L, Kizner L, et al. Novacor left ventricular assist system (vs.) HeartMate vented electric left ventricular assist system as a long-term mechanical circulatory support device in bridging patients: a prospective study. *J Thorac Cardiovasc Surg.* 2000;119:581–587.
16. Mussivand T, Hetzer R, Vitali E, et al. Clinical results with an ePTFE inflow conduit for mechanical circulatory support. *J Heart Lung Transplant.* 2004;23:1366–1370.
17. Miller LW, Pagani FD, Russell SD, et al. Use of a continuous-flow device in patients awaiting heart transplantation. *N Engl J Med.* 2007;357:885–896.
18. Pagani FD, Miller LW, Russell SD, et al. HeartMate II Investigators. Extended mechanical circulatory support with a continuous-flow rotary left ventricular assist device. *J Am Coll Cardiol.* 2009;54:312–321.
19. Slaughter MS, Rogers JG, Milano CA, et al. Advanced heart failure treated with continuous-flow left ventricular assist device. *N Engl J Med.* 2009;361:2241–2251.
20. Park SJ, Milano CA, Tatooles AJ, et al. Slaughter MS; HeartMate II Clinical Investigators. Outcomes in advanced heart failure patients with left ventricular assist devices for destination therapy. *Circ Heart Fail.* 2012;5:241–248.
21. Jorde UP, Kushwaha SS, Tatooles AJ, et al. Results of the destination therapy post-Food And Drug Administration approval study with a continuous flow left ventricular assist device: a prospective study using the INTERMACS registry (Interagency Registry for Mechanically Assisted Circulatory Support). *J Am Coll Cardiol.* 2014;63:1751–1757.
22. Frazier OH, Myers TJ, Gregoric ID, et al. Initial clinical experience with the Jarvik 2000 implantable axial-flow left ventricular assist system. *Circulation.* 2002;105:2855–2860.
23. Kohno H, Matsumiya G, Sawa Y, et al. The Jarvik 2000 left ventricular assist device as a bridge to transplantation: Japanese Registry for Mechanically Assisted Circulatory Support. *J Heart Lung Transplant.* 2018;37;71–78.
24. Goldstein DJ. Worldwide experience with the MicroMed DeBakey ventricular assist device as a bridge to transplantation. *Circulation.* 2003;108(suppl II):II272–7.
25. Wieselthaler GM, O Driscoll G, Jansz P, et al. Initial clinical experience with a novel left ventricular assist device with a magnetically levitated rotor in a multi-institutional trial. *J Heart Lung Transplant.* 2010;29:1218–1225.
26. Strueber M, O'Driscoll G, Jansz P, et al. Multicenter evaluation of an intrapericardial left ventricular assist system. *J Am Coll Cardiol.* 2011;57:1375–1382.
27. Aaronson KD, Slaughter MS, Miller LW, et al. Use of an intrapericardial, continuous-flow, centrifugal pump in patients awaiting heart transplantation. *Circulation.* 2012;125:3191–3200.
28. Strueber M, Larbalestier R, Jansz P, et al. Results of the post-market Registry to Evaluate the HeartWare Left Ventricular Assist System (ReVOLVE). *J Heart Lung Transplant.* 2014;33:486–491.
29. Rogers JG, Pagani FD, Tatooles AJ, et al. Intrapericardial left ventricular assist device for advanced heart failure. *N Engl J Med.* 2017;376:451–460.
30. Milano CA, Rogers JG, Tatooles AJ, et al. HVAD: The ENDURANCE supplemental trial. *JACC Heart Fail.* 2018;6:792–802.
31. Esmore D, Kaye D, Spratt P, et al. A prospective, multicenter trial of the VentrAssist left ventricular assist device for bridge to transplant: safety and efficacy. *J Heart Lung Transplant.* 2008;27:579–588.
32. Esmore D, Spratt P, Larbalestier R, et al. VentrAssist left ventricular assist device: clinical trial results and Clinical Development Plan update. *Eur J Cardiothorac Surg.* 2007;32:735–744.
33. Morshuis M, El-Banayosy A, Arusoglu L, et al. European experience of DuraHeart magnetically levitated centrifugal left ventricular assist system. *Eur J Cardiothorac Surg.* 2009;35:1020–1028.
34. Moazami N, Steffen RJ, Naka Y, et al. Lessons learned from the first fully magnetically levitated centrifugal LVAD trial in the United States: the DuraHeart trial. *Ann Thorac Surg.* 2014;98:541–548.
35. Mehra MR, Naka Y, Uriel N, et al. A fully magnetically levitated circulatory pump for advanced heart failure. *N Engl J Med.* 2017;376:440–450.
36. Mehra MR, Goldstein DJ, Uriel N, et al. Two-year outcomes with a magnetically levitated cardiac pump in heart failure. *N Engl J Med.* 2018;378:1386–1395.
37. Netuka I, Sood P, Pya Y, et al. Fully magnetically levitated left ventricular assist system for treating advanced HF. A multicenter study. *J Am Coll Cardiol.* 2015;66:2579–2589.
38. Krabatsch T, Netuka I, Schmitto JD, et al. HeartMate 3 fully magnetically levitated left ventricular assist device for the treatment of advanced heart failure -1 year results from the CE mark trial. *J Cardiothorac Surg.* 2017;12:23.
39. Schmitto JD, Pya Y, Zimpfer D, et al. Long-term evaluation of a fully magnetically levitated circulatory support device for advanced heart failure-two-year results from the HeartMate 3 CE mark study. *Eur J Heart Fail.* 2018 Jul 27. https://doi.org/10.1002/ejhf.1284. [Epub ahead of print].
40. Gustafsson F, Shaw S, Lavee J, et al. Six-month outcomes after treatment of advanced heart failure with a full magnetically levitated continuous flow left ventricular assist device: report from the ELEVATE registry. *Eur Heart J.* 2018 Aug 27. https://doi.org/10.1093/eurheartj/ehy513. [Epub ahead of print].
41. Rogers JG, Aaronson KD, Boyle AJ, et al. Continuous flow left ventricular assist device improves functional capacity and quality of life of advanced heart failure patients. *J Am Coll Cardiol.* 2010;55:1826–1834.
42. Petrucci RJ, Wright S, Naka Y, et al. Neurocognitive assessments in advanced heart failure patients receiving continuous-flow left ventricular assist devices. *J Heart Lung Transplant.* 2009;28:542–549.
43. Petrucci RJ, Rogers JG, Blue L, et al. Neurocognitive function in destination therapy patients receiving continuous-flow vs pulsatile-flow left ventricular assist device support. *J Heart Lung Transplant.* 2012;31:27–36.
44. Russell SD, Rogers JG, Milano CA, et al. Renal and hepatic function improve in advanced heart failure patients during continuous-flow support with the HeartMate II left ventricular assist device. *Circulation.* 2009;120:2352–2357.
45. Crow S, John R, Boyle A, et al. Gastrointestinal bleeding rates in recipients of nonpulsatile and pulsatile left ventricular assist devices. *J Thorac Cardiovasc Surg.* 2009;137:208–215.

46. John R, Kamdar F, Liao K, Colvin-Adams M, Boyle A, Joyce L. Improved survival and decreasing incidence of adverse events with the HeartMate II left ventricular assist device as bridge-to-transplant therapy. *Ann Thorac Surg*. 2008;86:1227–1234.
47. Stulak JM, Lee D, Haft JW, et al. Gastrointestinal bleeding and subsequent risk of thromboembolic events during support with a left ventricular assist device. *J Heart Lung Transplant*. 2014;33:60–64.
48. Healy AH, McKellar SH, Drakos SG, Koliopoulou A, Stehlik J, Selzman CH. Physiologic effects of continuous-flow left ventricular assist devices. *J Surg Res*. 2016;202:363–371.
49. Maltais S, Kilic A, Nathan S, et al. Gregoric I, and on behalf of the PREVENT study investigators. PREVENtion of HeartMate II pump thrombosis through clinical management: the PREVENT multi-center study. *J Heart Lung Transplant*. 2017;36:1–12.
50. Starling RC, Moazami N, Silvestry SC, et al. Unexpected abrupt increase in left ventricular assist device thrombosis. *N Engl J Med*. 2014;370:33–40.
51. Teuteberg JJ, Slaughter MS, Rogers JG, et al. The HVAD left ventricular assist device. Risk factors for neurological events and risk mitigation strategies. *JACC Heart Fail*. 2015;3:818–828.
52. Najjar SS, Slaughter MS, Pagani FD, et al. An analysis of pump thrombus events in patients in the HeartWare ADVANCE bridge to transplant and continued access protocol trial. *J Heart Lung Transplant*. 2014;33:23–34.
53. Estep JD, Starling RC, Horstmanshof DA, et al. Risk assessment and comparative effectiveness of left ventricular assist device and medical management in ambulatory heart failure patients: results from the ROADMAP study. *J Am Coll Cardiol*. 2015;66:1747–1761.
54. Starling RC, Estep JD, Horstmanshof DA, et al. Risk assessment and comparative effectiveness of left ventricular assist device and medical management in ambulatory heart failure patients: the ROADMAP study 2-year results. *JACC Heart Fail*. 2017;5:518–527.
55. Kirklin JK, Naftel DC, Stevenson LW, et al. INTERMACS database for durable devices for circulatory support: first annual report. *J Heart Lung Transplant*. 2008;27:1065–1072.
56. Kirklin JK, Pagani FD, Kormos RL, et al. Eighth annual INTERMACS report: special focus on framing the impact of adverse events. *J Heart Lung Transplant*. 2017;36:1080–1086.
57. Copeland JG, Smith RG, Arabia FA, et al. Investigators CardioWest Total Artificial HeartCardiac replacement with a total artificial heart as a bridge to transplantation. *N Engl J Med*. 2004;351:859–867.
58. Torregrossa G, Morshuis M, Varghese R, et al. Results with SynCardia total artificial heart beyond 1 year. *ASAIO J*. 2014;60:626–634.
59. Carpentier A, Latrémouille C, Cholley B, et al. First clinical use of a bioprosthetic total artificial heart: report of two cases. *Lancet*. 2015;386:1556–1563.
60. Latrémouille C, Carpentier A, Leprince P, et al. A bioprosthetic total artificial heart for end-stage heart failure: results from a pilot study. *J Heart Lung Transplant*. 2018;37:33–37.

Psychosocial and Quality of Life Issues in Mechanical Circulatory Support

Kathleen L. Grady, Mary Amanda Dew

KEY POINTS

Preimplantation Considerations
Psychosocial Outcomes During Mechanical Circulatory Support
Psychosocial Predictors of Clinical Outcomes During Mechanical Circulatory Support
Postimplantation and End-of-Life Considerations
Conclusions and Future Clinical and Research Directions

The use of mechanical circulatory support (MCS) as a long-term therapy for end-stage heart failure is associated with many psychosocial considerations for both patients and their families. These considerations span the process of care: they encompass factors including evaluation, informed consent, and decision-making before implantation; health-related quality of life (HRQOL) and behavioral outcomes during and after MCS implantation; impact of psychosocial factors on clinical outcomes after MCS implantation; and end-of-life concerns. Like many other medical interventions, the success of MCS is ultimately judged by its ability not only to prolong life but also to maximize psychosocial and physical well-being. Hence, it is critical for health care providers and researchers alike to understand the key psychosocial issues that emerge at each step in the process of MCS intervention, as well as the empirical evidence available regarding them. Better understanding of the issues and related evidence is important for improved education of patients and their families, especially since long-term MCS is a viable treatment option. It is also important for the development and evaluation of new strategies to maximize psychosocial outcomes in patients receiving MCS.

This chapter discusses the relevant psychosocial issues across the process of MCS intervention, organized according to the model depicted in Fig. 16.1. Issues are considered from the perspective of providing better clinical care, and research findings are noted that inform this care. In the final section of the chapter, the most pressing clinical and research concerns that must be addressed in future work on psychosocial factors in MCS are delineated. Throughout the chapter, although many psychosocial factors that are relevant to use of long-term MCS (i.e., MCS beyond the acute care setting) in all age groups are considered, the primary focus is on adult populations because of the increasing use of MCS in adults, either as a bridge to heart transplantation (BTT), bridge to transplantation candidacy (BTC), or permanent, "destination" therapy (DT).

PREIMPLANTATION CONSIDERATIONS

Whether patients receive long-term MCS is determined by multiple medical and psychosocial factors. Medical indications for MCS are discussed elsewhere in this book; reviewed here are the range of psychosocial factors that appear to influence access to and patient preferences for this treatment. Then, among patients undergoing evaluation for MCS, the psychosocial issues that must be assessed in determining eligibility for MCS implantation are delineated, and procedures for ensuring patient informed consent for this treatment option are discussed.

Disparities in Access to Mechanical Circulatory Support

Disparities in access to health care, including organ transplantation, have been well documented; there are enduring worldwide disparities based on race/ethnicity, sex, geographic region, and socioeconomic status.[1–3] Evidence suggests that similar psychosocial disparities exist for access to care for advanced heart disease, including MCS. Some disparities specific to MCS may have reflected technological limitations. For example, the larger fully implantable pulsatile devices that predominated in the 1990s and early 2000s were not compatible with female patients' typically smaller body habitus. However, despite the smaller size of current MCS devices, the proportion of MCS recipients who are women continues to underrepresent the proportion of women with advanced heart disease who could benefit from this therapy.[4]

Joyce and colleagues[5] provided the most comprehensive analysis to date of not only sex-related but also other psychosocial disparities in access to MCS. They examined a large national database on interventions used for patients aged 18 to 85 years hospitalized from 2002 to 2003 for congestive heart failure or cardiogenic shock. Patients with diagnoses that represented clear contraindications to MCS implantation were excluded. Results indicated that, even after controlling for severity of medical comorbidities, patients who were older than 65 years, female, and/or African American were less likely to receive MCS. There were also marked geographic variations, with patients from the western United States showing the highest likelihood of receiving MCS relative to all other regions. Geographic disparities have been similarly noted in other countries and have been attributed to patient mix, referral patterns, and the regional distribution of centers that perform MCS implanation.[6]

However, at least in the United States, Joyce and colleagues[5] found no evidence that regional differences in MCS implantation rates varied by patient medical factors, and such differences were maintained

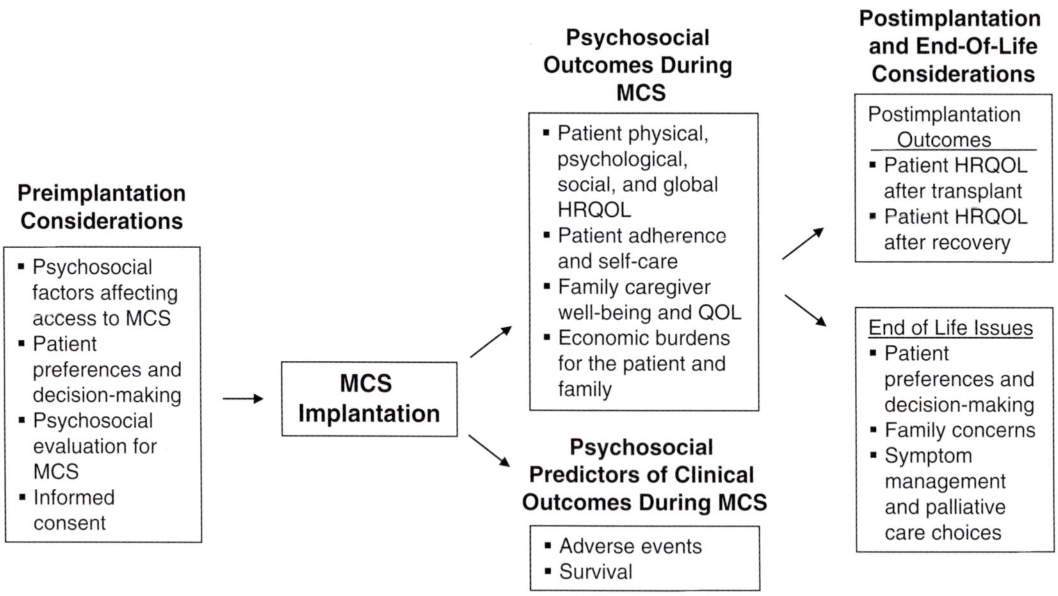

Fig. 16.1 Psychosocial factors at each stage of the mechanical circulatory support *(MCS)* process. *HRQOL*, Health-related quality of life; *QOL*, quality of life.

even after controlling for the distribution of academic medical centers (which were more likely than nonacademic centers to use MCS). Furthermore, the strong evidence of race disparities in this study was also independent of patient medical factors and other factors, including whether patients were admitted to an academic center. Interestingly, neither insurance status nor average income in the communities where patients resided affected their likelihood of receiving MCS. Neither characteristic affected the association of race with receipt of MCS.

The race and sex disparities in MCS uncovered to date likely stem from multiple factors, including referral practices and biases, uneven application of evidence-based guidelines, and patient preferences for care.[2,7] Patient preferences are addressed later; noted here is that further work is needed to delineate the underlying causes of unequal access to MCS so that appropriate steps can be taken to reduce or eliminate them. At least in the more general context of care for heart failure and cardiovascular disease, there is growing evidence that interventions that facilitate care provider adherence to clinical practice guidelines and algorithms can reduce some disparities in treatments offered to patients.[2,8]

Informed Consent

Informed consent is a process, not an event, followed by documentation of that process (i.e., signing of a consent form). This process has four basic elements: (1) decision-making capacity of the patient or surrogate, (2) disclosure of sufficient details of the proposed treatment by the physician, (3) demonstration of understanding of the disclosed information by the patient or surrogate, and (4) voluntary agreement to the treatment.[9] Importantly, this process is patient centric.

Decision-Making Capacity

Clinicians are responsible for ensuring decision-making capacity. The decision-making capacity of patients with advanced heart failure may be impaired due to mild cognitive decline, low health literacy, numeracy, and moods/emotions.[10,11] It is incumbent upon clinicians to screen for these impairments in at-risk patients and integrate strategies to address them. Informed consent may also be challenging if the patient's decision-making capacity is compromised (e.g., due to reduced level of consciousness or moderate to severe cognitive impairment) and the burden of consent falls to the next-of-kin, which is less than ideal. Families may experience decisional conflict and uncertainty about the best course of action especially if surgical risks are high and outcomes are uncertain and may be poor. Use of temporary MCS as a possible bridge to longer-term MCS or transplantation may provide time to stabilize the patient, evaluate next steps, and allow the family, and possibly the patient, time to consider options.[12] Advance directives can provide guidance for family members who must make emergent decisions regarding treatment options on behalf of a critically ill family member.

Informing Patients, Caregivers, and Families About Treatment Options

Informing patients with advanced heart failure (i.e., stage D heart failure) and their families about therapeutic options necessarily includes discussing the patient's current medical condition and disclosing risks, benefits, self-care, effect on lifestyle, financial costs, caregiver burden, and end-of-life considerations of the current medical plan. Conversations to inform patients about their current medical condition would include discussing advanced heart failure and its natural history (i.e., the trajectory of advanced heart failure and poor prognosis), the patient's current health status and prognosis, likelihood of increasing symptom burden and declining functional status, poor quality of life, caregiver burden, the potential for frequent hospital readmissions, and increasing costs of care.[12] Discussion of the current medical treatment plan typically includes optimization of heart failure therapies[13] and ongoing management of comorbidities. It is important that patients understand the risks and benefits of medical therapy, as well as the plan for continued care, which could include supportive care (e.g., palliative care and hospice). As the patient's heart failure worsens, discussion of new treatment options may be considered.

For patients who are hospitalized with acute heart failure, particularly if hospitalizations are recurrent, discussions would include modifications to the treatment plan (e.g., initiation of intravenous diuretics for refractory fluid retention, use of inotropes, and dose reduction or withdrawal of neurohormonal antagonists to manage symptomatic hypotension, azotemia) and use of temporary support (e.g., intraaortic balloon pumping or short-term percutaneous or extracorporeal support) in the event of refractory cardiogenic shock.[10,13]

Surgical treatment options (e.g., MCS), which are reasonable to consider for an individual patient, may also be discussed. When discussing the option of MCS, it is important to discuss benefits and risks for the specific device being recommended for implantation (overall and specific to the hospital where the device will be implanted) and the implant strategy (i.e., BTT, BTC, or DT). Potential benefits of improvement in survival, quality of life, and function need to be balanced with possible risks, including device-related adverse events such as bleeding, neurological events, pump thrombosis, and infections, as well as possible worsening of serious concurrent comorbidities or development of new life-threatening comorbid conditions.[14,15] Although, to some extent, risks will be patient specific, results from large published MCS trials should be included in these discussions. In addition, potential improvement in heart failure symptoms (e.g., decreased shortness of breath, peripheral edema, and fatigue), possible development of new MCS-related symptoms (e.g., bleeding, dizziness, and pain), and potential psychological morbidities (e.g., anxiety and depression) need to be discussed with patients.[16,17] Length of hospitalization, recovery, and hospital readmission after MCS implantation are also important topics.[14] Regarding implant strategy, patients need to understand that a given strategy might change after surgery. For example, patients who receive an implant as BTT and experience a catastrophic device-related complication may be removed from the waiting list for heart transplantation and the MCS device would remain in place until the end of the patient's life. On the other hand, patients may receive MCS as DT, but contraindications to transplantation may be reversed with device therapy, and listing for transplantation may then become an option. Finally, a discussion of device durability and the option of device replacement, if beneficial and desirable, is important at the time of initial implantation.[13]

Discussions regarding self-care and changes in lifestyle should include the topics of device management and troubleshooting, driveline dressing changes, permitted activities (e.g., return to work, home management, and driving), and activities that may not be permitted (e.g., immersion in water such as swimming). In addition, following a "heart-healthy" diet and being active, including participating in a formal rehabilitation program or home exercise program, are important topics of discussion. Furthermore, patients need to learn about important safety issues in the home environment and community, such as power supply, telephone services, and a plan for urgent/emergent return to the hospital. Financial costs associated with MCS implantation (including at the time of implantation and after discharge) are also important topics of discussion with patients and their families when deciding on therapeutic options.

Discussing end of life is difficult, but necessary, in the context of informing patients about MCS as a treatment option. When and how much information to share about end of life are individualized and based on patient characteristics (including patient preferences and goals), clinical risk factors (e.g., high surgical risk), and implant strategy. For example, a less detailed discussion of end of life may be undertaken for patients receiving MCS as BTT, whereas more information may be appropriate for patients who receive implantation as BTC or DT. An end-of-life conversation, at the appropriate time, includes a discussion of anticipated end-of-life trajectories, availability of hospice, and device deactivation.[14,18]

It is generally expected that patients on MCS will have caregivers in order to be discharged from the hospital.[12,19] Most caregiving for patients with major chronic illnesses is performed by family members.[20] Thus, caregivers and family members need to be informed about MCS, so that they can learn about the caregiving role (e.g., performing driveline dressing changes, troubleshooting device malfunction, providing transportation to follow-up appointments and tests, initiating plans for emergency return to the hospital for device-related complications, and often providing emotional support). Caregivers and family members also need to be informed about the possible impact of caregiving on their lives. For example, many device programs require that a device-trained person remain close to the patient at all times, which may be challenging if the device-trained person is also employed. Multiple caregivers may help mitigate this challenge. Finally, caregivers also need to be informed that they may experience psychological sequelae, which will be discussed in the section on family caregiver well-being and quality of life.

Understanding of Treatment Options

Challenges abound in determining patient understanding of discussions on treatment options. A variety of strategies have been used, including decision-making worksheets, more informative consent forms, standardized education, decision aids, and written tests and elicitation of oral feedback, which may simply be asking a patient to repeat what (s)he heard a clinician say.[9] Discussions with multidisciplinary team members (e.g., cardiologists, surgeons, ventricular assist device coordinators, palliative care teams, psychologists, dietitians, and social workers) are beneficial as each team member focuses on different aspects of informing patients about MCS. Additionally, advanced heart failure patients considering MCS are often encouraged to visit with a current MCS patient, to learn about MCS from a "lived experience" perspective. Participation in support groups, when available, is also highly encouraged. Written information and videos regarding device management, troubleshooting, and dressing change procedures, as well as illustrations of the device, are important educational supplements during the informed consent process. Patients also may want to see the actual hardware and accessories. It is important to recognize the possibility of influence or bias (i.e., bias toward accepting MCS therapy), without adequate discussion of risks, alternative options, and caregiver considerations when sharing information.[21]

Agreement to Treatment Options

Finally, agreement to a treatment option assumes voluntariness that is free from manipulation or coercion (i.e., the decision is made autonomously). This final element of informed consent is predicated on the first three elements (i.e., decision-making capacity, full disclosure of treatment options, and understanding).

After being fully informed of available therapeutic options, some patients with advanced heart failure choose medical therapy, which may be viewed as a refusal of lifesaving therapy. Patients with decision-making capacity who understand the risks and benefits of medical therapy and the consequences of refusing MCS device implantation are, of course, free to make this choice. Understanding patient values, preferences, goals, culture, and background may help to clarify the patient's choice of continuing medical therapies or undergoing MCS implantation.[10]

Patient and Family Preferences and Decision-Making

With the shift from physician- to patient-centric informed consent, advanced heart failure patient decision-making regarding the treatment options of continuing medical therapies or agreeing to MCS implantation requires not only that clinicians fully inform patients about treatment options but also that patients share their values and preferences for treatment with clinicians, hence the term "shared decision-making." Shared decision-making has four components: (1) at minimum, two participants (i.e., a clinician and patient), (2) sharing of information by both participants, (3) consensus building about the preferred treatment, and (4) agreement on the treatment to be implemented.[11] These components are the pillars of shared decision-making and as a whole, can build trust, enhance readiness for decision-making, align treatment options with desired outcomes, and reduce the potential for and resolve conflict.[10] Given the complexities and trajectory of advanced heart failure and high-stakes nature of MCS, ideally, shared decision-making is an iterative process that evolves over time, as the patient's condition changes and patient values, preferences, and goals are clarified.[10] The value of the iterative nature of this process is also supported by literature that suggests that advanced heart failure patient preferences for desired outcomes can change over time.[22]

Sharing of information is predicated on effective communication between participants that is clear and accurate. Sometimes, patients have preexisting notions or do not understand information being shared (e.g., about their health status and prognosis), which can result in misconceptions. In a study of ambulatory patients with heart failure, patients overestimated their life expectancy compared with model-based predictions for survival, using the Seattle Heart Failure Model.[23] Furthermore, greater disease severity (i.e., higher New York Heart Association [NYHA] class and lower ejection fraction) was independently related to overestimation of life expectancy. Reasons for this discordance in heart failure patient versus model estimates of survival were not clear but may have included inadequate communication between clinicians and patients, patient-specific factors (e.g., hope and optimism), and language or cultural barriers.[23] The researchers suggested that a better understanding of prognosis and life expectancy may be important to decision-making about advanced cardiac therapies, including MCS. In follow-up, this research team conducted a qualitative, descriptive study using semistructured interviews with patients diagnosed with heart failure ($n = 24$) to explore their perceptions of model-based survival estimates.[24] They determined that the majority of these patients wanted individualized prognostic survival estimates (preferably early in their disease history), recognized the uncertainty associated with these estimates, and viewed these estimates as providing hope and control rather than provoking anxiety.[24]

Similarly, heart failure patients need to communicate their values, preferences, and goals. Regarding the option of MCS, clinicians might ask specific questions, such as "What do you hope to get from MCS surgery?" "What are you willing to give up when you get MCS surgery?" Ask-tell-ask is one of many useful communication techniques that can be used to engage patients and families in shared decision-making conversations.[25]

There is a growing body of evidence about shared decision-making in patients with advanced heart failure who are considering MCS as a treatment option. McIlvennan and colleagues[26] explored the decision-making processes of advanced heart failure patients considering MCS by conducting in-depth interviews with 22 patients ($n = 15$ who had DT MCS implantation and $n = 7$ who declined device implant). The majority of those agreeing to MCS implant used an "automatic" decision process, while some agreeing to implant and all decliners used a more "reflective" process. Patients using an "automatic" decision process cited fear of dying and wanting to live as long as possible, noting that they "had no choice." DT MCS decision-making with minimal deliberation has been reported by other researchers.[27] In contrast, decliners often reflected on the meaning of their lives, indicated that they did not fear death, but saw it as an option, and considered options based on their preferences for quality versus quantity of life. In a qualitative study of DT MCS decision-making and implications for caregivers ($n = 17$), researchers reported that caregivers often placed the needs of their loved one ahead of their own needs, and some caregivers indicated that they felt pressure to make a decision quickly.[28]

Decision aids, designed to improve patient decision-making,[29] are available for use with patients considering both medical and surgical treatment options. Thompson and colleagues[30] reported on the creation of decision aids for patients considering DT MCS. Using International Patient Decision Aid Standard guidelines,[31] they created both paper and video DT MCS decision aids and tested them for acceptability (i.e., readability, bias, and usability). These decision aids were recently assessed by this team for effectiveness in a multisite randomized trial of 248 patients who were considering the option of DT MCS.[32] Allen and colleagues[32] determined that these decision aids improved patient knowledge and concordance between stated values and treatment choice at 1 month after implantation but did not improve concordance between stated values and actual treatment at 6 months.

An understanding of patient decision-making can also be gained through examining regret. Regret is "remorse or distress over a decision."[33] In a study of decision-making regarding MCS implantation, Blumenthal-Barby and colleagues[27] interviewed MCS candidates and MCS patients and their caregivers (overall $n = 45$) and reported low levels of decisional regret, indicating that most patients and caregivers made decisions that were consistent with their values.

Psychosocial Evaluation for Mechanical Circulatory Support

Earlier, the issue of psychosocial disparities in access to MCS was addressed—that is, the issue of who is evaluated for device implantation. Although disparities in *access* are inherently unfair and unethical, MCS programs must legitimately weigh psychosocial as well as medical factors for each candidate for MCS therapy to appropriately *select* patients mostly likely to benefit from device implantation. Psychosocial factors must also be examined to determine whether psychological, behavioral, or other psychosocial interventions might usefully be offered to patients to increase their chances of favorable outcomes after MCS implantation.

The specific components of the psychosocial evaluation have received limited attention in the MCS literature. This is in contrast to the extensive scrutiny that other medical factors have received as potential criteria for the selection of patients for MCS.[12] In general, the factors typically evaluated in potential transplantation candidates are also viewed as important for the evaluation of candidates for MCS.[34–37] These elements are listed in Table 16.1 and include lifetime mental health and substance use histories; past and current level of adherence to medical regimens; cognitive status and ability to give informed consent; social history and current status, including financial circumstances; the availability of a primary family caregiver and general support from the family; and knowledge about current illness and treatment options.

An additional element that requires special consideration in MCS candidates concerns patients' understanding of and capacity (both physical and cognitive) to operate the MCS device.[12,37] Moreover, the safety of the home environment must be considered, and factors including whether reliable electricity is available and whether the home is accessible by health care personnel must be determined. Assessment of these issues can be critical for decisions about patient educational needs, for patient/family preparation for patients to live outside of the hospital with MCS, and ultimately, for decisions about patients' eligibility for MCS.

Among the remaining elements, psychiatric and substance use history, general cognitive status, medical adherence history, and the presence of a family caregiver are most often noted as important for team decisions about patients' need for psychosocial interventions or referrals for additional more extensive evaluation (regarding psychiatric or cognitive status, for example).[34–37] These factors are also critical for team decisions about patient eligibility for MCS. For example, patients must have the cognitive capacity to understand the risks and benefits associated with MCS and any other treatment options. They must also have strong social supports: the presence of a family caregiver and

TABLE 16.1 Components of the Psychosocial Evaluation of Candidates for Mechanical Circulatory Support

Component	Areas Addressed
Mental health history and current status	Mood and anxiety disorders; suicidal ideation or past attempts; psychosis; personality disorders; treatment history
Substance use history and current status	Quantity, frequency, duration, and recency of use of alcohol, tobacco, and other substances; diagnosable disorder and level of impairment in daily life; treatment and rehabilitation history
Adherence history and current status	Adherence to components of previous and current treatment regimens for heart disease or other chronic health conditions; understanding of rationale for current regimen
Cognitive functioning and capacity	Orientation in person, time, and place; appearance and affect; evidence of impairments that would affect capacity to understand what will be required for care during MCS and (if relevant) after transplantation; capacity to give informed consent
Social history and current status	Demographics, including employment and financial circumstances; marital status; living arrangements; coping strategies for managing health issues; religious beliefs and orientation; concurrent stressors (work related, home related, other); literacy and health literacy
Family caregiver availability and general family supports	Presence of a family member to provide care and assistance on a daily basis; emotional supportiveness of family or close friends; understanding by family of patient's health situation
Understanding of current illness and treatment options	Perceptions of medical condition; perceptions of health-related impairments in daily life; understanding of the risks and benefits of MCS; understanding of the transplant process (if relevant); attitudes and expectations about MCS, including preferences and goals
Capacity to operate MCS device	Understanding of basic device operation; physical and cognitive capacity to operate the device and respond to alerts/alarms; safety of the home environment for MCS operation

MCS, Mechanical circulatory support.

availability of other supports from the family and friends are essential for guaranteeing that patients can be safely discharged to home after device implantation. Strong caregiver availability and support may mitigate potential limitations that patients may have in other areas. For example, patients with limitations in their ability to operate the MCS device may be acceptable candidates if they have extensive supports and assistance for daily functioning.

When considering psychosocial factors as eligibility criteria, it is important to distinguish whether patients are being considered for BTT, BTC, or DT. If MCS is to be used for BTT, the psychosocial criteria for transplantation candidacy would be relevant, albeit with some modifications. For example, a greater emphasis is usually placed on ensuring the availability of a family caregiver during the period of MCS, compared with the family caregiver requirements typical for transplantation eligibility. In addition, although abstinence from substance use is often important for MCS eligibility, the required duration of abstinence may be less than that typical for transplantation candidates, most often because of the urgent need for MCS. The duration requirement might instead affect whether the MCS device is implanted as BTC versus BTT. Thus, if a patient could not meet transplantation eligibility criteria regarding duration of abstinence before MCS implantation (e.g., due to medical urgency) or needed to demonstrate an enduring ability to adhere to treatment requirements, the psychosocial evaluation might result in a patient receiving MCS as BTC. Once the duration criteria are met, the patient might transition to BTT. In this regard, it is noteworthy that patients defined as BTC based on the Interagency Registry for Mechanically Assisted Circulatory Support (INTERMACS) database between 2006 and 2011 were considerably more likely to have current substance use/abuse at the time of implantation than were BTT patients.[38]

It has been argued that patients being considered for DT may require a somewhat different approach in the application of any psychosocial criteria, compared to BTT and BTC patients.[35] DT patients are, by definition, not candidates for heart transplantation. Thus, the psychosocial criteria applied for heart transplantation eligibility—which evolved in response to the need to maximize the utility of scarce donor organs—may be only partially relevant. Because MCS devices are not in short supply, there may be few compelling reasons to deny patients DT based on factors that would generally preclude transplantation candidacy (e.g., continued substance use).[13,35] For patients being considered for DT, the goal of applying psychosocial criteria should be to determine if patients are able, when drawing on the full range of resources that can be mustered for them, to live with MCS and manage (usually with family caregiver assistance) their complex care regimen at home. A complication, however, in "relaxing" the application of psychosocial criteria for DT patients is that some of these patients may in fact ultimately be considered for transplantation. Under such circumstances, patients would require a new evaluation of their psychosocial eligibility for transplantation, and the psychosocial standards more typically applied for transplantation candidacy then would become relevant.

PSYCHOSOCIAL OUTCOMES DURING MECHANICAL CIRCULATORY SUPPORT

Psychosocial outcomes after MCS encompass all components of patient HRQOL, as well as behavioral outcomes related to medical adherence and self-care.[39] HRQOL is multifaceted and includes physical functional well-being, emotional and social functioning, and global quality of life perceptions. In the following sections, evidence regarding patient HRQOL and behavioral outcomes is considered, and evidence concerning family caregiver well-being is summarized. Finally, the economic burdens experienced by patients and families are important issues to address insofar as the financial costs associated with MCS ultimately may affect access to this treatment and preferences for it versus other intervention strategies.

Patient Health-Related Quality of Life

Physical Functional Health-Related Quality of Life

Over the past 20 years, there has been consistent evidence that both objective measures (e.g., exercise capacity) and subjective measures of physical functioning (e.g., perceived functional status) improve with MCS. Such improvements were noted with the earlier pulsatile devices and continue to be observed with the smaller continuous-flow devices in use today.[17,40–44] Once patients have recovered from the immediate effects of implantation, the majority become fully ambulatory and are able to engage in routine activities of daily living.[45–49] Regardless of whether they received implantation as BTT or DT, they showed marked improvements over their preimplantation baseline in functional status (e.g., NYHA class and distance traveled in the 6-minute walk test) and physiologic parameters (e.g., mean oxygen consumption levels, resting cardiac output, and mean arterial pressure).[44–48,50–56] Reviews of the literature indicate that, among patients receiving MCS implantation, objectively assessed functional status and patients' perceptions of physical well-being are better than those of individuals receiving optimal medical management.[17,40–42] Nevertheless, MCS patients' physical functioning, on average, remains poorer than that observed after heart transplantation, no matter whether it is assessed by subjective perceptions or objective performance measures.[57,58]

An important issue is whether and how patients' physical functional HRQOL continues to change over time after implantation. Among patients receiving MCS as BTT, Grady and coworkers[59] found reductions in self-reported bothersome physical symptoms as early as 2 weeks after implantation, and recent reviews including studies of both BTT and DT cohorts document sustained or continued gains in patient-reported overall physical functioning and satisfaction with physical status across the first 1 to 2 years postimplantation.[17,40] With regard to objective indices of physical functioning, it appears that improvement plateaus after the first several months postimplantation, although exercise-based interventions appear modestly successful at further improving these outcomes.[60]

Despite the physical functional HRQOL benefits, MCS recipients remain impaired, on average, relative to normative, "healthy" populations.[44] Furthermore, patients on MCS report significant physical functional difficulties and concerns in some areas. They frequently describe the onset of new physical symptoms after implantation, arising primarily from device-related adverse events. The majority of MCS recipients experience adverse events, the most common of which are bleeding, infections, and neurological events.[17,61] These events frequently lead to rehospitalizations, with attendant physical deconditioning and functional decline. Complications such as stroke can lead to permanent physical disability, as well as shortened survival time.[46,62–64] Patients report significant worries about the risk for these complications and resulting physical impairments.[41,65–67] With respect to device-related symptoms, patients frequently report pain at the driveline exit site and difficulties sleeping due to the position of the driveline and may have concerns about and reduced satisfaction related to sexual activity due to worries about disrupting the positioning of the driveline.[65–70] These subjectively reported symptoms can be objectively documented. For example, Casida and colleagues[69,70] found that MCS patients not only reported poor sleep quality but also had marked sleep disruptions based on actigraphy.

Finally, it is noteworthy that studies reporting improvements in physical functional HRQOL over time focus on patients who are able to provide ongoing HRQOL data. The risk for morbidities and mortality in MCS patients remains high. Patients who are too ill or become too ill to provide HRQOL data are not captured in most studies' analyses, and thus, physical functional HRQOL levels described among patients at 1 to 2 years postimplantation may be biased.[17,40,41] The most accurate conclusion from work to date may be that physical functional HRQOL *can* show dramatic, sustained gains over time among patients on MCS, although this potential may not be achieved by all patients. Continued advances in MCS technology and patient medical management strategies may ensure that increasing proportions of patients experience these gains. Regarding patient management, it appears essential that MCS programs either provide their own exercise and rehabilitation services or overcome insurance-related or other barriers to referral of patients to external cardiac rehabilitation programs.[44]

Psychological Health-Related Quality of Life

Psychological HRQOL encompasses emotional well-being as well as cognitive functioning. HRQOL in this domain improves with MCS, although the improvements are less striking than those observed in the physical functioning domain.[41,43] With respect to emotional well-being, small case series and qualitative reports suggest that some patients' preimplantation psychological distress levels do not abate or are high after MCS implantation.[71–73] However, reports of larger cohorts (either with the earlier pulsatile devices or with continuous-flow devices) have noted that, on average, levels of depression and anxiety-related symptoms show significant and clinically significant reductions from before to after device implantation.[47,48,52,74–77] These improvements in psychological well-being have been observed even after controlling for factors such as patients' age and severity of illness at the time of device implantation.[47,75,76] Among patients able to be reassessed over time, the improvements in distress levels appear to continue or are at least maintained during the first year of MCS.[52,76,78] Among patients on BTT MCS, once they recover from the initial effects of device implantation, their emotional well-being is better and shows greater improvement from baseline (presurgical) levels compared to patients receiving optimal medical management without MCS.[48,52] However, their psychological HRQOL appears poorer than that of heart transplant recipients[41,79] and is lower than normative levels in healthy populations.[41,79,80]

The occurrence of adverse events during MCS appears to have major impact on patients' psychological HRQOL, and psychological distress is strongly linked to worries over the potential for adverse events or recurrences of those events.[66,67,72] The presence of a diagnosable psychiatric disorder, including mood and anxiety disorders, is common in patients on MCS, with up to 80% experiencing at least one episode of disorder during MCS.[34,73,81,82] Commonly reported psychological stressors include concerns about device malfunction and failure.[65–67,72]

The sensitivity of psychological HRQOL to adverse events postimplantation (and in BTT patients, the uncertainty regarding whether and when transplantation will occur) has led to consensus recommendations that patients on MCS should be routinely monitored for psychiatric symptoms.[12] Moreover, given effective treatments for many psychiatric disorders, it is important to promptly initiate treatment with psychotropic medications and other psychological and behavioral interventions for mental health problems once these conditions are identified.[12,34]

Although there is little empirical work past the first 1 to 2 years of MCS, case reports and small case series indicate that as the duration of support lengthens, patients whose emotional well-being improved initially during MCS may go on to show pronounced declines in psychological status. These declines appear closely linked to physical health declines.[41,73,83,84] For example, Tigges-Limmer and colleagues[84] report the suicide of a patient on MCS at approximately 3 years postimplantation after a period of marked deterioration in his physical health, and despite intensive psychiatric treatment.

Cognitive functioning is also an integral component of psychological HRQOL in patients on MCS, and cognitive status has an important impact on patients' ability to function independently. Although cognitive impairments are common in patients with end-stage heart disease, including those awaiting heart transplantation, there has been limited examination of how cognitive functioning is affected by treatment with MCS.[12,85] However, because neurologic events during MCS remain relatively prevalent and can be devastating, MCS patients are at risk for new, irreversible cognitive impairments.[83,85] Whether these impairments are linked to the MCS per se or are complications associated with cardiac surgery can be difficult to determine. Nevertheless, new cognitive impairments remain problematic in the MSC population.

It is therefore noteworthy that some reports have documented statistically significant, although mild, improvements in several domains of cognitive functioning (e.g., visuospatial and executive function) across the first 6 to 8 months in patients receiving BTT MCS and across as long as 24 months after patients received DT MCS.[86,87,88] These reports noted no significant declines in any domain evaluated. These results are encouraging, although they must be tempered by the fact that, as noted earlier, patients who were too ill could not be reassessed. Thus, the findings may reflect the levels of cognitive functioning attainable in the absence of major neurologic insult.

Social Health-Related Quality of Life

Social functioning has presented assessment challenges in patients on MCS, perhaps because of the wide array of activities and concerns encompassed within this domain. Rather than systematic assessment, the literature is characterized by anecdotal and relatively general comments that patients receiving MCS are able to perform regular activities of daily living, engage in various leisure activities (e.g., going to restaurants, gardening, and engaging in sports), travel, return to work or school, or otherwise have an "active lifestyle."[89,90]

The few studies that have empirically examined patients' ability to perform activities of daily living (including outcomes in both patients receiving pulsatile support and those with continuous flow devices) find that functioning improves from preimplantation to postimplantation[61] and show continued gains with time.[47,49,78] However, satisfaction with functioning and with social relationships appears to remain stable or may even decline with time. For example, Grady and colleagues[78] observed that by the end of the first year of MCS, satisfaction with interpersonal relationships declined somewhat, and patients reported increased limitations in their ability to engage in social interactions. There have been few recent comparisons of social functioning in MCS patients versus patients receiving medical management alone, transplant recipients, or normative samples. It appears that social functioning is better in MCS recipients than in medically managed patients[48,57] but may be poorer than that in transplant recipients.[57,91]

Additional qualitative studies shed light on why social functioning may not show the large and sustained gains noted in other areas of HRQOL, such as physical functioning, and may appear poorer than for transplant recipients. Such work reveals the importance that patients place on structuring their daily lives so as to maintain a sense of control over their general ability to function and interact with others, and they focus on normalizing their lives through specific routines and activities.[71] Nevertheless, patients may come to realize that, despite their improved physical status, they are in fact unable to resume social roles that they once had (e.g., returning to work) and that the ever-present device limits feelings of "normalcy."[66,92] Many patients dislike the need to rely on others for assistance with daily activities and wish that they could achieve more complete independence during MCS.[66,72] Patients may feel limited by factors such as restrictions on driving, which promote continued dependence on others.[42,66]

On the other hand, qualitative studies have noted that patients may experience social benefits that were unexpected and positive, including deeper intimate connections with their sexual partners.[92] It was noted earlier that patients may have concerns about their physical ability to engage in sexual activity, but this must be balanced against findings that MCS recipients may feel emotionally closer to their partners, as well as to other family members, after they recover from implantation surgery.[43,92] At the same time, body image—including distress over one's surgical scars and seeing the device driveline—is also an important issue as patients attempt to return to daily activities and interactions with others.[66,72]

Global Health-Related Quality of Life

Particularly in recent clinical trials and large series of patients on MCS, only global indices, rather than domain-specific evaluations of HRQOL, are reported. Thus, patients may be asked to complete multi-item measures that include items reflecting the full range of HRQOL (usually in the context of living with heart disease), and then a global score is computed. Alternatively, patients may be asked simply to rate their overall HRQOL. Either way, the result is a composite view that has the advantage of reflecting the "big picture" from the patient's perspective, but that has the disadvantage of not allowing for the identification of specific areas that might be uniquely problematic for patients on MCS.

With this caveat in mind, it is noteworthy that global HRQOL generally has been found to show (1) clinically significant improvements from preimplantation to postimplantation in patients receiving both BTT and DT,[a] (2) sustained or continued improvements over time during MCS, at least during the first several years of support,[b] and (3) large advantages relative to equally ill patients who did not receive MCS.[52,57,58] Nevertheless, global HRQOL in MCS patients appears poorer than that observed in transplant recipients.[57]

Given the evidence that there are important HRQOL domain-specific limitations and concerns linked to MCS, it is essential to supplement global HRQOL information with specific examination of patient self-reports in the separate physical functional, psychological, and social domains. In addition, the factors that may contribute to global HRQOL perceptions may differ from those that are the strongest determinants of domain-specific HRQOL. For example, Brouwers and colleagues[80] found that the important correlates of mental/emotional HRQOL (e.g., female sex, and being unemployed) were not significant correlates of patients' perceived global HRQOL or their physical functional HRQOL.

Patient Medical Adherence and Self-Care

Adherence to the postimplantation medical and self-care regimen is a domain of psychosocial outcomes distinct from patient HRQOL. Most MCS recipients are discharged to home, where they are expected to engage in a variety of self-care and monitoring activities, including those related to basic device management, medication taking, and lifestyle requirements (e.g., smoking cessation), and they must participate in required clinical follow-up.[96,97]

Several qualitative reports delineate patients' concerns and worries about their abilities to engage in self-care but suggest that feelings of confidence and self-efficacy for performing such activities increase with duration of MCS.[66,72,92] The literature on self-care and adherence to the MCS regimen is small. However, there is evidence that patients' perceptions of their ability to engage in self-care can improve with MCS implantation,[47,61,78] although this is not always observed.[48] Casida and colleagues[98] examined adherence to the postimplantation regimen, reporting that adherence levels were high and did not vary by duration of MCS. Independence in self-care (i.e., ability to manage requirements without caregiver assistance) appeared to be slightly higher in patients who had MCS for longer durations, although the differences were not significant. Greater adherence was associated with better global HRQOL.

[a] References 47–49, 52, 56, 57, 64, 93.
[b] References 45, 46, 56, 61, 93–95.

Family Caregiver Well-Being and Quality of Life

The impact of MCS extends well beyond the patient, to encompass the primary family caregiver and other family members. Given family caregivers' role in assisting and providing emotional support to MCS recipients, it is important to understand both the benefits and burdens experienced by family members in order to develop educational strategies and to implement interventions to minimize strain on the family.

A recent review summarized both the growing qualitative and quantitative literatures on family caregiver outcomes.[99] Three central findings were noted. First, caregivers experience significant psychological distress that may be as high as or higher than that observed in MCS recipients. This distress is related to concerns about the patient, concerns about the caregiver's ability to assist the patient, and worries about the caregiver's ability to maintain employment and other social roles. Second, caregivers report considerable burden in providing care to the MCS recipient. This burden can be associated with feelings of social isolation and may lead to declines in caregivers' physical health and well-being. Third, caregivers develop new coping strategies and approaches to manage the tasks they have adopted in caring for the MCS recipient. The use of such strategies may mitigate caregivers' psychological distress.

Many of the studies included in the review by Cicollini and colleagues[99] were cross-sectional reports. A recent prospective study therefore adds to these findings by showing that, while MCS recipient global HRQOL and depression and anxiety symptoms showed significant improvement from preimplantation to postimplantation, their family caregivers' global HRQOL worsened and the caregivers' levels of depression and anxiety showed no change.[74] This report followed patient-caregiver dyads only through the first 3 months postimplantation; it would be important to determine if trends for these HRQOL indicators changed with longer follow-up. Other caregiver outcomes, including perceived caregiving burden, were not examined.

Economic Burdens for the Patient and Family

Given the prevalence of heart failure in the United States, it is not surprising that the economic burden of heart failure is substantial.[100] Costs of heart failure can be especially high for patients with advanced heart failure who become refractory to medical therapies and undergo MCS implantation either as BTT or DT. Seo et al.[101] conducted a systematic review of the cost effectiveness of MCS as BTT versus heart transplantation without a bridge, reporting that overall, posttransplant survival and adverse events did not differ between groups, and use of MCS as BTT may be cost-effective, especially for patients with prolonged wait times who are at risk for poor outcomes while awaiting transplant. Using Markov modeling, Rogers et al.[102] determined that compared to medically managed advanced heart failure patients, the 5-year costs of continuous-flow MCS as DT were higher ($62,856 vs. $360,407, respectively). Notably, these authors suggest that MCS costs have decreased from costs associated with first-generation devices, due to improved survival, decreased costs of implantation, and improved functional ability of patients. At 5 years, gain in quality-adjusted life years was also higher in the MCS group (1.87) versus the medically managed group (0.37).[102] Rogers et al.[102] concluded that, overall, the cost-effectiveness of continuous flow DT MCS has improved.

While cost-effectiveness has improved, other studies suggest that MCS is probably still not cost-effective, as per generally accepted thresholds, and that refinement of patient selection, reduction in device/surgical costs, improvement in MCS technology, reduction in adverse events, and improvement in quality of life are needed to further enhance cost-effectiveness.[103–105] Selection criteria that incorporate both need and potential risk for poor outcomes after surgery can contribute to reduced costs of care. The US Centers for Medicare and Medical Services developed "acceptance criteria" as part of the Joint Commission advanced disease-specific care certification requirements for DT MCS (Box 16.1).[85] Lastly, guidelines for care of patients with MCS may help to reduce adverse events and improve outcomes and thus potentially reduce costs of care.[12]

BOX 16.1 Requirements Specific to Ventricular Assist Device Destination Therapy

Acceptance Criteria

- Patients who have an anticipated survival benefit
- Patients with New York Heart Association functional classification class IV heart failure symptoms who have failed to respond to optimal medical management
- Patients with a demonstrated functional limitation with a peak oxygen consumption of 14 mL/kg/min or less
- Patients with a continued need for intravenous inotropic therapy
- Patients who have been evaluated for heart transplant and were not selected as candidates

Individualized costs specific to patients and families deserve comment. It is imperative to discuss costs (both inpatient and outpatient) with patients and families before implant. Depending on insurance and governmental coverage plans, many patients and families may not be able to bear the economic burden of MCS. Discussion of potential cost and the individual patient's insurance coverage for MCS is greatly aided by a knowledgeable social worker and/or financial clearance officer of the program. After implantation, patients and families may experience significant economic stress and burden, especially if family members are expected to function as caregivers yet must also work. Thus, economic burden can be related to the direct costs of medical care and indirect costs of potentially lost wages.

Studies in the heart failure literature suggest that enhancing patient self-care is related to a reduction in heart failure hospitalizations and all-cause hospitalizations, although there was little or no actual measurement of self-care.[106,107] Another study demonstrated that patient self-care was related to direct heart failure inpatient costs.[108] Evidence of this relationship has not been found in the MCS literature. However, strategies to enhance MCS patient self-care and effective caregiver assistance may contribute to safe (and perhaps early) discharge to the community and reduce the incidence of hospital readmission, which would ultimately contribute to cost savings. An understanding of the relationships among MCS patient self-care, caregiver assistance, and costs of care is needed.

PSYCHOSOCIAL PREDICTORS OF CLINICAL OUTCOMES DURING MECHANICAL CIRCULATORY SUPPORT

Earlier, the psychosocial factors that are routinely assessed in psychosocial evaluations of candidates for MCS were discussed. Their assessment is important in part because of growing evidence showing that these factors predict postimplantation morbidities and mortality. Illustrative findings include the following:

- MCS recipients with a preimplantation history of *nonadherence to medical directives* are at higher risk for adverse events, such as pump thrombosis.[109]
- A preimplantation history of *depression* is associated with higher postimplantation risks for infections and rehospitalizations.[110,111]
- Preimplantation *tobacco use* and *alcohol/drug abuse* increases the risk for use of these substances postimplantation.[112] Moreover,

smoking tobacco increases the risks for postimplantation morbidities, including pump thrombosis and gastrointestinal bleeding,[109,113] as well as mortality.[114] Alcohol and drug abuse increases the risks for postimplantation driveline infections and rehospitalizations[111,112] and mortality.[112]

- Patients with stronger *social supports* before MCS implantations have a lower postimplantation mortality risk.[115] MCS recipients whose primary family support person exits the caregiver role have a higher 30-day hospital readmissions rate.[116]
- Patients with lower *global HRQOL* before implantation have poorer survival postimplantation[47]; those rated lower *across elements of the pre-MCS psychosocial evaluation* are at greater risk for rehospitalization after implantation.[117]

POSTIMPLANTATION AND END-OF-LIFE CONSIDERATIONS

Compared with the range of psychosocial issues considered before and during MCS, more limited attention has been directed to outcomes beyond the period of MCS or at the terminal phases of such support. For BTT patients or for patients able to recover and found not to require transplantation, outcomes after explantation comprise a critical component of the cost-benefit analysis of MCS. For all patients on MCS, psychosocial issues that arise at the end of life also deserve careful attention, not only from the standpoint of preparing patients and their families but also to educate health professionals about issues of concern in this patient population.

Postimplantation Outcomes

Patient Health-Related Quality of Life After Heart Transplantation

Two psychosocial issues have been considered in patients transplanted after MCS. The first concerns whether transplantation provides further HRQOL benefits to MCS recipients (who have already likely attained significant HRQOL gains during MCS). A cross-sectional comparison of posttransplant HRQOL in BTT patients versus patients currently on MCS indicated a trend for HRQOL advantages in the transplant recipients.[91] More definitive evidence comes from longitudinal studies: by 3 months after transplantation, objectively assessed physical functional capacity (i.e., exercise capacity) exceeded that observed in the same patients at 3 months after MCS implantation.[118] Similar advantages were seen in a study of patient-reported physical and psychological HRQOL.[119] However, social HRQOL did not show further gains, and transplantation was associated with heightened self-reported stress related to adherence and self-care activities.[91] Grady and colleagues[119] speculated that new medical regimen requirements may contribute to transplant recipients' greater perceived stress. In patients formerly on MCS, qualitative studies also note a shift in focus after transplantation from daily life with heart failure to the need to learn new, permanent routines.[72]

A second issue for posttransplantation HRQOL outcomes concerns how BTT patients' outcomes compare with those of transplant recipients who did not require MCS. Dew and coworkers[120,121] found that during the first year of posttransplantation, BTT patients and those who had not required MCS showed similar and significant improvements in physical functional HRQOL. Psychological HRQOL was also similar and was either stable or improved in both groups. However, the posttransplantation cognitive status of the BTT patients was significantly poorer, and BTT patients (particularly those with poorer cognitive status) were less likely to return to employment. Whether there are HRQOL differences beyond the first year posttransplantation is unclear. One report found no differences in psychological HRQOL between patients who had and patients who had not required MCS before transplantation,[79] while another study noted that BTT patients had better posttransplantation HRQOL in some physical and psychological areas.[122] Neither study examined HRQOL controlling for posttransplant medical complications, which may have contributed to the differences between these studies' findings.

Bunzel and associates[65] studied not only transplant recipients who had been BTT but also their spouses. Interestingly, although no BTT patients developed posttraumatic stress disorder (PTSD) after transplantation, over one-fourth of the spouses developed PTSD. However, without any non-BTT comparison group of heart recipients and caregivers, it is difficult to infer that stressors related to MCS led to caregiver PTSD, and there may have been other transplantation-related factors that triggered this disorder. PTSD has been observed at about the same rate in other samples of caregivers to heart transplant recipients, independent of whether the recipients had required MCS.[123] Nevertheless, Bunzel and colleagues' work[65] points to the need for a better understanding of caregiver as well as MCS patient outcomes after transplantation.

Patient Health-Related Quality of Life After Recovery From Mechanical Circulatory Support

The same psychosocial concerns about posttransplantation outcomes are relevant to patients on MCS who recover sufficiently that their device can be explanted. To date, however, there has been very limited consideration of this group—most likely because recovery and explantation remain rare.[60] Nevertheless, outcomes appear promising, particularly for objectively assessed physical functional capacity. For example, recent work indicates that explanted patients can achieve capacity levels similar to healthy controls.[124] Impact on patient-reported HRQOL is less clear. One report of a small case series of explanted patients found that their HRQOL showed very few impairments.[125] A second study identified nonsignificant trends indicating more favorable HRQOL in explanted patients (who were generally within 1 year of explant) than in patients who continued on MCS.[91] A report examining patients several years after explant found that they showed better psychological but not physical HRQOL compared to heart recipients never requiring MCS. However, their HRQOL levels resembled those of BTT patients who had received transplants.[122] A qualitative report noted that explanted patients were particularly likely to appreciate the greater independence they now had in their daily lives, and they felt that the sense of uncertainty experienced during MCS had been removed.[72] Quality-of-life concerns or benefits among caregivers to these individuals have not been identified.

Palliative Care, Hospice, and End-of-Life Considerations

Palliative Care and Hospice Consultation

Palliative care aims to enhance patient quality of life and reduce suffering through treatment of symptoms and initiation of interventions that address physical, psychosocial, and spiritual needs, as well as support families.[14] The palliative care service is often consulted during evaluation for MCS, especially DT MCS, at which time they may participate in shared health care decision-making. Importantly, palliative care is provided concurrently with disease-modifying medical and surgical therapies.[13] When MCS patients experience serious adverse events and increasing symptoms after device implantation, palliative care interventions may be increasingly integrated into care.[126] For MCS patients who are nearing the end of life, it is reasonable to initiate a referral to hospice services, so that collaboratively with MCS team members, a plan for end-of-life care can be developed.[126,127] End-of-life care planning includes symptom relief and providing patient comfort measures and supportive care, as well as helping family members with coping and anticipatory grief counseling and initiating a conversation about elective device deactivation to allow for a natural death.[128]

Discontinuation of Mechanical Circulatory Support

When therapies prolong life but do not reverse the underlying medical condition, the American Medical Association has concluded that the therapy may be withdrawn if it serves the best interests of the patient.[129] Withdrawal of life-sustaining therapy is "the cessation and removal of an ongoing medical therapy with the explicit intent not to substitute an equivalent alternative treatment; it is fully anticipated that the patient will die following the change in therapy."[130] Withdrawal of life-sustaining therapy (i.e., device deactivation) is discussed with patients and families as part of the consent process, as previously described, and again when the prognosis and burden of continued device use outweigh the benefits.[14] Conversations with patients and families about device deactivation should include informing them about the patient's current condition and prognosis, alternatives to withdrawal of MCS, and the anticipated consequences of device deactivation (i.e., death).[128] The decision to withdraw treatment belongs ultimately to the patient or, if the patient is no longer capable of making informed decisions to withdraw treatment, a surrogate.[131] Bioethicists, mental health professionals, and the hospice team may be helpful to patients and families as they consider device withdrawal, especially when there are differences of opinion between patients and families or among family members about whether to withdraw MCS.

Device deactivation may be done in the hospital or home, once the patient and family have made their decision and are ready to proceed. The MCS team, unit staff, if the patient is hospitalized, and hospice team should also be in agreement with the plan for device deactivation. It can be difficult for health care professionals to face these patient and family decisions, and they may not always agree with each other.[132] This might especially be the case if the patient and/or family has decided that the suffering and the burden of care outweigh the benefits but the care providers (e.g., MCS team) may not yet see it this way. Conflict among staff about the plan for device deactivation should be discussed among staff with the goal of reaching agreement and formulating a plan to proceed.[133] Bioethicists may be helpful to this process through educating and reassuring staff that an ethical choice has been made. Deactivation is performed by MCS clinicians who know how to stop the device, silence alarms, monitor the patient's condition until death, and disconnect the equipment, as well as palliative care clinicians who can manage symptoms and provide comfort and support to the family.[127,128] A debriefing among staff after device deactivation may help individuals deal with their feelings about MCS withdrawal.[133] Institutions may consider developing hospital policies surrounding device withdrawal in collaboration with MCS and hospice teams and bioethicists.

CONCLUSIONS AND FUTURE CLINICAL AND RESEARCH DIRECTIONS

MCS, as a therapeutic option, generally improves HRQOL in patients from before to after implantation but can nonetheless be adversely affected by many other factors, including complications associated with MCS. Understanding "life on a device" provides clinicians with important information with which to educate patients and their families during the informed consent process and shared decision-making. After MCS, studies of HRQOL have provided information regarding benefits and potential risk factors for poor HRQOL outcomes that can guide clinicians in developing strategies to improve outcomes.

The literature on shared decision-making, psychosocial outcomes, and end of life regarding MCS is increasing; more research is needed. Areas have been highlighted wherein more evidence exists (e.g., decision-making and HRQOL) and those areas with a paucity of evidence (e.g., postimplantation HRQOL outcomes). Of course, no matter what the evidence is with devices in use today, the psychosocial literature needs to keep pace with the evolution of MCS, as new risks and challenges are identified with new technology. Furthermore, measures currently used to assess HRQOL after MCS implantation are generic and heart failure specific and do not address the unique burdens of MCS, lacking the sensitivity and precision to address the myriad effects of MCS on patients' lives.[16] Clearly, opportunities abound for the future study of decision-making regarding MCS, psychosocial evaluation for MCS, HRQOL during and long-term after implantation, and end-of-life considerations.

REFERENCES

1. Institute of Medicine. *How Far Have We Come in Reducing Health Disparaties? Progress Since 2000: Workshop Summary*. Washington, DC: National Academies Press; 2012.
2. Okwuosa IS, Lewsey SC, Adesiyun T, Blumenthal RS, Yancy CW. Worldwide disparities in cardiovascular disease: challenges and solutions. *Internat J Cardiol.* 2016;202:433–440.
3. Dew MA, DiMartini AF. Transplantation. In: Friedman HS, ed. *The Oxford Handbook of Health Psychology*. New York: Oxford University Press; 2011:522–559.
4. Cook JL, Grady KL, Colvin M, et al. Sex differences in the care of patients with advanced heart failure. *Circ Cardiovasc Qual Outcomes.* 2015;127:S56–S59.
5. Joyce DL, Conte JV, Russell SD, et al. Disparities in access to left ventricular assist device therapy. *J Surg Res.* 2009;152:111–117.
6. Insam C, Paccaud F, Marques-Vidal P. The region makes the difference: disparities in management of acute myocardial infarction within Switzerland. *European J Prev Cardiol.* 2014;21:541–548.
7. McIlvennan CK, Lindenfeld J, Kao DP. Sex differences and in-hospital outcomes in patients undergoing mechanical circulatory support implantation. *J Heart Lung Transplant.* 2017;36:82–90.
8. Walsh MN, Yancy CW, Albert NM, et al. Equitable improvement for women and men in the use of guideline-recommended therapies for heart failure: findings from IMPROVE HF. *J Cardiac Fail.* 2010;16:940–949.
9. Hall D, Prochazka AV, Fink AS. Informed consent for clinical treatment. *Can Med Assoc J.* 2012;184(5):533–540.
10. Allen L, Stevenson L, Grady K, et al. Decision-making in advanced heart failure: a scientific statement from the American Heart Association. *Circ.* 2012;125(15):1928–1952.
11. Matlock DD, McGuire WC, Magid M, Allen L. Decision making in advanced heart failure: bench, bedside, practice, policy. *Heart Fail Rev.* 2017;22:559–564.
12. Feldman D, Pamboukian SV, Teuteberg J, et al. The 2013 International Society for Heart and Lung Transplantation Guidelines for Mechanical Circulatory Support: executive summary. *J Heart Lung Transplant.* 2013 Feb;32(2):157–187.
13. Yancy CW, Jessup M, Bozkurt B, et al. 2013 ACCF/AHA guideline for the management of heart failure: a report of the American College of Cardiology Foundation/American Heart Association Task Force on practice guidelines. American College of Cardiology Foundation/American Heart Association Task Force on Practice Guidelines. *Circ.* 2013 Oct 15;128(16):e240-327.
14. Rizzieri AG, Verheijde JL, Rady MY, et al. Ethical challenges with the left ventricular assist device as a destination therapy. *Philos Ethics Humanit Med.* 2008;3:20.
15. Kirklin J, Naftel D, Pagani F, et al. Long-term mechanical circulatory support (destination therapy): on track to compete with heart transplantation? *J Thorac Cardiovasc Surg.* 2012;144:584–603.

16. Grady KL, Magasi S, Hahn EA, McGee EC, Yancy C. Health-related quality of life in mechanical circulatory support: development of a new conceptual model and items for self-administration. *J Heart Lung Transplant.* 2015;34:1292–1304.
17. McIlvenan C, Magid KH, Ambardekar A, Thompson J, Matlock DD, Allen LA. Clinical outcomes after continuous-flow left ventricular assist devices: a systematic review. *Circ Heart Fail.* 2014;7:1003–1013.
18. Goldstein NE, May CW, Meier DE. Comprehensive care for mechanical circulatory support: a new frontier for synergy with palliative care. *Circ Heart Fail.* 2011;4:519–527.
19. Peura JL, Colvin-Adams M, Francis GS, et al. Recommendations for the use of mechanical circulatory support: device strategies and patient selection: a scientific statement from the American Heart Association. *Circ.* 2012 Nov 27;126(22):2648–2667.
20. Farran C. Family caregiving intervention research: where have we been? Where are we going? *J Gerontol Nurs.* 2001;27:38–45.
21. Iacovetto MC, Matlock DD, McIlvennan CK, et al. Educational resources for patients considering a left ventricular assist device: a cross-sectional review of Internet, print, and multimedia materials. *Circ Cardiovasc Outcomes.* 2014;7:905–911.
22. Stevenson LW, Hellkamp AS, Leier CV, et al. Changing preferences for survival after hospitalization with advanced heart failure. *J Am Coll Cardiol.* 2008;52:1702–1708.
23. Allen LA, Yager JE, Funk MJ, et al. Discordance between patient-predicted and model-predicted life expectancy among ambulatory patients with heart failure. *JAMA.* 2008;299(21):2533–2542.
24. Narayan M, Jones J, Portalupi L, McIlvennan C, Matlock D, Allen L. Patient perspectives on communication of individualized survival estimates in heart failure. *J Cardiac Fail.* 2017;23:272–277.
25. Goodlin S, Quill T, Arnold R. Communication and decision-making about prognosis in heart failure care. *J Cardiac Fail.* 2008;14:106–113.
26. McIlvennan C, Allen L, Nowels C, Brieke A, Cleveland J, Matlock D. Decision making for destination therapy left ventricular assist devices "There was no choice" versus "I thought about it an awful lot." *Circ Cardiovasc Qual Outcomes.* 2014;7:374–380.
27. Blumenthal-Barby JS, Kostick K, Delgado E, et al. Assessment of patients' and caregivers' informational and decisional needs for left ventricular assist device placement: implications for informed consent and shared decision making. *J Heart Lung Transplant.* 2015;34:1182–1189.
28. McIlvennan C, Jones J, Allen L, et al. Decision-making for destination therapy left ventricular assist devices: implications for caregivers. *Circ Cardiovasc Qual Outcomes.* 2015;8:172–178.
29. O'Connor AM, Wennberg JE, Legare F, et al. Toward the "tipping point": Decision aids and informed patient choice. *Health Aff.* 2007;26:716–725.
30. Thompson JS, Matlock D, McIlvennan C, Jenkins A, Allen L. Development of a decision aid for patients with advanced heart failure considering destination therapy left ventricular assist device. *J Am Coll Cardiol Heart Fail.* 2015;3:965–976.
31. https://decisionaid.ohri.ca/. Accessed 11/30/17.
32. Allen LA, McIlvennan CK, Thompson JS, et al. Effectiveness of an intervention supporting shared decision making for destination therapy left ventricular assist device: the DECIDE-LVAD randomized clinical trial. *J Am Med Assoc Int Med.* 2018;178(4):520–529.
33. Brehaut JC, O'Connor AM, Wood TJ, et al. Validation of a decision regret scale. *Med Decis Making.* 2003;23(4):281–292.
34. Caro MA, Rosenthal JL, Kendall K, et al. What the psychiatrist needs to know about ventricular assist devices: a comprehensive review. *Psychosomatics.* 2016;52:229–237.
35. Eshelman AK, Mason S, Nemeh H, et al. LVAD destination therapy: applying what we know about psychiatric evaluation and management from cardiac failure and transplant. *Heart Fail Rev.* 2009;14:21–28.
36. Petty M, Bauman L. Psychosocial issues in ventricular assist device implantation and management. *J Thorac Dis.* 2015;7:2181–2187.
37. Dew MA, DiMartini AF, Dobbels F, Grady KL, Jowsey-Gregoire SG, Kaan A, Kendall K, Young QR, Abbey SE, Butt Z, Crone CC, De Geest S, Doligalski CT, Kugler C, McDonald L, Ohler L, Painter L, Petty MG, Robson D, Schlöglhofer T, Schneekloth TD, Singer JP, Smith PJ, Spaderna H, Teuteberg JJ, Yusen RD, Zimbrean PC. The 2018 ISHLT/APM/AST/ICCAC/STSW recommendations for the psychosocial evaluation of adult cardiothoracic transplant candidates and candidates for long-term mechanical circulatory support. *J Heart Lung Transplant.* 2018;37:803–823.
38. Teuteberg JJ, Stewart GC, Jessup M, et al. Implant strategies change over time and impact outcomes: insights from the INTERMACS (Interagency Registry for Mechanically Assisted Circulatory Support). *J Am Coll Cardiol Heart Fail.* 2013;1:369–378.
39. Cupples S, Dew MA, Grady KL, et al. Report of the Psychosocial Outcomes Workgroup of the Nursing and Social Sciences Council of the International Society for Heart and Lung Transplantation: present status of research on psychosocial outcomes in cardiothoracic transplantation: review and recommendations for the field. *J Heart Lung Transplant.* 2006;25:716–725.
40. Abshire M, Dennison Himmelfarb CR, Russell SD. Functional status in left ventricular assist device-supported patients: a literature review. *J Cardiac Fail.* 2014;20:973–983.
41. Brouwers C, Denollet J, de Jonge N, Caliskan K, Kealy J, Pedersen SS. Patient-reported outcomes in left ventricular assist device therapy: a systematic review and recommendations for clinical research and practice. *Circ Heart Fail.* 2011;4:714–723.
42. MacIver J, Ross HJ. Quality of life and left ventricular assist device support. *Circ.* 2012;126:866–874.
43. Rosenberger EM, Fox KR, DiMartini AF, Dew MA. Psychosocial factors and quality-of-life after heart transplantation and mechanical circulatory support. *Curr Opin Organ Transplant.* 2012;17:558–563.
44. Hayward CS, Fresiello L, Meyns B. Exercise physiology in chronic mechanical circulatory support patients: vascular function and beyond. *Curr Opin Cardiol.* 2016;31:292–298.
45. Pagani FD, Miller LW, Russell SD, et al. Extended mechanical circulatory support with a continuous-flow rotary left ventricular assist device. *J Am Coll Cardiol.* 2009;54:312–321.
46. Slaughter MS, Rogers JG, Milano CA, et al. Advanced heart failure treated with continuous-flow left ventricular assist device. *N Engl J Med.* 2009;361:2241–2251.
47. Grady KL, Naftel DC, Myers S, et al. Change in health-related quality of life from before to after destination therapy mechanical circulatory support is similar for older and younger patients: analyses from INTERMACS. *J Heart Lung Transplant.* 2015;34:213–221.
48. Stehlik J, Estep JD, Selzman CH, et al. Patient-reported health-related quality of life is a predictor of outcomes in ambulatory heart failure patients treated with left ventricular assist device compared with medical management: results from the ROADMAP study (Risk assessment and comparative effectiveness of left ventricular assist device and medical management). *Circ Heart Fail.* 2017;10:e003910.
49. Weerahandi H, Goldstein N, Geffman LP, et al. Pain and functional status in patients with ventricular assist devices. *J Pain Symptom Management.* 2016;52:483–490.
50. Bogaev RC, Pamboukian SV, Moore SA, et al. Comparison of outcomes in women versus men using a continuous-flow left ventricular assist device as a bridge to transplantation. *J Heart Lung Transplant.* 2011;30:515–522.
51. Miller LW, Pagani FD, Russell SD, et al. Use of a continuous-flow device in patients awaiting heart transplantation. *N Engl J Med.* 2007;357:885–896.
52. Rose EA, Gelijns AC, Moskowitz AJ, et al. Long-term use of a left ventricular assist device for end-stage heart failure. *N Engl J Med.* 2001;345:1435–1443.
53. Allen JG, Weiss ES, Schaffer JM, et al. Quality of life and functional status in patients surviving 12 months after left ventricular assist device implantation. *J Heart Lung Transplant.* 2010;29:278–285.
54. Haft J, Armstrong W, Dyke DB, et al. Hemodynamic and exercise performance with pulsatile and continuous-flow left ventricular assist devices. *Circ.* 2007;116(suppl 11):I8–I15.
55. Rogers JG, Butler J, Lansman SL, et al. Chronic mechanical circulatory support for inotrope-dependent heart failure patients who are not transplant candidates: results of the INTrEPID Trial. *J Am Coll Cardiol.* 2007;50:741–747.
56. Rogers JG, Aaronson KD, Boyle AJ, et al. Continuous flow left ventricular assist device improves functional capacity and quality of life of advanced heart failure patients. *J Am Coll Cardiol.* 2010;55:1826–1834.

57. Emin A, Rogers CA, Banner NR; Steering Group, UK Cardiothoracic Transplant Audit. Quality of life of advanced chronic heart failure: medical care, mechanical circulatory support and transplantation. *Eur J Cardiothorac Surg*. 2016;50:269–273.
58. Pruijsten RV, Lok SI, Kirkels HH, et al. Functional and haemodynamic recovery after implantation of continuous-flow left ventricular assist devices in comparison with pulsatile left ventricular assist devices in patients with end stage heart failure. *Eur J Heart Fail*. 2012;14:319–325.
59. Grady KL, Meyer P, Mattea A, et al. Improvement in quality of life outcomes 2 weeks after left ventricular assist device implantation. *J Heart Lung Transplant*. 2001;20:657–669.
60. Ganga HV, Leung A, Jantz J, et al. Supervised exercise training versus usual care in ambulatory patients with left ventricular assist devices: a systematic review. *PLoS ONE*. 2017;12:e0174323.
61. Kirklin JK, Pagani FD, Kormos RL, et al. Eighth annual INTERMACS report: special focus on framing the impact of adverse events. *J Heart Lung Transplant*. 2017;36:1080–1086.
62. Harvey L, Holley C, Roy SS, et al. Stroke after left ventricular assist device implantation: outcomes in the continuous-flow era. *Ann Thorac Surg*. 2015;100:535–541.
63. Parikh NS, Cool J, Karas MG, et al. Stroke risk and mortality in patients with ventricular assist devices. *Stroke*. 2016;47:2702–2706.
64. Slaughter MS, Pagani FD, McGee EC, et al. HeartWare ventricular assist system for bridge to transplant: combined results of the bridge to transplant and continued access protocol trial. *J Heart Lung Transplant*. 2013;32:675–683.
65. Bunzel B, Laederach-Hofmann K, Wieselthaler G, et al. Mechanical circulatory support as a bridge to heart transplantation: what remains? Long-term emotional sequelae in patients and spouses. *J Heart Lung Transplant*. 2007;26:384–389.
66. Chapman E, Parameshwar J, Jenkins D, et al. Psychosocial issues for patients with ventricular assist devices: a qualitative pilot study. *Am J Crit Care*. 2007;16:72–81.
67. Dew MA, Kormos RL, Winowich S, et al. Human factors issues in ventricular assist device recipients and their family caregivers. *ASAIO J*. 2000;46:367–373.
68. Eckman PM, Dhungel V, Mandras S, et al. Sexual function after left ventricular assist device. *J Am Coll Cardiol*. 2013;61:2021–2022.
69. Casida JM, Brewer RJ, Smith C, Davis JE. An exploratory study of sleep quality, daytime function, and quality of life in patients with mechanical circulatory support. *Int J Artificial Organs*. 2012;35:531–537.
70. Casida JM, Davis JE, Brewer RJ, Smith C, Yarandi H. Sleep and daytime sleepiness of patients with left ventricular assist devices: a longitudinal pilot study. *Prog Transplant*. 2011;21:131–136.
71. Casida JM, Parker JA. A preliminary investigation of symptom pattern and prevalence before and up to 6 months after implantation of a left ventricular assist device. *J Artif Organs*. 2011;40:511–520.
72. Hallas C, Banner NR, Wray J. A qualitative study of the psychological experience of patients during and after mechanical cardiac support. *J Cardiovasc Nurs*. 2009;24:31–39.
73. Baba A, Hirata G, Yokoyama F, et al. Psychiatric problems of heart transplant candidates with left ventricular assist devices. *J Artif Organs*. 2006;9:203–208.
74. Bidwell JT, Lyons KS, Mudd JO, et al. Quality of life, depression, and anxiety in ventricular assist device therapy: longitudinal outcomes for patients and family caregivers. *J Cardiovasc Nurs*. 2017;32:455–463.
75. Grady LK, Naftel D, Stevenson L, et al. Overall quality of life improves to similar levels after mechanical circulatory support regardless of severity of heart failure before implantation. *J Heart Lung Transplant*. 2014;33:412–421.
76. Reynard AL, Butler RS, McKee MG, Starling RC, Gorodeski EZ. Frequency of depression and anxiety before and after insertion of a continuous flow left ventricular assist device. *Am J Cardiol*. 2014;114:433–440.
77. Yost G, Ghat G, Mahoney E, Tatooles A. Reduced anxiety and depression in patients with advanced heart failure after left ventricular assist device implantation. *Psychosomatics*. 2017;58:406–414.
78. Grady KL, Meyer PM, Dressler D, et al. Longitudinal change in quality of life and impact on survival after left ventricular assist device implantation. *Ann Thorac Surg*. 2004;77:1321–1327.
79. Heilmann C, Kaps J, Hartmann A, et al. Mental health status of patients with mechanical aortic valves, with ventricular assist devices and after heart transplantation. *Interact Cardiovasc Thorac Surg*. 2016;23:321–325.
80. Brouwers C, de Jone N, Caliskan O, Manintveld, et al. Predictors of changes in health status between and within patients 12 months post left ventricular assist device implantation. *Eur J Heart Fail*. 2014;16:566–573.
81. Brouwers C, Denollet J, Caliskan K, et al. Psychological distress in patients with a left ventricular assist device and their partners: an exploratory study. *Eur J Cardiovasc Nurs*. 2015;14:53–62.
82. Heilmann C, Kuipers N, Beyersdorf F, et al. Does listing for heart transplant for longer than 30 days before ventricular assist device implantation influence utilization of psychotherapeutic support and outcome? *Eur J Cardiothorac Surg*. 2012;41:1371–1376.
83. Badiye A, Munos-Mendoza J, Chaparro SV. Severing your lifeline: the impact of neuropsychiatric conditions after left ventricular assist device implantation. *Int J Artif Organs*. 2014;37:182–183.
84. Tigges-Limmer K, Schonbrodt M, Roefe D, et al. Suicide after ventricular assist device implantation. *J Heart Lung Transplant*. 2010;29:692–694.
85. Vitale CA, Chandekar R, Rodgers PE, Pagani FD, Malani PN. A call for guidance in the use of left ventricular assist devices in older adults. *J Am Geriatr Soc*. 2012;60:145–150.
86. Bhat G, Yost G, Mahoney E. Cognitive function and left ventricular assist device implantation. *J Heart Lung Transplant*. 2015;34:1398–1405.
87. Petrucci RJ, Wright S, Naka Y, et al. Neurocognitive assessments in advanced heart failure patients receiving continuous-flow left ventricular assist devices. *J Heart Lung Transplant*. 2009;28:542–549.
88. Petrucci RJ, Rogers JG, Blue L, Gallagher C, et al. Neurocognitive function in destination therapy patients receiving continuous-flow vs pulsatile-flow left ventricular assist device support. *J Heart Lung Transplant*. 2012;31(1):27–36.
89. Siegenthaler MP, Westaby S, Frazier OH, et al. Advanced heart failure: feasibility study of long-term continuous axial flow pump support. *Eur Heart J*. 2005;26:1031–1038.
90. Schmitto JD, Hanke JS, Rojas S. Circulatory support exceeding five years with a continuous-flow left ventricular assist device for advanced heart failure patients. *J Cardiothorac Surg*. 2015;10:107.
91. Wray J, Hallas CN, Banner NR. Quality of life and psychological well-being during and after left ventricular assist device support. *Clin Transplant*. 2007;21:622–627.
92. Abshire M, Prichard R, Cajita M, DiGiacomo M, Himmefarb CD. Adaptation and coping in patients living with an LVAD: a metasynthesis. *Heart Lung*. 2016;45:397–405.
93. Krabatsch T, Netuka I, Schmitto JD, et al. Heartmate 3 fully magnetically levitated left ventricular assist device for the treatment of advanced heart failure -1 year results from the CE Mark trial. *J Cardiothorac Surg*. 2017;12:23.
94. Park SJ, Milano CA, Tatooles AJ, et al. Outcomes in advanced heart failure patients with left ventricular assist devices for destination therapy. *Circ Heart Fail*. 2012;5:241–248.
95. Starling RC, Naka Y, Boyle AJ. Results of the post-U.S. Food and Drug Administration-approval study with a continuous flow left ventricular assist device as a bridge to heart transplantation. *J Am Coll Cardiol*. 2011;57:1890–1898.
96. Casida JM, Peters RM, Magnan MA. Self-care demands of persons living with an implantable left-ventricular assist device. *Res Theory Nurs Practice*. 2009;23:279–293.
97. Kato N, Jaarsma T, Ben Gal T. Learning self-care after left ventricular assist device implantation. *Curr Heart Fail Rep*. 2014;11:290–298.
98. Casida JM, Wu HS, Abshire M, Ghosh B, Yang JJ. Cognition and adherence are self-management factors predicting the quality of life of adults living with a left ventricular assist device. *J Heart Lung Transplant*. 2017;36:325–330.
99. Cicollini G, Cerratti F, della Pelle C, Simonetti V. The experience of family caregivers of patients with a left ventricular assist device: an integrative review. *Prog Transplant*. 2016;26:135–148.
100. Benjamin EJ, Blaha M, Chiuve S, et al. Heart disease and stroke statistics - 2017 update. A report from the American Heart Association. *Circ*. 2017;135(10):e146–e603.

101. Seo M, Zhao D, Byron M, et al. Long-term prognosis and cost-effectiveness of left ventricular assist device as bridge to transplant: a systematic review. *Intl J Cardio.* 2017;235:22–32.
102. Rogers JG, Bostic RR, Tong KB, Adamson R, Russo M, Slaughter MS. Cost-effectiveness analysis of continuous-flow left ventricular assist devices as destination therapy. *Circ Heart Fail.* 2012;5:10–16.
103. Long EF, Swain GW, Mangi AA. Comparative survival and cost-effectiveness of advanced therapies for end-stage heart failure. *Circ Heart Fail.* 2014;7:470–478.
104. Nunes A, MacArthur R, Kim D, et al. A systematic review of the cost-effectiveness of long-term mechanical circulatory support. *Value in Health.* 2016;19:494–504.
105. Mehra M, Yoshifumi N, Uriel N, et al. A fully magnetically levitated circulatory pump for advanced heart failure. *N Engl J Med.* 2017;376:440–450.
106. McAlister FA, Stewart S, Ferrua S, et al. Multidisciplinary strategies for the management of heart failure patients at high risk for admission: a systematic review of randomized trials. *J Am Coll Cardiol.* 2004;44:810–819.
107. Jovcic A, Holroyd-Leduc JM, Straus SE. Effects of self-management intervention on health outcomes of patients with heart failure: a systematic review of randomized controlled trials. *BMC Cardiovasc Disord.* 2006;6:43.
108. Lee C, Carlson B, Riegel B. Heart failure self-care improves economic outcomes, but only when self-care confidence is high. *J Card Fail.* 2007;13:S75.
109. Kirklin JK, Naftel DC, Pagani FD, et al. Pump thrombosis in the Thoratec HeartMate II device: an update analysis of the INTERMACS Registry. *J Heart Lung Transplant.* 2015;34:1515–1526.
110. Gordon RJ, Weinberg AD, Pagani FD, et al. Prospective, multicenter study of ventricular assist device infections. *Circ.* 2013;127:691–702.
111. Snipelsky D, Stulak JM, Schettle SD, et al. Psychosocial characteristics and outcomes in patients with left ventricular assist device implanted as destination therapy. *Am Heart J.* 2015;170:887–894.
112. Cogswell R, Smith E, Hamel A, et al. Substance abuse at the time of left ventricular assist device implantation is associated with increased mortality. *J Heart Lung Transplant.* 2014;33:1048–1055.
113. Singh G, Albeldawi M, Kalra SS, Mehta PP, Lopez R, Vargo JJ. Features of patients with gastrointestinal bleeding after implantation of ventricular assist devices. *Clin Gastroenterol Hepatol.* 2015;13:107–114.
114. Copeland JG, Smith RG, Bose RK, Tsau PH, Nolan PE, Slepian MJ. Risk factor analysis for bridge to transplantation with the CardioWest total artificial heart. *Ann Thorac Surg.* 2008;85:1639–1644.
115. Bruce CR, Minard CG, Wilhelms LA, et al. Caregivers of patients with left ventricular assist devices: possible impacts on patients' mortality and Interagency Registry for Mechanically Assisted Circulatory Support – defined morbidity events. *Circ Cardiovasc Qual Outcomes.* 2017;10:e002879.
116. Koeckert M, Vining P, Reyentovich A, et al. Caregiver status and outcomes after durable left ventricular assist device implantation. *Heart Lung.* 2017;46:74–78.
117. Maltby MC, Flattery MP, Burns B, Salyer J, Weinland S, Shah KB. Psychosocial assessment of candidates and risk classification of patients considered for durable mechanical circulatory support. *J Heart Lung Transplant.* 2014;33:836–841.
118. Pruijsten RV, de Jone N, Kirkels JH, et al. Left ventricular assist device: a functional comparison with heart transplantation. *Netherlands Heart J.* 2008;16:41–46.
119. Grady KL, Meyer PM, Dressler D, et al. Change in quality of life and psychological well-being during and after left ventricular assist device implantation to after heart transplantation. *J Heart Lung Transplant.* 2003;22:1254–1267.
120. Dew MA, Kormos RL, Winowich S, et al. Quality of life outcomes after heart transplantation in individuals bridged to transplant with ventricular assist devices. *J Heart Lung Transplant.* 2001;20:1199–1212.
121. Dew MA, Myaskovsky L, Switzer GE, et al. Profiles and predictors of the course of psychological distress across four years after heart transplantation. *Psychol Med.* 2005;35:1215–1227.
122. George RS, Yacoub MH, Bowles CT, et al. Quality of life after removal of left ventricular assist device for myocardial recovery. *J Heart Lung Transplant.* 2008;27:165–172.
123. Dew MA, Myaskovsky L, DiMartini AF, et al. Onset, timing and risk for depression and anxiety in family caregivers to heart transplant recipients. *Psychol Med.* 2004;34:1065–1082.
124. Jakovljevic D, Yacoub MH, Schueler S, et al. Left ventricular assist device as a bridge to recovery for patients with advanced heart failure. *J Am Coll Cardiol.* 2017;69:1924–1933.
125. Birks EJ, Tansley PD, Hardy J, et al. Left ventricular assist device and drug therapy for the reversal of heart failure. *N Engl J Med.* 2006;355:1873–1884.
126. Sagin A, Kirkpatrick J, Pisani B, Fahlberg B, Sundlof A, O'Connor N. Emerging collaboration between palliative care specialists and mechanical circulatory support teams: a qualitative study. *J Pain Symptom Management.* 2016;52:491–497.
127. Whelan D, Goodlin S, Dickinson M, et al. End-of-life care in patients with heart failure. *J Cardiac Fail.* 2014;20:121–134.
128. Wiegand DL, Kalowes PG. Withdrawal of cardiac medications and devices. *AACN Adv Crit Care.* 2007;18(4):415–425.
129. American Medical Association. *Opinion 2.20. Withholding or Withdrawing Life-Sustaining Medical Treatment.* AMA Code of Medical Ethics, Council on Ethical and Judicial Affairs of the American Medical Association. Available at www.ama-assn.org/ama/pub/physician-resources/medical-ethics/code-medical-ethics/opinion220.page; Accessed 12.06.11.
130. Prendergast TJ, Claessens MT, Luce JM. A national survey of end-of-life care for critically ill patients. *Am J Respir Crit Care Med.* 1998;158:1163–1167.
131. *Deciding to Forego Life-Sustaining Treatment: A Report on the Ethical, Medical, and Legal Issues in Treatment Decisions.* Washington, DC: U.S. Government Printing Office; 1983.
132. McIlvennan C, Wordingham S, Allen L, et al. Deactivation of left ventricular assist devices: differing perspectives of cardiology and hospice/palliative medicine clinicians. *J Cardiac Fail.* 2017;23:708–712.
133. MacIver J, Ross HJ. Withdrawal of ventricular assist device support. *J Palliat Care.* 2005;21(3):151–156.

17

Left Ventricular Assist Device in Special Population of Patients

Yakov L. Elgudin, Soon J. Park

KEY POINTS

Case Presentation
Introduction
Modification in Surgical Technique
Potential Patient Population
Summary

CASE PRESENTATION

A 73-year-old retired psychiatrist presents with advanced congestive heart failure (HF) (New York Heart Association [NYHA] class IV). He was healthy until about 3 years ago. On evaluation, he is found to have restrictive cardiomyopathy (RCM) due to senile cardiac amyloidosis. He also develops acute worsening of his chronic renal dysfunction. He is in atrial fibrillation, and his right heart catheterization reveals severe biventricular failure (right atrium [RA], 22 mm Hg; pulmonary artery [PA], 51/28 mm Hg; pulmonary capillary wedge pressure [PCWP], 33 mm Hg; cardiac output [CO], 1.82 L/min). His echocardiogram reveals a very small left ventricular (LV) cavity (LV end-diastolic dimension [LVEDD], 26 mm; LV end-systolic diameter [LVESD], 19 mm), with normal LV ejection fraction (52%). He successfully undergoes HeartMate II left ventricular assist device (LVAD) implantation with improvement in forward blood flow and end-organ function (Fig. 17.1).

INTRODUCTION

The field of mechanical cardiac support has made significant advances since early 2000s, and the pumping mechanism of the native heart can now be effectively replaced with an LVAD. Substantial evidence exists that mechanical circulatory pumps can improve quality of life and longevity for those with end-stage dilated cardiomyopathy. However, similar mechanical options have not been widely used for patients with RCM. The existing pioneering experience for use of mechanical circulatory support in RCM will be reviewed and the potential benefits of employing LVAD in patients with failing Fontan circulation are explored.

Most patients with advanced HF have a significantly dilated left ventricle (LV) from the process of chronic remodeling. They face a very poor quality of life and exceedingly high mortality. The initial National Institutes of Health project goal of replacing the failing human heart with a total artificial heart (TAH) has proven much more challenging, and utilization of TAH in the clinical setting is rather limited to date. However, the field of LVAD has evolved rapidly over the past few decades. The initial construct of LVAD as a volume displacement pump mimicking the mechanism of the natural heart has now been nearly completely replaced by durable pumps. It is remarkable how these pumps transform the lives of those facing imminent death from advanced dilated cardiomyopathy, mostly ischemic or idiopathic, into vibrant individuals. Yet, those with RCM continue to suffer and face exceedingly high mortality. For instance, a young gentleman with familial hypertrophic cardiomyopathy (HCM) was rapidly deteriorating while awaiting heart transplantation. His LV cavity was nearly obliterated by a severely thickened LV, and he was struggling to maintain adequate forward flow by compensating his very small stroke volume with severe tachycardia. His impending demise compelled the application of a continuous-flow LVAD in this uncharted clinical arena. The surgical technique was modified to compensate for small LV cavity, and the LVAD pump speed had to be adjusted carefully under echocardiographic guidance. Application of successful support in this particular patient was very encouraging, and it opened up the possibility of LVAD support for those suffering from advanced HF due to various causes other than dilated cardiomyopathy.

Topilsky et al.[1] reported the first series on LVAD support and included eight study patients (four HCM and four RCM); outcomes were compared to 75 contemporaneous control patients with either idiopathic or ischemic dilated cardiomyopathy. As expected, baseline parameters associated with LV geometry significantly differed: LVEDD, 52.5 ± 6 mm vs. 68.6 ± 8 mm ($P<0.0001$); septal wall thickness, 16 (12, 19) mm vs. 10 (8.5, 11) mm ($P=0.0003$); and LV ejection fraction, 21% (20%, 36%) vs. 17% (15%, 22%) ($P=0.0087$). Study patients had higher central venous pressure (CVP) (18 [15, 20] mm Hg vs. 12 [9, 15] mm Hg, $P=0.03$) and lower pump flow (4.3 [3.8, 4.5] L vs. 5.2 [4.7, 5.5] L, $P=0.001$) postoperatively. The operative mortality was comparable (12.5% vs 9.3%, $P=0.8$). The actuarial 1-year survival rate was also comparable (87.5% [95% confidence interval, 52.9%–97.8%] vs. 73.2% [95% confidence interval, 60%–85%]), and this compared very favorably to 12.1% (95% confidence interval, 0%–55.2%, $P=0.1$) for those historically managed medically. This early experience demonstrated the feasibility of supporting patients with nondilated RCM or HCM in a clinically meaningful manner.

Swiecicki et al.[2] reported their experience using LVAD to support nine patients with cardiac amyloidosis. All patients had NYHA functional class IV symptoms, and the majority required inotropic and/or intraaortic balloon pump support prior to their LVAD implantation. LVAD implantation resulted in adequate forward blood flow for all patients. Seven out of nine patients were discharged from the hospital. Three patients succumbed to death at 59, 251, and 1111 days following surgery. Four patients were alive with a follow up of 16–24 months.

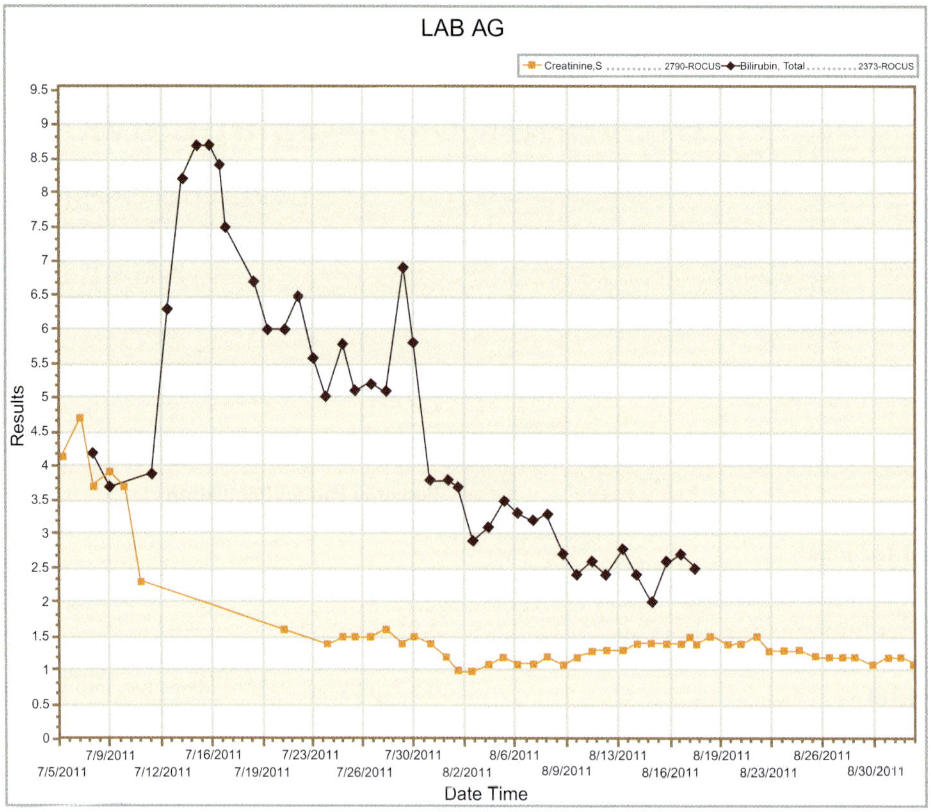

Fig. 17.1 Laboratory indicators of end-organ function before and after left ventricular assist device implantation in the case example.

Grupper et al.[3] reported their expanded LVAD experience involving 28 patients with RCM. The underlying etiologies for RCM included amyloidosis (10 patients), HCM (eight patients), sarcoidosis (five patients), chemotherapy/radiation (four patients), and Fabry disease (one patient). Their baseline echocardiography demonstrated a small LV cavity (LVESD, 46.8 ± 12.3 mm; LVEDD, 53.7 ± 11.3 mm), and right ventricular (RV) dysfunction was present in 82% of patients. Their Interagency Registry for Mechanically Assisted Circulatory Support profiles were one in seven patients, 2 in 19 patients, and three in two patients. LVAD was implanted as destination therapy (DT) in 11 and as bridge to transplantation (BTT) in 17 patients. Despite the technical challenges associated with a small LV cavity size and thickened LV wall, LVAD implantation was successful in all patients. RV failure requiring prolonged inotropic support occurred in 11 patients (39%), and the mean duration of support was 17 days. In-hospital mortality was 14%. Ten patients successfully proceeded to heart transplant, with no mortality, and their mean LVAD support duration was 472 (273–671) days. Of the remaining 18 patients who received LVAD as DT, the 1-year survival rate was 64%, and mean survival time was 651 (358–945) days. Neither the underlying etiology of RCM nor the LVAD indication (BTT/DT) influenced the survival outcome. However, those with a very small LV cavity (LVEDD <46 mm) had worse outcomes.

The three studies summarized here represent the evolution in expanding the application of LVAD therapy to a group of patients with RCM at Mayo Clinic. There seems to be objective evidence for survival benefit with LVAD implantation as compared to medical management for this group of patients.

MODIFICATION IN SURGICAL TECHNIQUE

During LVAD implantation, an inflow cannula inserted into the apex of the LV redirects blood to a pump and an outflow graft attached to the aorta delivers blood from the pump back into circulation. In some instances, the LV wall can be thick and the LV cavity small, making placement of an inflow cannula challenging. An approach used in our program to address LV geometry challenges in patients with HCM is first to arrest the heart with cardioplegia, which allows more precise execution of the surgery. After the intended location of inflow cannula placement is identified in the LV apex (Fig. 17.2A), a stab incision is made with an eleven blade from the epicardial surface into the LV cavity (see Fig. 17.2B). The tip of a Foley catheter treaded over the coring knife is inserted into the LV cavity (see Fig. 17.2C), and placement of the catheter in the LV cavity on transesophageal echocardiogram (TEE) is confirmed. The balloon of the catheter is inflated with 10 mL of saline solution. The catheter is gently pulled up, providing counter traction, and centered on the knife while the LV apex is cored (see Fig. 17.2D). Caution is exercised to avoid rupturing the balloon whose fragments can be lost in the LV cavity. Inspection of the LV cavity is important to ensure placement. In patients with HCM, excision of excess muscle circumferentially to create a space large enough to accommodate the inflow cannula may be necessary, whereas in patients with cardiac amyloidosis and friable myocardium that can tear easily, needles and sutures are handled carefully while affixing the inflow sewing ring (see Fig. 17.2E). Once the inflow cannula and ring are placed, the remaining implantation steps are completed. The inflow cannula is placed in the proper position running parallel to the septum and pointing toward the mitral valve, and this should be confirmed on TEE (Fig. 17.3).

Left Ventricular Assist Device Pump Speed Management

Nearly all patients with advanced HF due to dilated cardiomyopathy have biventricular failure. While the failing LV is the prevailing problem, the RV is adversely affected by increased afterload secondary to pulmonary hypertension. LVAD is effective in reducing LV congestion and substantially reduces secondary pulmonary hypertension. As a result, RV function improves with afterload load reduction in

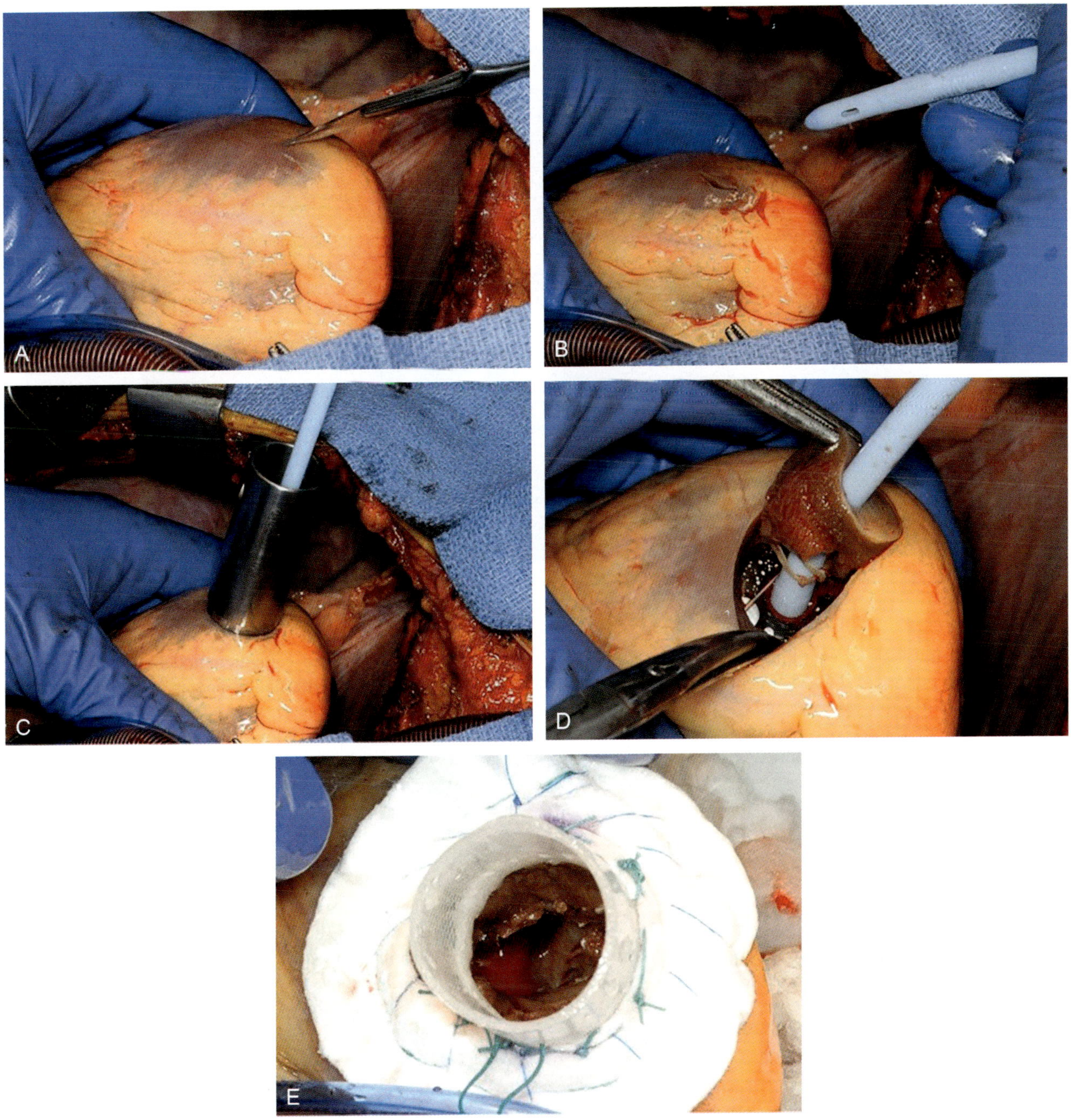

Fig. 17.2 (A) Location of inflow cannula placement. (B) Stab incision with an eleven blade. (C) Tip of a Foley catheter treaded over the coring knife. (D) Cored left ventricular apex. (E) Sutured inflow sewing ring.

the pulmonary vasculature. The incidence of RV failure requiring prolonged inotropic support following LVAD implantation is approximately 10%.

In patients with RCM, RV failure/dysfunction may be worse than in those with dilated cardiomyopathy since the infiltrative process can also directly affect the RV. Nearly 40% of these patients require prolonged inotropic support during the hospital stay following LVAD implantation. LVAD pump speed is adjusted to reduce LV end diastolic pressure (LVEDP) in an attempt to minimize secondary pulmonary hypertension for the failing RV. Echocardiography is important in determining the appropriate LVAD pump speed. The position of the interatrial septum should be concave into the left atrium, and the mitral deceleration time should be prolonged to reflect low LVEDP. The LV cavity may look small, but there should be unobstructed and continuous laminar flow into the inflow cannula. Echocardiographic images of a small LV cavity are a striking contrast to that of dilated cardiomyopathy. LVAD suction events due to inflow cannula obstruction have not been observed despite small LV cavity sizes. If the LVAD pump speed is reduced due to concerns about obstruction, patients are likely in biventricular failure with a low forward flow state (Fig. 17.4). These patients may need to be supported like those with a single ventricle in Fontan circulation. Patients with failing Fontan circulation develop elevated end-diastolic pressure of the systemic ventricle. This results in elevated systemic venous pressure through pulmonary congestion. These patients then suffer from protein losing enteropathy (PLE)

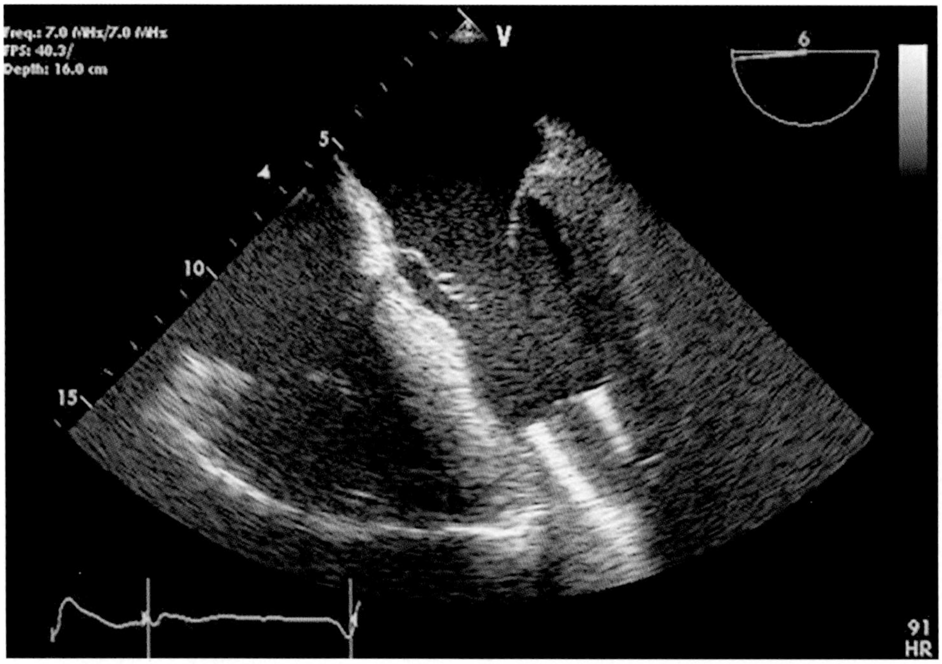

Fig. 17.3 Echocardiographic confirmation of proper left ventricular assist device inflow cannula placement. The inflow cannula runs parallel to the septum and points toward the mitral valve.

and a low cardiac output state. Low filling pressure of the systemic ventricle is critically important for well-functioning Fontan circulation. Similarly, LV filling pressure needs to be kept low in those with severe RV dysfunction. The underlying etiology for RCM may continue to progress, and LVAD may become less effective in providing forward flow. For those with no further therapeutic options, LVAD may provide some meaningful extra time with patients' loved ones. For others, heart transplant, chemotherapy, and/or autologous stem cell transplant may provide more durable benefit.

POTENTIAL PATIENT POPULATION

LVAD technology continues to evolve. It is anticipated that newer LVAD devices will become smaller in size, decrease the incidence of hemolysis, and be more durable. As a result, patient populations who can benefit from LVAD support will likely expand. It seems to make physiologic sense to apply LVAD in those with failing Fontan circulation. Frazier et al.[4] have reported one patient who was successfully supported by a ventricular assist device (VAD) for his failing single ventricle, albeit by a volume displacement VAD. Morales et al.[5] were the first to report success implanting a HM II LVAD in a 15-year-old patient with failing Fontan circulation and PLE. Lorts et al.[6] recently reported the first successful implantation of a third-generation LVAD, HeartMate 3 (HM3), in a 22-year-old patient with failing Fontan circulation who developed profound cardiogenic shock and required a veno-arterial extracorporeal membrane oxygenation support prior to implantation of the HM3 LVAD. This patient was eventually discharged from the hospital and followed for 3 months without incidence of stroke or bleeding. Improvements in LVAD technology, particularly pump size and hemocompatibility, will open new horizons in using VAD technology for the single-ventricle patient who has exhausted staged palliation options. Additionally, to date, LVAD has only been implanted to support a failing systemic ventricle. However, further miniaturization of pumps should allow for VAD implantation into a Fontan circuit itself to improve pulmonary blood flow.

Durham et al.[7] applied computer modeling to support systemic VAD support in those with failing Fontan physiology. Their model showed that LVAD support could reduce systemic venous congestion by 35% and increase forward flow by 41% in this population. A clinical trial (The Destination Therapy Evaluation for Failing Fontan Study) VAD was proposed by an investigator but was subsequently withdrawn due to lack of enrollment (ClinicalTrials.gov Identifier NCT01149603).

In the United States, the prevalence of HF with preserved ejection fraction (HFpEF), relative to HF with reduced ejection fraction (HFrEF), is increasing at an alarming rate of 1%, and an overwhelming majority of these patients are over age 65 years, such that the number of HFpEF patients currently outnumbers those with HFrEF. This group found that quality of life and life expectancy in patients with HFpEF were worse than in those with HFrEF. Mortality in their sample was 30%–60% at 5 years, with high rates of recurrent hospitalizations for acute decompensated HF.[7] Diagnosis of HFpEF remains disputed, and understanding of its pathophysiology is still developing. It is currently understood as a disease of the microvasculature, with endothelial dysfunction and rarefication, yet epicardial coronary artery stenosis is present in over 50% of patients, which contributes to their worsening prognosis.[8] In early 2018, Nguyen et al.[9] reported that HFpEF is an independent risk factor for increased mortality, postoperative shock, and other adverse outcomes in patients after cardiac surgery. Unfortunately, no pharmacologic therapy, including neurohormonal antagonists, has demonstrated benefit in HFpEF, unlike in those with HFrEF. In the future, those with advanced HFpEF may constitute a large group of patients who could benefit from the use of implantable LVAD. The feasibility and efficacy of LVAD support in those with nondilated LVs have already been evaluated and proven in those with RCM.

SUMMARY

LVADs have changed the landscape of HF management for the better. Patients with end-stage dilated cardiomyopathy have an excellent chance of living meaningful lives free of debilitating HF symptoms and recurrent hospitalizations. Durable LVADs have also been successfully employed

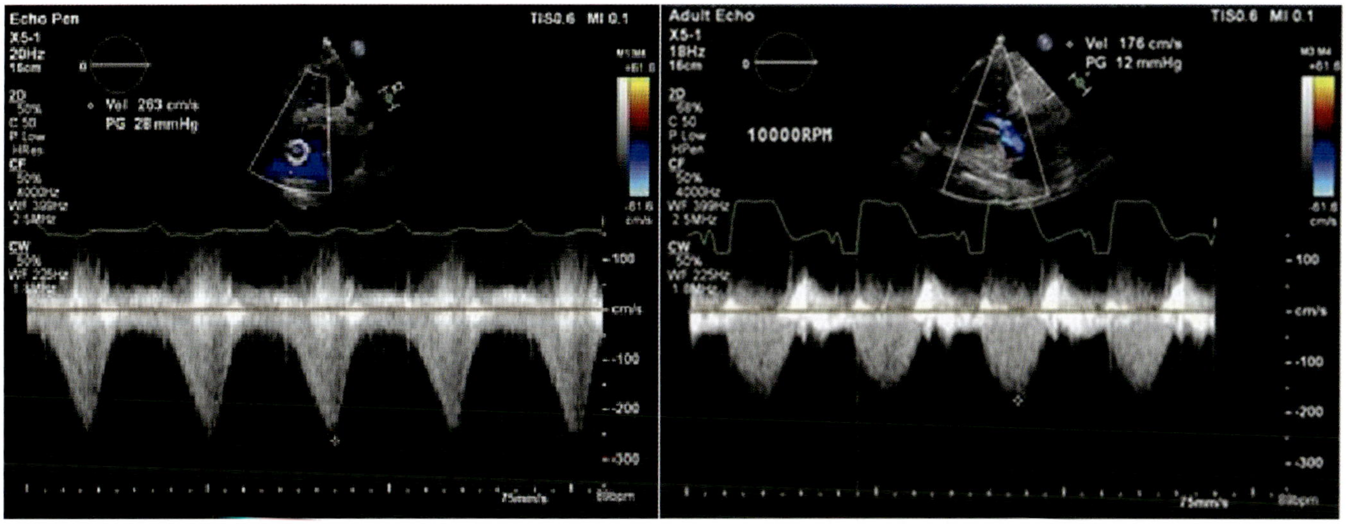

Fig. 17.4 Left ventricular assist device (LVAD) inflow velocity. A patient's LVAD pump speed was maintained at a lower setting with his small left ventricle cavity. He presented with fatigue and moderate to severe tricuspid regurgitation (TR). His flow velocity in the inflow cannula has a peak with high flow velocity during systole. At higher LVAD pump speed setting, the flow velocity has a blunted shape lower velocity during systole. His TR improved to moderate range.

in patients with RCM and relatively small LVs. However, there are still many patients with nondilated cardiomyopathy, including a vast population of patients with HFpEF, who do not currently have LVAD treatment options. These patients, in addition to a growing number of patients with failing Fontan, have the most need of critical improvements in LVAD pump size and hemocompatibility for expanded treatment options.

REFERENCES

1. Topilsky Y, Pereira NL, Shah DK, Boilson B, Schirger JA, Kushwaha SS, Joyce LD, Park SJ. Left ventricular assist device therapy in patients with restrictive and hypertrophic cardiomyopathy. *Circ Heart Fail*. 2011;4(3):266–275. https://doi.org/10.1161/CIRCHEARTFAILURE.110.959288. Epub 2011 Feb 8. PMID: 21303989. Select item 16855265.
2. Swiecicki PL, Edwards BS, Kushwaha SS, Dispenzieri A, Park SJ, Gertz MA. Left ventricular device implantation for advanced cardiac amyloidosis. *J Heart Lung Transplant*. 2013;32(5):563–568. https://doi.org/10.1016/j.healun.2013.01.987. Epub 2013 Mar 6. PMID: 23474361. Select item 21303989.
3. Grupper A, Park SJ, Pereira NL, Schettle SD, Gerber Y, Topilsky Y, Edwards BS, Daly RC, Stulak JM, Joyce LD, Kushwaha SS. Role of ventricular assist therapy for patients with heart failure and restrictive physiology: improving outcomes for a lethal disease. *J Heart Lung Transplant*. 2015 Aug;34(8):1042–1049. https://doi.org/10.1016/j.healun.2015.03.012. Epub 2015 Mar 26. PMID:25940074. Select item 23474361.
4. Frazier OH, Gregoric ID, Messner GN. Total circulatory support with an LVAD in an adolescent with a previous Fontan procedure. *Tex Heart Inst J*. 2005;32(3):402–404. PMID: 16392230. Select item 23804979.
5. Morales DLS, Adachi I, Heinle JS, Fraser CD. A new era: use of an intracorporeal systemic ventricular assist device to support a patient with a failing Fontan circulation. *J Thorac Cardiovasc Surg*. 2011 Sep 1;142(3).e138–40.
6. Lorts A, Villa C, Riggs KW, Broderick J, Morales DL. First use of HeartMate 3 in a failing Fontan circulation. *The Annals of Thoracic Surgery*. 2018; https://doi.org/10.1016/ J Thoracsur.2018.04.021.
7. Durham LA III, LA, Dearani JA, Burkhart HM, Joyce LD, Cetta Jr F, Cabalka AK, Phillips SD, Sundareswaran K, Farrar D, Park SJ. Application of computer modeling in systemic VAD support of failing Fontan physiology. *World J Pediatr Congenit Heart Surg*. 2011 Apr;2(2):243–248. https://doi.org/10.1177/2150135110397386. PMID: 23804979.
8. Roh Jason, Houstis Nicolas, Rosenzweig Anthony. Why don't we have proven treatment for HFpEF. *Circ Res*. 2017;120:1243–1245.
9. Lee S, Nguyen MD, Pierre Baudinaud MD, Alain Brusset MD, Florence Nicot MD, et al. Heart failure with preserved ejection fraction as an independent risk factor of mortality after cardiothoracic surgery. *J Thorac Cardiovasc Surg*. 2018;2:1–6.

18

Mechanical Circulatory Support in Pediatrics

Kyle William Riggs, David N. Rosenthal, David Luís Simón Morales

KEY POINTS

INTRODUCTION

Mechanical circulatory support (MCS) for pediatric patients has advanced enormously, since its first reported use in the 1950s by Gibbon, Kirklin, and Lillehei in the form of a cardiopulmonary bypass machine.[1,2] Kirklin and others were the first group to develop a pump oxygenator with a much smaller priming volume.[3] The rapid evolution of cardiopulmonary bypass continued for the next 20 years, including the refinement of deep hypothermic circulatory arrest in infants by Barratt-Boyes and Casteneda in the 1970s.[4,5] Over the ensuing decades, continued iterative improvements in cardiopulmonary bypass technology and operative techniques contributed to a significant reduction in mortality associated with pediatric cardiac surgery and paved the way for expanded indications for ventricular support in children with heart failure. While MCS is a remarkably diverse field with a multitude of devices, ventricular assist devices (VADs) are now a key component in the management of advanced pediatric heart failure. The early use of adult VADs in older, adult-sized adolescents demonstrated encouraging outcomes, but the development of the Berlin Heart EXCOR (Berlin Heart AG, Berlin, Germany) was the pivotal event that allowed for mechanical support in children of all sizes. Nonetheless, key technical challenges specific to pediatrics remain to this day, including pump design and the management of anticoagulation. Our understanding of the outcomes of MCS has also continued to grow, as there are now over 700 device placements at more than 40 hospitals documented in the Pediatric Registry for Mechanically Assisted Circulatory Support (PediMACS) database, allowing for detailed evaluation of this important group of patients.

HEART FAILURE IN CHILDREN

Although, worldwide, the major etiologies of heart failure in children include rheumatic heart disease, Chagas disease, cardiomyopathies, and congenital heart disease (CHD), in the United States, the most common causes of heart failure in children are dilated cardiomyopathy and CHD. Epidemiological studies estimate that pediatric dilated cardiomyopathy has a case incidence of ~400 cases per year in the US,[6,7] an estimated case prevalence of 6000 pediatric patients, and a median survival ranging from 7 to 18 years. It is important to note that not all of these patients have severe heart failure. According to the Organ Procurement and Transplantation Network, roughly 300 pediatric patients are listed annually for heart transplantation due to severe heart failure from dilated cardiomyopathy.[8] CHD constitutes a much more heterogeneous group of patients as the probability of heart failure varies greatly by specific lesion (Fig. 18.1).[9]

Single-ventricle lesions are a large contributor to the incidence of heart failure in the CHD population. It is estimated that over 2000 children are born annually with single-ventricle CHD, with approximately 300 CHD children undergoing heart transplantation.[8,10] Using national datasets, investigators have estimated that 14,000 pediatric heart failure hospitalizations occur annually with a 7.4% unadjusted mortality rate. Of these, 60%–70% are attributed to CHD.[11,12] Despite the greater prevalence of heart failure admissions for CHD, the vast majority of VADs (80%) are implanted in patients with cardiomyopathy.[13] High mortality associated with pediatric end-stage heart disease stems from directly related sequelae, such as low cardiac output, respiratory failure, malignant arrhythmias, stroke, thromboembolism, irreversible end-organ dysfunction, and infection.[14] This mortality has continued to improve over time with better medical care and advancing surgical repairs, including the use of MCS.[15]

Heart transplantation has become the standard of care for children with end-stage heart disease. Although survival has steadily improved after pediatric heart transplantation, donor availability leads to prolonged waitlist times, and mortality while listed continues to be a major challenge, with mortality rates approaching 20%.[16–18] However, recent studies have demonstrated a 50% reduction in waitlist mortality in pediatric patients receiving VAD support.[19,20] Zafar and colleagues found VADs to be an independent predictor of survival, whereas weight <10 kg, CHD diagnosis, extracorporeal membrane oxygenation (ECMO), mechanical ventilation, and renal dysfunction were all independent predictors of mortality on the waitlist. Evaluating the impact of age on this phenomenon, Law and colleagues showed that the VAD waitlist survival advantage was most profound in adolescent (>11 years) patients as compared with medical therapy. This is likely an effect of the

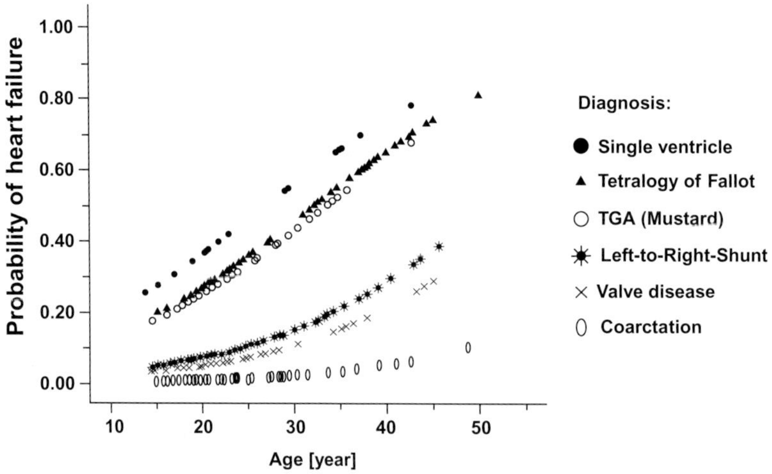

Fig. 18.1 Probability of heart failure over age and type of heart defect. Heart failure is seen in 20% of single ventricle patients by age 10 and rises 1.5% per year thereafter. *TGA*, Transposition of the great arteries. (Reprinted with permission from the American Journal of Cardiology.)

current stages of device development, with older patients being supported with third-generation VADs while pulsatile support or ECMO are the primary available options for smaller children. In this context, the National Heart, Lung, and Blood Institute (NHLBI) is funding development of the Jarvik 2015, a continuous-flow pediatric-specific device, which is beginning a clinical trial in patients 8–15 kg.

CURRENT DEVICES FOR PEDIATRIC CARDIAC SUPPORT

Extracorporeal Membrane Oxygenation

ECMO remains a common method of MCS for pediatric patients due to institutional familiarity and ability to rapidly initiate support. This familiarity has developed over 30 years, but improved outcomes have been limited, with nearly half of cardiac ECMO patients dying prior to discharge.[21] Although individual institutions have shown success and ECMO equipment has improved significantly, widespread success nationally as bridge-to-transplant support has not been realized. In addition, the incidences of mechanical, hemorrhagic, and neurologic complications all exceed 30%.

ECMO was initially used in pediatrics for primary respiratory failure with considerable success,[22,23] in contrast to adult ECMO for respiratory failure, in which a National Institutes of Health trial was halted due to the absence of a survival benefit.[24] The successful use of ECMO in pediatric respiratory disease is important for two reasons: (1) this finding highlighted the need for pediatric-specific investigations of new devices and (2) successful neonatal respiratory ECMO likely altered the course of development of mechanical cardiac support in children. With clinicians encouraged by its success in the area of respiratory support, ECMO for cardiac support became increasingly common despite its challenges, since it was all that was available for children with acute heart failure.

Initial reports of pediatric ECMO described its application primarily in postcardiotomy patients.[25–28] Survival rates for all pediatric patients supported for cardiac indications were nearly 50%, with significant complications of bleeding, thrombosis, and neurologic injury in over 30% of cases.[29–31] In 1992, Del Nido and colleagues described the use of ECMO in 33 patients for cardiac support after cardiac surgery.[32] Eleven of these patients were placed on support following cardiac arrest after an average of 65 minutes of cardiopulmonary resuscitation. Patients supported in this "rescue" fashion had a 64% early and 55% long-term survival rate despite the long duration of cardiopulmonary resuscitation. In addition, survival in this group was similar to that of the entire group. These findings led most centers with significant volumes of pediatric cardiac surgery to develop ECMO "rapid deployment" units.[33,34]

In cardiac surgery, ECMO has been used to maintain cardiorespiratory function until other cardiopulmonary derangements have been adequately treated, as a bridge to transplantation or as a bridge to long-term device placement.[32,35–40] Despite advancing VAD technology, ECMO remains the best support option for patients in cardiogenic shock requiring rapid support for cardiac arrest or to provide cardiopulmonary support as long as a pulmonary component is necessary. If a VAD is initially used, extracorporeal centrifugal pumps, such as the Pedi/CentriMag (Abbott, Lake Bluff, IL) or Jostra ROTAFLOW (MAQUET, Inc., Rastatt, Germany), lend themselves to the "splicing" of an oxygenator into the VAD circuit tubing if respiratory failure ensues.[41] Other novel techniques have been used to place a gas exchange membrane within an existing VAD circuit.[42,43] The most frequent potential contraindications to ECMO support are severe neurologic injury, prematurity and small size (<2 kg), active bleeding, irreversible disease, and noncardiac major structural and chromosomal abnormalities.[44] In general, successful arterial-venous ECMO support is usually for periods of less than 2 weeks, whether being used as a bridge to recovery or transplantation. Furthermore, ECMO support at time of heart transplantation is well recognized as one of the highest risk factors for posttransplant mortality, with 1- and 5-year survival reported at 61% and 35%, respectively, significantly lower than that of other pediatric heart transplant recipients whose median survival is >10 years.[45,46]

Left Ventricular Assist Devices

In addition to pulmonary function, ECMO supports both the right and left heart using a single cannulation strategy of systemic venous and arterial cannulation. Therefore, in the current era, most centers still rely on ECMO for all patients needing rapid or postcardiotomy support.

Nonetheless, it is clear that unchanged survival rates since 1985, high incidences of complications, and the inability to reliably and safely support children for longer than 2 weeks leave significant room for improvement. Over the same period of development of ECMO technology for children, ever-improving VAD technologies were being developed for long-term adult cardiac support. This technology has been carefully integrated into the care of children with heart failure as we await the development of better pediatric-specific devices.

Temporary Support Strategies

Regardless of device, temporary support has come to mean a quick and simple cannulation strategy for stabilization of cardiac function in (1) a patient thought to have an inflammatory etiology of heart failure (i.e., myocarditis or acute graft rejection) with an expectation to recover within 2 weeks and (2) as support for someone in cardiogenic shock as a bridge to a more durable device. Furthermore, temporary VAD support may provide a period to assess neurologic status or etiology of heart failure prior to placement of a durable VAD or performance of a heart transplant.[47] Typically, this has been accomplished with extracorporeal, centrifugal pumps such as the Centri/PediMag or the ROTAFLOW connected to temporary bypass cannulas placed centrally and off cardiopulmonary bypass.[48–50] It is the cannulation strategy rather than the choice of pump that best defines the type of support, as Berlin Heart cannulas placed on cardiopulmonary bypass can be used with extracorporeal, centrifugal pumps for extended periods of time as a bridge to transplant. This strategy also allows transition to other devices (e.g., Berlin Heart EXCOR) externally at the bedside and for pump exchange if thrombosis develops. This strategy is becoming increasingly popular, particularly in smaller patients presenting challenges with anticoagulation during their postoperative inflammatory state and for single-ventricle patients with pulmonary artery bands, large aortopulmonary collateralization, or shunted physiology. In these patients, the centrifugal mechanics of the pump make it ideal for rapidly accommodating changes in preload and flow without constant adjustment to the device parameters. Additionally, an oxygenator can be spliced into the circuit relatively easily to simulate ECMO, as can an ultrafiltration/dialysis system to provide renal support.[51] As these techniques in management and others are honed, evidence is accumulating that these historically "short-term" devices can safely support patients for longer periods of time than previously thought.[52]

Two other less commonly used temporary options are delivered percutaneously and are therefore less invasive. These include the TandemHeart (CardiaAssist, Pittsburgh, PA) and the Impella (Abiomed, Danvers, MA). Both devices require large vessels to accommodate the catheter dimensions, generally necessitating a body surface area (BSA) >1.3 m^2. The Impella is placed across the aortic valve under echocardiographic guidance to augment cardiac output with axial, continuous-flow support, while the TandemHeart has a venous cannula percutaneously placed through the atrial septum into the left atrium with arterial output to the femoral artery. Although little data exist regarding these devices in pediatrics, a single center reported that 10 Impella devices with a median implant time of 8 days (range, 1–21) supported eight patients (median age, 17 years; range, 6.5–25 years), with all discharged from the intensive care unit.[53] Five patients had posttransplant rejection or allograft vasculopathy causing heart failure, and four patients also required ECMO. Because the pediatric MCS field includes many children with multiple prior sternotomies, there was initial enthusiasm for the TandemHeart percutaneous system, but the fact that most movement, even for daily care (i.e., chest roentgenogram), often causes a change in location requiring repositioning has limited its use in the pediatric community.

Durable Strategies

As "adult" VADs became available over the past 20 years, they have been increasingly used in adolescents. Although covered in detail elsewhere in this text (see Chapter 10), durable VADs can be grouped broadly into two separate categories, pulsatile and continuous-flow pumps. Pulsatile pumps were the first VADs developed but have since given way to second- and third-generation continuous-flow pumps in the great majority of cases, with the exception of the Total Artificial Heart (SynCardia, Tuscon, AZ) and the pediatric-specific Berlin Heart EXCOR. In the PediMACS registry, among patients receiving a durable VAD, 94% of patients <20 kg receive a pulsatile, extracorporeal VAD, while 85% of those >20 kg get an intracorporeal, continuous-flow VAD, which in the past several years has increased to approximately 95%.

Continuous-flow devices. The HeartMate II (Thoratec) is an axial, continuous-flow pump approved for adults that can provide up to 10 L/min of cardiac output. When the HeartMate II pump was compared in a randomized fashion with the pulsatile HeartMate XVE (Thoratec) in a destination therapy population, it was found to have a significantly greater rate of "survival free from disabling stroke and reoperation to repair or replace the left VAD (LVAD) (62% vs. 7%)," with a 1-year survival of 68% versus 58% for the pulsatile pump.[54] With higher survival, better durability, and more functional capacity leading to a better quality of life, this device initiated the transition from pulsatile to continuous-flow technology in adult devices. This pump, along with others, has been used successfully in pediatric patients, although due to the device size, it is best suited for pediatric patients with a BSA ≥1.4 m^2 (~40–45 kg).[55,56] There are reports of pediatric patients discharged home on this device.[57] In a series of pediatric patients implanted with a HeartMate II, 95% were transplanted, recovered, or stable on the device at 6 months postimplantation, with 21% experiencing a bleeding complication, 7% suffering a stroke, and 11% developing sepsis.[58] In comparison to the HeartMate II, the HeartWare HVAD (Medtronic, MN) has a smaller device profile and is the most commonly used durable continuous-flow device in pediatric patients. More recently, the HeartMate 3 (Abbott, Lake Bluff, IL) has been used in children, making the HeartMate II more of historical significance in pediatric MCS.

The HeartWare HVAD, the most common intracorporeal continuous-flow device for children, was implanted in 192 pediatric patients (<19 years old) in the pediatric portion (PediMACS) of the Interagency Registry for Mechanically Assisted Circulatory Support (INTERMACS) from 2012 to 2017.[59] Within this review, the median BSA was 1.5 m^2 (range, 0.6–2.9 m^2), with 12 children weighing ≤20 kg, of whom 53% had CHD. The median duration of support was 2.8 months, with fewer infections (27% vs. 44%) and device malfunction/pump thrombosis (11% vs. 19%) compared with matched patients aged 19–30 years and a similar rate of major bleeds (23% vs. 23%) and stroke (10% vs. 12%) as the older patients. Importantly, there was no survival difference between the pediatric patients and young adults, while the rate of discharge on the device was 48% in children ≥20 kg. However, at 6 months, 59% of the pediatric patients were transplanted, with 32% alive on device compared with only 17% of the young adults transplanted with 77% alive on the device. These excellent outcomes were corroborated by a global report of 205 pediatric patients, with an 89% positive outcome at 1 year.[60] With outcomes comparable to those in adults, the HVAD is a great device option in children over 20 kg, with success also in some carefully selected patients below 20 kg.

With its Food and Drug Administration (FDA) approval for adults in late 2017, the HeartMate 3 has become an increasingly popular off-label intracorporeal continuous-flow device for pediatric patients. Its complete magnetic levitation technology provides frictionless rotor movement, with the goal of reducing hemolysis and thrombosis. Due to the magnetic levitation, it is slightly larger than the HVAD, although it has a shorter inflow cannula, which can be beneficial in pediatric patients with smaller ventricular cavities.[61] It is also thought to decompress the systemic ventricle better, which may be essential in supporting certain patient cohorts such as Fontan patients. Through the authors' personal communication (April 02, 2019, verbal communication with David Morales), we are aware of 32 pediatric implants of the HeartMate

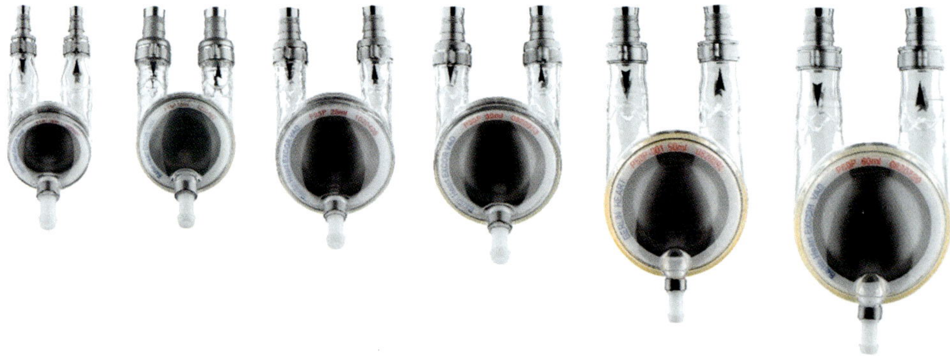

Fig. 18.2 The six available blood chamber sizes (10, 15, 25, 30, 50, and 60 mL) for the Berlin Heart EXCOR combined with multiple cannula options allow for its implantation in children of all sizes. (Courtesy Robert Kroslowitz, Berlin Heart, Inc., Berlin, Germany.)

3 and know data on 14 at six centers, primarily for dilated cardiomyopathy (93%). The median BSA was 1.8 m^2 (1.3–2.4 m^2), with support ranging from 5 to 315 days. Only one patient died on the device, and 36% were discharged home with currently no reports of stroke or pump thrombosis. The HeartMate 3 shows promise to be another excellent device to support pediatric patients, although longer follow-up and determination of the lower size limits must still be established.

Pulsatile devices. The total artificial heart (TAH) is the only currently available pulsatile MCS device for adults and it has also been employed in pediatric patients. The original TAH was conceived by Robert Jarvik in 1982 as the Jarvik 7 and has also had several other names, including the Symbion, Cardiowest, and currently the SynCardia TAH. It was first approved for bridge to transplantation in 2004. Since the development of the Freedom driver (~6 kg portable driver), the number of implants has tripled, with over 40% of the >2000 implants in the past 7 years. The TAH has offered life-sustaining support to a number of pediatric patients who could not be adequately supported with a VAD. Issues with multiple congenital defects requiring repair prior to LVAD support (i.e., intraventricular shunts, semilunar valve insufficiency, etc.), primary cardiac arrhythmias, and ventricular clots are uniquely resolved by replacement of the ventricles and atrioventricular valves with the device. Furthermore, the TAH is suited for specific patient populations, including those with chronic rejection after orthotopic heart transplantation (as the TAH allows for cessation of immunosuppression), late failing Fontan circulations, or chronic biventricular failure in the setting of an LVAD; cancer patients; or those with multiple defects that would require repair prior to VAD placement.[62] The device has biventricular, pneumatic compression chambers, which are implanted in the thoracic cavity in place of the native ventricles. The TAH is capable of providing supraphysiologic cardiac output with the differentiating ability to do so with a minimal central venous pressure that is nearly impossible to achieve with a VAD or even with a newly transplanted heart. This has allowed for recovery of other end organs (e.g., kidney or liver) thought not to be salvageable. The 70 cc TAH is available for use in patients with a BSA >1.7 m^2. Because of improving results and increasing use in patients with congenital defects and in pediatric patients, a 50 cc device was developed and is being evaluated in an FDA trial for use in patients with a BSA between 1.2 and 1.85 m^2 or for those in whom fit can be demonstrated by virtual implantation. This is the first time virtual fit has been allowed to be a criterion by the FDA, which is a result of work done by a few programs in the pediatric VAD community.[63] This software has shown that the device could be fit in 33% more patients than using BSA-derived criteria alone. As shown through personal communication with SynCardia (December 03, 2018, email communication with David Morales), the new device has been implanted >70 times, with a particular increase in congenital defect (4%–9% of implants), pediatric (4%–13%), and female (12%–70%) patients, making it a promising option for a selected pediatric population.

The Berlin Heart EXCOR is a paracorporeal, pulsatile, pneumatically compressed volume displacement pump. It is available in 10-, 15-, 25-, 30-, 50-, and 60-mL blood chamber sizes (Fig. 18.2). Use of customized polyurethane valves has allowed for the manufacturing of smaller blood pump sizes than have been used in "adult" pumps. Furthermore, a bedside driver unit, which is under development, will be available in 2019 and would allow better mobilization and the potential for pediatric patients to be discharged home with the EXCOR for the first time ever in North America. Its first reported successful use as a bridge to transplantation occurred in 1990,[64] with subsequent worldwide experience in more than 2000 patients at >100 centers. The longest known support is 877 days before successful transplantation.[65] The experience at the Berlin Heart Institute (Berlin, Germany) has been extensively reported.[66–68] The initial outcomes of 28 patients are displayed in Fig. 18.3, with 13 dying and 13 bridging to transplantation with 5 early posttransplantation deaths.[69] By 2000, survival had improved significantly, with a 74% survival rate to transplant or discharge. The authors also attributed this improvement to better decision-making, which entailed earlier implantation prior to irreversible organ failure, newer cannulas, switching from atrial cannulation to apical cannulation of the left ventricle, standardization of anticoagulation regimens, and a decrease in biventricular assist support.

The device was first used in North America in 2001 and was widely used by 2006. The initial multicenter experience with the EXCOR reported on 73 patients who had a 77% positive outcome.[70] In 2008, the FDA approved the device for an Investigational Device Exemption (IDE) trial, which enrolled 48 patients in two study arms for smaller and larger patients.[71] Several single-center reports describe many successful outcomes with great variation in the need for LVAD versus biventricular assist device (BiVAD) support, and ultimately, the IDE study confirmed the Berlin Heart EXCOR to be better than ECMO.[70,72–75] Enrolled contemporaneously with the IDE trial, the outcomes of all 204 children who underwent EXCOR implantation in North America (including those ineligible for the IDE trial) were reported as the real-world application of the device.[76] The investigators described a successful outcome in 75% of patients, with only one death due to device malfunction. Predictors of early mortality (<2 months) included lower weight, higher bilirubin, and BiVAD support. The most common cause of death was stroke in 33% of patients, most commonly thromboembolic. More recently, posttransplant survival analysis has shown no difference between patients bridged with a Berlin Heart EXCOR and patients with no device, with 94% 30-day, 90% 1-year, and 72% 5-year survival.[77] Similar outcomes were noted

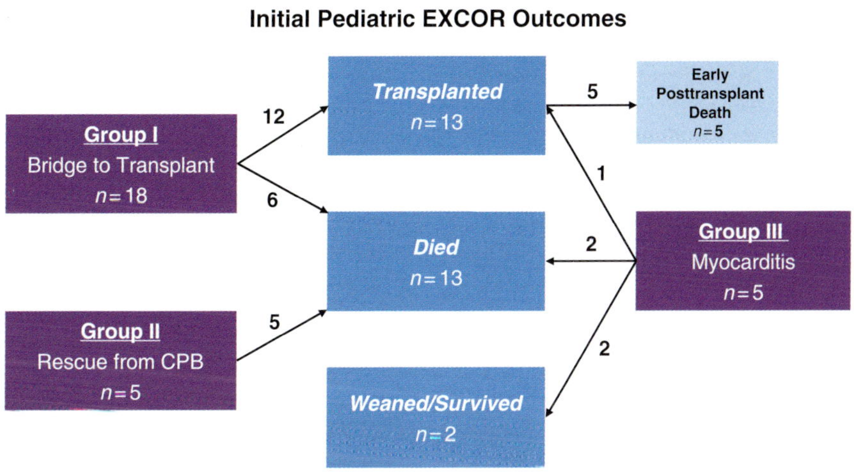

Fig. 18.3 Outcomes of the first 28 patients undergoing Berlin Heart EXCOR implantation grouped by indication for ventricular assist. *CPB*, Cardiopulmonary bypass.

in CHD patients bridged to transplantation, and findings in both series suggested that patients who would have been high-risk transplant candidates (i.e., ventilated, renal insufficiency) were made better candidates with VAD therapy.[78]

Pediatric Device Initiatives

With increased use of the Berlin Heart in North America, the U.S. Department of Health and Human Services identified pediatric MCS as a critical unmet need for pediatric patients. Because of the relatively small numbers of children requiring support compared with the adult market, industry investment was lacking. This prompted the development of a $22 million NHLBI initiative, the Pediatric MCS Program, to promote research and development of mechanical support devices specifically for small children. These awards (2004–2009) led to significant scientific advances culminating in the development of five novel pediatric circulatory support devices. These include a smaller version of the Jarvik 2000 (Jarvik Heart, NY) continuous-flow pump; a smaller pulsatile pump based on the Pierce-Donachy design of the Thoratec PVAD (Penn State Pediatric VAD; Pennsylvania State University–Hershey Medical Center, Hershey, PA); an adult catheter-based pump modified for extracardiac, intrapericardial use (Cleveland Clinic PediPump; Cleveland, OH); an implantable, fully magnetically levitated mixed flow pump (PediaFlow; University of Pittsburgh, Pittsburgh, PA); and a paracorporeal integrated pump oxygenator (Ension pCAS; Ension, Inc., Pittsburgh, PA).[79] Although all of these pumps saw successful animal experimentation and $23 million additional dollars were allocated for further funding, only the Jarvik 2015 is still undergoing testing and is currently in a safety-only FDA trial. The final device design is an intracorporeal, axial continuous-flow device the size of an AA battery for use in children 8–20 kg.

In addition to device development, the NHLBI has recognized the importance of rigorous data collection after approval of a device. INTERMACS has been a pivotal development for the adult MCS field, as has the pediatric-specific PediMACS portion, which now has over 700 device implants (January 12, 2019, verbal communication with PediMACS executive committee). Another recently established network, Advanced cardiac therapies improving outcomes network (ACTION), is a learning network of over 25 pediatric centers focused on improving the quality of care and outcomes for pediatric MCS through real-time sharing of data and management strategies.[80] Together, these networks and registries will be pivotal for researchers looking to optimize VAD care for pediatric patients, especially since individual center volume per year is low (< 10 per year).

BRIDGE-TO-TRANSPLANTATION

An increasing percentage of pediatric heart transplants (currently over 40%) are being performed in patients bridged with VAD support,[81] and current practice is demonstrating excellent waitlist survival while on VAD support with improvement in other end-organ function prior to transplantation. All of this is translating into excellent posttransplantation survival. Comparing posttransplantation outcomes between patients bridged to transplantation with VADs and those with no pretransplantation VAD support, Sutcliffe and colleagues[82] found no difference in 1-year posttransplantation survival (96% vs. 93%), infection (81% vs. 79%), or rejection (71% vs. 74%). Also, they noted that the VAD cohort had greater requirements for inotrope and ventilator support, along with increased liver and renal dysfunction at device implantation. By transplant, both liver and renal dysfunction had normalized in VAD patients and there was substantial decrease in the number of patients requiring inotropic support (94%–33%) and mechanical ventilation (44%–11%). Further evidence for VAD support improving renal function was shown in a PediMACS review of 150 patients with renal dysfunction (estimated glomerular filtration rate <90 mL/min/1.73 m^2), which found that estimated glomerular filtration normalized in 67% of patients by 1 month postimplantation.[83] In patients with renal dysfunction, an average improvement from 62.4 mL/min/1.73 m^2 to 107.7 ml/min/1.73^2 was associated with VAD support. This is important since renal dysfunction is highly associated with poor posttransplantation survival.[84,85] This renal improvement is seen as early as 1 week postimplantation and generally reaches a plateau at about 1 month.

Discharge from the hospital prior to transplantation may be an indicator of overall wellness and therefore may be associated with better posttransplantation survival. Additionally, hospital discharge has been associated with a lower cost of care while bridging patients to transplantation, which makes a continuous-flow device more desirable in a patient where discharge is possible.[86] Furthermore, the authors are aware of impending reports demonstrating that a period of time, generally ~2 months from time of VAD implantation, allows for improvement in numerous end-organ functions (i.e., respiratory, renal, functional, etc.) and is associated with improved posttransplantation survival as compared with less than 2 months of support. This is of critical importance, since patients "limping" to transplantation with other end-organ dysfunction consistently demonstrate worse posttransplantation survival, if they reach transplantation at all.[87,88] Overall, VADs of all types have continued to improve patient survival to transplantation and are now being examined for the potential to improve posttransplantation survival as well.

MANAGEMENT OF PEDIATRIC PATIENTS RECEIVING CARDIAC ASSIST DEVICE THERAPY

Cardiac support in children presents particular challenges beyond those seen in adults. Because of their size, devices must be smaller than those used in adults, which adds to the biomechanical complexity. In addition, whereas the majority of adults (>99%) in need of these services have normal anatomical cardiac and arteriovenous anatomy, the anatomy in children who are candidates for VAD support is frequently complex, since over 20% of VADs are placed in children with CHD. To compound this, the number of children requiring these devices is far smaller than the number of adults, resulting in a prolonged learning curve for each device. This is why ACTION, a multiinstitutional learning network, is such an important addition for improving VAD therapy in the field.

Indications for Mechanical Circulatory Support in Children

As mentioned previously, the general indications for cardiac support in children are primarily bridge to transplantation and, occasionally, bridge to recovery (6%) and, even less commonly, destination therapy (2%).[13] Although chronic care in children is limited, the fact that 50% of children with commonly used continuous-flow devices are discharged home means the line between bridge to candidacy and chronic support is becoming less clear. Although the use of the HeartMate 3 in adults has shown equivalent survival at 2 years to heart transplantation, minimization of complications remains an important hurdle for chronic VAD therapy. There is occasionally a role for destination therapy in certain pediatric cohorts (i.e., Duchene muscular dystrophy, cancer patients, obesity, etc.) who are thought not to be good transplant candidates and in patients with complex CHD for whom heart transplantation is not an option secondary to chronic medical conditions. It is possible in this group that destination therapy will improve end-organ function sufficiently to allow select patients to eventually undergo transplantation.

Acute pediatric heart failure most commonly arises postcardiotomy, induced by prolonged ischemic cardiac arrest, ventricular distention, residual defects, or as an exacerbation of preexisting (but often undiagnosed) myocardial dysfunction. Other cohorts include patients with structurally normal hearts presenting with acute myocarditis, decompensated cardiomyopathy, acute graft rejection, and those with CHD with long-standing myocardial dysfunction who decompensate secondary to a stressor (i.e., respiratory infection, arrhythmia, etc.).[89] Because of the short-term nature of successful ECMO support, initiation of MCS was historically reserved for those patients in extremis with fulminant cardiovascular collapse and impending cardiac arrest, and often only after cardiac arrest. However, with improving devices and MCS experience, it has become clear that implanting devices prior to major patient decompensation allows for the best survival while on circulatory support.[90] This is best demonstrated by the near 50% mortality of INTERMACS level I patients in critical cardiogenic shock undergoing VAD implantation compared with all other levels (Fig. 18.4).[13]

Early initiation of mechanical support may avoid the excessive use of pharmacologic agents (catecholamines) that increase myocardial oxygen demands while also increasing the workload of the heart (systemic and pulmonary vascular resistance). These additional stresses can compound the ongoing myocardial injury. Mechanical support reduces myocardial work while increasing myocardial oxygen delivery. These benefits are enhanced by the frequent ability to wean the patient from pharmacologic support and mechanical ventilation and improve other end-organ function.[82,83,89] Conditions that still benefit from the rapid initiation of ECMO with transition to temporary or durable support include patients with impending arrest not amenable to the timeframe required for VAD support, cardiac arrest, and those children presenting with heart failure and significant difficulty to ventilate.

Timing of Support and Device Selection

The field of VAD support has conclusively decided and demonstrated that the early implementation of VAD support, before end-organ deterioration,

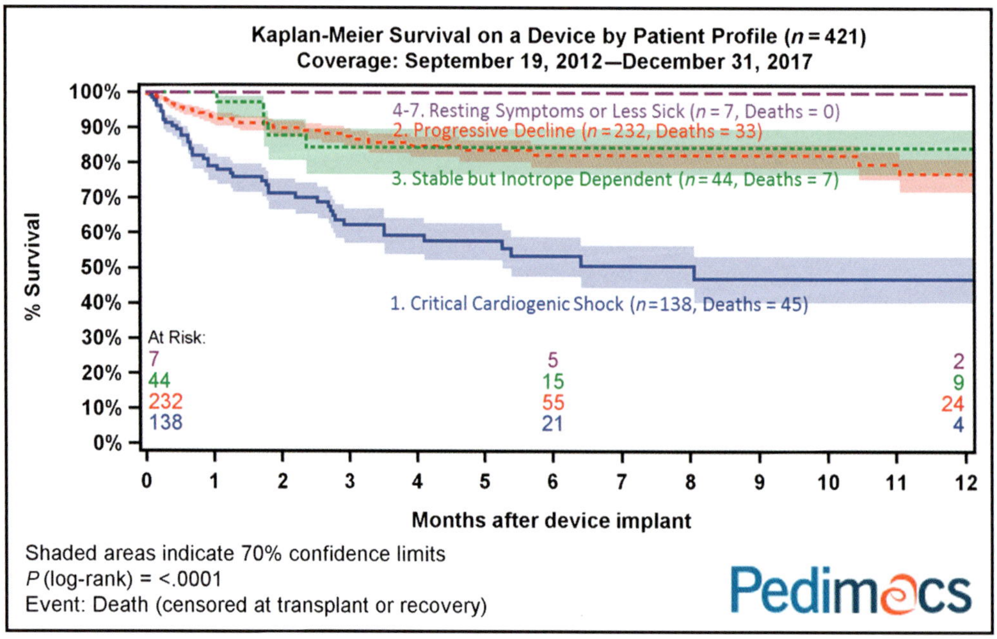

Fig. 18.4 Actuarial patients' survival in months after ventricular assist device implantation by severity of illness. (From Annals of Thoracic Surgery. 2019;107(4):993–1004).

leads to significantly better outcomes, and this has been corroborated in children by multiple studies.[13,66,91,92] Nonetheless, evidence of end-organ injury should be considered a relative indication for VAD placement and should be a cause for caution when considering heart transplantation, as it is associated with worse posttransplantation survival. Furthermore, significant cardiogenic shock should be considered a contraindication to durable devices, and these patients should undergo temporary VAD support to improve their candidacy for durable support.

Overall, indications for initiation and type of mechanical support are becoming better defined, as displayed in Fig. 18.5. ECMO would seem warranted for those patients who acutely collapse or have the need for pulmonary support. A temporary device strategy is warranted in those who have a condition thought to be rapidly reversible over the course of days (e.g. arrhythmia, postcardiotomy or posttransplantation, and myocarditis). In some institutions, this might be best performed with ECMO, while in others, a greater familiarity with temporary VADs might tip the balance toward this approach. The projected inability to wean from support in days (<2 weeks) or a chronic heart failure patient who is worsening in the absence of contraindications (e.g., severe neurologic injury and unrecoverable concomitant illness) should be considered an indication for durable VAD placement. Clinicians should consider VAD support in severe heart failure patients in whom another end-organ system begins to be threatened because of poor perfusion (i.e., the need for intubation due to cardiac failure; escalating or high doses of inotropic support; poor peripheral perfusion as evidenced by acidosis or base deficit, low mixed venous saturation, and cool extremities; and/or the onset of end-organ failure [renal or hepatic failure]).

OTHER TOPICS IN PEDIATRIC MECHANICAL CIRCULATORY SUPPORT

Biventricular Assist Device Support

Biventricular assist device support has decreased over time with experience in the adult population to less than 10% per the INTERMACS

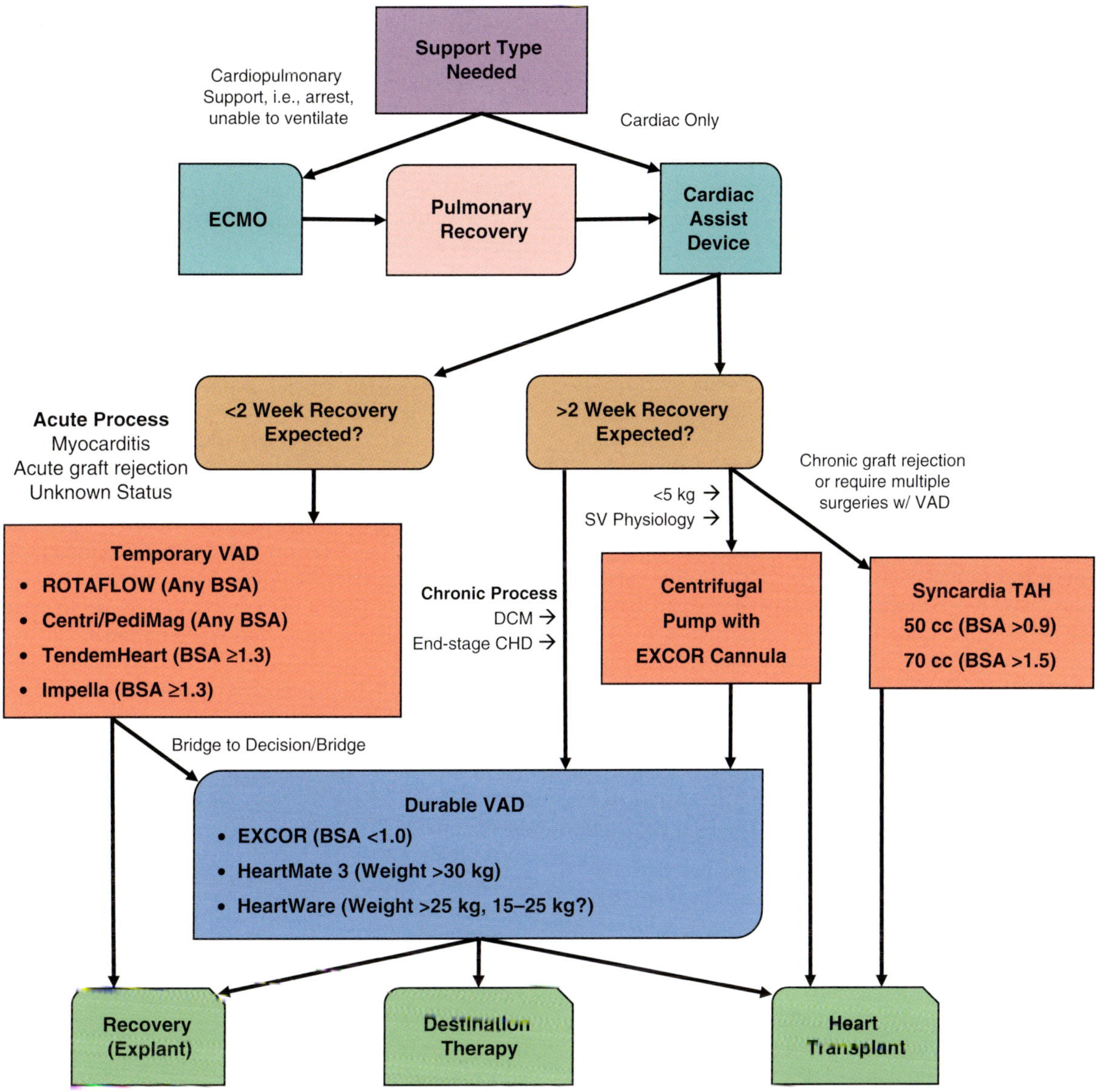

Fig. 18.5 Flow diagram for mechanical circulatory support decision making in pediatrics. *BSA*, Body surface area; *CHD*, congenital heart disease; *DCM*, dilated cardiomyopathy; *ECMO*, extracorporeal membranous oxygenation; *SV*, single ventricle; *TAH*, total artificial heart; *VAD*, ventricular assist device.

registry and has been associated with improved outcomes.[93,94] It is intuitive that biventricular support might magnify certain risks over LVAD support alone. Most notably in pediatrics, bleeding and infectious complications may increase because of the necessity of placing more equipment and having more exit sites in a small pediatric patient. As the pediatric VAD field has gained experience, the use of BiVAD therapy has decreased from over 50% to less than 20% in the current era with the expected improvement in survival. The Berlin Heart Institute pointed to the decreased reliance on biventricular support, from 68% to 33%, as their experience progressed as one reason for their significantly improved outcomes.[66] In the early North American experience, studies reported BiVAD use from 39% to 56% of the time as compared with 15% of the patients in the most recent PediMACS report.[13,55,95,96] A study of the Berlin Heart EXCORs in North America focused on BiVADs confirmed that this device strategy had a higher mortality than LVAD support but was unable to identify a specific cohort of patients who benefit from BiVAD support.[97] This is surprising, as most experts agree that around 10% or less of patients probably would benefit from biventricular support over LVAD support. Unlike many studies in adults that have focused on the hemodynamic and echocardiographic findings to determine who would be better served with BiVAD support, the need for biventricular support in pediatrics is likely associated with etiology of heart failure (e.g., arrhythmias, biventricular restrictive disease, and certain congenital defects) and timing of support, not preoperative hemodynamics or laboratory values.

At this time, most centers place an LVAD and attempt to wean from cardiopulmonary bypass. Once the patient is weaned and on LVAD support, right ventricular function and geometry are monitored in the operating room by transesophageal echocardiography, invasive pulmonary artery monitoring, and right ventricular or central venous pressure, as is gas exchange and lung compliance. Specific perioperative maneuvers can reduce the need for BiVAD support, including limiting circulating volume, reducing myocardial edema/cytokine overload via ultrafiltration, limiting bleeding/blood products, and always aggressively supporting the right heart in the immediate postimplantation period with inhaled nitric oxide and milrinone and/or epinephrine. Nonetheless, marked deterioration of right ventricular function necessitates placement of a right VAD (RVAD), although returning to the operating room to place an RVAD significantly decreases the chance of survival. Intensive care unit management is somewhat different with BiVADs versus LVAD only. Usually, no inotropes are required, nor is pharmacologic or electrical control of the heart rhythm. With LVAD use alone, careful attention must be paid to right ventricular output to ensure adequate filling of the LVAD. Right ventricular filling and function may be negatively affected by pericardial effusion, compression of the right ventricle by the LVAD outflow cannula (especially with the EXCOR), and ventricular septal orientation. With BiVAD support, the RVAD settings generally are made to ensure slightly less flow than for the LVAD to avoid producing undesired elevations in left atrial pressure leading to pulmonary congestion.

Congenital Heart Disease

MCS in patients with CHD presents several additional challenges and has continued to be associated with worse outcomes compared with patients with cardiomyopathy.[13,55,70,96] VAD support as a "salvage" operation following a failed palliation and ECMO presents a high risk for transition to VAD therapy as a bridge-to-transplantation strategy, and it remains unclear if this offers much of a survival benefit, especially in single-ventricle patients. Furthermore, unique anatomy (particularly transposition of the great arteries and single-ventricle circulations), mixed circulations, and shunts pose significant challenges with regard to the placement of VADs and the management of their care postoperatively.

Single-Ventricle Support

Although it is simplest to group patients on the single ventricle pathway as single-ventricle hearts (SVHs), from a clinical and outcomes-based research standpoint, they are best considered distinct pathophysiologic cohorts based on stage of palliation as either pre-bidirectional Glenn (BDG), post-BDG (prior to Fontan), or post-Fontan. As is the case in all VAD placement, but particularly in these populations, timing of initiation of support and patient selection are paramount to achieving good outcomes.

The Berlin Heart EXCOR has found little success in pre-BDG patients. Nine patients from the North American Berlin Heart EXCOR experience were SVH undergoing implantation prior to BDG, of whom eight died.[98] The survivor had previously undergone a Damus-Kaye-Stansel procedure at 19 months of age, making him an anomaly within the pre-BDG SVH group. Additionally, there is yet to be a report of a neonatal Norwood patient successfully bridged through transplantation and discharged home with a Berlin Heart EXCOR, emphasizing that this is an extremely challenging population to treat with MCS. Overall, they appear to be a group that is better supported by veno-arterial ECMO (VA-ECMO), which has been reported to yield a hospital discharge rate as high as 50%.[99] An emerging strategy of connecting Berlin Heart EXCOR cannulas to extracorporeal continuous-flow VADs has shown early success as it is able to readily adjust to the constantly changing Q_p:Q_s in shunted physiology and provide a cardiac index over 4 L/min/m^2.[100] Still, Berlin Heart EXCOR cannulas are not preferable in infants under 3 kg, where shunts and bypass cannulas are likely the better strategy.

Further analysis of the North American experience showed better outcomes in SVH patients after BDG, with 7 of 12 successfully bridged to transplantation with a Berlin Heart EXCOR.[98] Other reports demonstrate equally good survival with the Berlin Heart EXCOR, whereas hospital discharge after VA-ECMO has been reported at 41%.[101–103] Peripheral ECMO, which is via the cervical vessels because of patient size, usually is not well tolerated in BDG circulation because the heart is inadequately decompressed and secondary neurological complications develop. If peripheral cannulation is necessary, it should rapidly be converted to central ECMO or VAD support. It is important to bear in mind that there is usually a different physiology with late BDG failure as opposed to postcardiotomy rescue failure; the former is more common and usually systemic ventricular failure, while the latter is often a pulmonary vasculature issue. Therefore, BDG patients less commonly undergo "salvage" VAD operations, which contributes to the improved outcome over Stage I patients. However, there are opinions that BDG patients are challenging to support because the augmented decompression of the heart favors blood from the inferior vena cava more than that through the Glenn, resulting in cyanosis and poor perfusion at times. Somewhat surprisingly, post-BDG patients developing heart failure often have frequently changing Q_p:Q_s as well, with unexpectedly high cardiac index requirements because they often present in chronic heart failure leading to significant aorto-pulmonary collaterals. This again makes the combination of Berlin Heart EXCOR cannulas with centrifugal pumps a desirable option.

Analysis of post-Fontan MCS is complicated by multiple causes of heart failure (often a mixture of systolic and diastolic failure), complex comorbidities, and an array of potential circulatory support devices.[104] Although MCS is not always the right answer for these patients, after sufficient diagnostic work-up and an understanding if Fontan circulation failure is dominated by right or left sides issues, VAD support can

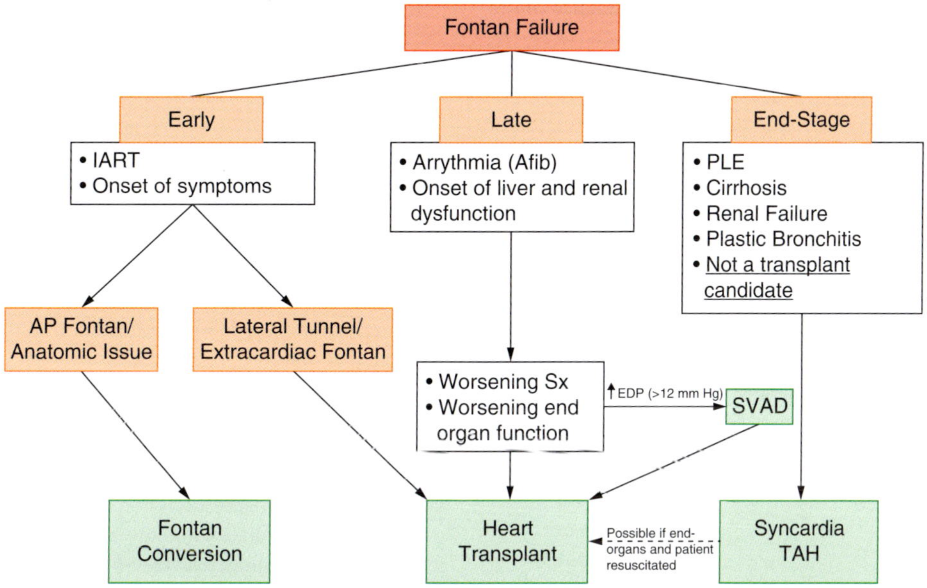

Fig. 18.6 Management flow diagram for the failing Fontan circulation. *AP*, Atriopulmonary; *EDP*, end-diastolic pressure; *IART*, intraatrial reentrant tachycardia; *PLE*, protein-losing enteropathy; *SVAD*, single-ventricle assist device; *Sx*, symptoms; *TAH*, total artificial heart.

successfully bridge many patients to transplantation or possibly serve as destination therapy. The ideal Fontan circulation VAD candidate has late systolic dysfunction with an elevated end-diastolic pressure (>12–14 mm Hg). If both are not present, the patient likely has predominantly right-sided failure, a common issue nonetheless, and will not benefit from VAD placement. Placing a VAD without knowing the end-diastolic pressure via a catheterization will result in inconsistent outcomes, which have marred much of the experience up to now. A simplistic management plan is demonstrated by Fig. 18.6.

As always, timing is essential, and ideally, VAD support should be instituted prior to the development of liver cirrhosis, protein losing enteropathy, renal insufficiency, and plastic bronchitis. With that in mind, VAD support can reverse end-organ dysfunction and improve a patient's transplant candidacy and potentially posttransplantation survival.[105] However, many of these complications are right sided in nature; therefore, a systemic VAD alone will not necessarily improve these issues. As mentioned previously, the TAH, which has been implanted in five Fontan patients, can provide supraphysiologic cardiac output with a central venous pressure <5 mm Hg, which could be of major benefit in Fontan patients with venous congestion and a chronically elevated central venous pressure. There are now over 15 publications reporting on more than 36 Fontan patients (nine through correspondence with the authors) who have undergone VAD or TAH implantation with more than two-thirds having positive outcomes.[61,98,105–116] With all of the complexities of the failing Fontan physiology and available support options, it is imperative to take a systematic approach to device and patient selection.

Adult Congenital Heart Disease

Adults with CHD represent a larger population than children with CHD and comprised 3.3% of the adults undergoing heart transplantation from 2009 to 2014, a rising number.[117,118] This population can also benefit from MCS, both as bridge to transplantation and as destination therapy. A 2017 review of durable VAD use in the INTERMACS registry identified 126 of 16,182 patients (<1%) as having CHD, of whom 17 were considered single-ventricle patients and 45 had a systemic morphological right ventricle.[119] In contrast, more than 20% of children supported with VADs or TAHs have CHD. These adults with CHD were younger and therefore more likely to be listed as bridge to transplantation (45%). There was more biventricular/TAH support in this population at 21%, which carried higher mortality and echoed similar challenges faced in the pediatric congenital heart population. The most promising finding from this analysis was that even though VAD therapy was less often used in this cohort, adult CHD patients receiving only an LVAD experienced similar survival as non-CHD patients, and ventricular morphology had no impact on survival. Another study of the INTERMACS database found that these patients had the same incidence of adverse events and showed the same improvement in functional status and quality of life after implantation as seen in non-CHD patients.[120] Adult CHD patients presenting with end-stage heart failure is an ever-expanding cohort who can be consistently and successfully managed with VAD support as bridge to transplantation with excellent outcomes, or for chronic therapy perhaps as experience and devices improve.

Adverse Events

Previously, the incidence of adverse events was best estimated from various single-center and small database reviews, with infection rates from 39% to 52%, bleeding from 22% to 33%, and neurologic complications from 13% to 27%.[55,95,96,121] As more robust registries have been created, such as PediMACS, adverse events continue to be significant, as demonstrated by a review of 432 device implantations in 364 pediatric patients, which found 58% of patients experiencing at least one major adverse event.[13,122] VAD type and patient age were important factors in adverse event incidence, with 68% of patients under 5 years old experiencing major events compared with 53% in the older cohort. When stratified by device type, implantable continuous-flow devices had the fewest infections, while paracorporeal continuous-flow devices had the most with paracorporeal pulsatile flow devices in between. The same held true for neurologic events. Additionally, bleeding, infection, and stroke occurred most frequently in the first 3 months after device implantation for all devices. The same report noted that just over 50% of patients with an intracorporeal continuous-flow device were discharged home.

A 2018 review of the Texas Children's Hospital experience found neurologic events to be similar among patients implanted with the Berlin Heart EXCOR at 29%, the HeartMate II at 18%, and the HVAD at 34% in 103 patients.[123] However, when analyzed by time from implantation, Berlin Heart EXCOR has the highest event rate (17.8 per 100 patient-months), but this was significantly lower and on par with the HeartMate II and HVAD in pediatric patients under 10 kg. A multicenter review of the HeartWare pediatric experience comparing outcomes to young adults actually found lower rates of infection of 27% versus 44% and device malfunction/thrombosis of 11% versus 19% in pediatric patients. Incidence of major bleed was 23% and stroke was 10% in the children, which was similar to the young adults.[59] Notably, in the 12 children under 20 kg, there were no bleeding events, only 17% developed infection, and 8% suffered a stroke, but 50% had some type of neurological event. Overall, these results are outstanding and demonstrate that with device and anticoagulation improvements, children can be supported by VADs with a reasonable rate of adverse events.

Anticoagulation

Children have unique physiologic issues that affect the dosing, metabolism, and complications of most drugs. In addition, few drugs have been studied as extensively in the pediatric population as in the adult population. These factors present unique challenges for anticoagulation of pediatric patients. Marked differences exist in both the procoagulation and anticoagulation pathways between children and adults. These differences also continually change until adulthood. Andrew and colleagues examined these differences in premature and term infants in the first 6 months of life and in children 1 through 16 years of age.[124–126] In infants, contact and vitamin K–dependent factors are at 70% of the levels found in the adult population. The coagulation inhibitors antithrombin III and proteins C and S are also low at birth. In newborns and children to 16 years of age, the capacity to generate thrombin is both decreased and delayed, although these changes are less notable in older children. Various genetic mutations, including the prothrombotic mutations factor V Leiden and the prothrombin gene; deficiencies of antithrombin, protein C, and protein S; as well as hyperhomocysteinemia and dysfibrogenemia, may also affect the infant patient.[127] All of these changes may alter the therapeutic effects of anticoagulation in children.[128] Central venous catheters are recognized as the single greatest risk factor for the development of thromboses in children,[129–131] associated with 90% of neonatal venous thromboses and over 66% of childhood thromboses.[130,132] Infection also plays a significant role in prothrombotic processes in children.[127] Neonatal platelets are hyporeactive to thrombin, epinephrine/adenosine diphosphate, and thromboxane, whereas the bleeding time is decreased because of increased red cell size and hematocrit and increased levels of von Willebrand factor.[132] It is not surprising, given this background, that the placement of a significant surface area of artificial material into the bloodstream of a critically ill child, while simultaneously administering anticoagulants, would be a difficult clinical scenario in which to control and thus reliably balance the incidence of thrombosis versus bleeding.

Anticoagulation for pediatric MCS has traditionally involved management with heparin while on ECMO, although new targets are constantly being sought (i.e., isolated inhibition of factor XII, etc.). Management of anticoagulation for long-term support devices presents a unique set of challenges, with more emphasis on platelet activation.[133] It may also be advantageous to switch from a continuous intravenous infusion (i.e., heparin) to anticoagulants that are dosed intermittently (i.e., warfarin, low-molecular-weight heparin, and antiplatelet agents) because this aids in patient mobility and decreases infectious risks. Oral management of coagulation with warfarin can be difficult, particularly in younger children, because of variable intake and absorption of the drug with frequent gastrointestinal issues or if unable to take pills. For these reasons, low-molecular-weight heparin may be a more acceptable substitute in children, although it does require twice-daily subcutaneous injections. The use of the direct thrombin inhibitor bivalrudin has been gaining popularity in smaller infants and those on temporary devices, though there is little published about the outcomes of this strategy. However, through ACTION, a standardized protocol for bivalrudin administration has been established in the vast majority of institutions placing VADs in pediatric patients. A recent modification to the Edmonton Guideline instituted at Stanford for their Berlin Heart EXCOR patients in 2012 increased the overall level of anticoagulation, which resulted in an 84% decrease in stroke and a 50% decrease in pump exchange in their institution. Notably, their protocol used the same lovenox dosing with aspirin titrated to 30 mg/kg/day and dipyridamole to 15 mg/kg/day. In addition to those medications common to both protocols, Stanford titrated clopidogrel up to 1 mg/kg/day (one dose) and dosed prednisone as needed for fibrinogen levels >600 mg/dL or other signs of inflammation.[134] As demonstrated by this protocol, laboratory monitoring of the activity of the coagulation system is complex and difficult to interpret. This is frequently done in conjunction with the hematology service. Prior to ACTION, there were sparse agreed-upon guidelines for anticoagulation regimens in pediatric MCS, including the goal level of anticoagulation required, the medicinal strategy for anticoagulation, and how to measure the levels of anticoagulation.[134,135] However, the future is bright now that this active learning network is standardizing these practices over programs that account for the vast majority of VAD therapy in the USA.

CONCLUSION

Patients with CHD are experiencing better survival now than ever before with improving operative techniques and perioperative management, which is resulting in a growing population of children and young adults with heart failure. Additionally, cardiomyopathy causes a significant amount of pediatric heart failure and currently still accounts for the majority of MCS devices being placed. Mechanical support options for these young patients have rapidly expanded over the past decade with the adaptation of adult devices and continued research into pediatric-specific devices. Although anticoagulation strategy, stroke, and other adverse events remain challenging in young patients, well-selected patients do extremely well with continuous-flow devices and can do well with pulsatile devices as well. The maturation of the field regarding timing of device placement has been the largest factor in the improved outcomes. While very few pediatric patients are receiving VADs as destination therapy, VADs have greatly increased patient survival to transplantation and show great promise for the future, as data registries allow better scrutiny of outcomes and pediatric specific devices come to fruition to meet current challenges.

REFERENCES

1. Gibbon JH. Application of a mechanical heart and lung apparatus to cardiac surgery. *Minn Med.* 1954;37(3):171–185.
2. Lillehei CW, Varco RL, Cohen M, et al. The first open heart corrections of tetralogy of Fallot. A 26 31 year follow-up of 106 patients. *Ann Surg.* 1986;204(4):490–502.
3. Kirklin JW, Dushane JW, Patrick RT, et al. Intracardiac surgery with the aid of a mechanical pump-oxygenator system (gibbon type): report of eight cases. *Proc Staff Meet Mayo Clin.* 1955;30(10):201–206.

4. Barratt-Boyes BG, Neutze JM. Primary repair of tetralogy of Fallot in infancy using profound hypothermia with circulatory arrest and limited cardiopulmonary bypass: a comparison with conventional two stage management. *Ann Surg*. 1973;178(4):406–411.
5. Castaneda AR, Lamberti J, Sade RM, Williams RG, Nadas AS. Open-heart surgery during the first three months of life. *J Thorac Cardiovasc Surg*. 1974;68(5):719–731.
6. Wilkinson JD, Westphal JA, Bansal N, Czachor JD, Razoky H, Lipshultz SE. Lessons learned from the Pediatric Cardiomyopathy Registry (PCMR) Study Group. *Cardiol Young*. 2015;25(S2):140–153.
7. Bharucha T, Lee KJ, Daubeney PEF, et al. Sudden death in childhood cardiomyopathy. Results from a long-term national population-based study. *J Am Coll Cardiol*. 2015;65(21):2302–2310.
8. Colvin-Adams M, Smith JM, Heubner BM, et al. OPTN/SRTR 2013 annual data report: heart. *Am J Transplant*. 2015;15(suppl 2):1–28.
9. Norozi K, Wessel A, Alpers V, et al. Incidence and risk distribution of heart failure in adolescents and adults with congenital heart disease after cardiac surgery. *Am J Cardiol*. 2006;97(8):1238–1243.
10. Hoffman JIE, Kaplan S. The incidence of congenital heart disease. *J Am Coll Cardiol*. 2002;39(12):1890–1900.
11. Rossano JW, Kim JJ, Decker JA, et al. Prevalence, morbidity, and mortality of heart failure–related hospitalizations in children in the United States: a population-based study. *J Card Fail*. 2012;18(6):459–470.
12. Nandi D, Lin KY, O'Connor MJ, et al. Hospital charges for pediatric heart failure related hospitalizations from 2000 to 2009. *Pediatr Cardiol*. 2016;37(3):512–518.
13. Blume ED, VanderPluym C, Lorts A, et al. Second annual Pediatric Interagency Registry for Mechanical Circulatory Support (Pedimacs) report: pre-implant characteristics and outcomes. *J Heart Lung Transplant*. 2018;37(1):38–45.
14. Rosenthal D, Chrisant MRK, Edens E, et al. International Society for Heart and Lung Transplantation: practice guidelines for management of heart failure in children. *J Heart Lung Transplant*. 2004;23(12):1313–1333.
15. Boneva RS, Botto LD, Moore CA, Yang Q, Correa A, Erickson JD. Mortality associated with congenital heart defects in the United States: trends and racial disparities, 1979–1997. *Circulation*. 2001;103(19):2376–2381.
16. McDiarmid SV, Cherikh WS, Sweet SC. Preventable death: children on the transplant waiting list. *Am J Transplant*. 2008;8(12):2491–2495.
17. Almond CSD, Thiagarajan RR, Piercey GE, et al. Waiting list mortality among children listed for heart transplantation in the United States. *Circulation*. 2009;119(5):717–727.
18. Rossano JW, Dipchand AI, Edwards LB, et al. The Registry of the International Society for Heart and Lung Transplantation: Nineteenth Pediatric Heart Transplantation Report—2016; Focus Theme: Primary Diagnostic Indications for Transplant. *J Heart Lung Transplant*. 2016;35(10):1185–1195.
19. Zafar F, Castleberry C, Khan MS, et al. Pediatric heart transplant waiting list mortality in the era of ventricular assist devices. *J Heart Lung Transplant*. 2015;34(1):82–88.
20. Law SP, Oron AP, Kemna MS, et al. Comparison of transplant waitlist outcomes for pediatric candidates supported by ventricular assist devices versus medical therapy. *Pediatr Crit Care Med*. 2018;19(5):442–450.
21. Paden ML, Rycus PT, Thiagarajan RR. Update and outcomes in extracorporeal life support. *Semin Perinatol*. 2014;38(2):65–70.
22. Bartlett RH, Andrews AF, Toomasian JM, Haiduc NJ, Gazzaniga AB. Extracorporeal membrane oxygenation for newborn respiratory failure: forty-five cases. *Surgery*. 1982;92(2):425–433.
23. UK collaborative randomised trial of neonatal extracorporeal membrane oxygenation. UK Collaborative ECMO Trail Group. *Lancet*. 1996;348(9020):75–82.
24. Zapol WM. Extracorporeal membrane oxygenation in severe acute respiratory failure: a randomized prospective study. *JAMA*. 1979;242(20):2193.
25. Bartlett RH, Gazzaniga AB, Huxtable RH, et al. Extracorporeal membrane oxygenation (ECMO) in newborn respiratory failure: technical consideration. *Trans Am Soc Artif Intern Organs*. 1979;25:473–475.
26. Hardesty RL, Doob GM, Griffith BP, Borovetz HS. Clinical experience with pediatric microporous oxygenator for profound hypothermia. *Arch Surg*. 1980;115(11):1356–1358.
27. Hardesty RL, Griffith BP, Debski RF, Jeffries MR, Borovetz HS. Extracorporeal membrane oxygenation. Successful treatment of persistent fetal circulation following repair of congenital diaphragmatic hernia. *J Thorac Cardiovasc Surg*. 1981;81(4):556–563.
28. Trento A, Estner SM, Griffith BP, Hardesty RL. Massive hemoptysis in patients with cystic fibrosis: three case reports and a protocol for clinical management. :3.
29. Klein MD, Shaheen KW, Whittlesey GC, Pinsky WW, Arciniegas E. Extracorporeal membrane oxygenation for the circulatory support of children after repair of congenital heart disease. *J Thorac Cardiovasc Surg*. 1990;100(4):498–505.
30. Weinhaus L, Canter C, Noetzel M, McAlister W, Spray TL. Extracorporeal membrane oxygenation for circulatory support after repair of congenital heart defects. *Ann Thorac Surg*. 1989;48(2):206–212.
31. Kanter KR, Pennington G, Weber TR, Zambie MA, Braun P, Martychenko V. Extracorporeal membrane oxygenation for postoperative cardiac support in children. *J Thorac Cardiovasc Surg*. 1987;93(1):27–35.
32. del Nido PJ, Dalton HJ, Thompson AE, Siewers RD. Extracorporeal membrane oxygenator rescue in children during cardiac arrest after cardiac surgery. *Circulation*. 1992;86(5 suppl):II300–II304.
33. Duncan BW, Ibrahim AE, Hraska V, et al. Use of rapid-deployment extracorporeal membrane oxygenation for the resuscitation of pediatric patients with heart disease after cardiac arrest. *J Thorac Cardiovasc Surg*. 1998;116(2):305–311.
34. Jacobs JP, Ojito JW, McConaghey TW, et al. Rapid cardiopulmonary support for children with complex congenital heart disease. *Ann Thorac Surg*. 2000;70(3):742–750.
35. Kulik TJ, Moler FW, Palmisano JM, et al. Outcome-associated factors in pediatric patients treated with extracorporeal membrane oxygenator after cardiac surgery. *Circulation*. 1996;94(9 suppl):II63-II68.
36. Raithel SC, Pennington DG, Boegner E, Fiore A, Weber TR. Extracorporeal membrane oxygenation in children after cardiac surgery. *Circulation*. 1992;86(5 suppl):II305–II310.
37. del Nido PJ, Armitage JM, Fricker FJ, et al. Extracorporeal membrane oxygenation support as a bridge to pediatric heart transplantation. *Circulation*. 1994;90(5 Pt 2):II66–II69.
38. Fiser WP, Yetman AT, Gunselman RJ, et al. Pediatric arteriovenous extracorporeal membrane oxygenation (ECMO) as a bridge to cardiac transplantation. *J Heart Lung Transplant*. 2003;22(7):770–777.
39. Gajarski RJ, Mosca RS, Ohye RG, et al. Use of extracorporeal life support as a bridge to pediatric cardiac transplantation. *J Heart Lung Transplant*. 2003;22(1):28–34.
40. Kirshbom PM, Bridges ND, Myung RJ, Gaynor JW, Clark BJ, Spray TL. Use of extracorporeal membrane oxygenation in pediatric thoracic organ transplantation. *J Thorac Cardiovasc Surg*. 2002;123(1):130–136.
41. Huang S-C, Chi N-H, Chen C-A, et al. Left ventricular assist for pediatric patients with dilated cardiomyopathy using the Medos VAD cannula and a centrifugal pump. *Artif Organs*. 2009;33(11):1032–1037.
42. Camboni D, Philipp A, Haneya A, et al. Serial use of an interventional lung assist device and a ventricular assist device. *ASAIO J*. 2010;56(3):270–272.
43. Wermelt JZ, Honjo O, Kilic A, van Arsdell G, Gruenwald C, Humpl T. Use of a pulsatile ventricular assist device (Berlin Heart EXCOR) and an interventional lung assist device (Novalung) in an animal model. *ASAIO J*. 2008;54(5):498–503.
44. Rais Bahrami K, Van Meurs KP. ECMO for neonatal respiratory failure. *Semin Perinatol*. 2005;29(1):15–23.
45. Rossano JW, Cherikh WS, Chambers DC, et al. The Registry of the International Society for Heart and Lung Transplantation: Twentieth Pediatric Heart Transplantation Report—2017; focus theme: allograft ischemic time. *J Heart Lung Transplant*. 2017;36(10):1060–1069.
46. Wehman B, Stafford KA, Bittle GJ, et al. Modern outcomes of mechanical circulatory support as a bridge to pediatric heart transplantation. *Ann Thorac Surg*. 2016;101(6):2321–2327.
47. Riggs KW, Morales DLS. Pediatric mechanical circulatory support: a new era of "using the right tools, for the right job, at the right time." *J Thorac Cardiovasc Surg*. 2017.

48. John R, Long JW, Massey HT, et al. Outcomes of a multicenter trial of the Levitronix CentriMag ventricular assist system for short-term circulatory support. *J Thorac Cardiovasc Surg*. 2011;141(4):932–939.
49. Hirata Y, Charette K, Mosca RS, Quaegebeur JM, Chen JM. Pediatric application of the Thoratec CentriMag BiVAD as a bridge to heart transplantation. *J Thorac Cardiovasc Surg*. 2008;136(5):1386–1387.
50. Kouretas PC, Kaza AK, Burch PT, et al. Experience with the Levitronix CentriMag in the pediatric population as a bridge to decision and recovery. *Artif Organs*. 2009;33(11):1002–1004.
51. Jefferies JL, Morales DL. Mechanical circulatory support in children: bridge to transplant versus recovery. *Curr Heart Fail Rep*. 2012;9(3):236–243.
52. Lorts A, Eghtesady P, Mehegan M, et al. Outcomes of children supported with devices labeled as "temporary" or short term: a report from the Pediatric Interagency Registry for Mechanical Circulatory Support. (Pedimacs). *J Heart Lung Transplant*. [Internet]. [cited 2017 Nov 9]; Available from: https://www.sciencedirect.com/science/article/pii/S1053249817320909.
53. Parekh D, Jeewa A, Tume SC, et al. Percutaneous mechanical dirculatory support using Impella devices for decompensated cardiogenic shock: a pediatric heart center experience. *ASAIO J*. 2018;64(1):98–104.
54. Slaughter MS, Rogers JG, Milano CA, et al. Advanced heart failure treated with continuous-flow left ventricular assist device. *New Engl J Med*. 2009;361(23):2241–2251.
55. Blume ED, Naftel DC, Bastardi HJ, Duncan BW, Kirklin JK, Webber SA. Outcomes of children bridged to heart transplantation with ventricular assist devices: a multi-institutional study. *Circulation*. 2006;113(19):2313–2319.
56. Owens WR, Iii RB, Dreyer WJ, Price JF, Morales DLS. Initial clinical experience with the HeartMate II ventricular assist system in a pediatric institution. *Artif Organs*. 2010;34(7):600–603.
57. Morales DLS, Adachi I, Heinle JS, Fraser CD. A new era: use of an intracorporeal systemic ventricular assist device to support a patient with a failing Fontan circulation. *J Thorac Cardiovasc Surg*. 2011;142(3):e138–e140.
58. Cabrera AG, Sundareswaran KS, Samayoa AX, et al. Outcomes of pediatric patients supported by the HeartMate II left ventricular assist device in the United States. *J Heart Lung Transplant*. 2013;32(11):1107–1113.
59. VanderPluym CJ, Adachi I, Niebler R, et al. Outcomes of children supported with an intracorporeal continuous-flow left ventricular assist system. *J Heart Lung Transplant*. 2018;25.
60. Conway J, Miera O, Adachi I, et al. Worldwide experience of a durable centrifugal flow pump in pediatric patients. *Semin Thorac Cardiovasc Surg*. 2018;15.
61. Lorts A, Villa C, Riggs KW, Broderick J, Morales DL. First use of HeartMate 3 in a failing Fontan circulation. *Ann Thorac Surg*. 2018;9.
62. Villa CR, Morales DLS. The total artificial heart in end-stage congenital heart disease. *Front Physiol* [Internet]. 2017 May 9 [cited 2017 Nov 8];8. Available from: https://www.ncbi.nlm.nih.gov/pmc/articles/PMC5422510/.
63. Moore RA, Lorts A, Madueme PC, Taylor MD, Morales DLS. Virtual implantation of the 50cc SynCardia total artificial heart. *J Heart Lung Transplant*. 2016;35(6):824–827.
64. Warnecke H, Berdjis F, Hennig E, et al. Mechanical left ventricular support as a bridge to cardiac transplantation in childhood. *Eur J Cardiothorac Surg*. 1991;5(6):330–333.
65. Kilic A, Nelson K, Scheel J, Ravekes W, Cameron DE, Vricella LA. Outcomes of heart transplantation in small children bridged with ventricular assist devices. *Ann Thorac Surg*. 2013;96(4):1420–1427.
66. Hetzer R, Alexi-Meskishvili V, Weng Y, et al. Mechanical cardiac support in the young with the Berlin Heart EXCOR pulsatile ventricular assist device: 15 years' experience. *Semin Thorac Cardiovasc Surg Pediatr Card Surg Annu*. 2006;9(1):99–108.
67. Hetzer R, Dandel M, Knosalla C, et al. Left ventricular asses devices and drug therapy in heart failure. *New Engl J Med*. 2007;356(8):869–70; author reply 871-2.
68. Hetzer R, Potapov EV, Stiller B, et al. Improvement in survival after mechanical circulatory support with pneumatic pulsatile ventricular assist devices in pediatric patients. *Ann Thorac Surg*. 2006;82(3):917–24; discussion 924-925.
69. Hetzer R, Loebe M, Potapov EV, et al. Circulatory support with pneumatic paracorporeal ventricular assist device in infants and children. *Ann Thorac Surg*. 1998;66(5):1498–1506.
70. Morales DLS, Almond CSD, Jaquiss RDB, et al. Bridging children of all sizes to cardiac transplantation: the initial multicenter North American experience with the Berlin Heart EXCOR ventricular assist device. *J Heart Lung Transplant*. 2011;30(1):1–8.
71. Fraser CDJ, Jaquiss RDB, Rosenthal DN, et al. Prospective trial of a pediatric ventricular assist device. *New Engl J of Med*. 2012;367(6):532–541.
72. Humpl T, Furness S, Gruenwald C, Hyslop C, Arsdell GV. The Berlin Heart EXCOR pediatrics—The SickKids experience 2004–2008. *Artif Organs*. 2010;34(12):1082–1086.
73. Gandhi SK, Huddleston CB, Balzer DT, Epstein DJ, Boschert TA, Canter CE. Biventricular assist devices as a bridge to heart transplantation in small children. *Circulation*. 2008;118(14_suppl_1):S89–S93.
74. Brancaccio G, Amodeo A, Ricci Z, et al. Mechanical assist device as a bridge to heart transplantation in children less than 10 kilograms. *Ann Thorac Surg*. 2010;90(1):58–62.
75. Karimova A, Van Doorn C, Brown K, et al. Mechanical bridging to orthotopic heart transplantation in children weighing less than 10kg: feasibility and limitations. *Eur J Cardiothorac Surg*. 2011;39(3):304–309.
76. Almond CS, Morales DL, Blackstone EH, et al. Berlin Heart EXCOR pediatric ventricular assist device for bridge to heart transplantation in US children. *Circulation*. 2013;127(16):1702–1711.
77. Bryant R, Zafar F, Castleberry C, et al. Transplant survival after Berlin Heart EXCOR support. *ASAIO J*. 2017;63(1):80–85.
78. Eghtesady P, Almond CSD, Tjossem C, et al. Post-transplant outcomes of children bridged to transplant with the Berlin Heart EXCOR pediatric ventricular assist device. *Circulation*. 2013;128(11 suppl 1):S24–S31.
79. Baldwin JT, Borovetz HS, Duncan BW, Gartner MJ, Jarvik RK, Weiss WJ. The National Heart, Lung, and Blood Institute pediatric circulatory support program: a summary of the 5-year experience. *Circulation*. 2011;123(11):1233–1240.
80. Action Learning Network [Internet]. *Action Learning Network*. [cited 2018 Dec 10]. Available from: https://www.actionlearningnetwork.org/.
81. Morales DLS, Zafar F, Rossano JW, et al. Use of ventricular assist devices in children across the United States: analysis of 7.5 million pediatric hospitalizations. *Ann Thorac Surg*. 2010;90(4):1313–1319.
82. Sutcliffe DL, Pruitt E, Cantor RS, et al. Post-transplant outcomes in pediatric ventricular assist device patients: A PediMACS-Pediatric Heart Transplant Study linkage analysis. *J Heart Lung Transplant*. 2017;13.
83. Friedland-Little JM, Hong BJ, Gossett JG, et al. Changes in renal function after left ventricular assist device placement in pediatric patients: a Pedimacs analysis. *J Heart Lung Transplant*. 2018;37(10):1218–1225.
84. Schumacher KR, Almond C, Singh TP, et al. Predicting graft loss by 1 year in pediatric heart transplantation candidates: an analysis of the Pediatric Heart Transplant Study database. *Circulation*. 2015;131(10):890–898.
85. Almond CS, Gauvreau K, Canter CE, Rajagopal SK, Piercey GE, Singh TP. A risk-prediction model for in-hospital mortality after heart transplantation in US children. *Am J Transplant*. 2012;12(5):1240–1248.
86. Rossano JW, Cantor RS, Dai D, et al. Resource utilization in pediatric patients supported with ventricular assist devices in the United States: a multicenter study from the Pediatric Interagency Registry for Mechanically Assisted Circulatory Support and the Pediatric Health Information System. *J Am Heart Assoc* [Internet]. 2018 Jun 1 [cited 2018 Oct 31];7(11). Available from: https://www.ncbi.nlm.nih.gov/pmc/articles/PMC6015374/.
87. Rizwan R, Zafar F, Chin C, Tweddell J, Bryant III R, Morales D. Listing low weight or ill infants for heart transplantation: is it prudent? *Ann Thorac Surg*. 2018.
88. Davies RR, Russo MJ, Mital S, et al. Predicting survival among high-risk pediatric cardiac transplant recipients: An analysis of the United Network for Organ Sharing database. *J Thorac Cardiovasc Surg*. 2008;135(1):147–155.e2.
89. Cohen G, Permut L. Decision making for mechanical cardiac assist in pediatric cardiac surgery. *Semin Thorac Cardiovasc Surg Pediatr Card Surg Annu*. 2005;8(1):41–50.
90. Chaturvedi RR. Cardiac ECMO for biventricular hearts after paediatric open heart surgery. *Heart*. 2004;90(5):545–551.
91. Potapov EV, Stiller B, Hetzer R. Ventricular assist devices in children: current achievements and future perspectives. *Pediatr Transplant*. 2007;11(3):241–255.

92. Stiller B, Weng Y, Hübler M, et al. Pneumatic pulsatile ventricular assist devices in children under 1 year of age. *Eur J Cardiothorac Surg.* 2005;28(2):234–239.
93. Arabía FA, Milano CA, Mahr C, et al. Biventricular support with intracorporeal, continuous flow, centrifugal ventricular assist devices. *Ann Thorac Surg.* 2018;105(2):548–555.
94. Holman WL, Pae WE, Teutenberg JJ, et al. INTERMACS: Interval Analysis of Registry Data. *J Am Coll Surg.* 2009;208(5):755–761.
95. Sharma MS, Webber SA, Morell VO, et al. Ventricular assist device support in children and adolescents as a bridge to heart transplantation. *Ann Thorac Surg.* 2006;82(3):926–932.
96. Reinhartz O, Keith FM, El-Banayosy A, et al. Multicenter experience with the thoratec ventricular assist device in children and adolescents. *J Heart Lung Transplant.* 2001;20(4):439–448.
97. Zafar F, Jefferies JL, Tjossem CJ, et al. Biventricular Berlin Heart EXCOR pediatric use across the United States. *Ann Thorac Surg.* 2015;99(4):1328–1334.
98. Weinstein S, Bello R, Pizarro C, et al. The use of the Berlin Heart EXCOR in patients with functional single ventricle. *J Thorac Cardiovasc Surg.* 2014;147(2):697–705.
99. Pizarro C, Davis DA, Healy RM, Kerins PJ, Norwood WI. Is there a role for extracorporeal life support after stage I Norwood? *Eur J Cardiothorac Surg.* 2001;19(3):294–301.
100. Gazit AZ, Petrucci O, Manning P, et al. A novel surgical approach to mechanical circulatory support in univentricular infants. *Ann Thorac Surg.* 2017;104(5):1630–1636.
101. Niebler RA, Shah TK, Mitchell ME, et al. Ventricular assist device in single-ventricle heart disease and a superior cavopulmonary anastomosis. *Artif Organs.* 2016;40(2):180–184.
102. De Rita F, Hasan A, Haynes S, et al. Mechanical cardiac support in children with congenital heart disease with intention to bridge to heart transplantation. *Eur J Cardiothorac Surg.* 2014;46(4):656–662.
103. Jolley M, Thiagarajan RR, Barrett CS, et al. Extracorporeal membrane oxygenation in patients undergoing superior cavopulmonary anastomosis. *J Thorac Cardiovasc Surg.* 2014;148(4):1512–1518.
104. Horne D, Conway J, Rebeyka IM, Buchholz H. Mechanical circulatory support in univentricular hearts: current management. *Semin Thorac Cardiovasc Surg Pediatr Card Surg Annu.* 2015;18(1):17–24.
105. Arnaoutakis GJ, Blitzer D, Fuller S, et al. Mechanical circulatory support as bridge to transplantation for the failing single ventricle. *Ann Thorac Surg.* 2017;103(1):193–197.
106. Woods RK, Ghanayem NS, Mitchell ME, Kindel S, Niebler RA. Mechanical circulatory support of the Fontan patient. *Semin Thorac Cardiovasc Surg Pediatr Card Surg Annu.* 2017;20(Supplement C):20–27.
107. Hoganson DM, Boston US, Gazit AZ, Canter CE, Eghtesady P. Successful bridge through transplantation with Berlin Heart ventricular assist device in a child with failing Fontan. *Ann Thorac Surg.* 2015;99(2):707–709.
108. Poh CL, Chiletti R, Zannino D, et al. Ventricular assist device support in patients with single ventricles: the Melbourne experience. *Interact CardioVasc Thorac Surg.* 2017;25(2):310–316.
109. Halaweish I, Ohye RG, Si MS. Berlin Heart ventricular assist device as a long-term bridge to transplantation in a Fontan patient with failing single ventricle. *Pediatr Transplant.* 2015;19(8):E193–E195.
110. Jabbar AA, Franklin WJ, Simpson L, Civitello AB, Delgado RM, Frazier OH. Improved systemic saturation after ventricular assist device implantation in a patient with decompensated dextro-transposition of the great arteries after the Fontan procedure. *Tex Heart Inst J.* 2015;42(1):40–43.
111. Valeske K, Yerebakan C, Mueller M, Akintuerk H. Urgent implantation of the Berlin Heart EXCOR biventricular assist device as a total artificial heart in a patient with single ventricle circulation. *J Thorac Cardiovasc Surg.* 2014;147(5):1712–1714.
112. Mackling T, Shah T, Dimas V, et al. Management of single-ventricle patients with Berlin Heart EXCOR ventricular assist device: single-center experience. *Artif Organs.* 2012;36(6):555–559.
113. Cardarelli MG, Salim M, Love J, et al. Berlin Heart as a bridge to recovery for a failing Fontan. *Ann Thorac Surg.* 2009;87(3):943–946.
114. Russo P, Wheeler A, Russo J, Tobias JD. Use of a ventricular assist device as a bridge to transplantation in a patient with single ventricle physiology and total cavopulmonary anastomosis. *Paediatr Anaesth.* 2008;18(4):320–324.
115. Ricci M, Gaughan CB, Rossi M, et al. Initial experience with the TandemHeart circulatory support system in children. *ASAIO J.* 2008;54(5):542–545.
116. Prêtre R, Häussler A, Bettex D, Genoni M. Right-Sided Univentricular cardiac assistance in a failing Fontan circulation. *Ann Thorac Surg.* 2008;86(3):1018–1020.
117. Marelli AJ, Ionescu-Ittu R, Mackie AS, Guo L, Dendukuri N, Kaouache M. Lifetime prevalence of congenital heart disease in the general population from 2000 to 2010. *Circulation.* 2014;130(9): 749–756.
118. Doumouras BS, Alba AC, Foroutan F, Burchill LJ, Dipchand AI, Ross HJ. Outcomes in adult congenital heart disease patients undergoing heart transplantation: a systematic review and meta-analysis. *J Heart Lung Transplant.* 2016;35(11):1337–1347.
119. VanderPluym CJ, Cedars A, Eghtesady P, et al. Outcomes following implantation of mechanical circulatory support in adults with congenital heart disease: an analysis of the Interagency Registry for Mechanically Assisted Circulatory Support (INTERMACS). *J Heart Lung Transplant.* 2017;7.
120. Cedars A, Vanderpluym C, Koehl D, Cantor R, Kutty S, Kirklin JK. An Interagency Registry for Mechanically Assisted Circulatory Support (INTERMACS) analysis of hospitalization, functional status, and mortality after mechanical circulatory support in adults with congenital heart disease. *J Heart Lung Transplant.* 2018;37(5):619–630.
121. Deng MC, Edwards LB, Hertz MI, et al. Mechanical Circulatory Support Device Database of the International Society for Heart and Lung Transplantation: Third Annual Report—2005. *J Heart Lung Transplant.* 2005;24(9):6.
122. Rosenthal DN, Almond CS, Jaquiss RD, et al. Adverse events in children implanted with ventricular assist devices in the United States: data from the Pediatric Interagency Registry for Mechanical Circulatory Support (PediMACS). *J Heart Lung Transplant.* 2016;35(5):569–577.
123. Fraser CD, Chacon-Portillo MA, Zea-Vera R, et al. Ventricular assist device support: single pediatric institution experience over two decades. *Ann Thorac Surg.* 2018.
124. Andrew M, Paes B, Milner R, et al. Development of the human coagulation system in the healthy premature infant. *Blood.* 1988;72(5):1651–1657.
125. Andrew M, Paes B, Milner R, et al. Development of the human coagulation system in the full-term infant. *Blood.* 1987;70(1):165–172.
126. Andrew M, Vegh P, Johnston M, Bowker J, Ofosu F, Mitchell L. Maturation of the hemostatic system during childhood. *Blood.* 1992;80(8):1998–2005.
127. Hoppe C, Matsunaga A. Pediatric thrombosis. *Pediatr Clin North Am.* 2002;49(6):1257–1283.
128. Revel-Vilk S, Chan A, Bauman M, Massicotte P. Prothrombotic conditions in an unselected cohort of children with venous thromboembolic disease. *J Thromb Haemost.* 2003;1(5):915–921.
129. Andrew M, Marzinotto V, Pencharz P, et al. A cross-sectional study of catheter-related thrombosis in children receiving total parenteral nutrition at home. *J Pediatr.* 1995;126(3):358–363.
130. Massicotte MP, Dix D, Monagle P, Adams M, Andrew M. Central venous catheter related thrombosis in children: analysis of the Canadian Registry of Venous Thromboembolic Complications. *J Pediatr.* 1998;133(6):7.
131. Nowak-Göttl U, Dübbers A, Kececioglu D, et al. Factor V Leiden, protein C, and lipoprotein (a) in catheter-related thrombosis in childhood: a prospective study. *J Pediatr.* 1997;131(4):608–612.
132. Monagle P, Adams M, Mahoney M, et al. Outcome of pediatric thromboembolic disease: a report from the Canadian Childhood Thrombophilia Registry. *Pediatr Res.* 2000;47(6):763–766.
133. Houël R, Mazoyer E, Boval B, et al. Platelet activation and aggregation profile in prolonged external ventricular support. *J Thorac Cardiovasc Surg.* 2004;128(2):197–202.
134. Rosenthal DN, Lancaster CA, McElhinney DB, et al. Impact of a modified anti-thrombotic guideline on stroke in children supported with a pediatric ventricular assist device. *J Heart Lung Transplant.* 2017;36(11):1250–1257.
135. Cooper DS, Prêtre R. Clinical management of pediatric ventricular assist devices. *Pediatr Crit Care Med.* 2013;14(5 suppl 1):S27–S36.

Facilitating Myocardial Recovery

Emma Birks, Craig H. Selzman

KEY POINTS

Heart failure (HF) is characterized by a pathologic process known as remodeling that involves progressive enlargement (See Chapter 9) of the ventricle, reduction in contractility, and an increase in intracardiac pressures. These changes are associated with adverse cellular, structural, and functional changes in the myocardium (see Chapter 9). Historically, the remodeling process was considered largely irreversible once HF had been present for a period of time (years). However, patients with chronic advanced HF supported with a left ventricular assist device (LVAD) that provides near-total unloading of the ventricle can show a near-normalization of the structural abnormalities of the myocardium, or "reverse remodeling." These findings are often associated with significant recovery of the underlying cardiac function, sufficient to allow for removal of the LVAD (myocardial recovery or "remission" of end-stage HF). A cohort of patients now exist who have had their device removed and have had sustained recovery for many years. These patients can return to a normal quality of life, without requiring transplantation, thereby making the precious donor heart available for another needy individual.

Yet, despite significant reversal of structural changes in most patients after a period of mechanical support, only a small percentage of patients have had their LVADs removed. This observation is due to a number of reasons. First, reverse remodeling does not always equate with clinical recovery. Despite favorable cardiac structure, functional improvement may either lag or not occur (Fig. 19.1).[1] Second, while transplant has a defined benefit and well-known natural history, trepidation about recurrence of HF following LVAD removal is prevalent in those who care for these patients. Finally, many institutions do not actively search for myocardial recovery, and as such, it is underevaluated, underpromoted, and underestimated. Conversely, some institutions who have focused on promoting and testing for recovery and removing the pump when patients show significant improvement in underlying cardiac function have shown high rates of recovery. This enthusiasm was ignited following reports showing high rates of recovery and explantation using a prospective attempt combining LVAD support with aggressive adjuvant reverse remodeling drug therapy to concurrently promote recovery, along with regular testing of underlying myocardial function, followed by an additional strategy to sustain recovery. This approach was associated with a 70% recovery rate, with more than 3 years of follow-up.[2] Subsequently, increasingly more institutions are now adopting an aggressive approach of facilitating and testing for recovery and potential LVAD explantation.

This area of myocardial recovery from chronic HF is a relatively new, exciting, and developing field. However, many controversial and challenging questions persist: can chronic HF really reverse? Is there a state of irreversibility? How can clinicians test for recovery? Is the recovery sustainable? What are the markers and predictors of recovery? This chapter addresses these questions and presents the data available on the concept of myocardial recovery with LVAD support.

HISTORY OF RECOVERY AND DEVICE EXPLANTATION

LVADs provide profound pressure and volume unloading of the left ventricle (LV) while restoring systemic blood flow. In 1994, Frazier and colleagues[3] were the first to describe myocardial improvement in a study of 18 patients supported with the pneumatic vented electric HeartMate device (Thoratec Corp., Pleasanton, CA). Of the patients, 12 had nonischemic etiology and six had ischemic etiology of HF. In all cases, the investigators found that LVAD support resulted in a significant reduction in the cardiothoracic ratio (from 0.65 to 0.55, $P<0.003$), a decrease in LV end-diastolic dimension (LVEDD; from 7.0 to 5.5 cm, $P<0.05$), and a 43% improvement in LV ejection fraction (EF) from baseline by echocardiography. These patients also showed improved hemodynamics, including a reduction in pulmonary capillary wedge pressure (PCWP) and improvement in cardiac index. Histologic examination showed the mean area of attenuated myocytes to be reduced from 60% to 21% from the time of implantation compared to after mechanical circulatory support (MCS). This was the first report suggesting that significant improvement of cardiac structure and function was possible with LVAD support.

Levin and colleagues[4,5] measured the end-diastolic pressure-volume relationship (EDPVR) at the time of cardiac transplantation in patients treated with medical therapy versus patients bridged with LVAD support. EDPVRs of hearts from medically treated patients were shifted toward markedly larger volumes. In contrast, EDPVRs of hearts from LVAD-supported patients were similar to EDPVRs of normal hearts

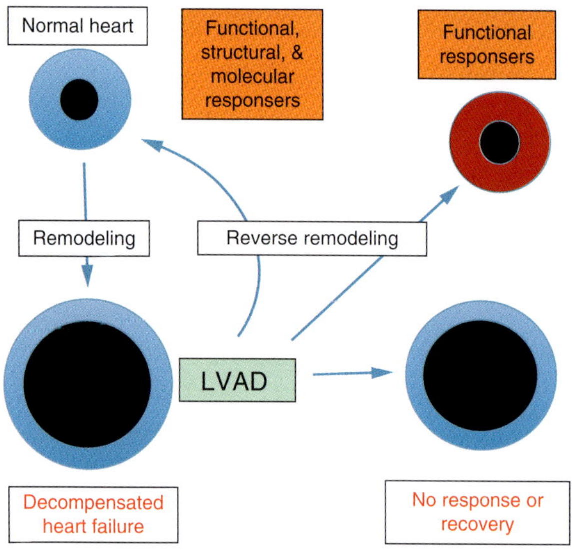

Fig. 19.1 Left ventricular assist devices *(LVADs)* are placed in patients with adverse pathologic remodeling and development of advanced heart failure. After implantation, the heart undergoes variable levels of reverse remodeling. If inadequate (nonresponder), then continued support and/or transplantation remain the mainstay of therapy. If cellular, metabolic, architectural, and functional reversal occurs to normal, then these patients exhibit myocardial recovery. Another, perhaps more common, group includes patients who demonstrate functional improvement, possibly without structural and/or molecular normalization. These latter two groups (in *orange*) are both considered "responders" to therapy and are candidates for consideration of LVAD removal. (From Selzman CH, Madden JL, Healy AH, et al. Bridge to removal: a paradigm shift for left ventricular assist device therapy. *Ann Thorac Surg*. 2015;99:360–367.)

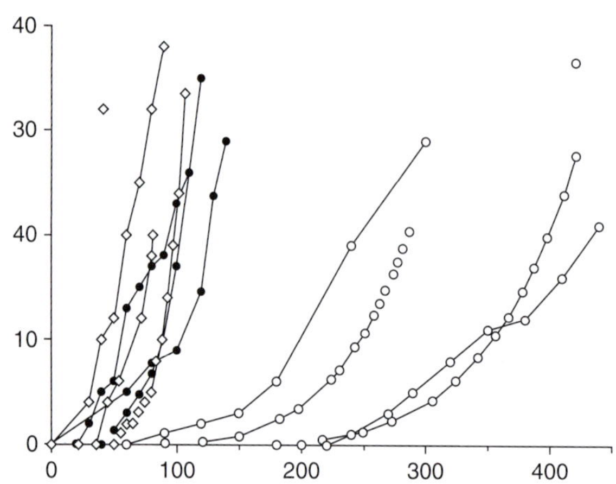

Fig. 19.2 Graph showing the end-diastolic pressure-volume relation (EDPVR) of hearts from medically treated patients with end-stage idiopathic cardiomyopathy (○), heart failure patients after prolonged left ventricular assist device (LVAD) support (•), and normal subjects (◇). Whereas the EDPVRs of hearts from medically treated patients were shifted far to the right of the normal hearts, EDPVRs from the LVAD groups were close to normal. *x* axis shows volume in milliliters; *y* axis, pressure in mm Hg. (From Levin HR, Oz MC, Chen JM, Packer M, Rose EA, Burkhoff D. Reversal of chronic ventricular dilation in patients with end-stage cardiomyopathy by prolonged mechanical unloading. *Circulation*. 1995;91:2717–2720.)

technically unsuitable for transplantation (Fig. 19.2). This study suggested that chronic hemodynamic unloading of sufficient magnitude and duration can result in reversal of chamber enlargement and normalization of cardiac structure, even in the most advanced stages of HF.

The first report of recovery and subsequent device explantation with LVAD support was in a series of five patients with advanced nonischemic HF (three with idiopathic dilated cardiomyopathy and two with postpartum cardiomyopathy).[6] In three of these patients, the LVAD was removed electively after the patients showed recovery of myocardial function. In the other two patients, it was removed because of device malfunction. One patient died of a noncardiac cause 10 days after LVAD removal, but the other four patients remained alive and well 35, 33, 14, and 2 months after LVAD removal.

Several subsequent reports showed recovery rates between 5% and 10% and impressive transplant-free survival rates near 70%, 5 years after explantation. One of the largest cohorts was derived from the large multicenter Thoratec Registry.[7] In this series, they reported that 22 of 281 (8.1%) patients with nonischemic cardiomyopathy underwent explantation, with 17 of the 22 (70%) patients alive and 16 in New York Heart Association (NYHA) class I and one in class II at latest follow-up. These patients had 86% and 77% transplant-free survival rates at 1 year and 5 years, respectively. Approximately 50% of the patients had proven myocarditis or postpartum cardiomyopathy as the cause of HF, a finding that has been true of several patients who have had recovery with LVAD support.

Another large series was reported by Mancini et al.[8] (Fig. 19.3), who observed in a retrospective review of 111 patients with LVAD support as bridge to transplant (BTT) (46% of whom had dilated cardiomyopathy) that only five (4.5% overall, but 9% of patients with nonischemic etiology) had sufficient myocardial recovery for the device to be explanted. Four of these five patients had nonischemic cardiomyopathy. Only one of the five patients who underwent explantation was alive with maintained LV function after 15 months of follow-up; one patient died of HF 3 months after explantation, one patient had sudden death, and two patients required LVAD reimplantation. These authors argued that significant recovery occurred in only a small percentage of patients and primarily in patients with nonischemic causes of HF. At the time, this study provided skepticism and slowed the belief that recovery was very likely.

A higher success of device removal and more sustained recovery has subsequently been reported by the Berlin group.[9,10] Their initial report showed that the first five patients who underwent explantation had sustained normal LV function for 51 to 592 days. A subsequent report in 2004 demonstrated that 32 of 131 (24%) patients with nonischemic HF had device explantation associated with a 5-year survival rate of 78.3% ± 8.1%. HF recurred in the first 3 years in 14 of the 31 patients whose devices were explanted, but only two patients died of HF after explantation. The other 12 patients with recurrent HF underwent successful transplantation. The patients whose devices were explanted had 69.4% and 58.2% freedom from recurrence of HF at 3 and 5 years, respectively. Several risk factors were associated with recurrence of HF after explantation, including a pre-explantation EF less than 45%, LVEDD greater than 55 mm, and history of HF greater than 5 years. Among patients who did not have these risk factors, none had HF recurrence during the first 3 years after explantation. By 2008, the Berlin group reported 81 patients weaned from LVADs, biventricular ventricular assist devices, and right ventricular assist devices (VADs) that had been implanted for terminal HF.[11] The investigators analyzed 35 BTT patients older than 14 years who had received an LVAD for nonischemic cardiomyopathy (excluding patients with myocarditis) who were able to undergo device explantation). Of the 35 patients, 30

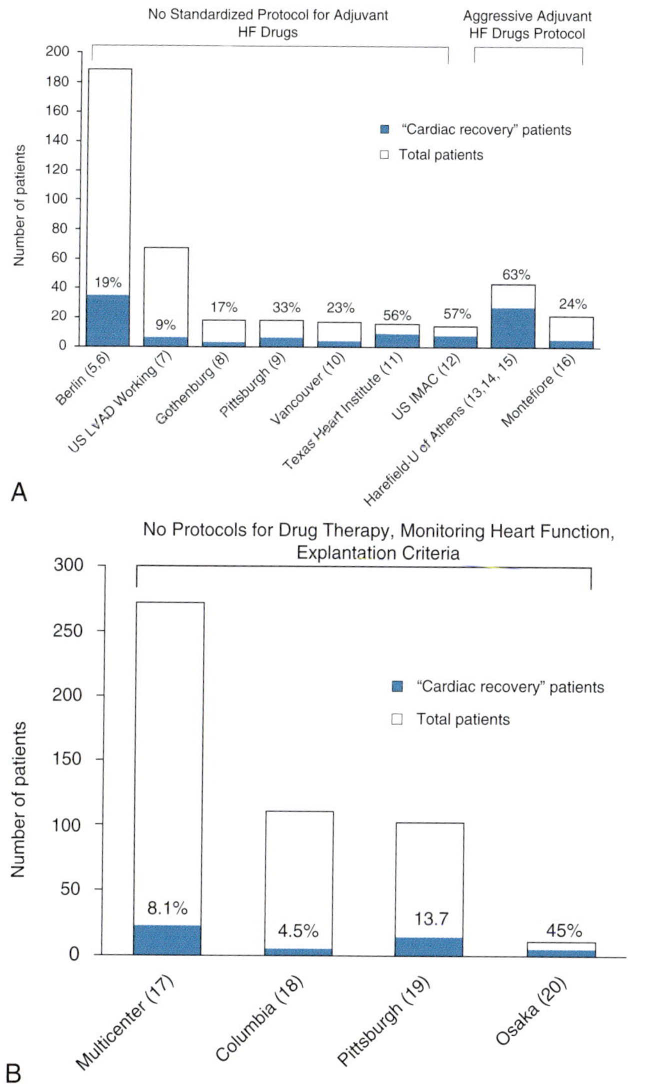

Fig. 19.3 Summary of published retrospective and prospective recovery studies. *HF*, Heart failure. (From Drakos SG, Mehra MR. Clinical myocardial recovery during long-term mechanical support in advanced heart failure: insights into moving the field forward. *J Heart Lung Transplant.* 2016;35:413–420.)

had the device explanted electively, and in the other five it was precipitated by pump-related complications. There were no established criteria to define recovery. In eight of the electively weaned patients, the LVAD was removed with a subnormal EF (30%–44%) and LVEDD of 56 to 60 mm. However, the overall 5- and 10-year survival rates after LVAD removal (including posttransplant survival for patients with HF recurrence) were 79.1% ± 7.1% and 75.3% ± 7.7%, respectively. At the end of the fifth post-weaning year, these patients had a 61.3% ± 9.0% probability of freedom from HF recurrence. The authors showed that if the patient remained stable 1 year after explantation, the probability of freedom from HF recurrence at the end of 5 and 10 years was 84.2% ± 8.4% and 61.8% ± 11.4%, respectively.

A critical observation from this cumulative series was that patients with long-term weaning stability had a shorter history of HF, were younger, and required a shorter duration of support.[12–14] One important advance in the approach pursued by the Berlin group was to begin to reduce pump speed and flow to examine native heart function 1 month after implantation, but as with all published reports on recovery up to this point, there was no standardized use of an oral HF drug regimen in these patients and no true off-pump testing (as will be described later).

Until recently, the only prospective serial study was a multicenter study of 67 patients (37 with nonischemic cardiomyopathy and 30 with ischemic cardiomyopathy) who had an LVAD placed for refractory HF carried out by a group of investigators at eight US LVAD centers, called the LVAD Working Group.[15] All patients received a HeartMate XVE device, which minimized the potential confounding effect of various types of support. The patients were to be placed on a regimen of oral HF drugs if tolerated after implantation. However, no target doses of the HF medications were defined, and investigators managed drug selection and dosing by physician preference rather than by protocol. As a result, the maximum doses achieved were highly variable among patients, or the drugs were not given, and no conclusion could be reached regarding the potential benefit of routine use of additional reverse remodeling oral HF drug therapy.

The Thoratec HeartMate XVE could be turned off from automatic pumping and hand pumped four to five times per minute to allow examination of native heart function over time. Not all of the centers in this study were experienced with "pump-off" studies, and they were not performed in all of the patients. Some patients had an echocardiogram at reduced, rather than zero, LVAD support (15 minutes after reducing the LVAD flow to 4 L/min). Patients with an EF greater than 40% at reduced or zero LVAD support underwent dobutamine echocardiography with simultaneous hemodynamic monitoring. Additional testing included cardiopulmonary exercise tests, but these were performed on full pump support in a subset of patients at one site only.

The echocardiograms (Fig. 19.4) showed that there was a fair amount of recovery of native cardiac function after 1 month of support, with EF increasing from a mean of 17% before LVAD implantation to an average of 34% ($P<0.001$), with reduction of LVEDD from 7.1 cm to 5.1 cm ($P<0.001$) and LV mass reduced from 320 g to 194 g ($P<0.001$). Peak VO_2 (peak rate of oxygen consumption) improved on LVAD support (13.7 ± 4.2 mL/kg/min vs. 18.9 ± 5.5 mL/kg/min at 30 vs. 120 days, respectively; $P<0.001$). Only six (9%) subjects underwent explantation for myocardial recovery, but there were no protocol-specified explantation criteria.

POSSIBLE EXPLANATIONS OF THE LOW RATE OF MYOCARDIAL RECOVERY

The MCS field has progressed significantly whereby the use of continuous-flow pumps is the norm. Yet, the prospects for recovery remain stagnant nearly two decades later. The general sense that myocardial recovery is more of an anecdote than a true phenomenon has historically been engrained within the annual Interagency Registry for Mechanically Assisted Circulatory Support (INTERMACS) reports. In each of the yearly publications, competing outcome curves consistently portray the rate of myocardial recovery at 1%–2%.[16] However, missing in these database reports is that few centers prospectively look for evidence of recovery. While one can argue about the pathophysiologic semantics of reverse remodeling, remission of HF, and myocardial recovery, the fundamental issue is that the clinician must look for recovery to find it.[1,17,18]

To address this issue further, the University of Utah group studied INTERMACS patients that were a priori designated as bridge to recovery (BTR). Within this cohort, six independent predictors of cardiac recovery were identified: age <50 years, nonischemic cardiomyopathy,

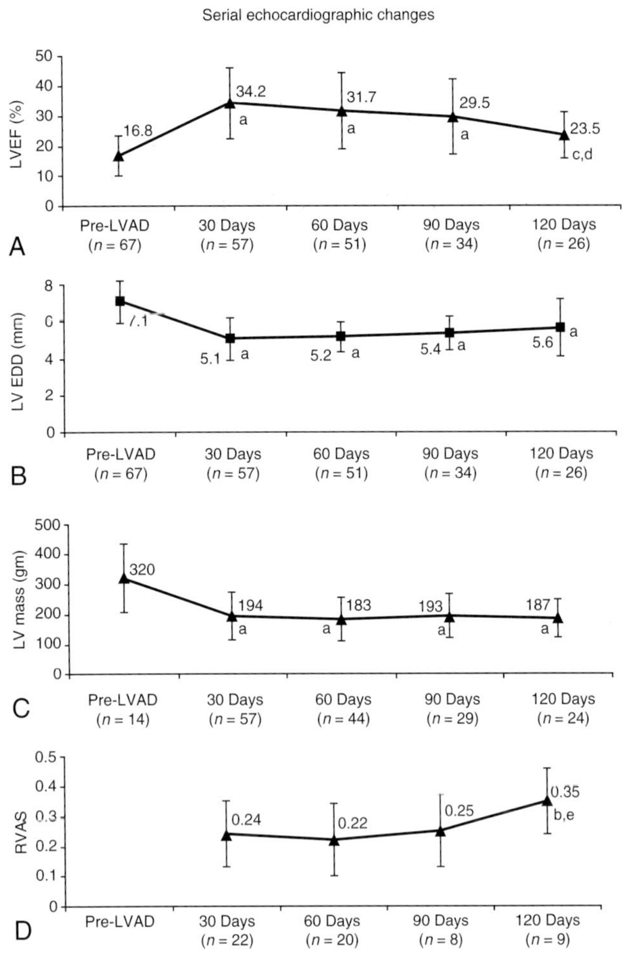

Fig. 19.4 Serial echocardiographic changes in left ventricular assist device (LVAD)-supported patients. Left ventricular ejection fraction *(LVEF)* (A), left ventricular end-diastolic diameter *(LVEDD)* (B), and left ventricular *(LV)* mass (C) were significantly improved vs. pre-LVAD. Right ventricular area shortening *(RVAS)* (D) was improved at 120 days vs. measurements at 30 and 60 days of support. Comparisons with pre-LVAD: $^{a}P<0.001$. Comparisons with 30-day values: $^{b}P<0.05$, $^{c}P<0.01$. Comparisons with 60-day values: $^{d}P<0.05$, $^{e}P<0.01$. (From Maybaum S, Mancini D, Xydas S, et al. Cardiac improvement during mechanical circulatory support: a prospective multicenter study of the LVAD Working Group. *Circulation*. 2007;115:2497–2505.)

time from cardiac diagnosis <2 years, absence of an implantable cardioverter defibrillator, serum creatinine level <1.2 mg/dL, and LVEDD <6.5 cm. On the basis of these results, the INTERMACS Cardiac Recovery Score was derived.[19] The score ranged from 0 to 9, and three groups with significantly different recovery potential were identified: a low probability group (0–3), an intermediate probability group (4 to 6), and a high probability group (7–9). Using this stratification methodology in the INTERMACS BTR population, evidence of recovery was seen in 0%, 4.9%, and 25.4% for patients in the low, intermediate, and high probability categories, respectively. In those patients not designated as BTR, the recovery rates were lower, but not negligible, in the three groups (low, 0.2%; intermediate, 1.3%; high, 8.1%). When applied to the Utah LVAD population, the score suggested a recovery rate of nearly 40% in the high probability group (Fig. 19.5). These results highlight the importance of prospectively testing for recovery. Summarily, the I-CAR score can potentially identify patients that programs could dedicate time, resources, and therapies to augment the chance for recovery and pump explantation.

Assessment of Myocardial Recovery

In most centers, LVADs are implanted either as a BTT or as destination therapy, and the underlying myocardial function is not retested. Regular evaluation of myocardial function following device implantation is essential during the recovery process. Most of the early weaning protocols did not assess the true native myocardial function because they were based on measurements taken while the device was operating at full support. Echocardiographic studies, cardiopulmonary exercise testing, and right and left heart catheterization methods have now been described that can be performed safely and regularly, with the pump providing negligible or no forward flow, to monitor and detect recovery.

The ultimate goal of removing an LVAD depends upon a safe, accurate, and reproducible method of monitoring myocardial recovery. Patients should be studied during a period of limited or no LVAD support to test the true underlying cardiac function. It is important to perform echocardiographic, functional, and hemodynamic tests before deciding whether to explant the pump. A method was developed at Harefield Hospital for off-pump echocardiographic assessment of patients on the pulsatile HeartMate XVE pump.[20] This protocol required administration of 10,000 units of unfractionated heparin 5 minutes before pump cessation, then acutely stopping the LVAD (while hand pumping for three bursts every 15 seconds to prevent stagnation of blood within the pump) and taking measurements of peripheral hemodynamics (e.g., blood pressure and heart rate) while echocardiographic parameters were obtained both at rest and whenever possible after exercise to test inotropic reserve. Pneumatic hand pumping was stopped while taking hemodynamic and echocardiographic measurements. Hemodynamic assessments were first done at baseline with the device on; then immediately after LVAD discontinuation; and at 5, 10, and 15 minutes after device cessation. Echocardiographic measurements were obtained at baseline and at 5 and 15 minutes after device cessation. If device cessation was tolerated for 15 minutes, a 6-minute walk (6MW) test was performed with repeat measurements afterward to determine the inotropic reserve. Echocardiographic measurements included LV end-systolic diameter (LVESD), LVEDD, and EF, along with a detailed assessment of valvular regurgitation (particularly mitral, which, if significant, could lead to overestimation of LV function and also result in recurrent HF by over reloading after explantation). Simultaneous hemodynamic measurements included systolic and diastolic blood pressure, mean arterial pressure (MAP), and heart rate. During the off-pump periods, patients were closely observed for symptoms such as dizziness, sweating, or palpitations. This series was the first time that these pumps had been turned completely off. Importantly, none of the patients experienced short-term or long-term adverse effects after the testing, and, in particular, no thromboembolic complications were seen. Initial device discontinuation was tolerated in 97.6% of patients.[20]

Inotropic reserve was defined as the change in hemodynamics and echocardiographic parameters after the 6MW test without any infusion with inotropic agents (Fig. 19.6). During these "off-pump" tests in all LVAD conditions, EF was significantly higher in the patients who subsequently recovered compared with the patients who did not. Similarly, the recovered group showed a significant increase in EF after the 6MW compared with the 15-minute off-pump test, suggesting the presence of inotropic reserve, but there was no significant change in EF in the nonrecovered group. Five minutes after device cessation, the LVESD and the LVEDD significantly increased in both groups. However, there was no further increase in ventricular dimensions in the recovered cohort whereas the nonrecovered group had progressive increase in LVEDD. Both the systolic blood pressure and the pulse pressure decreased significantly within 5 minutes after

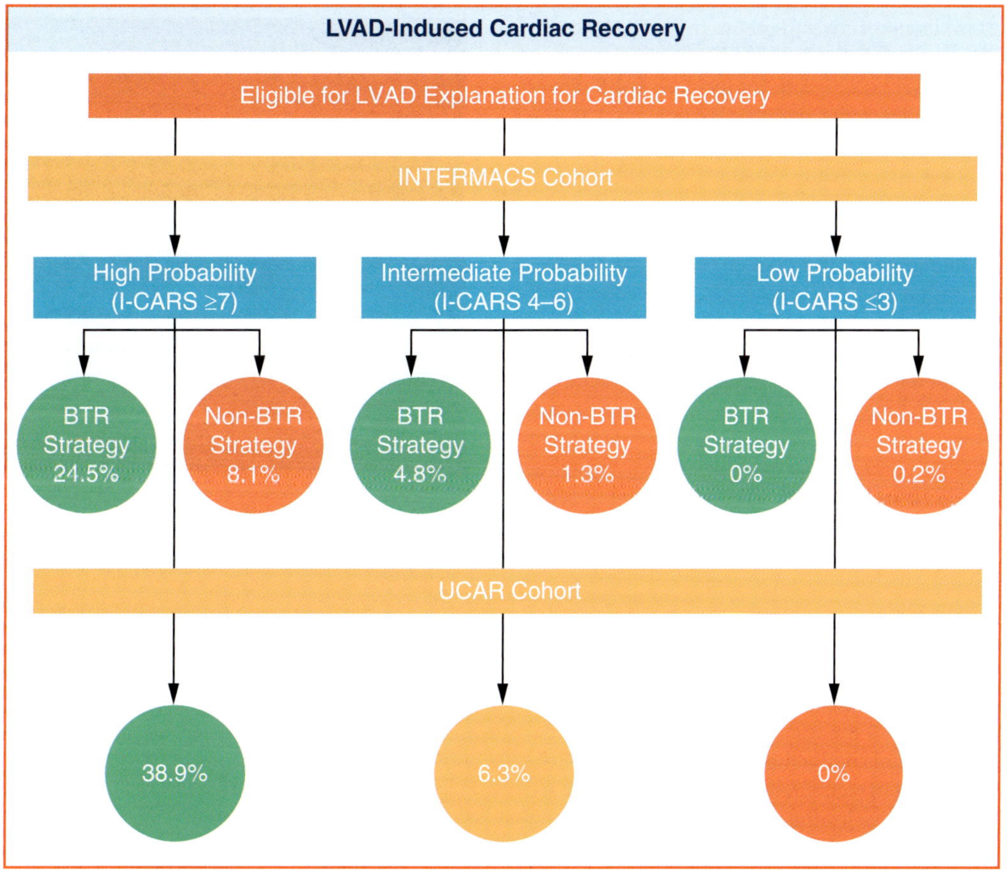

Fig. 19.5 Flowchart showing the outcome from a study evaluating the true incidence of cardiac recovery in patients from the Interagency Registry for Mechanically Assisted Circulatory Support *(INTERMACS)* who received a left ventricular assist device *(LVAD)*, some as an a priori bridge-to-recovery *(BTR)* strategy. A predictive model of cardiac recovery led to the creation of an INTERMACS Cardiac Recovery Score *(I-CARS)* denoting tiered probability of recovery, which was validated through a Utah Cardiac Recovery *(UCAR)* program cohort. (From Wever-Pinzon O, Drakos SG, McKellar SH, et al. Cardiac recovery during long-term left ventricular assist device support. *J Am Coll Cardiol.* 2016;68:1540–1553.)

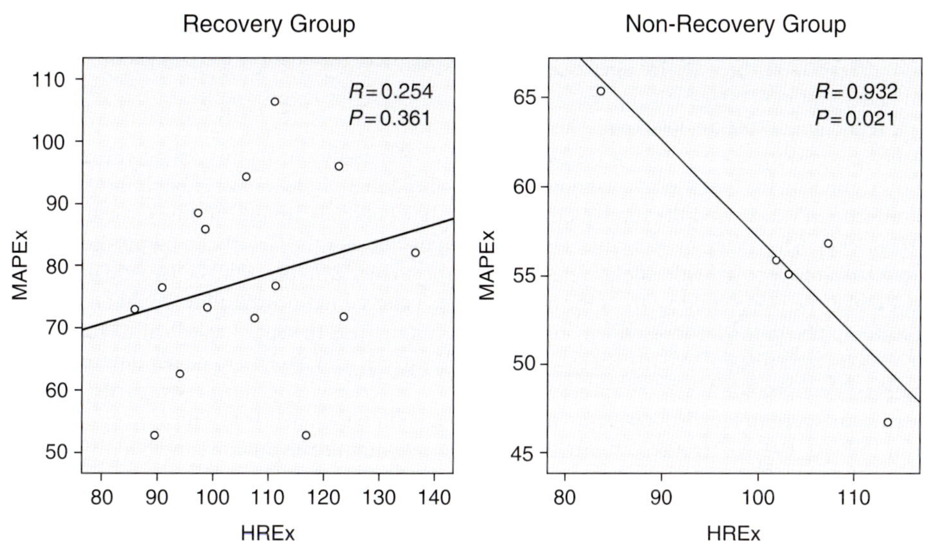

Fig. 19.6 *(Left)* Recovery group showing no correlation between heart rate *(HR)* and mean arterial pressure *(MAP)* after the 6-minute walk (6MW) test, suggesting that the rise in HR was independent of the MAP change and a true inotropic reserve response. *(Right)* Nonrecovered group showing a significantly negative correlation between HR and MAP after the 6MW, suggesting that the increase in the heart rate was compensatory for MAP reduction. *Ex*, exercise. (From George RS, Yacoub MH, Tasca G, et al. Hemodynamic and echocardiographic responses to acute interruption of left ventricular assist device support: relevance to assessment of myocardial recovery. *J Heart Lung Transplant.* 2007;26:967–973.)

turning the pump off in the nonrecovered group. In contrast, an improvement was noted in systolic blood pressure and pulse pressure in the recovered group as well as a significant increase in EF. These improvements suggest that inotropic reserve was preserved in the recovered group. In the nonrecovered group, there was an increase in heart rate, which appeared to be compensatory for a reduction in MAP (Fig. 19.6).

In this study, the strongest predictors of recovery were stable or increased MAP (60 mm Hg) and pulse pressure measured 15 minutes after pump deactivation or 6MW. An EF ≥53% after the 6MW was the strongest predictor of recovery with sensitivity and specificity of 93% and 80%, respectively (receiver operating characteristic curve area = 0.82). Except for the EF, none of the echocardiographic or hemodynamic parameters measured with the device on full support predicted recovery. This study demonstrated the safety and effectiveness of the previous protocol for monitoring myocardial recovery with the pulsatile HeartMate XVE LVAD. While admittedly historic in the era of continuous-flow pumps, this study demonstrated the importance of a standardized approach for searching for myocardial recovery.

In patients supported with a pulsatile-flow device, inflow and outflow valves prevent regurgitation of blood from the aorta to the LV during device deactivation. Hence, LV loading secondary to cessation of a pulsatile pump, such as the HeartMate XVE, reflects a physiologic response that reveals the true underlying function of the native LV. Reducing the speed of continuous-flow devices, such as the HeartMate II LVAD, can result in regurgitant volume flowing from the aorta to the LV, causing excessive loading and making assessment of the native LV function less reliable. With continuous-flow pumps, it is important to identify a speed at which there is no forward or backward flow so that the underlying myocardial function can be safely and effectively assessed. In addition, continuous-flow device patients are anticoagulated with warfarin, so supplemental heparin (5000–10,000 u) is required only if the international normalized ratio (INR) is subtherapeutic.

With regard to continuous-flow pumps, George and colleagues[21] performed a prospective study of flow across the HeartMate II LVAD in patients with idiopathic dilated cardiomyopathy. After ensuring an INR of ≥2.0, LV echocardiographic parameters and peripheral hemodynamics were measured serially at three device speed settings: the baseline device speed and 15 minutes after reducing the speed to 6000 rpm, with subsequent reduction to 5000 or 4000 rpm. The LVAD flow pattern was established by positioning a pulsed wave Doppler sample volume at the inflow cannula in the best possible window. Peak velocities in the forward direction ($Vmax_f$) and the reverse direction ($Vmax_r$) were assessed (Fig. 19.7). The changing velocities over the flow period in both the forward and the reverse directions were determined by tracing the areas under the Doppler curve from the leading edges of the velocity spectrum to obtain the forward velocity time integral (VTI_f) and reverse velocity time integral (VTI_r). There were no adverse events or symptomatic deterioration when the speed was reduced to 4000 rpm. Reducing the speed to less than 6000 rpm did not have a significant effect on LVEDD, LVESD, fractional shortening, or EF, suggesting that there is no need to reduce the speed of the device to less than 6000 rpm in the assessment of the native LV performance. As the LVAD speed was reduced to 6000 rpm, the blood volume through the inflow cannula decreased significantly, but further reductions in the LVAD speed did not change the inflow cannula blood volume significantly, confirming that speeds less than 6000 rpm were not needed to assess the underlying LV function and that this testing was safe. A summary of proposed low speed echo testing for the HeartMate II is shown in Fig. 19.8.

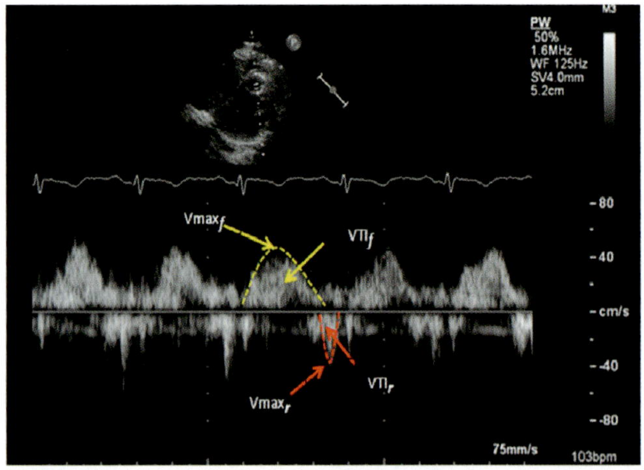

Fig. 19.7 Measurements taken from Pulsed Waved Doppler to quantify the forward and reverse flows. The positive spectrum represents forward flow and occurs in systole, whereas the negative spectrum represents the reverse flow and occurs in diastole. The spectra were quantified by measuring the peak velocity and their time integral. *$Vmax_f$*, Forward peak velocity; *$Vmax_r$*, reverse peak velocity; *VTI_f*, forward velocity time integral; *VTI_r*, reverse velocity time integral. (From George RS, Yacoub MH, Tasca G, et al. Hemodynamic and echocardiographic responses to acute interruption of left ventricular assist device support: relevance to assessment of myocardial recovery. *J Heart Lung Transplant*. 2007;26:967–973.)

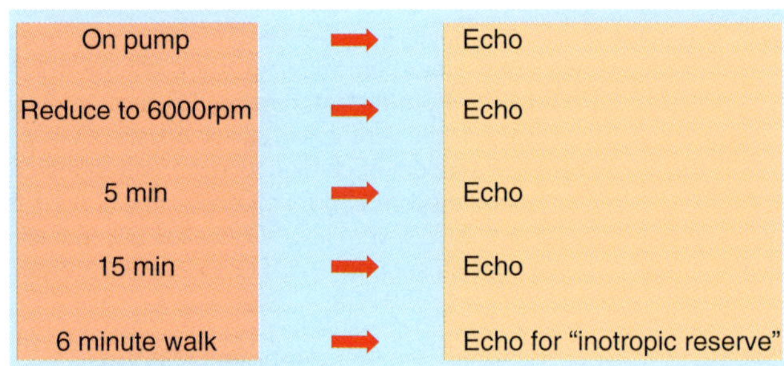

Fig. 19.8 Summary of the suggested course of a low speed echo.

Generally, during this testing, the continuous-flow pump is run at a speed that produces just enough forward flow to counteract the backflow (which is around 1 L/min), resulting in as close to no net flow as possible. For the HeartWare pump, the speed at which net neutral flow occurs is 1800 rpm. For the HeartMate 3 pump, the speed at which it is believed net neutral flow would be expected is 4000 rpm (Fig. 19.9 summarizes the speed at which to run the different pumps to assess recovery with as close to no net flow as possible).

Several investigators have reported more sophisticated echocardiographic parameters to assess recovery potential. Ferrari and colleagues[22] used a minimally invasive method to determine the predictive power of Emax, the slope of the LV end-systolic pressure-volume relationship, and an afterload-independent and preload-independent index of LV contractility. Contractile reserve, also known as inotropic reserve, refers to the objective quantification of LV contractility after either a pharmacologic or physiologic stress and is reduced in patients with ischemic or nonischemic cardiomyopathy. However, different indices have been used to determine contractile reserve. The most frequently used is the absolute change in EF after dobutamine infusion, although there is an inability to distinguish abnormalities in contractility from

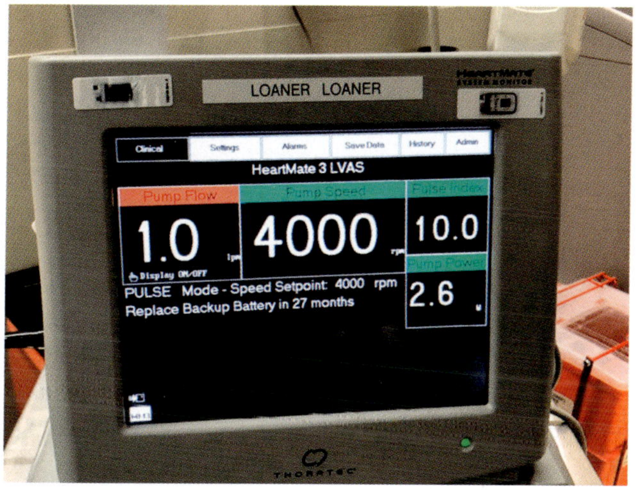

Fig. 19.9 HeartMate 3 testing in a patient at 4000 rpm, which generates the 1 L required to counteract the 1 L backflow from the pump to be able to test the underlying myocardial function at no net flow.

alterations in preload or afterload. Conventionally, an absolute increase in the EF by 5% during dobutamine infusion compared with resting indicates preservation of contractile reserve with a strong correlation to prognosis.[23,24]

By recording the hemodynamic response during dobutamine stress echocardiography, Khan and coworkers[25,26] evaluated 16 patients with increasing doses of dobutamine (from 5 μg/kg/min to 40 μg/kg/min). Hemodynamics and two-dimensional echocardiography were performed at each dose level. Dobutamine stress separated the study population into two groups: patients who had favorable responses to dobutamine (9 of 16) and patients who had unfavorable responses (i.e., experienced hemodynamic deterioration; 7 of 16). Favorable dobutamine responses were characterized by improved cardiac index, improved force-frequency relationship in the LV (dP/dt), improved LVEF, and decreased LVEDD. All nine favorable responders underwent LVAD explantation, and six survived for more than 12 months. Dobutamine stress echocardiography with hemodynamic assessment is also a useful tool in assessing physiologic improvement in myocardial function of patients with LVAD support.

Cardiopulmonary exercise testing with pump settings that provide net neutral flow is also an important component of the recovery testing process of underlying myocardial function. If the INR is greater than 2, then the speed of the device is reduced, and if the INR is less than 2, 5–10,000 units of unfractionated heparin is given 10 minutes before pump speed reduction. During the cardiopulmonary exercise test at reduced pump speed, patients are closely observed for symptoms, and measurements at rest and at peak exercise on a modified Bruce protocol are undertaken. Mancini and colleagues[8] also performed hemodynamic and metabolic measurements both at rest and at peak exercise (cycling) with optimal and reduced LVAD support without reported complications. Although it is important to perform cardiopulmonary exercise testing at net neutral flow speed in LVAD patients, the results are influenced by many other variables, such as the overall condition of the patient. Thus, it is typically used as additional information to help an explantation decision rather than critical information for that decision.

Cardiac power output (CPO) is a novel, central hemodynamic measure that has been suggested to be a direct and possibly the best indicator of overall cardiac function.[31] CPO is calculated as MAP × cardiac output/451, where MAP = [(systolic blood pressure – diastolic blood pressure)/3] + diastolic blood pressure. By incorporating both pressure and flow domains of the cardiovascular system, CPO is an integrative and unique measure of cardiac pumping capability. Resting and peak exercise CPOs have been shown to be powerful predictors of prognosis and mortality in patients with chronic HF and cardiogenic shock.[27,28] Patients with a peak CPO less than 2 W have a considerably higher mortality rate than do patients with a peak CPO greater than 2 W. Jakovljevic and associates[29] measured CPO in continuous-flow LVAD patients at net neutral flow during cardiopulmonary exercise testing and found CPO to be a useful and predictive marker of recovery.

Patients who tolerate LVAD flow reduction to minimal levels and show echocardiographic signs of recovery should also undergo right ± left heart cardiac catheterization. Important measurements to obtain include right atrial pressure, pulmonary artery pressure, PCWP, LV end-diastolic pressure (LVEDP), and cardiac output (both thermodilution and Fick). It is important to obtain these measurements both with the device on and after 15 minutes at net neutral flow speed. A left ventriculogram after the LVAD has been at low speed for 15 minutes also shows ventricular function well. An outflow graft angiogram may be used to verify device contribution to flow and/or regurgitant volumes at the speed at which the hemodynamics were measured (Fig. 19.10). The most important hemodynamic variables suggesting significant and sustained myocardial recovery with reloading after LVAD removal are stable or improved PCWP and cardiac output following reduction of the pump speed for 15 minutes.

OPTIMIZING MYOCARDIAL RECOVERY

With an armamentarium of tools to assess recovery, efforts must also be directed at optimizing myocardial recovery. Many patients simply have their devices placed, and therapies are focused on blood pressure control rather than reverse remodeling. The thought process is that the patient has failed advanced HF medical treatment and the machine will provide the output necessary for a patient with lifetime use, or if the patient is bridged to transplant, simply focus on the device rather than the heart. Using the LVAD as a platform to induce myocardial recovery and combining the unloading with other therapies to maximize recovery are likely to lead to a significant increase in the rate of recovery.

Indeed, just the mechanical unloading of the weakened ventricle may be a powerful tool to promote myocardial recovery. To understand

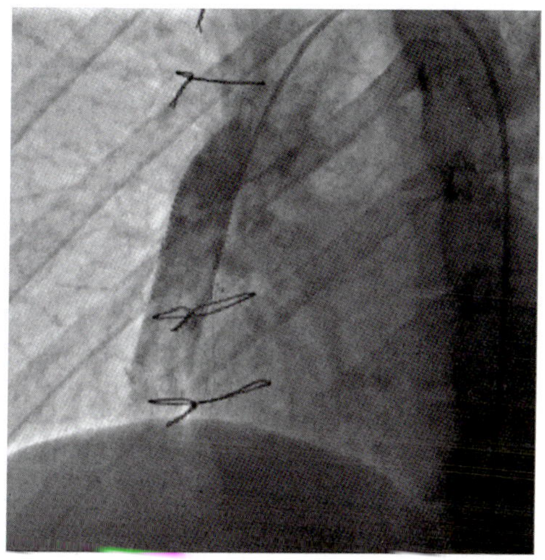

Fig. 19.10 A pigtail catheter directed into the outflow conduit of the device with contrast injected to ensure that there is no significant forward or backward flow in diastole and demonstrate that the testing speed is evaluating underlying myocardial function without excessive ventricular loading.

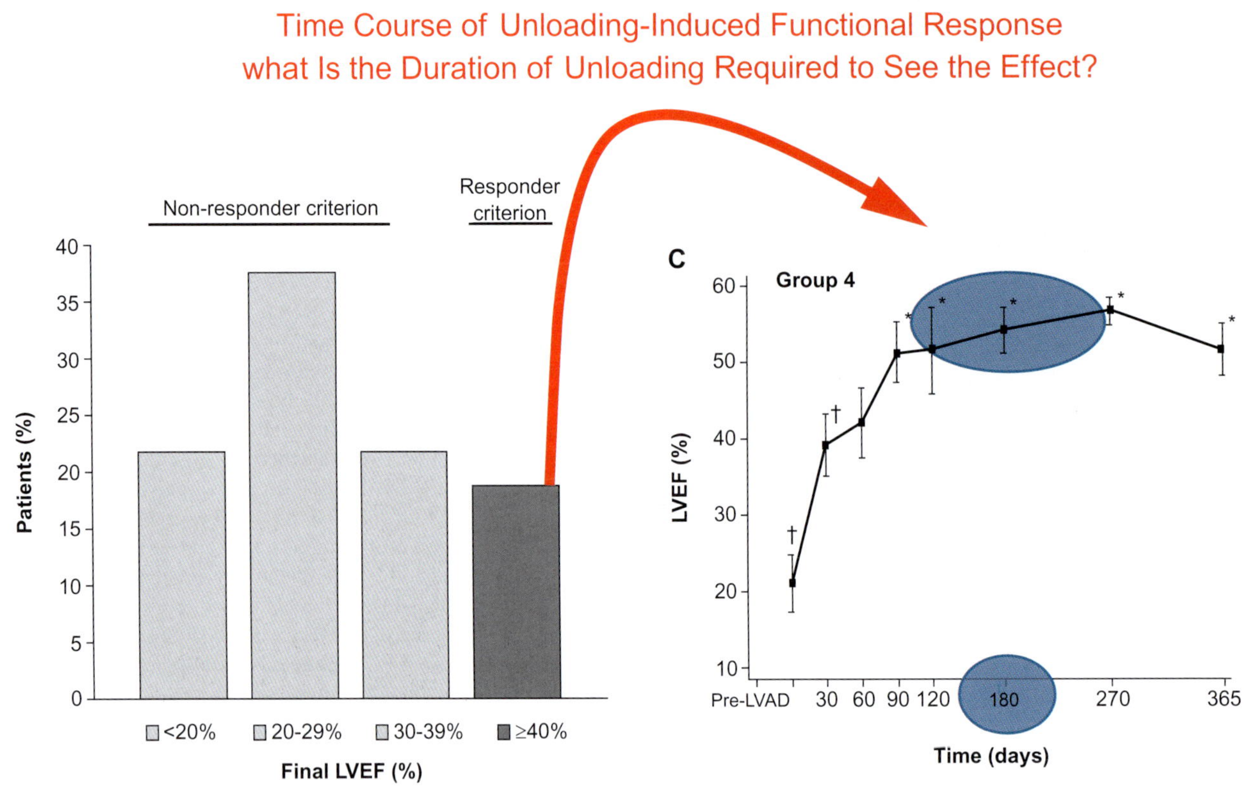

Fig. 19.11 Relative increase in left ventricular ejection fraction *(LVEF)* during turn-down echocardiography in patients supported with a left ventricular assist device. The time course of the "responders" is depicted in the second panel, demonstrating that the majority of patients have functional response within 6–9 months. (From Drakos SG, Wever-Pinzon O, Selzman CH, et al. Magnitude and time course of changes induced by continuous-flow left ventricular assist device unloading in chronic heart failure: insights into cardiac recovery. *J Am Coll Cardiol.* 2013;61:1985–1994.)

the influence of unloading alone, 81 continuous flow (CF)-LVAD patients with echocardiograms performed at reduced pump speed were followed.[30] Within this group, nearly 20% of patients had significant recovery of LV function (EF >40%). Importantly, most of the improvement in function occurred in the first 6 months after LVAD implantation (Fig. 19.11). Furthermore, these changes occurred both with and without aggressive neurohormonal blockade, with the latter approach being more favorable.[31] Finally, this phenomenon was not just in patients with dilated cardiomyopathies, but also, albeit with lower rates, in those with ischemic disease.[32,33] These studies are some of the largest to prospectively link mechanical unloading with functional recovery and provides the framework with which to build adjuvant medical strategies to enhance the frequency with which recovery takes place.

HAREFIELD PROTOCOL

A strategy was developed at Harefield Hospital that combined LVAD mechanical unloading with specific pharmacologic drugs known to enhance reverse remodeling in an attempt to maximize the incidence of recovery. This regimen consisted of an LVAD speed set for optimal unloading, combined with HF drugs known to enhance reverse remodeling (phase 1), followed by the administration of clenbuterol (phase 2) to improve the durability of recovery in these patients after explantation.[34] The other important part of this protocol was to systematically and regularly test underlying cardiac function in patients throughout the protocol with the pump off, or essentially off, at regular intervals to assess their response to treatment and guide therapy.

Harefield Protocol—Phase 1

The pharmacologic interventions of the first phase were designed to act on component parts of the myocardium, with the aim of reversing pathologic hypertrophy, remodeling, and normalizing cellular metabolic function. Reverse remodeling HF drugs were aggressively initiated immediately after weaning of inotropic support when there is adequate end-organ recovery and titrated to very high doses (targeted doses: lisinopril, 40 mg daily; carvedilol, 25–50 mg twice daily; spironolactone, 25 mg daily; digoxin, 125 μg daily; and losartan, 100 mg daily). Patients had simultaneous increases in angiotensin-converting enzyme inhibitors (ACEIs), beta-1 and beta-2 blockers, and aldosterone inhibitors, followed by the angiotensin II antagonists, although the angiotensin-converting enzyme inhibition is the greatest priority in increasing the therapy.

The rationale of the first phase of this regimen was to combine mechanical unloading with drugs known to enhance reverse remodeling. Patients often did not tolerate large doses of ACEIs, beta blockers, aldosterone antagonists, and angiotensin II inhibitors while in severe HF because of renal failure or hypotension. However, once patients achieved good cardiac output and adequate blood pressure and renal function from LVAD support, they tolerated HF drugs well. ACEI (and angiotensin II inhibition) was a crucial part of this strategy and was used along with the aldosterone antagonist to reduce fibrosis.

The specific benefits of neurohormonal inhibition by using ACEIs with VAD support have been extensively demonstrated. Klotz and colleagues[35] showed that prolonged mechanical hemodynamic unloading increased myocardial tissue levels of angiotensin II with concomitant increases in collagen cross-linking and myocardial stiffness. Elevated serum levels of angiotensin II can be reduced by blocking the renin-angiotensin-aldosterone system with an ACEI. These investigators examined the myocardium of patients before and after LVAD support in patients treated with or without ACEI therapy during LVAD support. After LVAD, tissue angiotensin II levels were significantly reduced in the ACEI group but increased in control subjects. Similarly, cross-linked collagen decreased during LVAD support in the ACEI group, as did LV mass and myocardial stiffness. Myocardial tissue levels of total, soluble, and insoluble cross-linked collagen significantly increased during LVAD support in the control group.[36]

The same group also investigated paired LV myocardial samples obtained from 20 patients before and after LVAD support. Pre-LVAD renin levels were 100 times greater than in normal controls.[37] In patients not receiving ACEIs, LVAD support reversed this. Myocardial aldosterone levels decreased in parallel with cardiac renin in the non-ACEI group. Cardiac norepinephrine increased sevenfold in patients not treated with ACEI, possibly owing to the increase in angiotensin II. ACEI therapy prevented these changes; renin and aldosterone remained high, and no increase in norepinephrine occurred. Thus, while LV unloading lowers myocardial renin and aldosterone, it allows cardiac angiotensin generation to increase, stimulating the sympathetic nervous system, which ACEIs prevent, supporting the rationale for use of ACEI.

Harefield Protocol—Phase 2

It seemed logical that cardiac muscle "atrophy" (observed with isolation and lack of mechanical work) would be a possible consequence of a period of LVAD myocardial unloading and that a lack of preload and mechanical work of the ventricle may partially explain the lack of durability of myocardial recovery observed previously in some other studies. Although the concept of LVAD-induced atrophy has since been disputed,[38] it was hypothesized that to achieve consistent successful device explantation, a period of reverse remodeling and regression of pathologic myocardial hypertrophy should be followed by attempts to produce beneficial "physiological hypertrophy," with additional beneficial effects at the level of the cardiomyocyte and matrix. Clenbuterol induces a type of myocardial hypertrophy associated with improved systolic and diastolic function, with increased sarcoplasmic reticulum calcium content, histological prevention of fibrosis, normal collagen levels, and enhanced expression of contractile genes.[39,40] This improved contractility without fibrosis is often referred to as physiological hypertrophy.

In the Harefield protocol, the second stage of pharmacologic therapy was instituted after maximal regression in the LVEDD had been achieved while the LVAD was in place. When the LVEDD was less than 60 mm on low speed testing, the initial nonselective beta blocker carvedilol was switched to a beta-1 selective adrenergic receptor blocker (e.g., bisoprolol or metoprolol), leaving beta-2 receptors unblocked for clenbuterol. Clenbuterol was added to all phase 1 drugs at an initial dose of 40 μg twice daily and then titrated to a target dose of 700 μg three times daily. The dose was adjusted to maintain the resting heart rate at less than 100 beats/min.

The rationale for using clenbuterol, a beta-2 agonist, as the phase 2 pharmacotherapeutic target is multifactorial. Clenbuterol is known to induce physiologic, rather than pathologic, myocardial hypertrophy. This form of hypertrophy is associated with improved systolic and diastolic function, prevention of fibrosis, and enhanced expression of contractile genes.[41,42] Clenbuterol also has other positive actions on cardiac function. As a selective beta-2-adrenergic receptor agonist, it is a potent synthetic analog to epinephrine; induces insulin like growth factor 1, through which skeletal muscle hypertrophy is mediated; and reduces adverse signaling patterns mediated through beta-1 receptors, including apoptosis.[43] Because most negative effects of beta stimulation seem to be beta-1 receptor mediated, administration of beta-1 antagonists in conjunction with beta-2 agonists such as clenbuterol seemed safe and appropriate.

Harefield Protocol Prospective Trial—Pulsatile Pump

Using this strategy of combining optimal LVAD unloading with reverse remodeling therapy, followed by clenbuterol administration, two prospective studies were performed at Harefield Hospital in London in patients with nonischemic cardiomyopathy receiving an LVAD.[2,44] The first prospective study consisted of 20 patients who received a pulsatile HeartMate XVE LVAD as BTT. Patients with myocarditis (proven on histologic examination of the large transmural core of myocardial tissue removed for insertion of the apical cannula) were excluded so as to focus on patients with chronic HF. The average age of the patients was 37.6 ± 13.7 years (range, 15–57 years), and the mean duration of HF was 4.5 ± 4.5 years. All patients had deteriorating NYHA class IV HF despite inotropic support at the time of VAD implantation.

Echocardiography was performed weekly after implantation for the first month and monthly thereafter. After week 4, studies were performed both on- and off-pump (as described above) at 5 minutes and 15 minutes, and after a 6-minute walk (if tolerated), to determine inotropic reserve. When the patients were able to walk 450 m in 6 minutes with the device off, with no deterioration of the echocardiographic measurements, formal cardiopulmonary exercise tests were performed monthly with the device on and off.

Cardiac catheterization was performed before explantation, right-sided and left-sided pressures and cardiac output were measured (with the device on and off for 15 minutes), and a left ventriculogram was obtained with the device off. Explantation was considered if the following criteria were met (measured with the LVAD off for 15 minutes): LVEDD <60 mm, LVESD <50 mm, and EF >45%; a LVEDP (or PCWP) <12 mm Hg; resting cardiac index >2.8 L/min/m^2; and maximal oxygen consumption (VO_2 max) >16 mL/kg/min and an increase in minute ventilation (V_E) relative to the production of carbon dioxide (VCO_2) (V_E/VCO_2 slope) <34.

Lisinopril, spironolactone, and losartan were restarted after explantation with the same high target doses, but clenbuterol was discontinued. Carvedilol was restarted in place of bisoprolol. Of the 15 patients who received a complete course of the combination therapy, 11 (73%) had sufficient recovery to meet the explantation criteria. For the explanted patients, the mean duration of support was 320 ± 186 (range, 63–603) days. For the explanted patients, the LVEF (with the pump off for 15 minutes) was 64% ± 8% before explantation compared with 12% ± 6% before implantation (P = 0.001), the LVEDD was 55.9 ± 8.3 mm compared with 75.1 ± 16.3 mm (P = 0.002), and the LVESD was 39.6 ± 6.5 mm compared with 66.9 ± 16.3 mm (P = 0.002). Before explantation, the VO_2 max (with the pump off) was 20.7 ± 6.1 mL/kg/min, with a VE/VCO_2 slope of 32.5 ± 7.9. Cardiac catheterization before explantation (with the pump off) showed a PCWP of 9.0 ± 4.1 mm Hg (compared with 23.8 ± 9.7 mm Hg on inotropic therapy before implantation; P = 0.004), cardiac output of 5.4 ± 1.2 L/min, cardiac index of 2.8 ± 0.7 L/min/m^2, and pulmonary artery oxygen saturation of 66.9% ± 4.8%.

Although the numbers were too small for meaningful analysis, age, LV dimensions, and the duration of HF were not determinants of recovery. Of five patients with an LVEDD of greater than 80 mm, four recovered. The actuarial survival rate 1 year and 4 years after explantation was 90.9% and 81.8%, respectively. One patient died of intractable arrhythmia 24 hours after explantation without evidence of

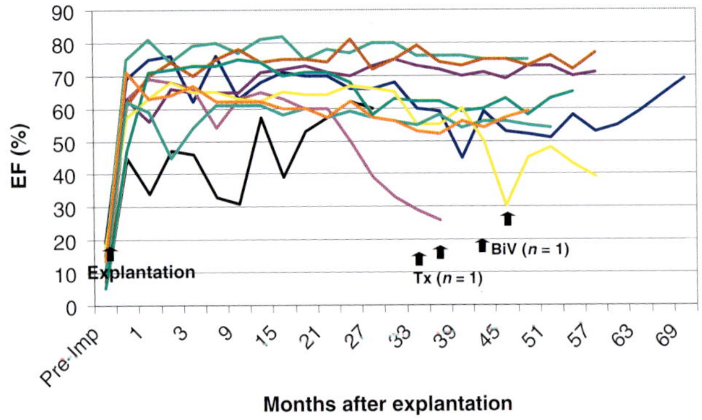

Fig. 19.12 Ejection fraction *(EF)* before implantation *(Pre-Imp)* and after explantation in the first Harefield study. (From Birks EJ, Tansley PD, Hardy J, et al. Left ventricular assist device and drug therapy for the reversal of heart failure. *N Engl J Med.* 2006;355:1873–1884.)

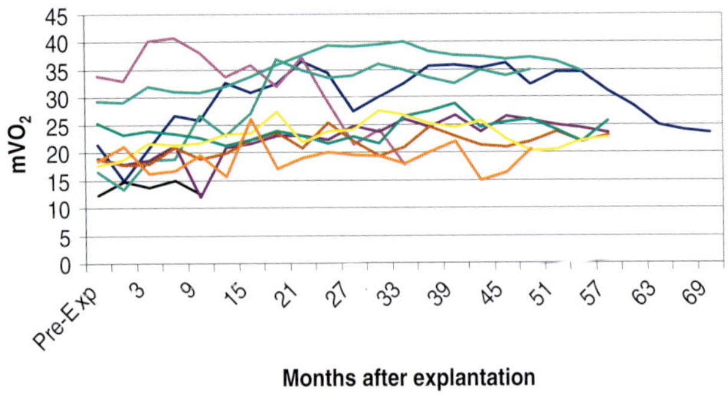

Fig. 19.13 Maximal oxygen consumption *(mVO_2)* with exercise before *(Pre-Exp)* and after explantation in the HeartMate I explanted patients. (From Birks EJ, Tansley PD, Hardy J, et al. Left ventricular assist device and drug therapy for the reversal of heart failure. *N Engl J Med.* 2006;355:1873–1884.)

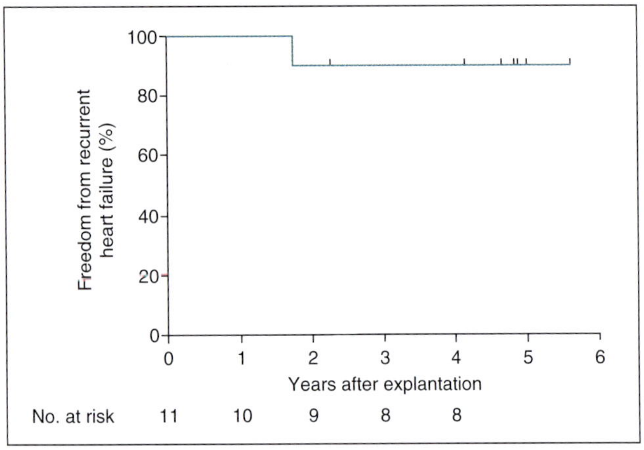

Fig. 19.14 Cumulative rate of freedom from recurrence of heart failure among the surviving patients who underwent explantation. (From Birks EJ, Tansley PD, Hardy J, et al. Left ventricular assist device and drug therapy for the reversal of heart failure. *N Engl J Med.* 2006;355:1873–1884.)

deteriorating ventricular function, and another died of lung carcinoma 27 months after explantation. The minimum period of follow-up after explantation was approximately 4 years (range, 1519–2058 days; mean, 1799 ± 153 days). At a mean follow-up of 59 ± 5 months, EF was 64% ± 12%, LVEDD was 59.4 ± 12.1 mm, LVESD was 42.5 ± 13.2 mm, and mean VO_2 max was 26.3 ± 6.0 mL/kg/min (Figs. 19.12 and 19.13). All surviving patients continued to be in NYHA class I except one, in whom HF recurred and who underwent successful transplantation 33 months after explantation. Among the surviving patients, the cumulative rate of freedom from recurrence of HF 1 year and 4 years after explantation was 100% and 88.9%, respectively (Fig. 19.14).

Among the patients whose devices were successfully explanted, hemodynamic testing 1 year after explantation showed a PCWP of 9.5 ± 6.2 mm Hg, LVEDP of 9.3 ± 5.5 mm Hg, cardiac output of 4.9 ± 2.1 L/min, cardiac index of 2.4 ± 1.2 L/min/m^2, and pulmonary artery oxygen saturation of 73.5% ± 32%. The quality of life as assessed by the Minnesota Living With Heart Failure Score in these patients at 3 years was near-normal. The longest follow-up now is of a patient 18 years after explantation.

Harefield Protocol Prospective Trial—Continuous-Flow Pump

Following this study, there was a transition from volume displacement, pulsatile-flow LVADs to the newer continuous-flow designs. Although more durable, the hydrodynamic characteristics of pulsatile-flow and continuous-flow VADs vary markedly, and it was unknown whether the latter would be as effective in promoting myocardial recovery and whether, despite superior outcomes with the continuous-flow design, there is similar or reduced LV unloading. Maximal reduction of wall stress seems a potentially important goal, and in theory, continuous-flow pumps might achieve less reduction in LVEDP than the pulsatile-flow pumps. However, the ability to adjust pump speed and LV decompression might improve unloading. The secondary induction of ventricular arrhythmias with excessive speeds and reduction in LV size owing to physical contact of the LV wall with the inflow cannula of the device was also a concern that could limit maximal unloading. With continuous-flow devices, the characteristics of unloading are different, testing of underlying myocardial function is more complex, and optimizing medication was likely to be more difficult because of reduced pulse pressure.

As such, the next question was whether the profound pressure and volume unloading of the LV that occurs with LVAD was specific to the pulsatile-flow pumps or whether recovery can also occur with continuous-flow pumps. Theoretically, continuous-flow pumps might unload less, but they unload continuously, whereas pulsatile-flow pumps are asynchronous with the cardiac cycle and might intermittently load the ventricle.

Of the 15 patients receiving the combination therapy in the original Harefield study, one had a HeartMate II continuous-flow pump, which was explanted over 15 years ago. The protocol was subsequently successfully applied to a cohort of chronic HF patients, including one with a familial cardiomyopathy treated with the Jarvik 2000 LVAD.[45,46] The Jarvik pump is implanted in the LV cavity and is more difficult to remove without damaging the heart or ventricular function. For those who recovered, the graft was ligated, and the device remained inside the ventricle without any adverse sequelae for the patients. One patient is now alive and well over 5 years after ligation of the graft and discontinuation of the device.

A second trial with the Harefield Recovery Protocol was conducted between February 2006 and January 2009 in 20 prospective patients with dilated nonischemic cardiomyopathy receiving a continuous-flow pump as BTT.[44] The study used the same drug regimen and protocol as the first study (see Table 19.1), with only the substitution of the pulsatile-flow HeartMate XVE LVAD for the continuous-flow HeartMate II LVAD. Again, none of the patients had histologic evidence of acute myocarditis, and the study was aimed to test the reversibility of advanced chronic HF.

TABLE 19.1 Baseline Demographics, Clinical, Echo, and Laboratory Data of Patients in the Harefield HeartMate I and II Prospective Recovery Studies and the US Harefield Recovery Protocol Study

	Harefield HeartMate I Recovery Study	Harefield HeartMate II Recovery Study	US HARP Study
Total no. of patients	20	20	17
Age, mean ± SD (range), years	37.6 ± 13.7 (15–57)	35.2 ± 12.6 (16–58)	48 (31–60)
Sex	16 male; 4 female	16 male; 4 female	15 male; 2 female
Race	19 Caucasians; 1 black	17 Caucasians; 3 black	8 Caucasians; 6 black; 3 Hispanic
Heart failure history, mean ± SD (range), years	3.91 ± 4.6	3.2 ± 3.5	7.2 ± 4.3 (1–16.5)

HARP, Harefield Recovery Protocol.

Of the 20 patients with dilated cardiomyopathy receiving a HeartMate II as BTT who were enrolled in the study, 16 were men. Mean age was 35.2 ± 12.6 years, and all patients were in NYHA class IV with decompensating HF. Patients were receiving a mean of two inotropes, seven (35%) had intraaortic balloon pump support, two were mechanically ventilated, and two had hemofiltration devices. Four patients required temporary mechanical bridging support because they were considered too sick for initial implantation with a long-term device, three with a Levitronix device, and one with extracorporeal membrane oxygenation. Preoperative cardiac index was 1.39 ± 0.43 L/min/m^2, PCWP was 31.5 ± 5.7 mm Hg, pulmonary artery saturation was 43.7% ± 12.6%, creatinine was 1.8 ± 1.0 mg/dL, and bilirubin was 2.8 ± 1.5 mg/dL. Echocardiography showed preoperative LVEDD of 71.7 ± 8.9 mm, LVESD of 65.7 ± 7.7 mm, and EF of 14.6% ± 6.6%. Mean HF history was 3.2 ± 3.5 years (range, 1.5–132 months; median, 21 months) (Table 19.1). Three patients required right VAD at the time of LVAD implantation (Levitronix Centrimag) support for 24.3 ± 9.1 days. The cohort was followed until all patients underwent explantation or transplantation or remained listed at study termination. At the end of phase 1 therapy, 16 patients reached the study criteria to receive clenbuterol (end-diastolic diameter was <60 mm with the pump at 6000 rpm for 15 minutes).

As with the pulsatile-flow VAD study, echocardiograms were performed before implantation and monthly after implantation. Measurements were obtained with the LVAD at full speed initially, followed by a reduction of the pump speed to 6000 rpm. Echocardiographic measurements and images were repeated 5 minutes and 15 minutes after the speed was reduced to 6000 rpm. If reduction of LVAD support was tolerated for 15 minutes, a 6MW test was performed with the device operating at 6000 rpm, followed by repeated echocardiographic measurements to determine the LV response to exercise and inotropic reserve. When the patient achieved a 6MW distance of 450 m, a cardiopulmonary exercise test was performed monthly with the device on and again with the device at 6000 rpm.

Right and left heart cardiac catheterization was performed before implantation and explantation. Explantation was considered when the same criteria as mentioned previously were achieved with the LVAD at 6000 rpm for 15 minutes. These criteria were considered the minimum for explantation, and if the parameters were still improving, the combination therapy was continued until the maximum improvement had been achieved in each patient.

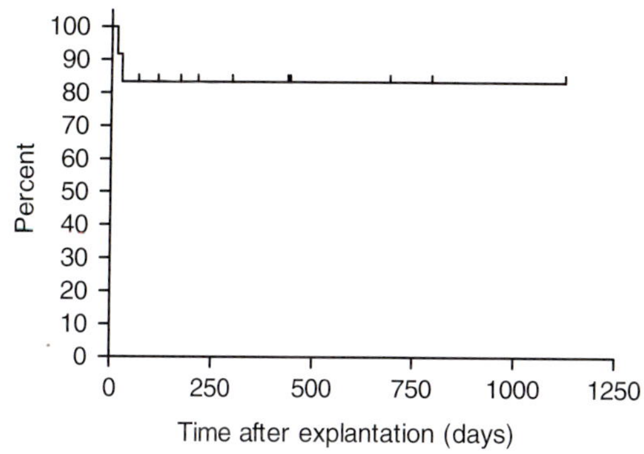

Fig. 19.15 Freedom from death or heart failure recurrence in the HeartMate II explanted patients.

Of the 20 patients, 12 (60%) showed sufficient recovery to meet the previously described explantation criteria and were explanted. For patients undergoing device explantation, the duration of LVAD support was 286 ± 97 days (range, 193–439). Actuarial survival after explantation was 83.3% at 30 days, 1 year, 2 years, and 3 years.

After a mean follow-up of 430.7 ± 337.1 days (range, 56–1112 days), all 10 surviving explanted patients remained in NYHA class I with a mean EF of 58.1% ± 13.8%, LVEDD of 59.0 ± 9.3 mm, LVESD of 4.2 ± 10.7 mm, and mVO_2 of 22.6 ± 5.3 mL/kg/min (Fig. 19.15). Mean creatinine was 1.3 ± 0.5 g/dL, and bilirubin was 1.1 ± 0.4 mg/dL. The cumulative freedom from death and recurrence of HF in the patients who underwent explantation was 83.3% at 30 days, 1 year, and 3 years (Fig. 19.15).

This prospective study showed that reversal of severe chronic HF secondary to dilated nonischemic cardiomyopathy could be achieved in a high proportion of patients using continuous-flow pumps combined with aggressive pharmacologic therapy. The rate and durability of recovery in this series using this strategy are significantly higher than previously reported. It is unclear what role clenbuterol played in the success of the combination therapy because it was initiated after the heart was mostly reverse remodeled and there was already significant improvement in myocardial function. Clenbuterol was intended to improve myocardial function further and, more importantly, to improve the durability of recovery. Importantly, this study showed that reverse remodeling could occur as effectively with the continuous-flow as with the pulsatile pumps.

U.S. Harefield Recovery Protocol Study

The success of the original Harefield study ignited enough interest to try to duplicate these results on a wider scale. The US Harefield Recovery Protocol (HARP) trial was a multicenter trial using a protocol that was essentially the same as the two Harefield Recovery studies (except patients were required to have a HF duration >1 year) and included the phase 1 uptitration to maximal recommended doses of an ACEI, beta blocker, angiotensin receptor blocker, aldosterone antagonist, and digoxin until the reduction in LVEDD afforded by the LVAD had plateaued at less than 6.0 cm. At that time, clenbuterol was started and uptitrated by protocol to target doses. Patients gave informed consent to be withheld from being on the active heart transplant waiting list for 6 months after LVAD implantation to evaluate adequately the potential for sufficient myocardial recovery unless a device complication required earlier transplantation.

Otherwise, the patients were managed exactly as the Harefield study with phase 1 drugs before the introduction of clenbuterol.

The HARP trial's protocol was designed for the HeartMate I device to replicate the initial Harefield publication. In total, there were 17 patients enrolled in the US study: 15 men and 2 women, including 8 whites, 6 blacks, and 3 Hispanics. Mean age was 48 years (range, 31–60 years). The mean HF duration was 7.2 years (median, 8.0 years; range, 1–16.5 years). The demographics of the US study cohort are shown in Table 19.1 compared with the Harefield cohort studied with the XVE device. A reduction in LVEDD and increase in EF were seen by the end of phase 1 of the trial (Figs. 19.16 and 19.17); EF increased from 21% before VAD implantation to 40% at the end of phase 1, and LVEDD decreased from 75 mm to 56 mm.

Overall, a large number of patients dropped out of the study by investigator decision, because of HeartMate XVE VAD-related complication, or severe right ventricular failure. Nine patients were withdrawn from the study, five before receiving any clenbuterol (because of right HF, two abdominal perforations due to the HM XVE, one HMXVE device complication, and one subdural hemorrhage) and four after receiving some clenbuterol (two because of HM XVE pump failure and pump exchange, one driveline infection, and one for administrative reasons). Consequently, very few patients reached target clenbuterol doses. One patient died of a cerebral hemorrhage during the study before receiving a dose of clenbuterol. Two patients were successfully recovered on the LVAD; only one underwent explantation and remained free of HF at latest follow-up. As mentioned, the near-total conversion from implantation of the larger pulsatile pumps such as the HeartMate XVE to the much smaller continuous-flow HeartMate II pumps made enrollment during the latter half of the study very difficult.[47]

The lack of perceived success of this trial was less about the therapy offered but more so related to trial activity, adherence to prespecified protocols, HeartMate XVE–related complications, and the general lack of enthusiasm at the time to implant the HeartMate XVE pump. Hence, a secondary HARP study using the HeartMate II device was discussed but ultimately was halted because of a lack of adequate supply of the oral formulation of clenbuterol. The oral tablet form is only 20 μg, and the target dose for the study was 2100 μg, or 100 tablets/day, which was difficult for reliable drug compliance. One patient with a HeartMate II was recruited in the United States to the second phase of the study before the trial was halted and this patient was successfully recovered and explanted and remains well and free from HF (E. Rame, personal communication) at latest follow-up.

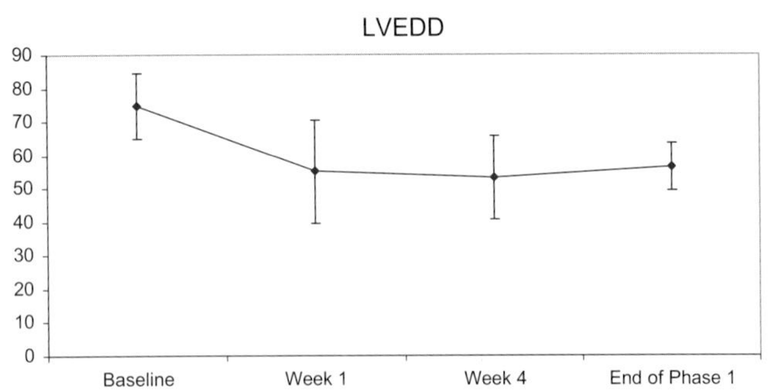

Fig. 19.16 Reduction in left ventricular end-diastolic diameter *(LVEDD)* after phase 1 therapy in the U.S. Harefield Recovery Protocol (HARP trial) (unpublished data).

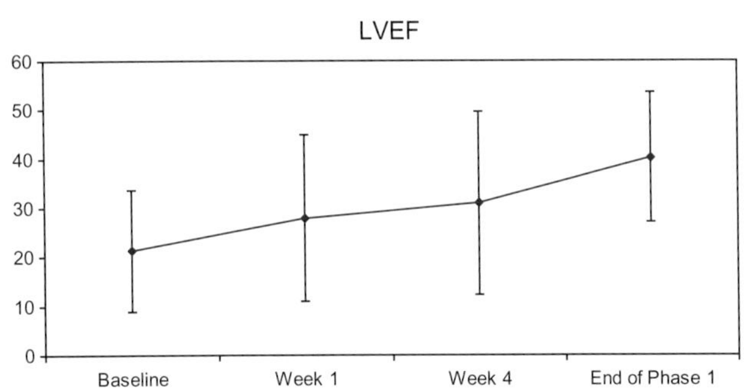

Fig. 19.17 Increase in left ventricular ejection fraction *(LVEF)* after phase 1 therapy in the U.S. Harefield Recovery Protocol (HARP trial) (unpublished data).

Remission From Stage D Heart Failure Study

As previously mentioned, the rationale for phase 2 intervention with clenbuterol remains enticing, yet its true influence remains uncertain. Indeed, in combination therapy trials, it remains unknown whether it was the optimization of the pump speed to enhance unloading, the additional high dose reverse remodeling drugs, the rigorous weaning and testing, or the clenbuterol itself that led to the much higher rate of recovery. To develop clarity around these questions, investigators renewed their focus on the phase 1 approach of aggressive reverse remodeling and optimizing pump speed combined with regular testing. The Harefield studies enrolled small groups of patients at a center dedicated to the pursuit of recovery. However, in theory, this approach could be done at any center, so the next step was to see if this approach can be successfully utilized at other centers to promote broad adoption of this strategy for recovery.

Other individual centers have taken a Harefield-like approach with regard to aggressive medical therapy and diligent testing with impressive results. The Montefiore group recently published their prospective use of three-step testing for select patients deemed as candidates for recovery. Restoration of myocardial function was assessed 4 weeks after patients reached maximally tolerated doses of HF medicines.[48] If echocardiography at rest and with diminished support ("turn-down") demonstrated an EF >40% (step 1), then they proceed to cardiopulmonary stress test (step 2) and right heart catheterization (step 3).[49] Of 34 patients, 21 subjects made it to step 1 testing, with 16 showing no evidence of improved function. Of the remaining five who "normalized" function, one elected to keep their LVAD, one had an exercise-induced increase in PCWP and not deemed an explant candidate, and three went on to explantation and are free from major HF events 3–5 years after explantation. While this study shows, much like Harefield or Berlin, that a single center can work toward LVAD-induced myocardial recovery, it remained to be seen if a uniform approach could be adopted across several institutions, a key component for a broader application.

RESTAGE-HF (Remission From Stage D Heart Failure) is a prospective, nonrandomized, multicenter study of 40 subjects with chronic advanced HF from nonischemic cardiomyopathy receiving the HeartMate II continuous-flow pump.[50] The six participating centers had previous experience in recovery and explanting LVAD patients.

The primary objective of the RESTAGE trial was to determine the proportion of subjects with sufficient improvement in ventricular function/remission from HF after undergoing a standardized LVAD plus pharmacologic recovery treatment and testing protocol to allow removal of the LVAD within an 18-month period. The secondary objectives were to determine the durability of sustained remission from HF following LVAD explantation at 12 months and up to 3 years as well as to determine the predictors of recovery.

The primary endpoint was predefined and statistically powered for the proportion of subjects treated with the standardized LVAD plus pharmacologic recovery protocol who experience LVAD removal and subsequent freedom from mechanical circulatory support or heart transplantation for 1 year post-LVAD removal to >10%, a liberal estimate of the proportion of subjects who would experience this outcome with usual clinical care. Qualifying criteria for LVAD removal were the following criteria measured at a pump speed of 6000 rpm (i.e., measured with no net flow):

1. LVEDD <60 mm, LVESD <50 mm, LVEF >45%, and
2. LVEDP or PCWP ≤15 mm Hg, and
3. Resting cardiac index >2.4 L/min/m^2
4. ±Maximal oxygen consumption with exercise (mVO_2) >16 mL/kg/min

Secondary endpoints included the proportion of evaluable subjects meeting explant criteria and subsequently explanted, the time course of reverse remodeling on an LVAD, the time course and sustainability of reverse remodeling following LVAD explantation, the predictors of recovery and device removal and changes in maximal and submaximal exercise capacity, renal and liver function, EF measured at 6000 rpm, and quality of life.

The inclusion criteria were all consecutive, eligible patients with nonischemic cardiomyopathy aged between 18 and 59 years implanted with a HeartMate II as either BTT or destination therapy with severe chronic HF (EF <25% and cardiomegaly) who were resistant to intensive medical therapy and requiring LVAD implantation. Subjects had enlarged ventricles but with a history of HF <5 years. Subjects were excluded if they had an LVEDD below normal (restrictive cardiomyopathy) or evidence of active acute myocarditis confirmed by histology. This was an attempt to focus on recovery from chronic HF, and subjects were also excluded if they had hypertrophic obstructive cardiomyopathy or sarcoidosis.

Aggressive pharmacologic management was started (consisting of the drugs used in the Harefield protocol) intended to enhance reverse remodeling. Five drugs were started early (the first initiated immediately following the weaning of inotropic support following implantation) and titrated to a MAP >60 mm Hg if the patient was asymptomatic with adequate potassium and renal function to achieve maximum doses as previously described.

In this protocol, the target dose of losartan was increased to 150 mg PO daily based on publication of the Effects of high-dose versus low-dose losartan on clinical outcomes in patients with heart failure (HEAAL) trial[51] (Table 19.2). There was a detailed protocol for their uptitration, with digoxin being started first once the patient was out of the operating room and then as soon as the patient was off inotropic support. Lisinopril was started at 2.5 mg qd. If tolerated based on renal function and symptoms, the dose was then doubled to up to a target dose of 20 mg bid. Carvedilol was started at 3.125 mg twice daily once the lisinopril had reached 7.5 mg bid and then intermittently titrated up with the lisinopril, reaching a max of 25 mg twice daily or three times daily if tolerated. Spironolactone 25 mg daily was started within the first 10 days after LVAD insertion. Losartan was added at 25 mg daily and increased by 25-mg increments to 150 mg daily as tolerated, once the patient was on lisinopril 20 mg twice daily, carvedilol 25 mg twice daily, and spironolactone at 25 mg daily. If tolerated, the carvedilol was increased to 50 mg bid.

Pump speed optimization was a protocolized priority in this trial. After implantation, prior to discharge or at the first outpatient visit after discharge, the pump speed was adjusted using echocardiographic guidance to achieve an LVEDD <6 cm or smaller (if possible) and mitral regurgitation (MR) <2 (if possible).

Recovery monitoring was standardized as summarized in Table 19.3. At 6 weeks, 4, 6, 9, and 12 months postimplantation, an echocardiographic examination at normal clinical pump speed was followed by repeat evaluations 5 and 15 minutes following speed reduction, and then again after the 6MW test at 6000 rpm. Once echocardiographic improvement was seen, cardiopulmonary exercise test was performed at 6000 rpm and a right and left heart catheterization was completed at the patient's normal speed and then with the speed at 6000 rpm for at least 15 minutes.

Following device explantation, lisinopril, spironolactone, carvedilol, digoxin, and losartan were restarted as soon as possible and uptitrated to the same target doses. The goal was to start and titrate the ACEI in priority over the beta blocker to prevent recurrent adverse reverse remodeling.

RESTAGE is ongoing, with complete enrollment of the entire 40 subject cohort.

TABLE 19.2 Target Pharmacological Therapy Used in the RESTAGE Trial

Drug Name	Maximum Dose	Frequency
Lisinopril	40 mg	Daily
Carvedilol	25 mg	Twice daily (three times if tolerated)
Spironolactone	25 mg	Daily
Digoxin	125 µg	Daily
Losartan	150 mg	Daily

RESTAGE, Remission From Stage D.

SURGERY FOR MYOCARDIAL RECOVERY

The Harefield and RESTAGE trials highlight the importance of medical therapy and routine assessments, but there are significant surgical issues that must be considered when adopting a recovery paradigm. While, to date, there are no protocolized algorithms, many recommendations can be made with regard to surgical strategies aimed towards bridging patients to recovery and pump removal.[1]

Insertion

While the variability of clinical presentation will often determine the specifics for surgical implantation, prospectively defining recovery as a goal implies the need to fix structural heart defects at the time of the initial implant. The most common scenario is related to valve disorders, and much has been written about management of concomitant valve disease with patients requiring VAD.[52–54]

Aortic valve competence is required for proper VAD function. Depending on the speed setting and level of unloading, continuous-flow LVADs result in aortic valves that are either closed or infrequently opening. This situation can provoke aortic valve commissural fusion, with subsequent development of aortic stenosis and/or aortic insufficiency (AI). Preexisting AI is known to worsen in the setting of VAD support, and it is recommended that AI be corrected at the time of VAD placement.[55,56] Some centers have taken an aggressive approach either by coapting the aortic leaflets or fully oversewing the valve.[57] Within the recovery paradigm, replacing an oversewn aortic valve at the time of LVAD explant is not desirable. Acknowledging a lack of data to support a particular approach, potential explant patients with indications for aortic valve intervention are best served with a bioprosthetic aortic valve replacement. This strategy would extend to patients who have an existing mechanical aortic valve or native valve aortic stenosis. One potential problem, however, is the tendency for bioprosthetic valves to fuse with long-term continuous-flow support.[58]

Management of tricuspid valve regurgitation (TR) is more controversial. Patients referred for VAD placement will often have biventricular dilation and subsequent development of MR and TR.[59] While TR is a marker for potential RV dysfunction, it is unclear if fixing TR at the time of VAD implantation results in improved outcomes. While TR has been associated with longer postimplantation inotropic

TABLE 19.3 Resting and Exercise Cardiac Function and Exercise Capacity Variables in Explanted Patients Compared to Those on Left Ventricular Assist Device and Heart Failure Patients

	Heart Transplant Candidates ($n = 24$)	LVAD Implanted ($n = 18$)	LVAD Explanted ($n = 16$)	Healthy Controls ($n = 97$)
Sitting rest				
Heart rate, beats/min	76.7 ± 19.7	72.6 ± 13.3	73.3 ± 6.2	65.7 ± 10.6
Stroke volume, mL	49.1 ± 12.3[a]	76.7 ± 17.0	71.1 ± 11.3	73.7 ± 18.0
Systolic BP, mm Hg	94.5 ± 17.5	95.3 ± 21.1	105.2 ± 15.8	123.3 ± 11.7[b]
Diastolic BP, mm Hg	61.4 ± 10.3	63.3 ± 17.9	70.9 ± 12.7	76.3 ± 9.1[c]
Mean arterial BP, mm Hg	74.4 ± 12.1	72.8 ± 15.6	85.5 ± 12.6	95.7 ± 8.98[c]
Cardiac output, L/min	3.53 ± 0.66[a]	5.5 ± 1.4	5.2 ± 0.8	4.87 ± 1.20
Cardiac power output, W	0.59 ± 0.16[a]	0.89 ± 0.23	0.94 ± 0.20	1.02 ± 0.22
Vascular resistance, dyn/s/cm^{-5}	1735 ± 357[a]	1143 ± 433	1351 ± 293	14,85 ± 509
Oxygen consumption, mL/min	314.4 ± 54.2	371 ± 47	407 ± 35	374 ± 43
Oxygen consumption, mL/kg/min	4.32 ± 0.92	4.74 ± 0.56	4.88 ± 0.09	3.63 ± 0.66
Peak exercise				
Heart rate, beats/min	101.9 ± 21.6[a]	142.3 ± 26.0[d]	162.8 ± 12.9	173.9 ± 16.7
Stroke volume, mL	82.9 ± 22.2	88.9 ± 16.8	90.6 ± 15.2[e]	116.9 ± 18.5[b]
Systolic BP, mm Hg	94.9 ± 16.3[a]	115.6 ± 25.0[d]	140.1 ± 21.9[e]	199.1 ± 18.4[b]
Diastolic BP, mm Hg	59.4 ± 10.1	72.0 ± 14.5	78.1 ± 12.6[e]	66.0 ± 14.3
Mean arterial BP, mm Hg	74.0 ± 11.8[a]	86.9 ± 17.9[d]	103.5 ± 18.2[e]	120.8 ± 11.0[b]
Cardiac output, L/min	8.12 ± 1.52[a]	12.4 ± 1.9[d]	14.7 ± 2.37[e]	20.3 ± 3.9[b]
Cardiac power output, W	1.31 ± 0.31[a]	2.37 ± 0.67[d]	3.45 ± 0.72[e]	5.36 ± 0.94[b]
Vascular resistance, dyn/s/cm^{-5}	758 ± 195[a]	569 ± 118	583 ± 159[e]	495 ± 116
Oxygen consumption, mL/min	916 ± 227[a]	1814 ± 422[d]	2511 ± 420[e]	3090 ± 740[b]
Oxygen consumption, mL/kg/min	12.0 ± 2.2[a]	20.5 ± 4.3[d]	29.8 ± 5.9[e]	36.4 ± 10.3
Arterial-venous oxygen difference, mL O_2/100 mL of blood	11.3 ± 2.5[a]	15.1 ± 4.1[d]	17.2 ± 2.3	18.2 ± 3.7
Respiratory exchange ratio	1.10 ± 0.15	1.13 ± 0.07	1.11 ± 0.07	1.11 ± 0.08

Values are mean ± SD.
BP, Blood pressure; *LVAD*, left ventricular assist device.
[a]$p < 0.05$ transplants vs. LVAD implanted, LVAD explanted, and controls.
[b]$p < 0.05$ controls vs. transplants, LVAD explanted, LVAD implanted.
[c]$p < 0.05$ controls vs. transplants and LVAD implanted.
[d]$p < 0.05$ LVAD implanted vs. LVAD explanted, and controls.
[e]$p < 0.05$ LVAD explanted vs. controls.
From Jakovljevic DG, Yacoub MH, Schueler S, et al. Left ventricular assist device as a bridge to recovery for patients with advanced heart failure. *J Am Coll Cardiol*. 2017;69:1924–1933.

support and length of hospital stay, tricuspid valve repair plus VAD implantation has shown similar outcomes compared to LVAD implantation alone.[59] This has led some to question whether repair is necessary. Although no firm recommendation regarding TR can be made for the potential removal patient, the general focus remains on repairing structural defects that could influence reverse remodeling, including that of the right ventricle.

Mitral regurgitation is common in patients with HF secondary to the deleterious effects of remodeling. In addition to annular dilation, ventricular enlargement displaces the papillary muscles, distorts their anatomy, and tethers chordal support of the valve.[60] One could argue that MR will improve with LVAD unloading on its own. Indeed, the decrease in LV dimensions will enhance leaflet coaptation. Unfortunately, some ventricles might not remodel sufficiently, while others may redilate after LVAD explantation.[13,61]

As such, a more aggressive approach to repair may be indicated. Mitral intervention, either with repair or replacement, at the time of LVAD will incrementally decrease pulmonary vascular resistance.[62] The Utah group and others have routinely used the transapical edge-to-edge approach to treat severe MR in LVAD patients.[63] Although traditional mitral valve repair approaches can be safely used, there is an obligate increase in operative time and dissection. The edge-to-edge technique is fairly straightforward and adds only minutes to the procedure. As a technical point, the repair is more easily performed prior to putting a rigid sewing ring on the apical defect. For example, with the HeartWare device, Utah will make the core, perform the repair, and then attach the sewing ring. The ability to expose the mitral leaflets is greatly enhanced in this manner. While the ease of the transapical repair is appealing, the approach to mitral repair is patient dependent, and there are no data to help guide its use. As another example, in a patient who has multiple factors favoring recovery, yet has a 4.8-cm mitral annulus, some would take a more traditional approach to repair with an annuloplasty ring inserted through a left atrial approach.

Explantation

Traditionally, LVAD removal is performed through a midline sternotomy with complete extirpation of the device and outflow graft. Cardiopulmonary bypass without cardiac arrest is used to repair the apical defect either primarily or with patch closure. The outflow graft is transected at the level of the aorta either with suture or vascular stapling device. However, redo-sternotomy and explantation can place a patient at risk for other morbidity that might jeopardize a recovering myocardium, including blood transfusions and direct cardiac injury. As such, most groups have adopted less invasive techniques for VAD removal. All approaches need to consider anatomic issues, including need for structural valve repair and presence of LV thrombus.

Multiple techniques have been described to facilitate VAD removal without requiring extensive surgical repair of the ventricle, thereby allowing minimally invasive approaches. These often require femoral-femoral bypass on either the beating or fibrillating heart. Even through a minithoracotomy, the apical defect can be fixed directly as with a linear aneurysmorrhaphy repair. With the more flexible sewing rings (e.g., Jarvik 2000), the closure can actually incorporate the sewing ring in this suture.

With the HeartWare LVAD, the sewing ring can be removed and repaired primarily, or a specially manufactured titanium plug (Fittkau GmbH, Berlin, Germany) can be directly inserted.[64,65] With the HeartMate II LVAD, a felt plug can be fashioned intraoperatively using a spare sewing ring. This plug is inserted into the attached sewing ring to completely fill the apical defect, thus eliminating the need for extensive ventricular repair and minimizing operative time.[66] In Utah, this felt plug was also wrapped with CorMatrix, a biologic material, with the aim of creating a more biocompatible interface. The pump can be removed and the plug inserted on the beating heart or on peripheral cardiopulmonary bypass.

While some might argue that leaving a stiff sewing ring on the apex of the heart will decrease apical involvement in contractile function, most explanted hearts will have a portion of the apex that is either akinetic or hypokinetic, even with a geometric repair. One potential advantage to leaving the sewing ring intact is if the patient were to require LVAD reimplantation. In this case, rather than exposing large portions of the apex to replace a sewing ring, the existing plug can be removed and the inflow cannula can be reinserted relatively easily.

Other minimally invasive techniques for VAD removal include leaving a portion or all of the inflow or outflow cannulas/grafts in situ. Here, separate small incisions may be utilized to avoid a midline sternotomy.[67] A subxiphoid and separate left and right anterior mini thoracotomies are used to access the VAD, the inflow cannula, and outflow graft. Cardiopulmonary bypass is established using femoral venous cannulation and cannulation of the VAD outflow graft. The inflow VAD cannula and VAD can then be removed. The outflow graft is oversewn near the bypass cannula leaving a small piece of outflow graft in situ.

Recently, even less invasive approaches for VAD removal have been described. With the HeartMate II LVAD, the inflow graft present in the articulating elbow can be exposed by mini-thoracotomy. This graft can then be clamped, divided, and oversewn. Alternatively, an endovascular stapling device has been used to transect this graft. As such, the entire inflow and outflow components of the device are left in situ.[68] Finally, some have even advocated simply dividing the driveline and leaving the entire pump in situ, ultimately allowing the pump to fully develop a contained thrombus.

Potential complications of leaving portions of the VAD grafts in situ include thromboembolic events or infections. Few data are available regarding the frequency of these complications. Residual graft infections have been described, but overall the limited available reports would suggest that infection or thromboembolic events are uncommon.[69] Outside of a few case reports, the fate of a retained LV inflow cannula, for example, is purely speculative.

Currently, the authors recommend approaching VAD removal in BTR patients using one of the described minimally invasive techniques to avoid the need for redo sternotomy and potentially avoid the need for cardiopulmonary bypass. This strategy is particularly useful for HeartMate II explants, but potentially more challenging with other durable LVADs. The exception would be the presence of significant device infection, in which case complete removal is generally recommended. The need for cardiopulmonary bypass should not dissuade attempts at LVAD explantation, as long as the patient is appropriately selected. There is much room for creativity in the surgical approaches for these patients. As our understanding and management of myocardial recovery improve, many of the surgical techniques will continue to evolve.

QUALITY OF LIFE AFTER LEFT VENTRICULAR ASSIST DEVICE EXPLANTATION

Quality of life, or "the functional effect of an illness and its consequent therapy as perceived by the patient," is also extremely important. Long-term quality of life was assessed in patients whose LVAD was explanted for myocardial recovery and compared with the quality of life of patients who received a VAD as BTT and patients who underwent direct transplantation.[70] This study comprised 72 patients—14 explanted patients (3.6 ± 1.9 years since LVAD removal), 29 BTT patients (3.3 ± 2.3 years since transplantation), and 29 directly transplanted patients (3.8 ± 0.6 years since transplantation). The total quality-of-life SF-36 score was higher in the explanted group compared with the other cohorts. In all but two of the domains of the SF-36 questionnaire, the scores were significantly better in the explanted group compared with both the BTT and the transplantation groups. Both physical and mental health dimensions were better in the explanted group compared with both the BTT and transplantation groups. This small study suggests that recovery patients who are explanted have a better quality of life than either BTT or transplant patients.

The improved quality of life in the BTR group could be related to better renal function, lack of immunosuppression-related complications, absence of rejection, less infection, and lack of coronary disease. Jakovljevic et al.[71] recently assessed the functional capacity of LVAD explanted patients (n = 16) who had received the Harefield protocol and were now an average of 3.3 ± 1.1 (range, 0.3–5.8) years after explantation, comparing it to that of patients on a continuous-flow LVAD (n = 18; 219 ± 87 days postimplantation), candidates on the heart transplant waiting list (HTx, n =24), and 97 healthy controls (Table 19.3).[71] Heart transplant and LVAD implanted patients performed a modified Bruce protocol, and LVAD explanted patients and healthy controls performed the Bruce protocol. Cardiac function was represented by peak exercise cardiac power output (CPO), and functional capacity, by peak exercise O_2 consumption. Peak exercise CPO was significantly higher in healthy controls and explanted LVAD patients compared with other patients (healthy, 5.35 ± 0.95 W; explanted, 3.45 ± 0.72 W; LVAD implanted, 2.37 ± 0.68 W; and HTx, 1.31 ± 0.31 W; P<0.05), as was peak O_2 consumption (healthy, 36.4 ± 10.3 mL/kg/min; explanted patients, 29.8 ± 5.9 mL/kg/min; implanted LVADs, 20.5 ± 4.3 mL/kg/min; and HTx 12.0 ± 2.2 mL/kg/min; P<0.05; Fig. 19.18). In the LVAD explanted group, 38% of the patients achieved peak CPO and 69% achieved peak O_2 consumption within the ranges of healthy controls. Hence, many explanted patients had cardiac and physical functional capacities within the normal range of healthy controls, and LVAD explanted patients demonstrated significantly better cardiac and functional capacities than did patients on LVAD support, providing longer-term data suggesting that the functional recovery described in their previous studies (Fig. 19.19) were sustained (Fig. 19.20).

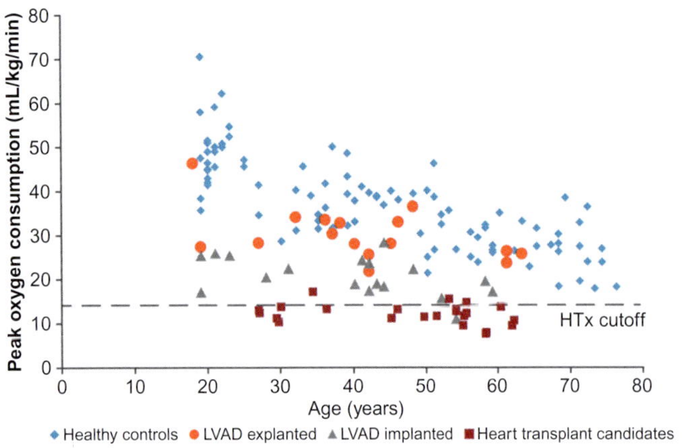

Fig. 19.18 Peak oxygen consumption in explanted left ventricular assist device *(LVAD)* patients compared to healthy controls, patients with an LVAD, and heart transplant candidates. (From Jakovljevic DG, Yacoub MH, Schueler S, et al. Left ventricular assist device as a bridge to recovery for patients with advanced heart failure. *J Am Coll Cardiol.* 2017;69:1924–1933.)

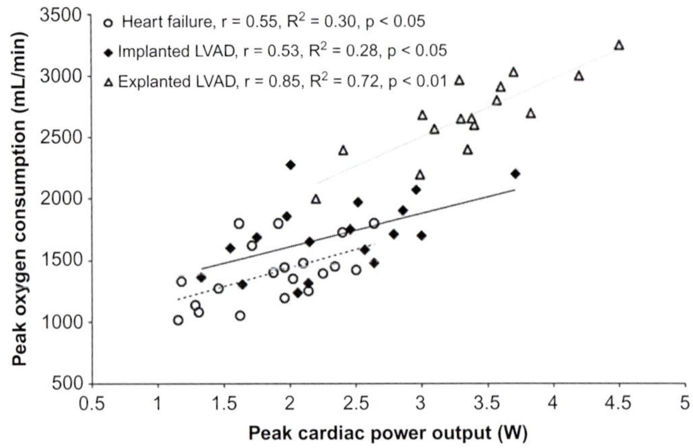

Fig. 19.19 Relationship between peak cardiac power output (reflecting pumping capacity) and peak oxygen consumption (reflecting functional capacity) in explanted patients compared to patients on left ventricular assist device *(LVAD)* support and patients with heart failure. (From Jakovljevic DG, Birks EJ, George RS, Trenell MI, Seferovic PM, Yacoub MH, Brodie DA. Relationship between peak cardiac pumping capability and selected exercise-derived prognostic indicators in patients treated with left ventricular assist devices. *Eur J Heart Fail.* 2011 Sep;13(9):992–999.)

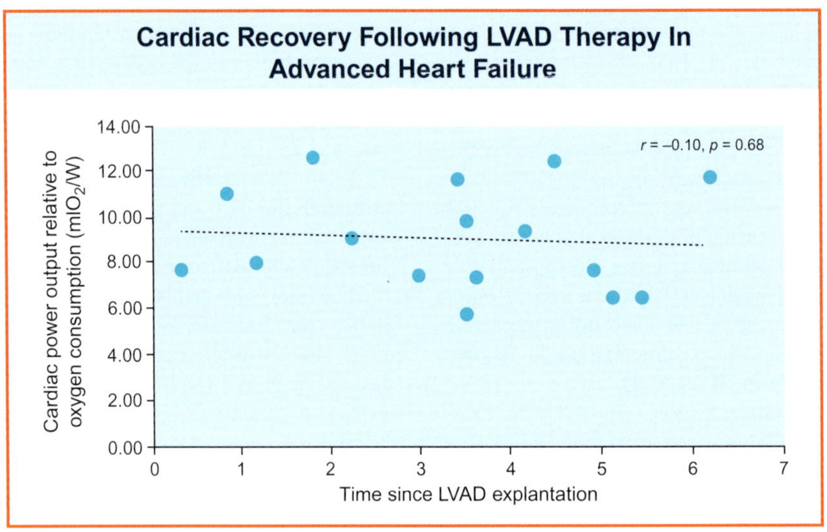

Fig. 19.20 Cardiac power output relative to oxygen consumption over time after explantation, showing sustained functional recovery. *LVAD*, Left ventricular assist device. (From Jakovljevic DG, Yacoub MH, Schueler S, et al. Left ventricular assist device as a bridge to recovery for patients with advanced heart failure. *J Am Coll Cardiol.* 2017;69:1924–1933.)

SUMMARY AND NEXT STEPS TO ENHANCE RATE OF RECOVERY

Using the Left Ventricular Assist Device as Myocardial Therapy

RESTAGE was designed to assess whether a standardized protocol of prospectively optimizing pump speed combined with an aggressive reverse remodeling pharmacological regimen together with regular testing of underlying myocardial function could lead to a high rate of significant recovery. The next steps are likely to focus on using this protocol as a "Stage 1" base that could be adopted by multiple centers.

A key piece that is missing in many LVAD-related trials is uniform utilization of the pump itself as a myocardial therapy. It is known that the pump can provide total-body therapy by restoring cardiac output and decreasing vascular congestion. Yet the way that patients are unloaded and, more importantly for the concept of recovery, how they are reloaded, remains undefined.

Intermittently decreasing the pump speed to allow increased ventricular preload, sufficient contractility to open the aortic valve, and increase myocardial work might be an alternative way to retrain the LV and cause physiologic hypertrophy in the future. Patients may benefit from defined periods of significantly reduced LVAD support, by engineered programs of reduced support. This concept has already been in place to some degree with the Jarvik ILS (Intermittent Low Speed) device (Jarvik Heart, NY). The Jarvik ILS feature significantly lowers the pump speed for 8 seconds every minute to allow the aortic valve to open and also results in intermittent reloading of the ventricle. The authors have used this technical feature to gradually reload the LV over several months to allow for reconditioning prior to explantation.[72]

The Texas Heart Institute has championed a strategy based on normalization of the cardiac cycle to guide eligibility for pump removal. Once hearts are adequately unloaded (dimensions within normal range and minimal MR), patients are serially evaluated at minimal pump speeds for normalization of aortic valve opening time. With this reconditioning approach, they have removed pumps from over 30 patients.[46,73]

Acknowledging that each patient has unique requirements for LVAD support based upon a variety of factors, an ideal recovery scenario would attempt to protocolize the reloading of the heart utilizing a stepwise approach. In a stepwise approach the "dose" of the LVAD will directly impact the loading conditions and environment for recovery. A more standardized approach becomes even more necessary when considering high-cost adjuvant drug trials. If there is no equipoise with the use of the pump in reloading, one will never know whether the true effect of recovery was from the management of the pump or the particular agent (i.e., see discussion regarding clenbuterol).

Using the Left Ventricular Assist Device as a Platform for Adjuvant Therapy

Within the context of the phase 2 approach to recovery, a variety of adjunctive agents could be used in combination with LVAD therapy. These clinical trials are difficult to design and are expensive, and the conclusions are limited by the inherent patient heterogeneity and small sample sizes. That said, the hemodynamic stability provided by the LVAD allows creative and innovative approaches.

Although several attempts at investigating the role of stem cells in LVAD patients have been abandoned by the National Heart and Lung Blood Institute (NHLBI) for administrative reasons, individual centers are injecting both autologous (ClinicalTrials.gov NCT00869024) and allogeneic mesenchymal stem cells (MSC) in LVAD patients (ClinicalTrials.gov NCT01759212). The National Institutes of Health–sponsored Cardiothoracic Surgery Network reported a 30-patient pilot trial of intramyocardial MSC injection at the time of LVAD placement. There were no safety issues, and potential efficacy signals were observed.[74] The follow-up MPC-LVAD 2 trial recently evaluated the efficacy and safety of intramyocardial injection of 150 million MPCs (compared to 25 million in the pilot trial) versus sham-control among 159 patients undergoing LVAD implantation. Although MPCs did not improve cardiac function as measured by temporary weaning from full LVAD support (the primary efficacy endpoint of the trial), a significant reduction in GI bleeding or epistaxis was observed in the MPC group, particular those with ischemic cardiomyopathies.[75] Future trials with precursor cells will focus on more functional endpoints and secondary dosing of MPCs. Importantly, adjuvant therapy studies are not limited to stem cells but also include therapies based on growth factors (e.g., SDF) and genes (e.g., *SERCA2a*).

While many deductive therapies can be envisioned, one cannot forget the unique nature of LVAD therapy that allows for inductive generation of novel therapies. The ability to obtain tissue both before (at the time of LVAD placement) and after (at the time of transplantation or explantation in a recovered patient) provides unique information, especially when combined with functional data. Indeed, a recovered patient provides a model to study the reversal of human HF with tissue and blood to reflect changes in the myocardium and circulation at the time of implantation and at the time of explantation (i.e., HF reversal) with parallel functional data. A vast amount of effort at the basic science level is examining novel pathways and molecular targets that might be years away but nevertheless fuel the excitement for this field.

Left Ventricular Assist Devices in the Future

With an aging population and a finite number of organs for transplant, it is likely that more HF patients who receive a VAD will undergo an aggressive attempt to induce recovery. The number of usable donor hearts has been declining worldwide, necessitating an alternative approach for these patients. Patients who do not respond to attempts at recovery will likely stay on the device for a prolonged period, and patients who develop VAD-related complications will undergo transplantation. Patients who can be explanted because of myocardial recovery should be—avoiding the need for immunosuppression and its associated complications and sparing the donor heart for another individual. Even if explanted patients should decompensate and require transplantation at a later stage, this approach is likely to extend their overall life span considerably. With time, our knowledge of the predictors of sustained recovery should be improved.

In summary, the ability to recover the LV, with the assistance of VADs to completely unload the heart, has been an area of interest for many years. Unfortunately, the percentage of patients who have had their LVAD removed successfully and sustained good ventricular function for a prolonged period (years) has been low—approximately 5% to 20% in most institutional series and much lower (around 1%) in the national US database INTERMACS. Success is primarily reported in younger patients with nonischemic etiology and typically acute HF from etiologies such as myocarditis, where the natural history of recovery is quite high. It is also likely to be the only select population in which most centers tend to monitor for recovery.

One of the main reasons for the low reported overall incidence of recovery in patients with chronic HF is probably the lack of belief that these patients can recover and the lack of testing for recovery. The vast majority of programs do not routinely test for or promote recovery, most do not optimize pump speed for unloading (many leave the aortic valve opening with partial unloading, sometimes wanting to retain some pulsatility), and most stop reverse remodeling HF drugs after implantation, believing them to have "failed" in that patient, only using them for hypertension control. A wider and more aggressive attempt to test for and promote recovery in a larger population of VADs is likely to result in a much higher incidence and a broader group of patients that can recover.

The answer to whether myocardial recovery is possible with periods of MCS used to be unknown because the question had never been studied in a rigorous manner, including use of protocols, employing aggressive oral HF drug therapy, and systematic weaning attempts to judge and assess for recovery. However, the more recent single-center studies followed by the RESTAGE-HF trial suggest that the recovery rate could be much higher. It is reproducible and has now been shown in several different centers and with several different devices. Durability of myocardial recovery has also been shown, and patients have a good quality of life. More widespread testing of myocardial function in patients treated with protocols that optimize unloading, combined with this aggressive pharmacological HF therapy, could dramatically increase the incidence of myocardial recovery and explantation seen.

REFERENCES

1. Selzman CH, Madden JL, Healy AH, et al. Bridge to removal: a paradigm shift for left ventricular assist device therapy. *Ann Thorac Surg*. 2015;99:360–367.
2. Birks EJ, Tansley PD, Hardy J, et al. Left ventricular assist device and drug therapy for the reversal of heart failure. *N Engl J Med*. 2006;355:1873–1884.

3. Frazier OH, Benedict CR, Radovancevic B, et al. Improved left ventricular function after chronic left ventricular unloading. *Ann Thorac Surg.* 1996;62:675–681, discussion 681–672.
4. Levin HR, Oz MC, Catanese KA, Rose EA, Burkhoff D. Transient normalization of systolic and diastolic function after support with a left ventricular assist device in a patient with dilated cardiomyopathy. *J Heart Lung Transplant.* 1996;15:840–842.
5. Levin HR, Oz MC, Chen JM, Packer M, Rose EA, Burkhoff D. Reversal of chronic ventricular dilation in patients with end-stage cardiomyopathy by prolonged mechanical unloading. *Circulation.* 1995;91:2717–2720.
6. Frazier OH, Myers TJ. Left ventricular assist system as a bridge to myocardial recovery. *Ann Thorac Surg.* 1999;68:734–741.
7. Farrar DJ, Holman WR, McBride LR, et al. Long-term follow-up of Thoratec ventricular assist device bridge-to-recovery patients successfully removed from support after recovery of ventricular function. *J Heart Lung Transplant.* 2002;21:516–521.
8. Mancini DM, Beniaminovitz A, Levin H, et al. Low incidence of myocardial recovery after left ventricular assist device implantation in patients with chronic heart failure. *Circulation.* 1998;98:2383–2389.
9. Dandel M, Weng Y, Siniawski H, Potapov E, Lehmkuhl HB, Hetzer R. Long-term results in patients with idiopathic dilated cardiomyopathy after weaning from left ventricular assist devices. *Circulation.* 2005;112:I37–I45.
10. Muller J, Wallukat G, Weng YG, et al. Weaning from mechanical cardiac support in patients with idiopathic dilated cardiomyopathy. *Circulation.* 1997;96:542–549.
11. Dandel M, Weng Y, Siniawski H, et al. Prediction of cardiac stability after weaning from left ventricular assist devices in patients with idiopathic dilated cardiomyopathy. *Circulation.* 2008;118:S94–S105.
12. Dandel M, Knosalla C, Hetzer R. Contribution of ventricular assist devices to the recovery of failing hearts: a review and the Berlin Heart Center Experience. *Eur J Heart Fail.* 2014;16:248–263.
13. Dandel M, Weng Y, Siniawski H, et al. Pre-explant stability of unloading-promoted cardiac improvement predicts outcome after weaning from ventricular assist devices. *Circulation.* 2012;126:S9–19.
14. Dandel M, Weng Y, Siniawski H, et al. Heart failure reversal by ventricular unloading in patients with chronic cardiomyopathy: criteria for weaning from ventricular assist devices. *Eur Heart J.* 2011;32:1148–1160.
15. Maybaum S, Mancini D, Xydas S, et al. Cardiac improvement during mechanical circulatory support: a prospective multicenter study of the LVAD Working Group. *Circulation.* 2007;115:2497–2505.
16. Kirklin JK, Pagani FD, Kormos RL, et al. Eighth annual INTERMACS report: special focus on framing the impact of adverse events. *J Heart Lung Transplant.* 2017;36:1080–1086.
17. Drakos SG, Kfoury AG, Stehlik J, et al. Bridge to recovery: understanding the disconnect between clinical and biological outcomes. *Circulation.* 2012;126:230–241.
18. Drakos SG, Mehra MR. Clinical myocardial recovery during long-term mechanical support in advanced heart failure: insights into moving the field forward. *J Heart Lung Transplant.* 2016;35:413–420.
19. Wever-Pinzon O, Drakos SG, McKellar SH, et al. Cardiac recovery during long-term left ventricular assist device support. *J Am Coll Cardiol.* 2016;68:1540–1553.
20. George RS, Yacoub MH, Tasca G, et al. Hemodynamic and echocardiographic responses to acute interruption of left ventricular assist device support: relevance to assessment of myocardial recovery. *J Heart Lung Transplant.* 2007;26:967–973.
21. George RS, Sabharwal NK, Webb C, et al. Echocardiographic assessment of flow across continuous-flow ventricular assist devices at low speeds. *J Heart Lung Transplant.* 2010;29:1245–1252.
22. Ferrari G, Gorczynska K, Mimmo R, et al. Mono and bi-ventricular assistance: their effect on ventricular energetics. *Int J Artif Organs.* 2001;24:380–391.
23. Kobayashi M, Izawa H, Cheng XW, et al. Dobutamine stress testing as a diagnostic tool for evaluation of myocardial contractile reserve in asymptomatic or mildly symptomatic patients with dilated cardiomyopathy. *JACC Cardiovasc Imaging* 2008;1:718–726.
24. Otasevic P, Popovic ZB, Vasiljevic JD, et al. Relation of myocardial histomorphometric features and left ventricular contractile reserve assessed by high-dose dobutamine stress echocardiography in patients with idiopathic dilated cardiomyopathy. *Eur J Heart Fail.* 2005;7:49–56.
25. Khan T, Delgado RM, Radovancevic B, et al. Dobutamine stress echocardiography predicts myocardial improvement in patients supported by left ventricular assist devices (LVADs): hemodynamic and histologic evidence of improvement before LVAD explantation. *J Heart Lung Transplant.* 2003;22:137–146.
26. Khan T, Okerberg K, Hernandez A, et al. Assessment of myocardial recovery using dobutamine stress echocardiography in LVAD patients. *J Heart Lung Transplant.* 2001;20:202–203.
27. Cotter G, Williams SG, Vered Z, Tan LB. Role of cardiac power in heart failure. *Curr Opin Cardiol.* 2003;18:215–222.
28. Fincke R, Hochman JS, Lowe AM, et al. Cardiac power is the strongest hemodynamic correlate of mortality in cardiogenic shock: a report from the SHOCK trial registry. *J Am Coll Cardiol.* 2004;44:340–348.
29. Jakovljevic DG, George RS, Donovan G, et al. Comparison of cardiac power output and exercise performance in patients with left ventricular assist devices, explanted (recovered) patients, and those with moderate to severe heart failure. *Am J Cardiol.* 2010;105:1780–1785.
30. Drakos SG, Wever-Pinzon O, Selzman CH, et al. Magnitude and time course of changes induced by continuous-flow left ventricular assist device unloading in chronic heart failure: insights into cardiac recovery. *J Am Coll Cardiol.* 2013;61:1985–1994.
31. Catino AB, Al-Sarie M, McCubrey R, et al. What is the role of standard heart failure drug therapy in the context of VAD-induced unloading of the failing human heart. *J Heart Lung Transplant.* 2015;34:S64.
32. Wever-Pinzon J, Al-Sarie M, Catino A, et al. Structural and functional myocardial improvement following continuous-flow mechanical unloading in chronic ischemic and non-ischemic cardiomyopathy. *J Heart Lung Transplant.* 2015;34. S1226-S1127.
33. Wever-Pinzon J, Selzman CH, Stoddard G, et al. Impact of ischemic heart failure etiology on cardiac recovery during mechanical unloading. *J Am Coll Cardiol.* 2016;68:1741–1752.
34. Yacoub MH. A novel strategy to maximize the efficacy of left ventricular assist devices as a bridge to recovery. *Eur Heart J.* 2001;22:534–540.
35. Klotz S, Foronjy RF, Dickstein ML, et al. Mechanical unloading during left ventricular assist device support increases left ventricular collagen cross-linking and myocardial stiffness. *Circulation.* 2005;112:364–374.
36. Klotz S, Danser AH, Foronjy RF, et al. The impact of angiotensin-converting enzyme inhibitor therapy on the extracellular collagen matrix during left ventricular assist device support in patients with end-stage heart failure. *J Am Coll Cardiol.* 2007;49:1166–1174.
37. Klotz S, Burkhoff D, Garrelds IM, Boomsma F, Danser AH. The impact of left ventricular assist device-induced left ventricular unloading on the myocardial renin-angiotensin-aldosterone system: therapeutic consequences? *Eur Heart J.* 2009;30:805–812.
38. Diakos NA, Selzman CH, Sachse FB, et al. Myocardial atrophy and chronic mechanical unloading of the failing human heart: implications for cardiac assist device-induced myocardial recovery. *J Am Coll Cardiol.* 2014;64:1602–1612.
39. Wong K, Boheler KR, Petrou M, Yacoub MH. Pharmacological modulation of pressure-overload cardiac hypertrophy: changes in ventricular function, extracellular matrix, and gene expression. *Circulation.* 1997;96:2239–2246.
40. Soppa GK, Smolenski RT, Latif N, et al. Effects of chronic administration of clenbuterol on function and metabolism of adult rat cardiac muscle. *Am J Physiol Heart Circ Physiol.* 2005;288:H1468–H1476.
41. Petrou M, Wynne DG, Boheler KR, Yacoub MH. Clenbuterol induces hypertrophy of the latissimus dorsi muscle and heart in the rat with molecular and phenotypic changes. *Circulation.* 1995;92:II483–489.
42. Wong K, Boheler KR, Bishop J, Petrou M, Yacoub MH. Clenbuterol induces cardiac hypertrophy with normal functional, morphological and molecular features. *Cardiovasc Res.* 1998;37:115–122.
43. Tevaearai HT, Eckhart AD, Walton GB, Keys JR, Wilson K, Koch WJ. Myocardial gene transfer and overexpression of beta2-adrenergic receptors potentiates the functional recovery of unloaded failing hearts. *Circulation.* 2002;106:124–129.

44. Birks EJ, George RS, Hedger M, et al. Reversal of severe heart failure with a continuous-flow left ventricular assist device and pharmacological therapy: a prospective study. *Circulation*. 2011;123:381–390.
45. Haj-Yahia S, Birks EJ, Rogers P, et al. Midterm experience with the Jarvik 2000 axial flow left ventricular assist device. *J Thorac Cardiovasc Surg*. 2007;134:199–203.
46. George RS, Khaghani C, Bowles CT, Khaghani A, Birks EJ. Sustained myocardial recovery 5 years after in situ disconnection of a Jarvik 2000 device. *J Heart Lung Transplant*. 2010;29:587–588.
47. Aaronson KD, Pagani FD, Maybaum SW, et al. Combination therapy with pulsatile left ventricular assst device, heart failure medication and clenbuterol in chronic heart failure: results from HARPS. *J Heart Lung Transplant*. 2011;30:S8–S9.
48. Formica P, Murthy S, Edwards P, Goldstein D, Maybaum S. A structured 3-step approach to evaluate cardiac recovery with continuous flow circulatory support. *J Heart Lung Transplant*. 2010;29:1440–1442.
49. Patel SR, Saeed O, Murthy S, et al. Combining neurohormonal blockade with continuous-flow left ventricular assist device support for myocardial recovery: a single-arm prospective study. *J Heart Lung Transplant*. 2013;32:305–312.
50. Birks EJ, Drakos SG, Selzman CH, et al. Remission from stage D heart failure (RESTAGE-HF): early results from a prospective multi-center study of myocardial recovery. *J Heart Lung Transplant*. 2015;34:S40–S41.
51. Konstam MA, Neaton JD, Dickstein K, et al. Effects of high-dose versus low-dose losartan on clinical outcomes in patients with heart failure (HEAAL study): a randomised, double-blind trial. *Lancet*. 2009;374:1840–1848.
52. John R, Naka Y, Park SJ, et al. Impact of concurrent surgical valve procedures in patients receiving continuous-flow devices. *J Thorac Cardiovasc Surg*. 2014;147:581–589, discussion 589.
53. Rao V, Slater JP, Edwards NM, Naka Y, Oz MC. Surgical management of valvular disease in patients requiring left ventricular assist device support. *Ann Thorac Surg*. 2001;71:1448–1453.
54. Ozturk P, Engin C, Ayik F, et al. Valvular procedures during ventricular assist device implantation. *Transplant Proc*. 2012;44:1732–1734.
55. Atkins BZ, Hashmi ZA, Ganapathi AM, et al. Surgical correction of aortic valve insufficiency after left ventricular assist device implantation. *J Thorac Cardiovasc Surg*. 2013;146:1247–1252.
56. Rajagopal K, Daneshmand MA, Patel CB, et al. Natural history and clinical effect of aortic valve regurgitation after left ventricular assist device implantation. *J Thorac Cardiovasc Surg*. 2013;145:1373–1379.
57. McKellar SH, Deo S, Daly RC, et al. Durability of central aortic valve closure in patients with continuous flow left ventricular assist devices. *J Thorac Cardiovasc Surg*. 2014;147:344–348.
58. Bonios MJ, Selzman CH, Gilbert EM, et al. Exertional angina due to fused aortic bioprosthesis during left ventricular assist device support: two cases and review of the literature. *ASAIO J*. 2017;63:e6–e9.
59. Piacentino V 3rd, Williams ML, Depp T, et al. Impact of tricuspid valve regurgitation in patients treated with implantable left ventricular assist devices. *Ann Thorac Surg*. 2011;91:1342–1346, discussion 1346–1347.
60. Selzman CH, Bhati RS, Sheridan BC, Stansfield WE, Mill MR. Surgical therapy for heart failure. *J Am Coll Surg*. 2006;203:226–239, quiz A259–260.
61. Kitada S, Kato TS, Thomas SS, et al. Pre-operative echocardiographic features associated with persistent mitral regurgitation after left ventricular assist device implantation. *J Heart Lung Transplant*. 2013;32:897–904.
62. Taghavi S, Hamad E, Wilson L, et al. Mitral valve repair at the time of continuous-flow left ventricular assist device implantation confers meaningful decrement in pulmonary vascular resistance. *ASAIO J*. 2013;59:469–473.
63. Russo MJ, Merlo A, Johnson EM, et al. Transapical approach for mitral valve repair during insertion of a left ventricular assist device. *ScientificWorldJournal*. 2013;2013:925310.
64. Sajjad M, Butt T, Oezalp F, et al. An alternative approach to explantation and exchange of the HeartWare left ventricular assist device. *Eur J Cardiothorac Surg*. 2013;43:1247–1250.
65. Schweiger M, Potapov E, Vierecke J, Stepanenko A, Hetzer R, Krabatsch T. Expeditious and less traumatic explantation of a heartware LVAD after myocardial recovery. *ASAIO J*. 2012;58:542–544.
66. Cohn WE, Gregoric ID, Radovancevic B, Frazier OH. A felt plug simplifies left ventricular assist device removal after successful bridge to recovery. *J Heart Lung Transplant*. 2007;26:1209–1211.
67. Haj-Yahia S, Birks EJ, Dreyfus G, Khaghani A. Limited surgical approach for explanting the HeartMate II left ventricular assist device after myocardial recovery. *J Thorac Cardiovasc Surg*. 2008;135:453–454.
68. Gonzalez-Stawinski GV, Mountis MM, Cohn WE, Frazier OH. Inflow graft interruption as a simple method for left ventricular assist device removal after successful bridge to recovery. *J Card Surg*. 2012;27:397–399.
69. Cohn WE, Fikfak V, Gregoric ID, Frazier OH. Retention of left ventricular assist device outflow grafts after transplantation. *J Heart Lung Transplant*. 2008;27:865–868.
70. George RS, Yacoub MH, Bowles CT, et al. Quality of life after removal of left ventricular assist device for myocardial recovery. *J Heart Lung Transplant*. 2008;27:165–172.
71. Jakovljevic DG, Yacoub MH, Schueler S, et al. Left ventricular assist device as a bridge to recovery for patients with advanced heart failure. *J Am Coll Cardiol*. 2017;69:1924–1933.
72. Healy AH, Koliopoulou A, Drakos SG, McKellar SH, Stehlik J, Selzman CH. Patient-controlled conditioning for left ventricular assist device-induced myocardial recovery. *Ann Thorac Surg*. 2015;99:1794–1796.
73. Frazier OH, Baldwin AC, Demirozu ZT, et al. Ventricular reconditioning and pump explantation in patients supported by continuous-flow left ventricular assist devices. *J Heart Lung Transplant*. 2015;34:766–772.
74. Ascheim DD, Gelijns AC, Goldstein D, et al. Mesenchymal precursor cells as adjunctive therapy in recipients of contemporary left ventricular assist devices. *Circulation*. 2014;129:2287–2296.
75. Yau TM, Pagani FD, Mancini DM, et al. Cardiothoracic Surgical Trials Network. Intramyocardial injection of mesenchymal precursor cells and successful temporary weaning from left ventricular assist device support in patients with advanced heart failure: a randomized clinical trial. *JAMA*. 2019;321:1176–1186.

20

The Critical Role of MCS Registries

Garrick C. Stewart, Lynne Warner Stevenson, James K. Kirklin

KEY POINTS

Origins of INTERMACS/PediMACS
INTERMACS Patient Profiles
Evolving Intent of Durable MCS Placement
Overall Outcomes
Adverse Events
Registry Comparison to Alternative Therapies
Impact of Registry Data on Clinical Use of VADs
Globalization of MCS Registries

ORIGINS OF INTERMACS/PEDIMACS

In The Artificial Heart: Prototypes, Policies, and Patients: Institute of Medicine Report from 1991, the committee opined that "maintaining a registry of mechanical circulatory support (MCS) recipients should be considered a routine aspect of this care."[1] With the approval of the HeartMate XVE (Thoratec, Pleasanton, CA) for reimbursement as long-term "destination therapy" (DT) by the Center for Medicare and Medicaid Services (CMS) in 2003, the stage was set for lifelong mechanical circulatory support uncoupled from cardiac transplantation. Subsequently, under the vision of Dr. John Watson and others at the National Heart, Lung, and Blood Institute (NHLBI), a Request for Proposals was assembled to create a national database for patients receiving this longer-term therapy. In June 2005, the Contract was awarded to the University of Alabama at Birmingham, with Dr. James Kirklin as principal investigator (PI) and Drs. David Naftel, Robert Kormos, and Lynne W. Stevenson as co-PIs. In 2011, under the contract renewal, Dr. Frank Pagani was added as a co-PI.

The Interagency Registry for Mechanically Assisted Circulatory Support (INTERMACS) was conceived as a unique joint effort between the NHLBI, CMS, the Food and Drug Administration, clinicians, scientists, and industry, thereby including the major stakeholders in this expensive, life-sustaining therapy. Over the next decade, INTERMACS investigators chronicled, analyzed, and facilitated the transition from bulky, flawed pulsatile technology to more durable revolutionary continuous-flow (CF) pumps (Table 20.1).[2,3] INTERMACS became a platform for progress—their investigators generating more than 80 publications, four NHLBI grants, and several grants from the American Heart Association. By the end of 2017, over 20,000 patients from more than 150 participating institutions had been entered into the database. As part of a long-term sustainability plan, with the conclusion of the NHLBI contract, ownership of INTERMACS transitioned to the Society of Thoracic Surgeons on January 1, 2018.

As part of the first NHLBI contract, INTERMACS was charged with creating a separate database within the INTERMACS platform that would focus on pediatric MCS. A separate database was created with variables and fields specific to the practice and clinical science of devices (both temporary and durable) for the infant, child, and teenager.[4] Data collection commenced on September 19, 2012. By the end of 2017, over 500 patients on support from 46 pediatric centers had been entered into the Pediatric Interagency Registry for Mechanical Circulatory Support (PediMACS) database.

INTERMACS PATIENT PROFILES

To track the national experience with ventricular assist devices, it became increasingly important to characterize clinical profiles at the time of implantation. The modern evolution of classifications for severity of disease is strongly impelled by the therapeutic options. When transplantation was the only approved therapy, the persistence of New York Heart Association (NYHA) Class IV symptoms at rest or minimal exertion was adequate to define Stage D, refractory heart failure (HF). For those patients deteriorating while awaiting transplantation, invasive hemodynamic parameters were used to guide therapy with short-term circulatory support such as intraaortic balloon counterpulsation, although benefit was difficult to establish in the absence of true control groups. As the benefits of durable devices extended into prolonged support outside of the hospital, they began to be considered for prevention as well as treatment of terminal hemodynamic decompensation leading to secondary organ dysfunction. When they were being used only as bridges to transplantation, the duration of support and device complications was relatively short for most patients.

Once the left ventricular assist device (LVAD) was approved for DT after the Randomized Evaluation of Mechanical Assistance for the Treatment of Congestive Heart Failure (REMATCH) trial, it became increasingly important to track the longer-term outcomes.[5] As major purposes of the registry included the refinement of patient and device selection and identification of best practices, it was considered essential to distinguish patients with various levels of compromise to standardize comparison of outcomes for different devices, different patients, and different implanting centers. Definition of NYHA Class IV was no longer adequate to distinguish these indications, and other states were informally proposed, such as "Class IV-B" and "Class V."

TABLE 20.1 Goals of the INTERMACS

- Facilitate refinement of patient selection to maximize outcomes with current and new device options
- Identify predictors of good outcomes as well as risk factors for adverse events after device implantation
- Develop consensus "best practice" guideline to improve clinical management by reducing short- and long-term complications of mechanical circulatory support device therapy
- Utilize registry information to guide improvements in technology, particularly as next-generation devices evolve
- Guide clinical testing and approval of new devices

INTERMACS, Interagency Registry for Mechanically Assisted Circulatory Support.

INTERMACS Profile definitions

Just prior to the inception of the INTERMACS, a consensus was reached regarding clinical descriptions of the severity of HF decompensation (Table 20.2).[6] The colloquial descriptor of "crash and burn" for Profile 1 described the patient on maximal inotropic support in whom survival was defined in hours. Profile 3 was defined as "stable on inotropes," which could be either in or out of the hospital, recognizing regional variation in availability of inotropic infusions at home. "Resting symptoms" daily despite high doses of diuretic therapy without any intravenous medications defined Profile 4, which are essentially chronic NYHA Class IV symptoms. Otherwise, the use of NYHA symptoms is problematic, as it depends on the degree of desired activities. The designations of "homebound" but comfortable at rest defined Profile 5 and "walking wounded" with limited

TABLE 20.2 INTERMACS Patient Profiles

INTERMACS Profile Description	Short-Hand	Timeframe for Intervention
Profile 1: Cardiogenic Shock Patients with life-threatening hypotension despite rapidly escalating inotropic support, critical organ hypoperfusion, often confirmed by worsening acidosis and/or lactate levels	"Crash and burn"	Definitive intervention needed within hours
Profile 2: Progressive Decline Patient with declining function despite intravenous inotropic support may be manifest by worsening renal function, nutritional depletion, inability to restore volume balance. Also describes declining status in patients unable to tolerate inotropic therapy.	"Sliding on inotropes"	Definitive intervention need within few days
Profile 3: Stable but Inotrope Dependent Patient with stable blood pressure, organ function, nutrition, and symptoms on continuous intravenous inotropic support (or a temporary circulatory support device or both) but demonstrating repeated failure to wean from support due to recurrent symptomatic hypotension or renal dysfunction.	"Dependent stability"	Definitive intervention elective over a period of weeks to few months
Profile 4: Resting Symptoms Patient can be stabilized close to normal volume status but experiences daily symptoms of congestion at rest of during ADLs. Doses of diuretics generally fluctuate at very high levels. More intensive management and surveillance strategies should be considered, which may in some cases reveal poor compliance that would compromise outcomes with any therapy. Some patients may shuttle between 4 and 5.	"Resting symptoms"	Definitive intervention elective over a period of weeks to few months
Profile 5: Exertion Intolerant Comfortable at rest and with ADL but unable to engage in any other activity, living predominantly within the house. Patients are comfortable at rest without congestive symptoms but may have underlying refractory elevated volume status, often with renal dysfunction. If underlying nutritional status and organ function are marginal, patient may be at more risk than Profile 4 and require definitive intervention.	"Exertion limited"	Variable urgency, depends on maintenance of nutrition, organ function, and activity
Profile 6: Exertion Limited Patient without evidence of fluid overload is comfortable at rest and with ADLs and minor activities outside the home but fatigues after the first few minutes of any meaningful activity. Attribution to cardiac limitation requires careful measurement of peak oxygen consumption, in some cases with hemodynamic monitoring to confirm severity of cardiac impairment.	"Walking wounded"	Variable, depends upon maintenance of nutrition, organ function and activity level
Profile 7: Advanced NYHA III A placeholder for more precise specification in the future, this level includes patients who are without current or recent episodes of unstable fluid balance, living comfortably with meaningful activity limited to mild physical exertion.	"Advanced NYHA III"	Transplantation of circulatory support may not currently be indicated

Modifiers for profiles: TCS—Temporary Circulatory Support, can modify only patients in hospital in Profiles 1–3. A—Arrhythmia, can modify any profile. Applies to recurrent ventricular tachyarrhythmias that have recently contributed substantially to clinical compromise. This includes frequent implantable cardioverter defibrillator shock or requirement for external defibrillator, usually more than twice weekly. FF—Frequent Flyer, can modify only outpatients, designating a patient requiring frequent emergency visits or hospitalization for diuretics, ultrafiltration, or temporary intravenous vasoactive therapy. A frequent flyer could be Profile 3 if at home and would rarely be Profile 7.

ADLs, Activities of daily living; *INTERMACS*, Interagency Registry for Mechanically Assisted Circulatory Support; *NYHA*, New York Heart Association.

activity outside the home defined Profiles 6 and 7. The least compromise was in Profile 7, which was added as a placeholder for patients comfortable with some limitation, without frequent exacerbations. At the time, this profile was not specified further, considering it to be outside the realm of imminent indications for mechanical circulatory support, but within the scope of potential candidates when the outcomes with devices have improved to offer a favorable benefit/risk option for patients who would likely be considered too well for transplantation. Minor amendments were made early after implementation to add the modifiers of arrhythmias contributing to decompensation (A—Arrhythmia) and frequent flyer for patients with recurrent decompensation from a more stable baseline (F—Frequent Flyer), which have been variably used. Later modification included the addition of TCS (Temporary Circulatory Support) to describe the patient whose clinical profile was assessed while on temporary circulatory support.

Relationship of INTERMACS Profiles to Outcomes

The first year's report of INTERMACS demonstrated the surprising finding that a substantial proportion of devices were being implanted in patients with Profile 1. In view of the obvious high risk from preoperative hypoperfusion and organ system compromise, it had been assumed that not many patients would have gone through a major surgical procedure from the "crash and burn" status, which instead represented 44% of all patients included in the first INTERMACS report (Table 20.3). Outcomes were significantly worse, with over 50% mortality at 1 year, compared with 35% for patients in Profile 2.[3] The best outcomes were in those patients who were stable on intravenous inotropic therapy at the time of device implantation (Fig. 20.1). One of the other notable features of the INTERMACS Profile 1 patients was the relatively higher rate of need for right ventricular support. This has particular relevance when considering whether Profile 1 patients are candidates for lifelong DT, for which the devices are approved for left ventricular support.

Over the following 10 years, the proportion of INTERMACS Profile 1 patients declined, with a corresponding increase in the proportion of Profile 3 patients. Although the indication for durable devices includes Class IV symptoms with peak oxygen consumption <12–14 mL/kg/min, this remains a small proportion of patients undergoing device therapy as of 2018. Although designed to track the outcomes for patients undergoing implantation of durable mechanical support, the INTERMACS profiles have provided useful calibration for other decisions. This was particularly important for patients undergoing urgent heart transplantation in Spain. Patients transplanted from Profile 1 had over 40% in-hospital mortality, which was more than 2-fold higher than from Profile 2 and over 4-fold higher for Profile 1 compared to Profile 3 or 4.[7] The excess mortality was attributed most often to primary graft failure and renal failure after transplantation. Comparison to contemporary outcomes with CF devices suggests that MCS offers better early outcomes than transplantation from a Profile 1 status. The INTERMACS profiles have provided further discrimination for outcomes in patients with ambulatory advanced HF followed in programs at centers that also have active MCS programs (Fig. 20.2).[8]

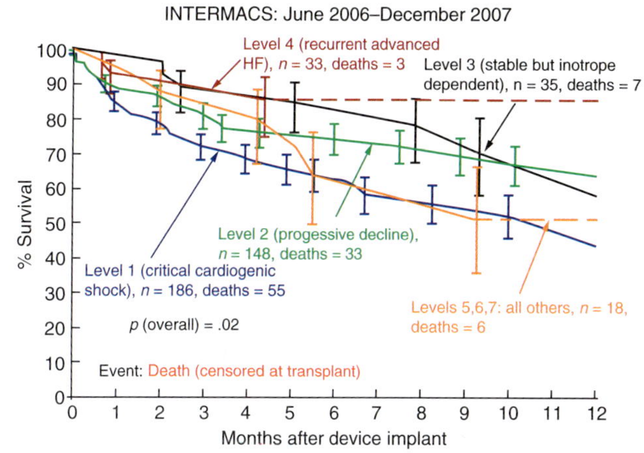

Fig. 20.1 Actuarial survival of patients implanted between June 2006 and December 2007 stratified by INTERMACS level at time of implant. The bars indicate ± 1 standard error. *HF*, Heart failure; *INTERMACS*, Interagency Registry for Mechanically Assisted Circulatory Support. (From Kirklin JK, Naftel DC, Stevenson LW, et al. INTERMACS database for durable devices for circulatory support: first annual report. *J Heart Lung Transplant* 2008;27:1065–1072.)

TABLE 20.3 Evolving INTERMACS Patient Profiles Across Implant Eras

Intermacs

CFLVAD IMPLANTS: APRIL 2008–DECEMBER 2017 FOLLOW-UP THROUGH JUNE 2018

	IMPLANT DATE ERA							
	2008–2010		2011–2014		2015–2017		TOTAL	
Patient Profile at Time of Implantation	*n*	Col %	*n*	Col %	*n*	Col %	*n*	Col %
1. Critical cardiogenic shock	394	15%	1154	14%	1104	15%	2652	14%
2. Progressive decline	1134	43%	3102	36%	2525	35%	6761	37%
3. Stable but inotrope dependent	627	23%	2706	32%	2742	38%	6075	33%
4. Resting symptoms	357	13%	1241	14%	800	11%	2398	13%
5. Exertion intolerant	77	3%	245	3%	94	1%	416	2%
6. Exertion limited	44	2%	86	<1%	29	<1%	159	<1%
7. Advanced NYHA Class 3	27	1%	37	<1%	9	<1%	73	<1%
Totals	2660	100%	8571	100%	7303	100%	18,534	100%

CFLVAD, Continuous-flow left ventricular assist device; *NYHA*, New York Heart Association.

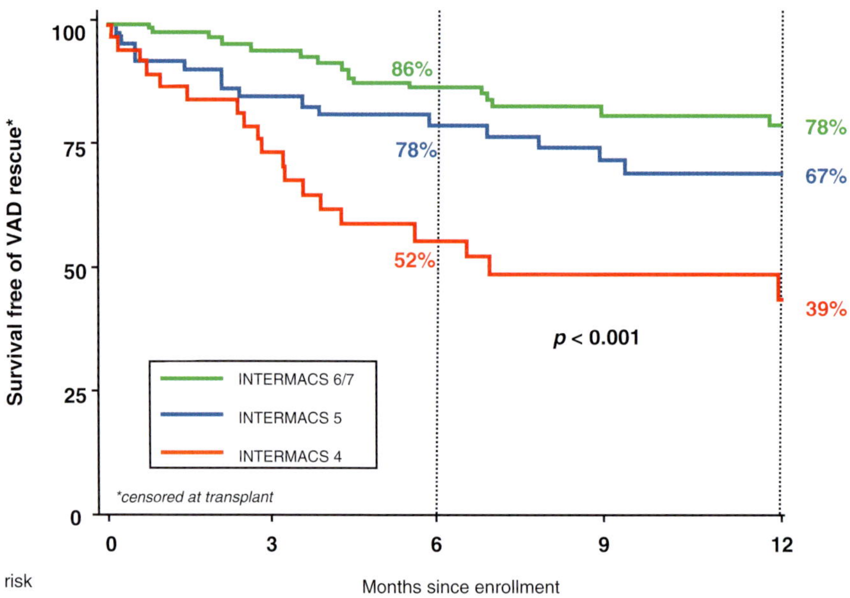

No. at risk			
INTERMACS 6/7	76	60	44
INTERMACS 5	53	40	31
INTERMACS 4	37	14	11

Fig. 20.2 Survival free of ventricular assist device *(VAD)* rescue according to Interagency Registry for Mechanically Assisted Circulatory Support *(INTERMACS)* profile among medically managed patients enrolled in the Medical Arm of Mechanically Assisted Circulatory Support screening pilot study. Estimated survival or VAD was modeled through 1 year using the Kaplan-Meier method with censoring at transplantation. Survival free of VAD rescue was significantly different according to INTERMACS profile ($P < 0.001$). (From Stewart GC, Kittleson MM, Patel PC, et al. INTERMACS (Interagency Registry for Mechanically Assisted Circulatory Support) profiling identifies ambulatory patients at high risk on medical therapy after hospitalizations for heart failure. *Circ Heart Fail.* 2016;9.)

EVOLVING INTENT OF DURABLE MCS PLACEMENT

First- and second-generation MCS devices were first approved as a bridge to transplantation (BTT) in part because transplant listed patients had a "bail-out option" in the event of device malfunction. Strategic designation for implant defined the Food and Drug Administration (FDA) indication for device therapy as well as CMS reimbursement. Additional device strategies used for FDA approval include lifelong DT and bridge to recovery. However, even in the early days of MCS, there was widespread recognition that many patients who were not actively listed for transplant at the time of implantation could potentially become transplant candidates following MCS due to improved end-organ function, reversal of pulmonary hypertension, and resolution of noncardiac comorbidities. Such patients have been referred to as bridge to decision (BTD), a designation that reflects the dynamic trajectory of real-world patients who require MCS and one that currently comprises a quarter of current registered implants in INTERMACS.

As the field has evolved from pulsatile to CF-LVADs, there has been a shift in implant strategy from BTT to BTD and, more recently, to DT or lifelong MCS. The use of LVADs as permanent replacement therapy in patients not listed for transplant increased over 10-fold since the approval of a CF device in early 2010 DT, a trend documented by INTERMACS.[9] Since 2011, DT has been the most common intent or strategy at the time of ventricular assist device (VAD) implantation. DT recipients represented 51% of all registered device implants by 2016, including over 70% of axial flow LVADs (Fig. 20.3).[10] Given ongoing donor organ scarcity and improving LVAD outcomes, recipients of LVAD therapy who are not transplant candidates at implantation are often being prepared for lifetime mechanical support.

Patients receiving LVAD for DT are older and have an accumulated burden of comorbid medication conditions such as chronic lung or kidney disease that would otherwise render them ineligible for transplant (Table 20.4). Patients receiving an implant strategy of DT have worse survival than BTT patients do, with 2-year survival of 69% for DT and 80% for BTT in CF MCS recipients (Fig. 20.4).[11] The Kaplan-Meier 5-year survival estimated for DT recipients of secondary generation MCS devices is 41%. In adjusted analyses of mortality after LVAD, DT recipients consistently demonstrate a 20% increased late hazard of death comparing to recipients of a bridging device.[11] The differences in outcomes between the sicker DT recipients and BTT patients are anticipated, but perhaps less than might be expected, due to the older age and higher burden of comorbidities. DT LVAD therapy has become a widely used, effective alternative to inotropic or palliative HF therapies and has uncoupled MCS use from donor organ supply.

Even as the transition of short-term support (BTT) to longer-term support (DT) was documented by INTERMACS, there was ongoing debate about whether the field of MCS should move beyond the artificial preimplant strategic distinctions contingent on transplant listing that were used to define reimbursement toward an MCS indication. From a regulatory and reimbursement standpoint, patients have been required to have their intended MCS strategy declared as either BTT or DT, yet INTERMACS has shown that nearly a quarter of current implants are instead the BTD when decision could not yet be

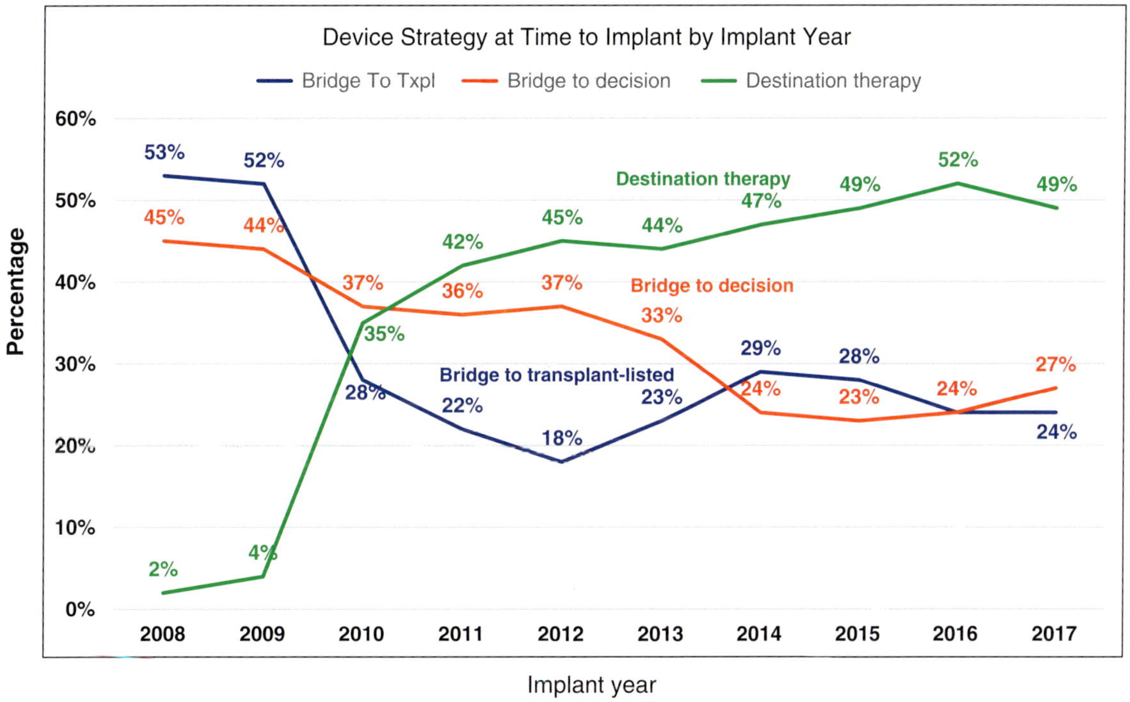

Fig. 20.3 Change in device indication over time in Society for Thoracic Surgery (STS) Intermacs. Frequency of patients implanted for destination therapy *(green)*, bridge to transplantation *(blue)*, and bridge to decision *(red)* between 2008 and 2017 are shown. *Txpl*, transplant. (From Kormos RL, Cowger J, Pagani FD, et al. The Society of Thoracic Surgeons—Intermacs database annual report: evolving indications, outcomes and scientific partnerships. *Ann Thorac Surg.* 2019.)

made regarding transplant. Although many BTD patients may eventually be listed for transplant, some never become eligible or develop complications on MCS that subsequently make them permanently ineligible for transplantation, effectively changing their strategy to long-term support. Analysis of INTERMACS data documented that comorbidities and social risks were more common as the perceived likelihood of transplant decreased. Patients who received an LVAD and were listed at implant (BTT) had superior survival compared to those designated as BTC or DT.[12] Even among those who were formally listed as BTT for transplant at the time of implantation, nearly 30% were still on LVAD support at 2 years. Furthermore, the strategic intent for a given patient continues to evolve over time. At 1 year, 15% of DT recipients had become potentially eligible for transplant. At 2 years, among BTT recipients still on support, 44% were no longer listed for transplant.[12] Regardless of initial implant strategy, patients often have a long duration of support and strategies change over time, challenging the regulatory categorization of LVAD recipient as either BTT or DT. There is significant regional variation in the duration of support and resultant change in eligibility, with the most consistent progression from LVAD to transplant being seen in regions with shortest waiting time for donor hearts. The Multicenter Study of MagLev Technology in Patients Undergoing Mechanical Circulatory Support Therapy with HeartMate 3 (MOMENTUM 3) trial of the third-generation magnetically levitated HeartMate 3 device removed this artificial strategic designation, an important constraint on previous trial designs.[13] Even after the device was proven to be safe and effective, when the manufacturer sought approval for short- and long-term support from a single trial with unified entry criteria without regard to transplant eligibility, the BTT/DT distinction has thus far remained necessary for regulatory and reimbursement structures.

OVERALL OUTCOMES

Survival

The INTERMACS has enrolled over 25,000 patients and counting, with 74% of devices CF-LVADs.[10] It is important to recognize that these outcomes include only those LVADs already approved and reimbursed in clinical use. Among registered CF-LVAD recipients, median duration of support was 20 months, representing over 31,500 patient-years of follow-up. In 2017, there was an equal split between axial flow (49%) and CF (51%) pumps registered.[10] One-year overall survival for isolated CF LVAD was 83% and 5-year survival was 46% in the most recent registry update using data through the end of 2017 (Fig. 20.5). One-year survivals for centrifugal and axial flow devices were 85% and 84%, respectively.[10] Among CF-LVAD implants listed for transplant (BTT), by 1 year, 53% were alive on the device, 34% had undergone transplantation, and 12% had died.[11] In the most recent era of pump implants from 2012 to 2017, most patients were implanted in Profiles 2–3 (Table 20.3).[10] Patients who require a right ventricular assist device (RVAD) for concomitant support (biventricular assist devices, or BiVADs) consistently demonstrate markedly reduced survival compared to isolated CF-LVAD recipients, with 1- and 5-year survival of 58% and 28%, respectively.[10]

The risk of death following MCS appears to track in three distinct phases: an early perioperative risk up to 3 months, a constant phase of risk, then a late risk phase. Characteristics associated with an increased early hazard of mortality included increasing recipient age, critical cardiogenic shock at time of LVAD implantation (Profile 1), evidence of right ventricular dysfunction (higher right atrial pressure, elevated serum bilirubin), renal dysfunction (dialysis within 48 hours of LVAD implantation), and previous or current need for a concomitant cardiac surgical procedure. History of medication noncompliance, older age,

TABLE 20.4 Device Recipient Comorbidities According to Implant Strategy

Intermacs

	CFLVAD IMPLANTS: APRIL 2008–DECEMBER 2017 FOLLOW-UP THROUGH JUNE 2018		
	OVERALL CFLVAD, *N* = 18,539		
Comorbidities Contraindications to Transplant	**Bridge to Decision (*n* = 5508)**	**Destination Therapy (*n* = 8033)**	**Bridge to Transplant Listed–Concerns (*n* = 4881)**
Advanced age	161 (2.9%)	2415 (30.1%)	39 (<1%)
Chronic renal disease	376 (6.8%)	1153 (14.4%)	621 (12.7%)
Currently smoking	386 (7.0%)	504 (6.3%)	28 (<1%)
Frailty	261 (4.7%)	490 (6.1%)	89 (1.8%)
Frequent ICD shocks	20 (<1%)	49 (<1%)	187 (3.8%)
History of alcohol abuse	198 (3.6%)	289 (3.6%)	184 (3.8%)
History of atrial arrhythmia	34 (<1%)	128 (1.6%)	762 (15.6%)
History of bone marrow TX	0 (0%)	3 (<1%)	3 (<1%)
History of drug use	260 (4.7%)	320 (4.0%)	174 (3.6%)
History of smoking	320 (5.8%)	610 (7.6%)	874 (17.9%)
History of solid organ cancer	107 (1.9%)	443 (5.5%)	89 (1.8%)
High BMI	774 (14.1%)	1223 (15.2%)	228 (4.7%)
Limited social support	255 (4.6%)	355 (4.4%)	59 (1.2%)
Other comorbidity	376 (6.8%)	669 (8.3%)	231 (4.7%)
Peripheral vascular disease	69 (1.3%)	330 (4.1%)	82 (1.7%)
Pulmonary disease	136 (2.5%)	460 (5.8%)	230 (4.7%)
Pulmonary hypertension	576 (10.5%)	1157 (14.4%)	593 (12.2%)
Repeated noncompliance	191 (3.5%)	282 (3.5%)	27 (<1%)
Severe diabetes	171 (3.1%)	513 (6.4%)	206 (4.2%)

Comorbidities that are contraindications to transplantation for bridge-to-decision patients and destination therapy patients are shown. Comorbidities are collected on the preimplantation form. Comorbidity data collection has evolved over the life of INTERMACS. This specific list of questions became available on the web-based data entry as of May 2, 2012 (version 3.0). So for this table, only primary continuous-flow implants from May 2, 2012, through December 31, 2017, have been included. Also, multiple comorbidities may be selected for a patient. The last column entitled "Bridge to Transplant Listed" will reflect the "concern" that was entered by the site.

BMI, Body mass index; *CFLVAD*, continuous-flow left ventricular assist device; *ICD*, implantable cardioverter defibrillator; *TX*, transplant.

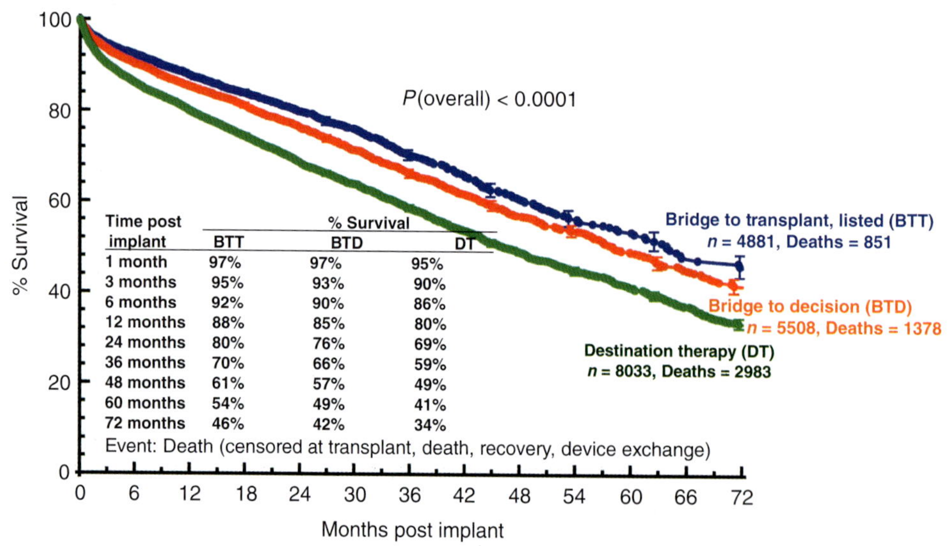

Fig. 20.4 Kaplan-Meier survival of continuous-flow left ventricular assist device recipients stratified by intention to treat at the time of implantation. (From Kirklin JK, Pagani FD, Kormos RL, et al. Eighth annual INTERMACS report: special focus on framing the impact of adverse events. *J Heart Lung Transplant* 2017;36:1080–1086.)

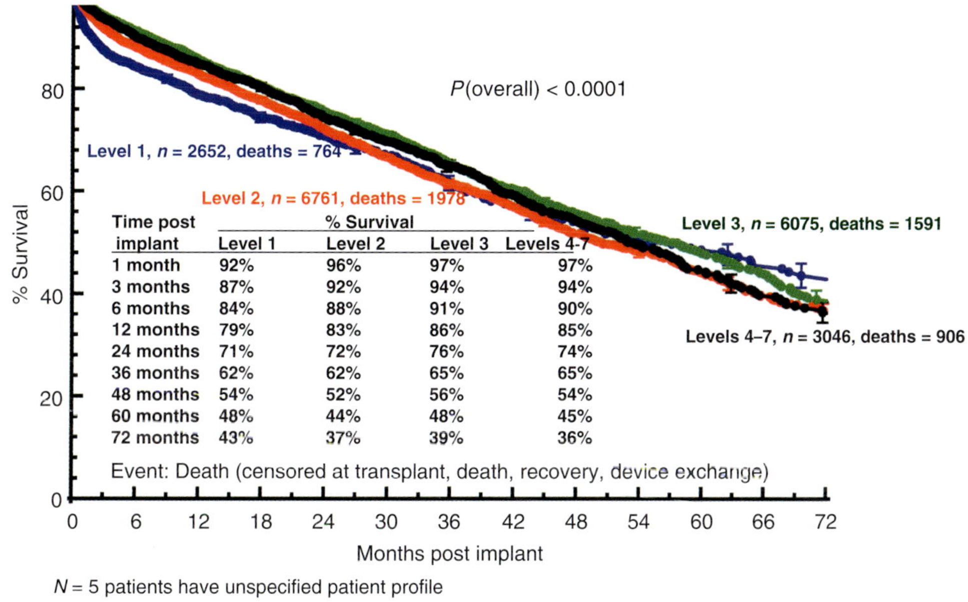

Fig. 20.5 Kaplan-Meier survival curves stratified by Interagency Registry for Mechanically Assisted Circulatory Support (INTERMACS) profile at the time of isolated continuous-flow left ventricular assist device (CFLVAD) implant. Average one-year survival is numerically lowest in patients undergoing implant as a Profile 1 or 2 but does not impact long term survival on device therapy relative to other profiles. (From Kormos RL, Cowger J, Pagani FD, et al. The Society of Thoracic Surgeons—Intermacs database annual report: evolving indications, outcomes and scientific partnerships. *Ann Thorac Surg*. 2019.)

and a higher implantation blood urea nitrogen level was associated with a strong constant hazard of mortality. Finally, the late hazard of mortality was influenced by higher body mass index, current tobacco use, presence of peripheral vascular disease, history of prior cardiac surgery before LVAD implantation, and higher preoperative right atrial pressure.[10]

Overall survival outcomes are worth noting for women and African American patients. Women represented just 21.3% of CF-LVAD in the most recent era (2012–2017) in INTERMACS.[10] This proportion is similar to MCS clinical trials, with 20% women enrolled in MOMENTUM 3 and among patients listed for transplant (25% women) in the United Network of Organ Sharing.[14,15] The lower frequency of MCS use in women has been attributed to the demographics of advanced systolic HF, which is dominated by ischemic cardiomyopathy. Ischemic etiologies of HF are more common in men in the age range where advanced therapies are most often considered. Analysis from INTERMACS revealed women to have an early hazard of death within the first 3 months of CF-VAD implantation (hazard ratio [HR], 1.47; $P < 0.001$).[10] There has also been concern about the potential for disparate outcomes according to race. In heart transplantation, there have been well-documented disparities in outcomes among African-American patients, with decreased graft survival compared with Caucasians.[16,17] However, in INTERMACS, African-American race has not been associated with an increased risk of death following MCS.[10]

In the rapidly evolving field of MCS, risk modeling for purposes of patient selection and recipient education is in a constant state of refinement. Large data repositories like INTERMACS track comprehensive preimplant variables and can inform patient selection. For example, INTERMACS has served as a real-world dataset to analyze the ability of the HeartMate Risk Score (HMRS) to discriminate outcomes beyond INTERMACS profile. The HMRS, a simple five-component clinical score, had modest discrimination for mortality in this large cohort of LVAD recipients (C-statistic: 0.62 for 90-day mortality; 0.60 for 2-year mortality).[18] Even so, patients in the high-risk HMRS group had a nearly three-fold increased 90-day mortality compared with the low-risk group and roughly two-fold increased 2-year mortality risk. More sophisticated risk models are now under construction using Bayesian network-based methods that incorporate modern machine learning algorithms. A recent report confirmed that the network model from the Cardiac Outcomes Risk Assessment project had superior performance in predicting survival compared with HMRS in the INTERMACS.[19] Next-generation network models can account for relationships between variables, although they require many more input variables that are currently available only in large registries.

Quality of Life

The advent of smaller CF pumps, with associated improvements in durability and clinical outcomes, allowed DT to become a sustainable treatment for advanced HF. Faced with a horizon of support measured in years rather than months, integration of health-related quality of life (HRQOL) into the assessment of MCS outcomes became an increasing priority.[20] This shift in implants from critical cardiogenic shock to more stable forms of advanced HF also highlighted the importance of understanding HRQOL both before and after implantation, since quality of life (QOL) consideration may be more important in elective MCS implant. Indeed, patients with HF consistently report that they care as much or more about its impact on QOL as on survival.[21] HRQOL assessment can allow us to define anticipated benefits in informed decision-making, refocus attention on patient-centered outcomes during long-term support, and facilitate analysis of the population benefits of MCS in the form of cost-effectiveness analysis.

Generic HRQQOL instruments (e.g., EuroQOL-5D) take into account a broad overview of illness and can be used to compare chronic illnesses in many populations receiving alternative treatments. By contrast, disease-specific questionnaires focus on relevant domains for a given disease but do not allow a comparison across conditions. When applied to assessment of HRQOL in MCS, HF-specific instruments will provide patients with important information about the extent to

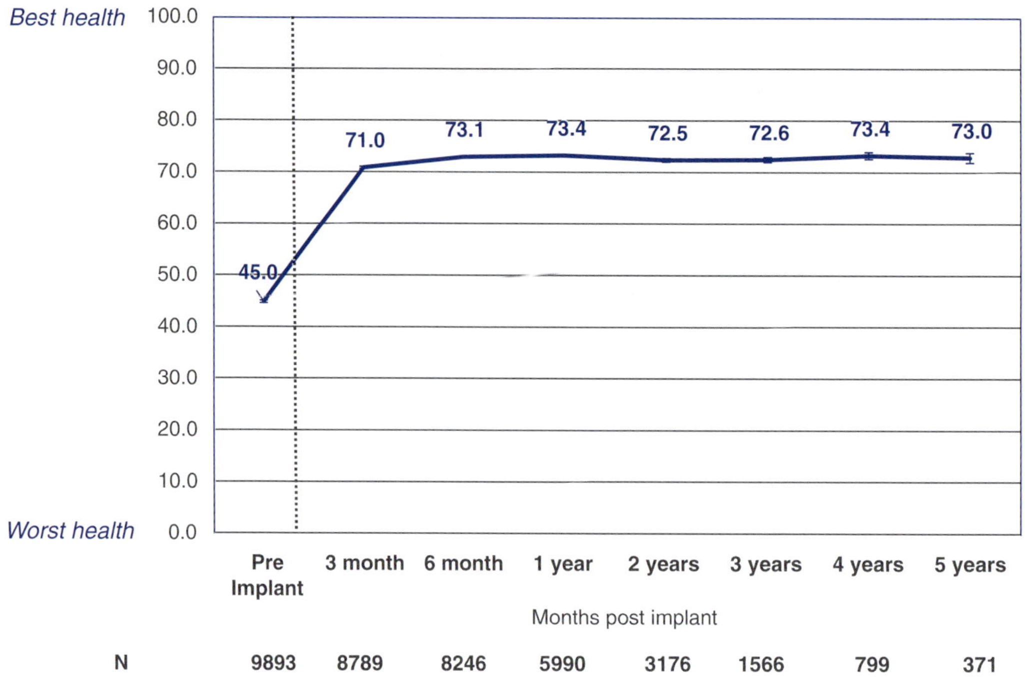

Fig. 20.6 Change in generic health-related quality of life following continuous-flow left ventricular assist device as measured by the EuroQOL-5D Visual Analog Scale. (From Kormos RL, Cowger J, Pagani FD, et al. The Society of Thoracic Surgeons—Intermacs database annual report: evolving indications, outcomes and scientific partnerships. *Ann Thorac Surg*. 2019.)

which HF symptoms will be relieved after MCS. In contrast, generic instruments will provide a view of overall QOL, including deficits in quality after MCS unrelated to HF symptoms. INTERMACS has been capturing comprehensive preimplant and serial assessment of both generic and HF-related QOL since 2012. Generic HRQOL was shown to be poor among patients across all INTERMACS Profiles 1–7 and improved to a similar level regardless of preimplant profile among those who remained on support at 6 months and 1 year.[22] The greatest improvements in HRQOL were within the first 3 months after implantation (Fig. 20.6). In addition, changes in HRQOL from before to after DT LVAD were similar in older and younger patients.[23] However, not all patients had the same improvement in HRQOL with MCS. Women surveyed reported significantly more problems regarding all dimensions of the EuroQOL-5D before implantation and significantly more problems regarding pain/discomfort and anxiety/depression at 3 and 6 months.[24] Additional factors associated with a decrease in HRQOL from before to 6 months after implantation included an adverse event within the first 6 months of implantation and residual NYHA Class 4 functional capacity.[24] There was also a considerable improvement in HF-specific measures after LVAD support (Fig. 20.7.) Among 1888 patients who underwent LVAD implantation between 2012 and 2014, 81.5% experienced moderate or large improvements in the HF-specific Kansas City Cardiomyopathy Questionnaire score, with good concordance with generic measures.[25] When patients in INTERMACS were queried about whether they were satisfied with their decision to receive a VAD, approximately 80% of responding patients indicated that they would recommend a VAD to someone based on their experience during the first 2 years.[11] As in most registries, there has been less consistency in obtaining patient-reported outcomes than in ascertaining survival. The conclusions are thus limited to patients who not only survived but also received and completed questionnaires, as shown in the declining numbers of patient responses over time.

ADVERSE EVENTS

Throughout the evolution of MCS, improvements in survival have been offset by concerns about adverse events. (See Chapter 13 for a comprehensive discussion of adverse events with durable MCS.) Common safety concerns with MCS include stroke, bleeding, device malfunction, and infection. Early in MCS, major clinical trials used variable adverse event definitions, largely due to differing manufacturers, indications, and target populations. Prior to INTERMACS, it was a challenge to make meaningful comparison between devices, centers, and patients.[26] INTERMACS standardized adverse event definitions in collaboration with FDA and industry so that the most important complications in approved devices could be tracked in real time. These adverse event definitions have allowed the development of performance measures for accreditation of device programs. Adverse event definitions have also evolved with changing incidence of device-related complications. The INTERMACS has developed updated definitions of right HF, device-related infection, and LVAD pump thrombosis, which have informed criteria for transplant listing status upgrade due to MCS complication.

Early Versus Late Adverse Events

The instantaneous risk of death is highest within the early postoperative phase, with multiorgan system failure and stroke the leading causes of death (Fig. 20.8). The occurrence of a major adverse event within the first 3 months also has a major impact on subsequent survival. INTERMACS has documented that bleeding as an adverse event reflects predominantly surgical bleeding during the first 3 months after gastrointestinal (GI) bleeding thereafter. After bleeding, infection is the most frequent adverse event in the first 3 months and the most common adverse event thereafter. Stroke persists as an important adverse event throughout the first year after implantation and beyond and is the leading cause of death late after CF-LVAD implantation. INTERMACS

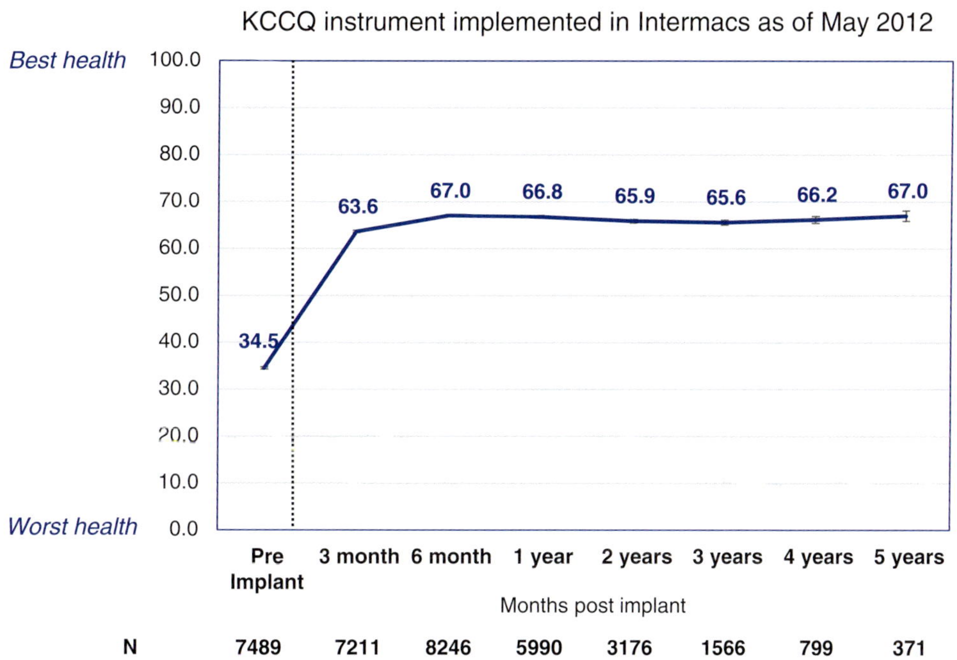

Fig. 20.7 Change in heart failure–specific quality of life following continuous-flow left ventricular assist device as measured by the Kansas City Cardiomyopathy Questionnaire *(KCCQ)* index score. (From Kormos RL, Cowger J, Pagani FD, et al. The Society of Thoracic Surgeons—Intermacs database annual report: evolving indications, outcomes and scientific partnerships. Ann Thorac Surg. 2019.)

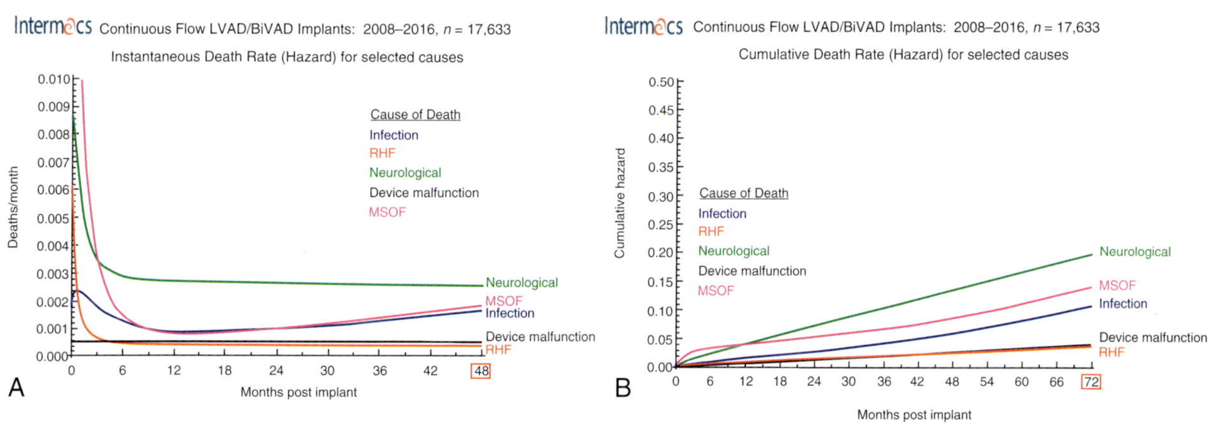

Fig. 20.8 (A) Hazard function curves indicating instantaneous risk of death over time for the major causes/modes of death. (B) Cumulative hazard function for major causes/modes of death. *BiVAD*, Biventricular assist device; *LVAD*, left ventricular assist device; *MSOF*, multiple system organ failure; *RHF*, right heart failure. (From Kirklin JK, Pagani FD, Kormos RL, et al. Eighth annual INTERMACS report: special focus on framing the impact of adverse events. *J Heart Lung Transplant.* 2017;36:1080–1086.)

has also registered differences in early (<3 months) and later (3–24 months) adverse events according to flow profile of CF-LVAD. Axial flow pumps have a significant higher rate of early and late GI bleeding, while centrifugal flow pumps have higher rates of stroke both in early (HR, 1.62; $P < 0.0001$) and late (HR, 1.47; $P < 0.0001$) stages, findings that are in concordance with clinical trials.[10,27] A detailed discussion of individual adverse events can be found in Chapter 13.

Freedom From Adverse Events and Patient Profile

Most patients receiving MCS will experience a major device-related adverse event such as bleeding, infection, device malfunction, or stroke (Fig. 20.9). In a composite of time to first major adverse event, patients with INTERMACS Profile 2–7 had greater freedom (30% at 1 year) compared to those in cardiogenic shock (Profile 1) at implantation (25% at 1 year).[11] Freedom from all-cause readmission was 30% at 1 month and 20% at 1 year.[10] When individual adverse events were analyzed by INTERMACS profile, severe right HF was highly correlated with patient profile, with patients in Profile 1 (cardiogenic shock) having a two-fold increase in risk compared to other profiles. Interestingly, when comparing patients with ambulatory Profiles 4–7 to those who are more critically ill in Profiles 1–3, there was no difference in the time to first pump-related infection, time to stroke, or time to first readmission.[11] The similarity of adverse event rates in Profiles 2–7 is sobering, as it suggests that overall adverse event rates will not necessarily be improved by placing VADs in "less sick" ambulatory advanced HF patients. Defining benchmark real-world adverse event rates in approved

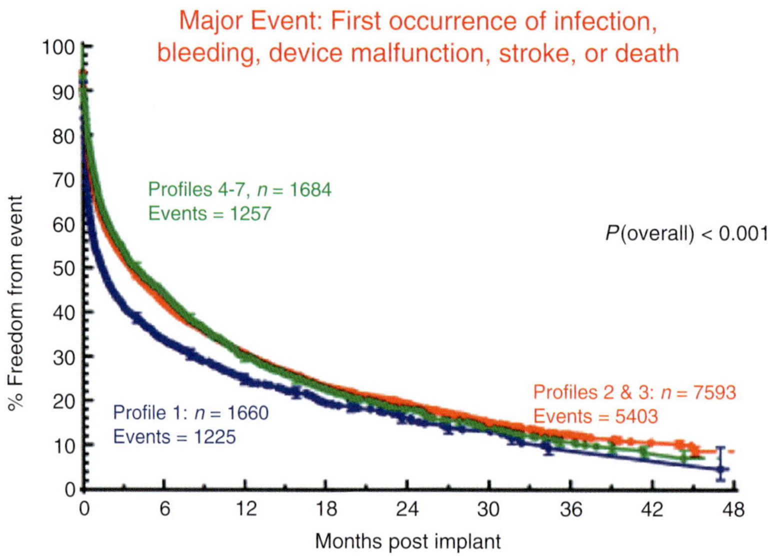

Fig. 20.9 Freedom from the combined major event of first infection, bleeding, device malfunction, stroke, or death. (From Kirklin JK, Pagani FD, Kormos RL, et al. Eighth annual INTERMACS report: special focus on framing the impact of adverse events. *J Heart Lung Transplant.* 2017;36:1080–1086.)

devices has informed preimplant education and consent, prepared patients and their families for life with MCS, and facilitated conversations about prognosis prior to implant and beyond.

REGISTRY COMPARISON TO ALTERNATIVE THERAPIES

Heart Transplant

The INTERMACS was designed to facilitate comparison to other alternative therapies, including transplant, investigational devices, and medical therapy. In many ways, the comparison of immediate MCS to listing for transplant with delayed MCS as needed for urgent bridge support is the most difficult because of the variable waiting time for a donor organ that does not apply to device therapy. Moreover, baseline profiles of illness are difficult to align since patients with evolving shock may not have time to wait for a transplant, and those patients with less severe illness have lower priority on the transplant waiting list. However, overall survival at 2 years is now similar between CF-LVAD and transplantation. Among BTT LVAD recipients, survival at 2 years is 80%, and in the International Society for Heart and Lung Transplantation (ISHLT) heart transplant registry, survival at 2 years is 83% in the most recent transplant era (2009–2016).[28] However, these crude survival rates do not take into account the morbidity of the transplant waiting list and the potential difference in HF-specific HRQOL with early MCS support compared with delayed MCS support. Even though most candidates supported with contemporary CF-LVADs generally have favorable waiting-list outcomes, survival and the likelihood of successful transplant worsen significantly once a serious LVAD-related complication has occurred. There is also concern about increased risk of primary graft dysfunction among patients supported with BTT LVAD, particularly those with increased time on MCS, renal dysfunction, and right ventricular failure.[29] Transplant candidates requiring temporary and biventricular support have the highest waitlist mortality, which has in turn has impacted listing criteria.[30] Complex decisions about when and how to support the failing heart in transplant-eligible patients will continue to be informed by registry comparisons.

Investigational Device Therapy and Registry Data

Approval of MCS devices for the BTT indication has never been supported by a randomized trial to a non-MCS therapy, since randomization is not reasonable in the face of progressive organ compromise and anticipated death. By 2010, two of the three devices were approved for the bridging indication without a control population and the third used a small historical control from the same institution.[31,32] The ADVANCE (Evaluation of the HeartWare Left Ventricular Assist Device for the Treatment of Advanced Heart Failure) trial of the HeartWare HVAD raised the standard for bridging approval by prospectively comparing outcomes with the new device compared to contemporary INTERMACS controls with other devices currently available for left ventricular support.[33] The criteria for entry into the investigational device trial were the same for selection of the control patients from the INTERMACS. However, adverse event reporting was not specifically aligned between the trial and registry and furthermore could not be specified by the brand of device used according to prior agreement. The challenge of using registry controls was also evident in the ADVANCE study after the level of illness at implantation was scrutinized. Profile 2 patients accounted for 52% of the control arm but only 24% of the investigational arm, with a conversely higher proportion of the more stable Profile 3 patients in the investigational arm (52%) compared to controls (21%), creating an unintended bias to less severe illness in the trial arm. Nevertheless, post hoc comparison indicated equivalent outcomes for each separate profile in the two arms of the study. The data from ADVANCE showed convincing noninferiority of the HVAD compared to contemporary axial flow LVAD therapy. By incorporating INTERMACS as a control group, the trial established a potential benchmark for approval of a 90% survival on device or transplantation by 1 year.[34]

Contemporary Medical Therapy

There are clear benefits for MCS implantation among eligible patients in Profile 1–2 compared to medical therapy.[5,35] Ambulatory patients in Profile 3 receiving continuous inotropic support have improving survival, but still only 50% per year, well below that offered by contemporary CF-LVAD therapy.[36] As a result, dependence on intravenous inotropic support as in INTERMACS Profile 3 has traditionally been considered the threshold that defines irreversible advanced HF and mandates consideration of advanced therapies. In the absence of this clear marker of severity, identifying which patients with advanced HF on oral therapies (INTERMACS Profile 4–7) would likely benefit from MCS becomes challenging. The largest potential impact of MCS on public health is for patients on oral HF therapies, well before the development of circulatory shock and end organ dysfunction, in whom support could be employed electively for long-term benefit with diminished perioperative risk. However, in 2015–2016, only 13% of device implantations in INTERMACS occurred in patients prior to inotrope dependence.[11] A lack of information on outcomes for patients with continued contemporary medical therapy has limited the ability to define and advance indications in the less sick advanced HF population. In this ambulatory population for whom death from HF is not imminent, shared decision-making about MCS requires more measured and individualized consideration of risk and benefit beyond survival. Integral to the original intent of INTERMACS was comparison between patients receiving approved LVADs and ambulatory patients living with advanced HF who were not receiving MCS. The field has struggled to identify ambulatory patients who are both sick enough and healthy enough to derive more benefit from MCS than from contemporary oral medical therapy, which itself is progressing rapidly. To remedy this knowledge gap, registries of ambulatory patients with advanced HF were developed with data fields that aligned with INTERMACS, including the Medical Arm for Mechanically Assisted Circulatory Support (MedaMACS) studies and the Registry Evaluation for Vital Information on VADs in Ambulatory Life (REVIVAL).

MedaMACS

In 2011–2012, the MedaMACS screening pilot registry enrolled 168 patients with advanced systolic HF who were not listed for transplant, selected using entry criteria that required a hospitalization for HF within the past year or another high-risk feature. MedaMACS was designed to generate a high-risk population of patients on oral medical therapy who could conceivably be considered for LVAD therapy, but eligibility for MCS was not required for entry. Only 47% of participants were alive with ongoing medical therapy at 1 year, and the risk of death or rescue LVAD therapy at 1 year was 61% in Profile 4 and 33% in Profile 5.[8] The registry documented a willingness of ambulatory patients to consider LVAD therapy prior to inotrope dependence and a significantly reduced generic HRQOL on medical therapy, particularly in Profile 4. These results supported the earlier use of elective LVAD in eligible patients with ambulatory NYHA Class IV (INTERMACS Profiles 4/5) HF, results in alignment with those of the industry-sponsored ROADMAP trial.[37]

The results from the screening pilot informed the MedaMACS study, which enrolled 161 outpatients between 2013 and 2015 from 11 MCS/transplant centers. Compared to the screening pilot, patients in MedaMACS had less advanced HF (32% Profile 5, 49% Profile 6) despite optimal oral medical therapy. Patients were followed prospectively for 2 years or until MCS, transplantation, or death. Because of aligned data fields, an intention-to-treat survival analysis was performed to compare outcomes for MedaMACS patients to a matched group of Profile 4–7 patients with LVADs from the INTERMACS. By 2 years after enrollment, 47% patients had experienced a primary endpoint, with 24% dying, 11% undergoing LVAD implantation, and 12% receiving a transplant.[38] Compared with 1753 contemporary patients with Profiles 4–7 receiving LVAD therapy, there was no overall difference in intention-to-treat survival between medical and LVAD therapy, but survival with LVAD therapy was significantly better than medical therapy among Profile 4–5 patients ($P = 0.0092$) (Fig. 20.10). Baseline HRQOL was lower among patients receiving LVAD than those enrolled on continuing oral medical therapy but increased after 1 year for survivors in both cohorts. These data highlighted that early referral to MCS programs is appropriate for patients with advanced systolic HF prior to inotrope dependence and offer data comparing real-world outcomes with ongoing medical therapy or elective LVAD implantation to informed sharing decisions about the timing of MCS.

REVIVAL

In 2015–2016, of the 5400 registered implants in INTERMACS, only 1.6% were in patients with Profiles 5–7 at the time of LVAD implantation.[11] Much of this reluctance stems from the unacceptably high adverse event rates across approved and investigational devices. Additional expansion of LVADs into ambulatory patients in INTERMACS Profile 5–7 HF will require not just improved technology with fewer adverse events but also better prognostic tools to identify those at greatest risk of dying without MCS and those who are most

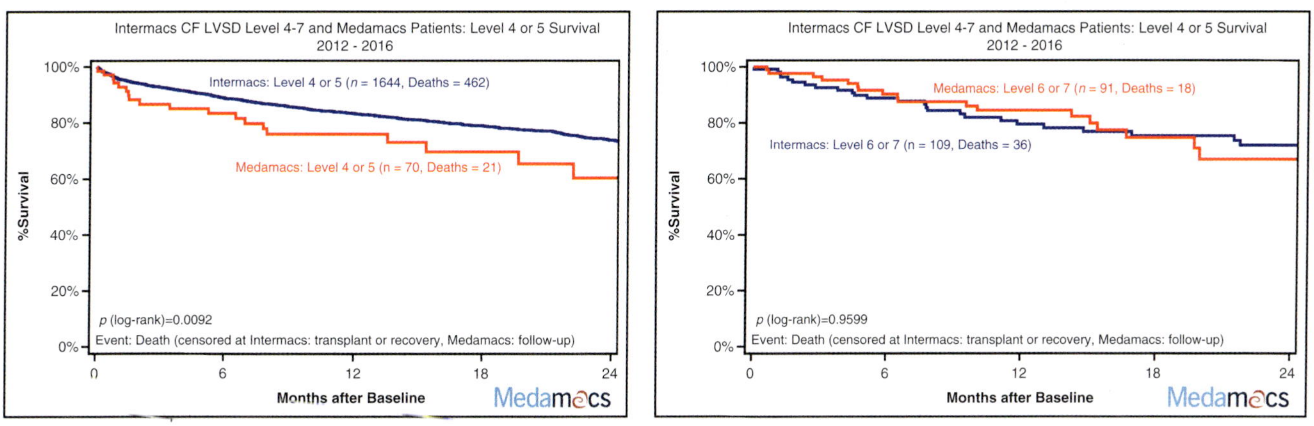

Fig. 20.10 Two-year survival with medical versus left ventricular assist device *(LVAD)* therapy stratified by Interagency Registry for Mechanically Assisted Circulatory Support patient profile at enrollment. (A) Kaplan-Meir survival suggested improved actuarial survival with LVAD versus medical therapy among Profile 4–5 patients. (B) Kaplan-Meier survival was similar with medical versus LVAD therapy among Profile 6–7 patients. Medical therapy patients were censored at the time of transplantation, LVAD placement, or last follow-up. Shaded areas represent 70% confidence intervals. *CF LVAD,* Continuous-flow left ventricular assist device. (From Ambardekar AV, Kittleson MM, Palardy M, et al. Outcomes with ambulatory advanced heart failure from the Medical Arm of Mechanically Assisted Circulatory Support (MedaMACS) Registry. *J Heart Lung Transplant* 2019.)

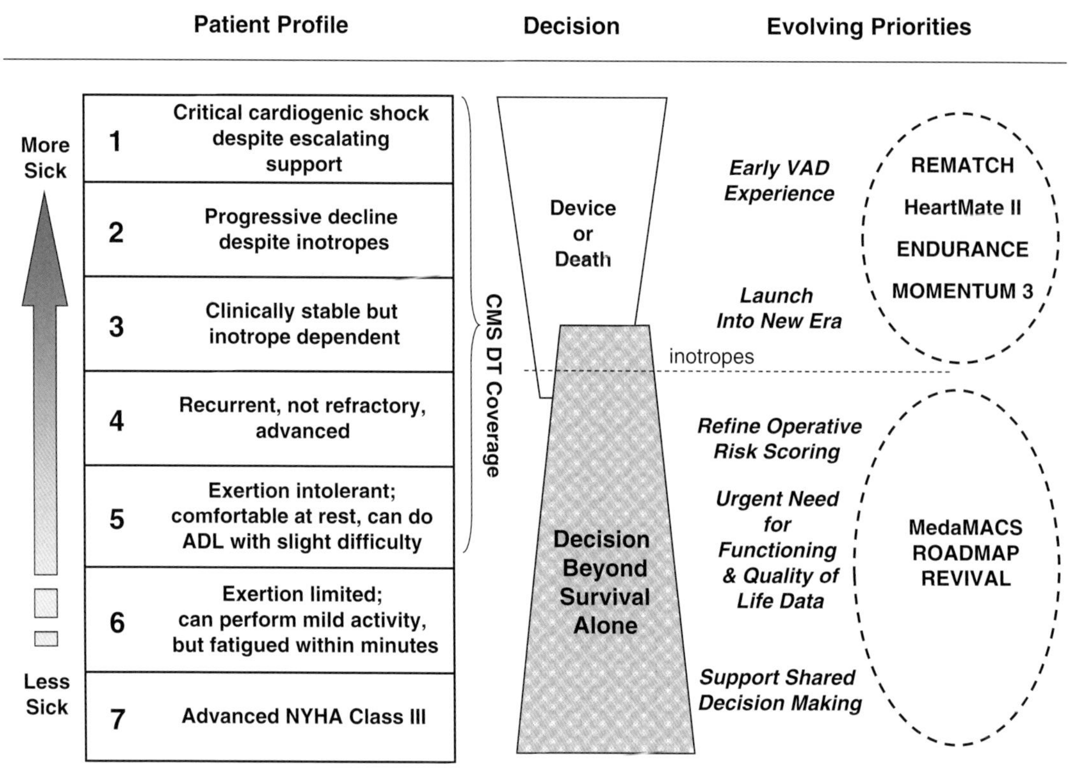

Fig. 20.11 Patient profiles and priorities for mechanical support in advanced heart failure. Interagency Registry for Mechanically Assisted Circulatory Support (INTERMACS) profiles integrate the severity and tempo of heart failure as a guide to outcomes after mechanical support. CMS services currently supports DT coverage patients on inotropes or those with severely reduced exercise capacity (Profiles 1–5). Decisions surrounding mechanical support differ according to the level of illness in the device recipient. Patients not facing imminent death may place greater emphasis on the device's impact on their functional capacity and quality of life. Priorities for both decision making and research have changed as use of VADs has expanded into the less sick patient profiles. The MedaMACS and REVIVAL registries will provide important context for the next wave of device studies in INTERMACS Profiles 4–7. *ADL*, Activity of daily living; *CMS*, Center for Medicare and Medicaid Services; *DT*, destination therapy; *ENDURANCE*, The HeartWare Ventricular Assist System as Destination Therapy of Advanced Heart Failure; *MedaMACS*, Medical Arm of Mechanically Assisted Circulatory Support; MOMENTUM 3, Multicenter Study of MagLev Technology in Patients Undergoing Mechanical Circulatory Support Therapy with HeartMate 3; *NYHA*, New York Heart Association; *REMATCH*, Randomized Evaluation of Mechanical Assistance for the Treatment of Congestive Heart Failure; *REVIVAL*, Registry Evaluation for Vital Information on VADs in Ambulatory Life; *VAD*, ventricular assist device. (Modified from Stewart GC, Stevenson LW. INTERMACS and MedaMACS: how will they guide future therapy? *Curr Cardiol Rep*. 2013;15:394.)

likely to have favorable outcome with VAD support (Fig. 20.11). Recent attention to adverse events on LVAD therapy—particularly to pump thrombosis and stroke—prevented equipoise for randomizing patients in NYHA Class III to medical versus currently approved device therapy.[39] The closing of the REVIVE-IT (Randomized Evaluation of VAD Intervention Before Inotropic Therapy) deprived the HF community of important information on a medically managed cohort in parallel to device therapy. Fortunately, the prospective registry intended to be part of the REVIVE-IT effort has been developed into the REVIVAL. REVIVAL is a prospective, observational multicenter patient cohort that has completed enrollment and follow-up of 400 patients with ambulatory advanced HF across 21 sites in the United States, with 92% of enrollees in Profiles 5–7. Overall 1-year combined rate of urgent transplantation, death, or durable MCS was 24%.[40] Unlike MedaMACS, REVIVAL also includes patients listed for transplant as Status 2 (former United Network of Organ Sharing Status definitions). This group was included as transplant candidates on oral medical therapy alone face a growing waitlist and difficult decisions about when and if to pursue MCS. By providing detailed information on patient-reported outcomes, prognosis, and dynamic clinical trajectories through serial evaluation, REVIVAL will determine the feasibility of identifying candidates for a trial of next-generation LVAD technology and other investigational therapies in NYHA Class III HF.

IMPACT OF REGISTRY DATA ON CLINICAL USE OF VADS

Through over a decade of the INTERMACS, the real-world tracking of MCS has shaped the clinical care of patients with MCS. The high risk of adverse events in critical cardiogenic shock patients facilitated earlier implantation prior to the development of end-organ dysfunction (Table 20.3). The registry has confirmed the effectiveness of DT LVAD in select patients and documented the expanded use of MCS for lifetime support. The continued risk of right ventricular failure as evidenced by higher mortality with both upfront biventricular assist device placement or delayed RVAD use has spurred development of right HF risk scores and influenced updated transplant waitlist priorities. The size of the INTERMACS has also allowed detailed analysis of MCS outcomes in forms of advanced HF less commonly treated with MCS, such as restrictive cardiomyopathy and adult congenital heart disease.[41,42] In both cases, the feasibility of contemporary LVAD therapy has been demonstrated, but outcomes with MCS in these subpopulations are worse compared to traditional systolic HF. These coupled data highlight the challenge of bridging such patients to transplant with current devices and informed the transition to the new heart transplant waitlist priority status levels, which now give upgraded priority to patients with restrictive cardiomyopathy and adult congenital heart disease.

INTERMACS has produced insights into the mechanism of post-LVAD complications. Examples include the paramount importance of intravascular hemolysis as a harbinger of LVAD pump thrombosis, the vulnerability of the driveline to infection in younger obese patients. Myocardial recovery to LVAD explantation has also been studied, with predictors of recovery being young age, nonischemic etiology, and limited use of preimplant HF medical therapy.[43] In addition to given insight into rare events, INTERMACS remains a platform for the evaluation of single-site performance and quality improvement projects. The data have also informed best practices, and registry participation has been required for DT program certification. INTERMACS data showed that implant volume impacted post-LVAD outcomes even after adjustment for preimplant patient features.[44] Medium-sized programs had better survival compared to small or very high-volume programs, suggesting a right sizing of LVAD program size.

Since all FDA-approved devices are included in INTERMACS, the registry can provide comparative data for device type selection in general

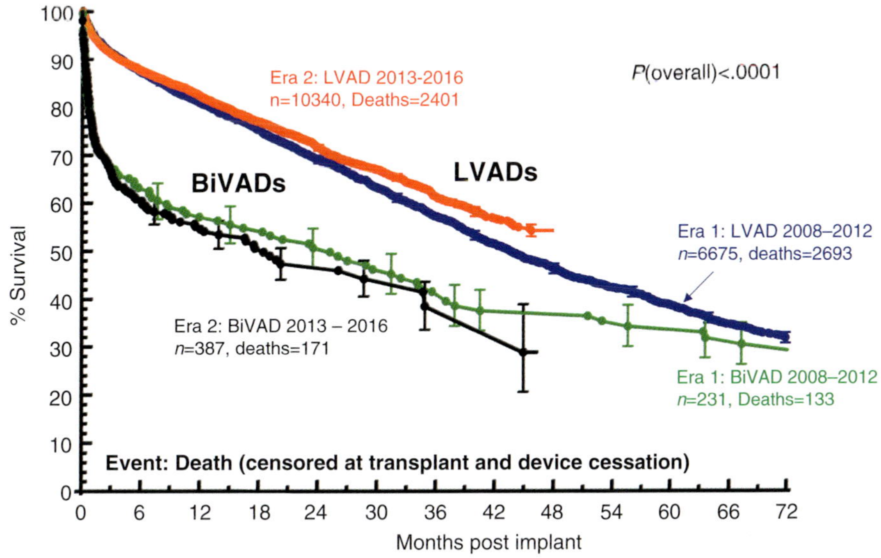

Fig. 20.12 Kaplan-Meier survival curves for LVAD and BiVAD recipients in the Interagency Registry for Mechanically Assisted Circulatory Support. *BiVAD*, Biventricular assist device; *LVAD*, left ventricular assist device. (From Kirklin JK, Pagani FD, Kormos RL, et al. Eighth annual INTERMACS report: special focus on framing the impact of adverse events. *J Heart Lung Transplant* 2017;36:1080–1086.)

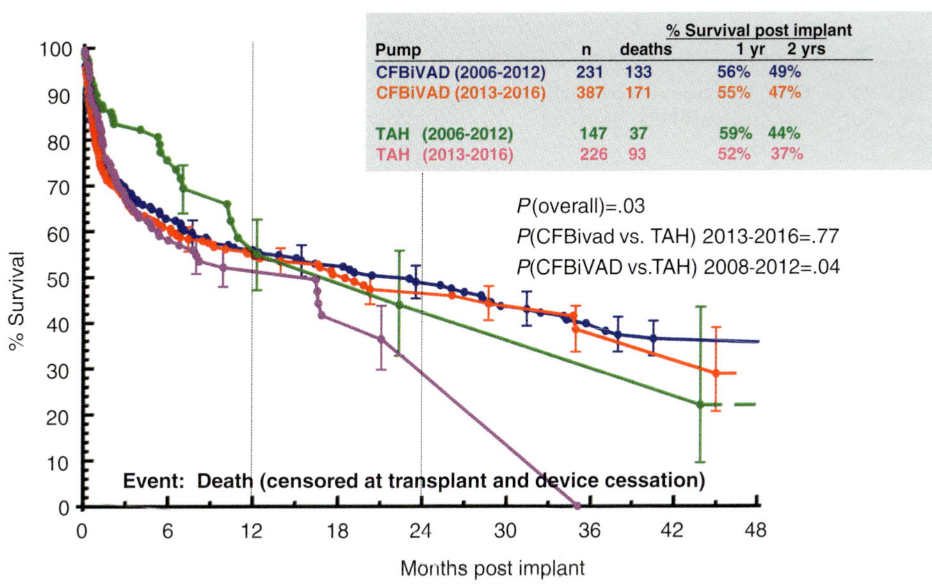

Fig. 20.13 Kaplan-Meier survival curves for LVAD, BiVAD, and TAH recipients in the Interagency Registry for Mechanically Assisted Circulatory Support. *BiVAD*, biventricular assist device; *CFBiVAD*, continuous-flow biventricular assist device; *LVAD*, left ventricular assist device; *TAH*, total artificial heart. (From Kirklin JK, Pagani FD, Kormos RL, et al. Eighth annual INTERMACS report: special focus on framing the impact of adverse events. *J Heart Lung Transplant*. 2017;36:1080–1086.)

usage. Although direct comparison between manufacturers has been prohibited by prior agreement, devices of different flow profiles (axial vs. centrifugal) or different configurations (LVAD vs. BiVAD, CF-BiVAD vs. total artificial heart) can be compared (Figs. 20.12 and 20.13). While there are statistically significant differences in the survival trajectory, survival is clinically comparable between the centrifugal and the axial flow devices: 84% vs. 85% at 1 year, 65% vs. 67% at 3 years, and 49% vs. 46% at 5 years.[10] The registry highlights the difference in adverse event between device types seen in clinical trials, with more GI bleeding in axial flow recipients and higher stroke rate with centrifugal flow. As the menu of durable MCS devices expands, INTERMACS will be an ever more important repository of postapproval device outcomes that will continue to inform device selection, configuration, and tracking of device-related adverse events. By integrated HRQOL and functional capacity assessments, INTERMACS can provide multiple outcomes of interest to inform patient-centered shared decision making, a key element of twenty-first century medicine that includes full disclosure of the anticipated risks and benefits of device therapy. Adverse event rates from INTERMACS were used to design the decision aid as part of a shared decision-making intervention for DT LVAD that improved patient decision quality as measured by patient knowledge and concordance between stated values and patient-reported treatment preference.[45]

GLOBALIZATION OF MCS REGISTRIES

The ISHLT carries a historical interest in MCS as a support system for patients on the heart transplant wait list. With the explosion of MCS after 2000, ISHLT began an international database for such devices. With the inception of INTERMACS, the ISHLT database was discontinued. However, interest was rekindled in 2010, and an international platform was created under the logo IMACS (ISHLT Mechanically Assisted Circulatory Support) registry, which began data collection in January 2013.[46] Multiple international collectives began contributing data, including "MACS" registries from Japan (JMACS) and Europe (EuroMACS), along with the United States (INTERMACS). This global collaboration has created a unique platform for risk-adjusted outcomes analytics for the international MCS community.[47]

REFERENCES

1. Institute of Medicine. The Artificial Heart: Prototypes, Policies, and Patients. Washington, DC: The National Academies Press. https://doi.org/10.17226/1820. 1991.
2. Kirklin JK, Naftel DC. Mechanical circulatory support: registering a therapy in evolution. *Circ Heart Fail.* 2008;1:200–205.
3. Kirklin JK, Naftel DC, Stevenson LW, et al. INTERMACS database for durable devices for circulatory support: first annual report. *J Heart Lung Transplant.* 2008;27:1065–1072.
4. Blume ED, Rosenthal DN, Rossano JW, et al. Outcomes of children implanted with ventricular assist devices in the United States: first analysis of the Pediatric Interagency Registry for Mechanical Circulatory Support (PediMACS). *J Heart Lung Transplant.* 2016;35:578–584.
5. Rose EA, Gelijns AC, Moskowitz AJ, et al. Long-term use of a left ventricular assist device for end-stage heart failure. *N Engl J Med.* 2001;345:1435–1443.
6. Stevenson LW, Pagani FD, Young JB, et al. INTERMACS profiles of advanced heart failure: the current picture. *J Heart Lung Transplant.* 2009;28:535–541.
7. Barge-Caballero E, Segovia-Cubero J, Almenar-Bonet L, et al. Preoperative INTERMACS profiles determine postoperative outcomes in critically ill patients undergoing emergency heart transplantation: analysis of the Spanish National Heart Transplant Registry. *Circ Heart Fail.* 2013;6:763–772.
8. Stewart GC, Kittleson MM, Patel PC, et al. INTERMACS (Interagency Registry for Mechanically Assisted Circulatory Support) profiling identifies ambulatory patients at high risk on medical therapy after hospitalizations for heart failure. *Circ Heart Fail.* 2016;9.
9. Kirklin JK, Naftel DC, Kormos RL, et al. The fourth INTERMACS annual report: 4,000 implants and counting. *J Heart Lung Transplant.* 2012;31:117–126.
10. Kormos RL, Cowger J, Pagani FD, et al. The Society of Thoracic Surgeons - Intermacs database annual report: evolving indications, outcomes and scientific partnerships. *Ann Thorc Surg.* 2019.
11. Kirklin JK, Pagani FD, Kormos RL, et al. Eighth annual INTERMACS report: special focus on framing the impact of adverse events. *J Heart Lung Transplant.* 2017;. https://doi.org/10.1016/j.healun.2017.07.005.
12. Teuteberg JJ, Stewart GC, Jessup M, et al. Implant strategies change over time and impact outcomes: insights from the INTERMACS (Interagency Registry for Mechanically Assisted Circulatory Support). *JACC Heart Fail.* 2013;1:369–378.
13. Mehra MR, Naka Y, Uriel N, et al. A fully magnetically levitated circulatory pump for advanced heart failure. *N Engl J Med.* 2016;.
14. Hsich EM, Starling RC, Blackstone EH, et al. Does the UNOS heart transplant allocation system favor men over women? *JACC Heart Fail.* 2014;2:347–355.
15. Mehra MR, Naka Y, Uriel N, et al. A fully magnetically levitated circulatory pump for advanced heart failure. *N Engl J Med.* 2017;376:440–450.
16. Morris AA, Kransdorf EP, Coleman BL, Colvin M. Racial and ethnic disparities in outcomes after heart transplantation: a systematic review of contributing factors and future directions to close the outcomes gap. *J Heart Lung Transplant.* 2016;35:953–961.
17. Allen JG, Weiss ES, Arnaoutakis GJ, et al. The impact of race on survival after heart transplantation: an analysis of more than 20,000 patients. *Ann Thorac Surg.* 2010;89:1956–1963. discussion 1963-4.
18. Adamo L, Tang Y, Nassif ME, et al. The HeartMate risk score identifies patients with similar mortality risk across all INTERMACS profiles in a large multicenter analysis. *JACC Heart Fail.* 2016;.
19. Loghmanpour NA, Kanwar MK, Druzdzel MJ, Benza RL, Murali S, Antaki JF. A new Bayesian network-based risk stratification model for prediction of short-term and long-term LVAD mortality. *ASAIO J.* 2015;61:313–323.
20. Grady KL, Warner Stevenson L, Pagani FD, et al. Beyond survival: recommendations from INTERMACS for assessing function and quality of life with mechanical circulatory support. *J Heart Lung Transplant.* 2012;31:1158–1164.
21. Lewis EF, Johnson PA, Johnson W, Collins C, Griffin L, Stevenson LW. Preferences for quality of life or survival expressed by patients with heart failure. *J Heart Lung Transplant.* 2001;20:1016–1024.
22. Grady KL, Naftel D, Stevenson L, et al. Overall quality of life improves to similar levels after mechanical circulatory support regardless of severity of heart failure before implantation. *J Heart Lung Transplant.* 2014;33:412–421.
23. Grady KL, Naftel DC, Myers S, et al. Change in health-related quality of life from before to after destination therapy mechanical circulatory support is similar for older and younger patients: analyses from INTERMACS. *J Heart Lung Transplant.* 2015;34:213–221.
24. Grady KL, Sherri W, Naftel DC, et al. Age and gender differences and factors related to change in health-related quality of life from before to 6 months after left ventricular assist device implantation: findings from Interagency Registry for Mechanically Assisted Circulatory Support. *J Heart Lung Transplant.* 2016;35:777–788.
25. Nassif ME, Spertus JA, Jones PG, et al. Changes in disease-specific versus generic health status measures after left ventricular assist device implantation: insights from INTERMACS. *J Heart Lung Transplant.* 2017;36:1243–1249.
26. Stewart GC, Stevenson LW. INTERMACS and MedaMACS: how will they guide future therapy? *Curr Cardiol Rep.* 2013;15:394.
27. Milano CA, Rogers JG, Tatooles AJ, et al. HVAD: the ENDURANCE supplemental trial. *JACC Heart Fail.* 2018;6:792–802.

28. Khush KK, Cherikh WS, Chambers DC, et al. The International Thoracic Organ Transplant Registry of the International Society for Heart and Lung Transplantation: thirty-fifth adult heart transplantation report-2018; focus theme: multiorgan transplantation. *J Heart Lung Transplant.* 2018;37:1155–1168.
29. Truby LK, Garan AR, Givens RC, et al. Ventricular assist device utilization in heart transplant candidates: nationwide variability and impact on waitlist outcomes. *Circ Heart Fail.* 2018;11.
30. Wever-Pinzon O, Drakos SG, Kfoury AG, et al. Morbidity and mortality in heart transplant candidates supported with mechanical circulatory support: is reappraisal of the current united network for organ sharing thoracic organ allocation policy justified? *Circulation.* 2013;127:452–462.
31. Miller LW, Pagani FD, Russell SD, et al. Use of a continuous-flow device in patients awaiting heart transplantation. *N Engl J Med.* 2007;357:885–896.
32. Frazier OH, Rose EA, McCarthy P, et al. Improved mortality and rehabilitation of transplant candidates treated with a long-term implantable left ventricular assist system. *Ann Surg.* 1995;222:327–336. discussion 336-8.
33. Aaronson KD, Slaughter MS, Miller LW, et al. Use of an intrapericardial, continuous-flow, centrifugal pump in patients awaiting heart transplantation. *Circulation.* 2012;125:3191–3200.
34. Stevenson LW, Hunt SA. A bridge far enough? *Circulation.* 2012;125:3069–3072.
35. Stevenson LW, Miller LW, Desvigne-Nickens P, et al. Left ventricular assist device as destination for patients undergoing intravenous inotropic therapy: a subset analysis from REMATCH (Randomized Evaluation of Mechanical Assistance in Treatment of Chronic Heart Failure). *Circulation.* 2004;110:975–981.
36. Hashim T, Sanam K, Revilla-Martinez M, et al. Clinical characteristics and outcomes of intravenous inotropic therapy in advanced heart failure. *Circ Heart Fail.* 2015;8:880–886.
37. Estep JD, Starling RC, Horstmanshof DA, et al. Risk assessment and comparative effectiveness of left ventricular assist device and medical management in ambulatory heart failure patients: results from the ROADMAP study. *J Am Coll Cardiol.* 2015;66:1747–1761.
38. Ambardekar AV, Kittleson MM, Palardy M, et al. Outcomes with ambulatory advanced heart failure from the Medical Arm of Mechanically Assisted Circulatory support (MedaMACS) Registry. *J Heart Lung Transplant.* 2019. in press.
39. Pagani FD, Aaronson KD, Kormos R, et al. The NHLBI REVIVE-IT study: understanding its discontinuation in the context of current left ventricular assist device therapy. *J Heart Lung Transplant.* 2016;35:1277–1283.
40. Aaronson KD, Stevenson LW, Pagani FD, et al. Identifying ambulatory advanced heart failure patients at high risk for death, LVAD or transplant at 1 year: how did the REVIVAL eligibility criteria perform? *J Heart Lung Transplant.* 2018;37:S195–S196.
41. Cedars A, Vanderpluym C, Koehl D, Cantor R, Kutty S, Kirklin JK. An Interagency Registry for Mechanically Assisted Circulatory Support (INTERMACS) analysis of hospitalization, functional status, and mortality after mechanical circulatory support in adults with congenital heart disease. *J Heart Lung Transplant.* 2018;37:619–630.
42. Patel SR, Saeed O, Naftel D, et al. Outcomes of restrictive and hypertrophic cardiomyopathies after LVAD: an INTERMACS analysis. *J Card Fail.* 2017;23:859–867.
43. Topkara VK, Garan AR, Fine B, et al. Myocardial recovery in patients receiving contemporary left ventricular assist devices: results from the Interagency Registry for Mechanically Assisted Circulatory Support (INTERMACS). *Circ Heart Fail.* 2016;9.
44. Cowger JA, Stulak JM, Shah P, et al. impact of center left ventricular assist device volume on outcomes after implantation. An INTERMACS Analysis. *JACC Heart Fail.* 2017;5:691–699.
45. Allen LA, McIlvennan CK, Thompson JS, et al. Effectiveness of an intervention supporting shared decision making for destination therapy left ventricular assist device: the DECIDE-LVAD Randomized Clinical Trial. *JAMA Intern Med.* 2018;178:520–529.
46. Kirklin JK, Mehra MR. The dawn of the ISHLT Mechanical Assisted Circulatory Support (IMACS) Registry: fulfilling our mission. *J Heart Lung Transplant.* 2012;31:115–116.
47. Kirklin JK, Cantor R, Mohacsi P, et al. First annual IMACS report: a global International Society for Heart and Lung Transplantation Registry for Mechanical Circulatory Support. *J Heart Lung Transplant.* 2016;35:407–412.

21

Regulatory and Reimbursement Landscape for Mechanical Circulatory Support

Donald A. Middlebrook, Robin Bostic, Tina Cady Ivovic

KEY POINTS

Introduction
History of Medical Device Regulations
Global Reimbursement
Regulatory Pathways for Mechanical Circulatory Support Devices
Reimbursement Pathways for Mechanical Circulatory Support Devices
Mechanical Circulatory Support Device Total Product Life Cycle
Creating Reimbursement for Left Ventricular Assist Devices
Postmarket Studies/Surveillance
Device Tracking
Mechanical Circulatory Support Device Registries
Mechanical Circulatory Support Device Corrections and Removals (Recalls)
Obsolescence
Lessons Learned
Conclusions

INTRODUCTION

A regulatory/reimbursement product plan should be created simultaneously, early in the product development cycle, with the concept of developing ongoing evidence to support appropriate device use. If each is treated separately and implemented linearly rather than collectively, significant market access delays and restrictions can be anticipated. Outlining clinical study protocols with regulatory agencies and payers is necessary to demonstrate whether the product is not only safe and effective but also reasonable and necessary, providing value to the health care system. An evidence development strategy sensitive to the needs of regulators, payers, and providers—when successfully implemented—allows patients faster access to life-saving technologies. This chapter provides global historical content impacting our current regulatory/reimbursement environment and defines the necessary course to patient access. The case study of mechanical circulatory support provides many elements of a successful regulatory/reimbursement evidence-based strategy.

HISTORY OF MEDICAL DEVICE REGULATIONS

Within the realm of US Medical Device Regulation and Reimbursement, medical devices went largely uncontrolled from a regulatory standpoint until the late 1930s, when Congress enacted the Federal Food, Drug, and Cosmetic Act of 1938.[1] This established the Food and Drug Administration (FDA) as a separate law enforcement agency to regulate mainly drugs but also medical devices and required they be proven safe before they could be marketed. Until 1938, medical devices were developed and marketed in an unregulated way, including eyeglasses (1752), the stethoscope (1815), the x-ray machine (1895), the electrocardiogram device (1903), and the world's first cardiac pacemaker (1936).[2] In the early 1950s came the first use of a mechanical heart manufactured by General Motors, and by the late 1960s, the world saw its first heart-lung bypass machine and mechanical artificial heart. Developments in medical devices and surgical procedures led to the first heart transplant (1967), performed by a South African surgeon Dr. Christiaan Barnard. The patient, a 53-year-old man, died 18 days later, but this event started what is now regarded as one of greatest medical achievements of our time, made possible by the advancement of medical devices.

In 1966, another regulatory milestone was established under the authority of the US FDA called the Fair Packaging and Labeling Act.[3] This act required all US foods, drugs, cosmetics, and medical devices in interstate commerce to be honestly and informatively labeled. Furthering the regulation of medical devices, the US Legislature passed the Medical Device Amendments Act of 1976[4] to establish a classification and control process to ensure the safety and effectiveness of medical devices. The amendments also required manufacturers of medical devices to register with the FDA, follow quality control procedures, and established premarket-approval (PMA) requirements for certain types of medical devices. It was not until the early 1990s when the next milestone relative to regulation of medical devices occurred. The US Legislature passed the Safe Medical Device Act of 1990,[5] requiring nursing homes, hospitals, and other facilities that use medical devices to report to the FDA incidents that suggested that a medical device probably caused or contributed to the death or serious injury of a patient. The Act also required manufacturers to conduct postmarket surveillance on permanently implanted medical devices whose failure might cause serious harm or death and to establish methods for tracing and locating patients depending on such devices. It also authorized the FDA to order medical device product recalls and other actions.

In 1997, after complaints of a slow medical device approval process from medical device manufacturers, the Legislative branch enacted the Food and Drug Modernization Act[6] to accelerate review of medical devices. The Modernization Act exempted premarket regulatory requirements for all Class I medical devices (low risk) that are not intended for critical human health. In 2002, the Legislature passed the Medical Device User Fee and Modernization Act,[7] which mandated fees to medical device companies for evaluation or approval of medical devices. Provisions were also established for medical device manufacturing inspections by accredited third parties and new requirements emerged for single-use medical devices. Then, in 2005, the Medical Device User Fee and Stabilization Act[8] was passed, which amended the original Medical Device User Fee and Modernization Act of 2002. This allowed the FDA to change how it uses the user fees and requires development of better regulatory systems to support effective and timely product reviews and also allowed it to enact new regulatory reforms, all aimed at bringing safe and effective devices to market sooner.

Finally, there are two additional pieces of legislation aimed at aiding in the FDA's goals to protect and promote public health while providing timely access to safe and effective medical devices; the FDA Amendments Act of 2007[9] and the FDA Safety and Innovation Act of 2012.[10] Both these legislative acts reauthorized user fees to provide resources to the FDA, aimed at timely review and approval of medical devices. These include improvements in the approval submission review process, codification of the use of interactive reviews to speed the review process, better FDA guidance development, and authorized FDA resources for improvements in reviewer training and review performance tracking.

Fig. 21.1 is a timeline of regulatory milestones from the inception of regulation through the current day.

History of Reimbursement in the United States

In 1965, the Federal Government created the Medicare program to combat the difficulties that people over 65 years had in getting private health insurance coverage. Remaining relatively static until the late 1990s, in the early 2000s, the program experienced a myriad of changes, including a name change. Previously called the Health Care Financing Administration, the Agency under the Department of Health and Human Services was renamed the Centers for Medicare and Medicaid Services (CMS). Along with this name change came several changes in Medicare benefits and the associated payment structures, which have evolved to shift away from fee for service to a more quality- and value-based payment system through legislative changes.[11–14]

Throughout this evolution, Medicare has become both the most transparent and the most influential payer in the United States. The payment systems, decisions, and policies from Medicare often influence the decisions and policies of private payers and other governmental programs.

Naturally, private or commercial payers continue to provide insurance coverage, mainly for employed Americans and their families. After World War II, President Truman lobbied for universal health care coverage, but the appetite of the Federal Government to fund such an endeavor was not there and the proposal failed as it was seen by many Americans as a form of socialism. Labor unions took over the charge and campaigned for employer-sponsored health insurance, which grew steadily from the 1940s and by 1960 had grown to nearly 145 million people covered.[15]

European Medical Device Regulations

Until the mid-1980s, each European country had its own approach to regulating medical device use. This made commercialization of medical devices within Europe very difficult for device manufacturers because each country had their own set of regulatory requirements. Some were less stringent and some were extremely complex, making it difficult for patients to access new technologies as they were developed. To remove individual country barriers within Europe, the New Approach to device regulations and the Global Approach to conformity assessments were developed.[16] Medical devices that are granted market access using the New Approach can be recognized by the Conformité Européenne (CE) Mark. New Approach directives were harmonized across European Union (EU) member states, which allowed device manufacturers to comply with a single set of requirements to market devices within the EU. Approximately 20 New Approach directives came into force during the mid-1980s, resulting in the creation of a single European market for devices by December 1992. The Global Approach supplemented the New Approach by defining the basis for Conformity Assessment Procedures within the New Approach directive but does not give conformity assessment details; those are described in the directives themselves—*The Guide to the Implementation of Directives Based on the New Approach and the Global Approach*.[17]

The EU has an open medical device regulatory system that is transparent, based on harmonized standards and spans all EU member states. Medical devices sold within the EU must meet the health and safety requirements set forth in the EU medical devices directives. These directives consolidate the EU regulatory requirements under one system, meaning that if a medical device receives CE Mark designation in one member state, it can be sold in all EU member states.

This standard-based framework has remained intact and relatively unchanged since its inception. However, in 2017, two new regulations on medical devices[18] were adopted by the EU and entered into force in mid-2017. These two new directives will replace existing directives and will begin to be enforced after a transitional period of 3 years. These new directives contain a series of important improvements to modernize the current system, including stricter controls on high-risk medical devices, greater definition of oversight of the Notified Bodies that perform the conformity assessments, improved transparency, a

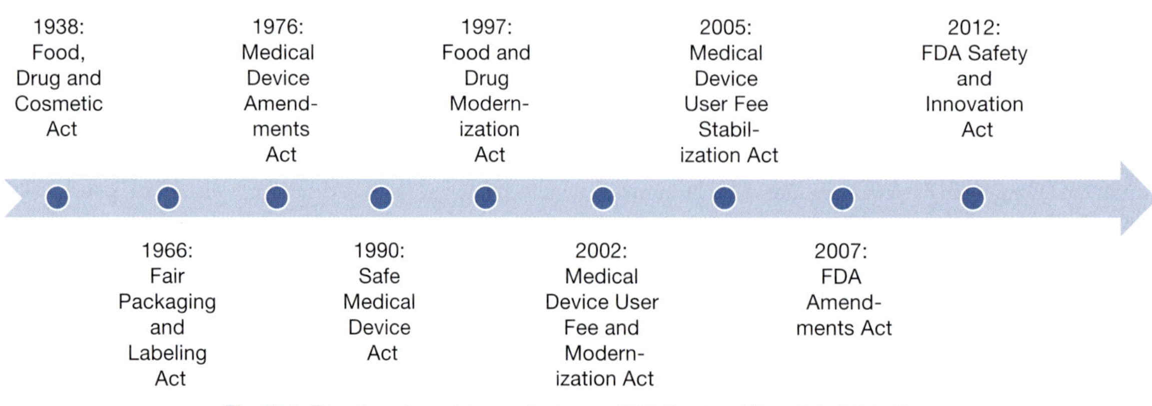

Fig. 21.1 Timeline of regulatory milestones. *FDA*, Food and Drug Administration.

tracking system for implantable medical devices, and reinforcement of rules governing clinical evidence that a medical device is safe for its intended use.

In summary, since the mid-1980s, medical devices placed on the market within the European community must bear the CE Mark indicating that the product complies with the applicable EU regulations and enables the commercialization of medical devices in 32 European countries.

Medical Device Regulations in Rest of World Markets

Countries such as Australia, Canada, Israel, Japan, New Zealand, Switzerland, South Africa, and member countries of the EU or of the European Economic Area[19] have established a regulatory framework for approval and use of medical devices. Often, the approval process allows the leverage of experiences and regulatory approvals within other established markets such and the United States and EU. Others require specific clinical evidence within the country before regulatory approvals can be achieved. Many countries simply have not addressed the development of regulatory controls, and despite the efforts of organizations such as the World Health Organization, the International Medical Device Regulators Forum, and the Global Harmonization Task Force, a single specific set of non–country-specific standards for the regulatory control of medical devices remains elusive. However, work toward this goal continues on many fronts.

GLOBAL REIMBURSEMENT

At this point in time, there is no global reimbursement pathway. Each country establishes medical coverage, creates adequate codes, and assigns a payment group for devices. However, there are country clusters with similar mechanisms in establishing reimbursement. Table 21.1 attempts to unify a noncentralized approach by country groupings.

TABLE 21.1 Device Reimbursement by Payment Clusters and Market Access Requirements

Cluster by Payment Type	Country	Dominant Market Access Requirements
Diagnostic Related Group (DRG)	Germany, Italy, Austria, Switzerland, Poland, Czech Republic	CE Mark and positive guidelines
Global budget	Canada, Scandinavian countries, Spain	CE Mark, hospital or regional budgets available for innovation, critical role of local providers and societies
Regional budget	China	NMPA (previously CFDA) approval, strong clinical claims, critical role of local providers and guidelines
Medicare budget	United States	FDA approval, reasonable and necessary, NCD with CED, clinical revenue during IDE trial
Payment categories	Japan	PMDA approval, clinical outcomes in Japanese patients, healthcare reform with focus on value underway
Listing with positive HTA	United States (private), France, United Kingdom, Australia (private), Belgium, Netherlands, Korea	Regulatory approval, strong clinical claims, cost-effectiveness, affordability, HTA, brand-specific lists, positive guidelines

CE, Certification mark; *CED*, Coverage With Evidence Development; *FDA*, Food and Drug Administration; *HTA*, Health Technology Assessment; *NCD*, National Coverage Determination; *NMPA*, National Medical Products Administration (previously known as *CFDA* [China Food and Drug Administration]); *PMDA*, Pharmaceuticals and Medical Devices Agency.

REGULATORY PATHWAYS FOR MECHANICAL CIRCULATORY SUPPORT DEVICES

Today's mechanical circulatory support (MCS) include devices for acute temporary support, short-term support or bridge to transplant (BTT), long-term support or destination therapy (DT), and total artificial heart (TAH). For the purpose of illustrating the total product life cycle for MCS devices, we have chosen to focus on BTT and DT support devices as these are highly complex and used worldwide. The regulatory pathway to commercial approval for a MCS device is dependent largely on its intended use. Today, there are two primary intended uses for MCS devices, although this is evolving and may someday be reduced to a single intended use for advanced heart failure patients with hemodynamic compromise requiring MCS. The first is short-term MCS for advanced heart failure patients who are refractory to medical treatment and in need of hemodynamic stabilization either as BTT or for myocardial recovery, and the second is for DT where the patient's options for either recovery or heart transplant are unlikely due to age, malignancy, or morbidity.

In the United States, MCS devices are considered Class III devices (regulatory classification) and require a PMA application from the FDA before commercialization can be granted. In the EU, MCS devices are also considered Class III medical devices and require approval of a Design Dossier from an EU Member State–appointed Notified Body before the MCS device can be commercially approved and placed onto the market. Significant preclinical design verification and validation (V&V) testing, animal testing, and data from prospective controlled human clinical evaluations are required to support the safe and effective use determination made by these regulatory bodies to gain commercial approval.

In major global markets, regulatory systems are used to establish medical device classification (Class I, II, or III)[20] based on their function and intended use. Less critical medical devices (Class I) such as syringes, tongue depressors, and wheelchairs may be exempt or have the least burdensome premarket regulatory requirements. More complex medical devices (Class II) such as catheters and ventilators may have standards or controls that must be met to ensure their safety and effectiveness prior to PMA. The highest regulatory classification for medical devices (Class III) is reserved for those that support or sustain human life, are of substantial importance in preventing impairment of health, or present a high risk of injury or illness to patients. Medical devices in this highest regulatory classification include breast implants, knee replacements, pacemakers and, of course, MCS devices. Because of the high-risk, life-sustaining nature of these devices, the regulatory pathway to market approval is also the most comprehensive and rigorous. Most medical devices in this category require valid scientific evidence to support that they are safe and effective for their intended use. Usually, this comes from demonstrating that the medical device conforms to required standards and performing extensive, lengthy, and costly prospective controlled clinical trials.

REIMBURSEMENT PATHWAYS FOR MECHANICAL CIRCULATORY SUPPORT DEVICES

Establishing reimbursement early in product development is essential for patient access. Although reimbursement is composed of coverage, coding, and payment, coverage—the conditions under which a product or service will be paid for—is the essential first step that drives ultimate access for patients and ideally is gained prior to the assignment of administrative codes or assignment into payment structures.

Before the launch of any MCS device, a comprehensive analysis of each of these reimbursement drivers is essential to market success. The primary path to payer coverage of a product, procedure, or service occurs when a product is deemed a "reasonable and necessary" medical treatment, but payers demand a further level of evidence to show *effectiveness* (does it work in the real world?) and *efficiency* (does it provide a better value?). The Advanced Medical Technology Association, an industry group representing medical technology manufacturers, has reported that CMS takes an average of 2 to 5 years to create coverage for a new product, with private insurers' timeframes varying widely.[21] The earlier the coverage process is initiated, the sooner reimbursement will be established. Perhaps most importantly, this 2- to 5-year anticipated timeframe for coverage can be reduced if a reimbursement plan is implemented early. When developing a reimbursement plan, the following questions should be asked and planned for accordingly:

1. Where will this product fit in the larger health care arena?
2. Will this product meet not only the US FDA "safe and effective" standards required for regulatory approval but also payers "reasonable and necessary" and likely "effective and efficient" requirements?
3. How can the reimbursement adequately cover the cost?

Where Will It Fit?

There are three broad categories in which the technology or procedure could fit (Table 21.2):

1. Similar to another product already on the market (a me too device)?
2. An expansion or different use of an existing technology?
3. Truly new and innovative?

Naturally, reimbursement is easiest to obtain with "me too" products because coverage, coding, and payment have been defined for the predicate product or products. In this case, the primary task is to ensure it fits within the structures created for the predicate product; in other words, it can be included under any existing coverage policies and is identified by using the existing technology codes, and the existing code(s) trigger appropriate payment.

TABLE 21.2 Reimbursement Analysis: Implications of Product Fit

	Similar to Another Product	Expansion of Existing Technology	Truly New and Innovative
Reimbursement components that must be developed	Confirm existing code and inclusion for coverage of this product	Alter coverage, coding, and payment to include this product	Create new coverage, coding, and payment structure for this product
Scientific evidence required	Usually FDA approval with same indications suffice for inclusion in existing coverage	Publication of controlled studies (usually one to two)	Publication of controlled studies (usually two to four) and cost-effectiveness data (publications or registry or both) data
Typical timeline after FDA approval	6 months to 1 year	1–2 years	2–5 years

FDA, Food and Drug Administration.

"Indication expansion" of an existing technology often requires altering coverage, coding, and payment to address the new indication. Published studies supporting the proposed expanded indication and revisions of established medical policy are necessary to create additional coverage. Codes may need to be revised, including new code descriptions, which can trigger different payment rates.

If the product is a new and innovative technology, as the first MCS device was a new reimbursement structure must be constructed and implemented to address coverage, coding, and payment.

Wherever the product "fits," a reasonable timeline for developing and implementing the reimbursement plan must be anticipated. If coverage, coding, and payment already exist for a similar product, 6 to 12 months is currently typical for getting this product positioned within the existing category. To modify existing or to obtain new administrative codes used to identify the product or service to payers—whether related to physician procedures (Current Procedural Terminology), the procedure to implant the device (International Classification of Diseases-10), or to the device itself (Healthcare Common Procedural Coding System)—the process usually takes approximately 1 to 2 years from the product's launch. For new technologies, historically, it has taken 2 to 5 years to create national medical coverage or to substantially expand existing guidelines, and code creation follows along a similar path.

MECHANICAL CIRCULATORY SUPPORT DEVICE TOTAL PRODUCT LIFE CYCLE

The Total Product Life Cycle (TPLC) is a conceptual framework for assessing any product or service.[22] It is often used by medical device regulators in the context of a regulatory paradigm to guide the regulation of market-driven evolution of medical devices from conception, through premarket development, to widespread market use, and finally to obsolescence and replacement by subsequent generations of products.[23] MCS devices are particularly unique in that they have one of the most challenging and potentially long lasting TPLCs of any medical device in its category. The aspects of the MCS TPLC and the regulatory and reimbursement considerations along the way are discussed in the next sections.

Design

Mechanical blood pumps are complex, electromechanical devices that must take over the workload of a weakened human heart to sustain human life for lengthy periods of time and, in many cases, for the rest of the patient's life. Therefore, the device design is critical and must take into consideration not only ease of surgical placement, device electrical interactions, and emission effects with other medical devices but also human factors related to power, control, and situational awareness. In addition to design factors, and because the regulatory burden is so high, the requirements that must be met and documented to ultimately demonstrate preclinical and clinical safety must be taken into consideration at the earliest possible point in the design process.

Once the MCS device concept is established, prototyping begins. This is a rapid phase of iteration where the design evolves many times before the final configuration is chosen. It can be said that it is better to fail early and often in this phase because mistakes and design modifications in later stages of the TPLC become very costly and time-consuming, jeopardizing the MCS development project altogether. For planning purposes, it can be expected that this phase of the TPLC will take 1–3 years to complete. Users' needs are of paramount importance in this phase and often involve outside expert advisory committees (clinicians, outside user communities, and patients) to help the MCS device developer meet the complex requirements associated with these medical devices. Rapid engineering feedback and design iteration are characteristics of this phase of the TPLC. Once the MCS device design is frozen, the next phase of the TPLC can begin, which is the preclinical engineering test phase.

Preclinical Testing

Preclinical testing is one of the most important and time-consuming phases of the TPLC for an MCS device. In general, MCS device developers should plan 4–5 years to complete this phase of the TPLC. A V&V master plan is first developed to define the testing requirements and the order in which they must be completed. A failure in this phase may mean an easy fix or may require a complete redesign, so this phase is one of the highest risk categories in the TPLC. Consideration must be given to material science, toxicity, biocompatibility, device characterization, limit testing, electrical safety, packaging, shelf life, software, reliability, sterilization, hazard analysis, manufacturability, human factor testing, and product quality requirements. Preclinical animal testing is also an important consideration in this phase and protocols should be developed based on prior experience, information within standards, and feedback gained from discussions with regulatory bodies. All preclinical testing should take into consideration the duration of intended use of the MCS device. In general, the longer the intended use, the longer the tests for safety and reliability should be conducted during preclinical testing.

It is usually early in this phase of the TPLC where there is the first opportunity to meet with regulators to discuss both design V&V requirements and plans for preclinical animal testing. In the United States, the MCS device developers may choose to request a presubmission meeting[24] with the FDA to discuss and receive informal input on the preclinical testing strategy. If the developer is in the EU, they may choose to meet with their EU Member State Accredited Notified Body who will ultimately evaluate the design, perform a conformity assessment, review and approval the premarket safety and effectiveness data, and authorize the MCS device to be CE Marked, allowing commercial placement onto the EU market. There are two points in the TPLC where presubmission meetings can be useful, one is to discuss the preclinical V&V requirements, including in vivo animal testing, and the other is to review the clinical trial strategy, analysis plan, and study protocol. Since the preclinical testing depends heavily upon whether the MCS device developer has performed sufficient testing to begin human clinical trials, it makes sense that these topics are discussed with the device regulators in two separate and distinct time points within the TPLC.

Clinical Testing

The study design used to support safety and effectiveness for an MCS device should be carefully considered. A good study design developed collaboratively with study investigators is likely to produce the best possible outcomes. A poor study design can cause lack of interest, failure to complete the study, and possibly uninterpretable data, causing a loss of time and resources and rendering the MCS device unapprovable. One example of a successfully designed MCS device clinical trial is the MOMENTUM 3 study of the HeartMate 3.[25] This was a prospective, randomized controlled trial that not only enrolled the largest number of patients of any previous MCS device study but also completed the enrollment in record time—a good example of what a collaborative effort with clinicians and regulators can mean in the execution of the clinical testing phase of the TPLC.

Efforts must be made upfront to design the trial so as to clearly demonstrate the MCS device is fit for its intended use. Other factors to be taken into consideration include study size, target patient population, duration of support, surgical considerations, statistical analysis, follow-up intervals, independent oversight committees, overall cost, and other factors that may be important for proper reimbursement once regulatory approvals are secured. In general, the clinical testing phase of the TPLC will take 3–5 years to complete. Some of the early MCS trials took twice as long to complete but less was known then compared with now, where device safety and performance characteristics are much more understood.

Sometimes, with a novel new MCS device or study design, it may be necessary to conduct a pilot study prior to beginning a pivotal trial, to better define the patient population, intended use, or appropriate outcome measures. If the MCS device is an iterative version based on historical previous devices and the intended use and patient populations are well known, a pilot phase can be incorporated into the pivotal study design.[25]

Just as with preclinical testing, the MCS device developers should plan to meet with the appropriate regulatory bodies to gain feedback on the proposed study design prior to submitting the application to begin the formal clinical trial. In the United States, the FDA regulates medical devices. To initiate a clinical trial for a Class III high-risk, life-sustaining medical device such as an MCS device, you must first get FDA approval. The regulatory process for gaining FDA approval to begin clinical trials is known as Investigational Device Exemption (IDE).[26] There are two categorizations for an IDE device: Category A (Experimental) or Category B (Nonexperimental/Investigational). IDE Category B allows CMS to cover both routine care items and services as well as the cost of the investigational device itself when specific criteria are met, while devices assigned to Category A are only eligible for payment of the routine services, not the device under investigation. Left ventricular assist devices (LVADs) have always been assigned Category B, and so all costs have been covered during the trials by Medicare and many commercial payers.

An IDE allows the MCS device developer to evaluate the safety and performance of the MCS device in a clinical trial environment. Once the MCS device developer has an approved IDE from the FDA, it can begin the process of gaining the necessary study site approvals so that enrollment can begin.

It is at this point the regulatory and reimbursement pathways must align. Prior to the IDE submission to the FDA, it is imperative that the CMS is engaged to determine not only if the study will be reimbursed but also if the endpoints will support the Medicare requirement that the device not only be safe and effective but also medically necessary and clinically beneficial with the Medicare population. As of January 1, 2015, sponsors requesting Medicare reimbursement during the clinical trial—which can include payment for the cost of the device—must submit a request for review and approval of IDE studies.[27] Once CMS has approved the clinical trial and the protocol has been accepted by the FDA, enrollment can begin.

Commercial payers have specific policies regarding coverage of any clinical trial. For example, the majority of Blue Cross Blue Shield plans do not reimburse the cost of the device but will cover the routine care surrounding the procedure, but some commercial payers will reimburse for the device as well as the hospitalization. It is important to gain commercial payers input prior to initiating a clinical trial so that the payers' concerns can be addressed prior to starting the trial, thus allowing for evidence development that can assist in creation or expansion of existing medial policies.

During an IDE study, if a need arises to implant an MCS device in a particular patient who may not qualify for the FDA-approved study, most likely due to the study's inclusion/exclusion criteria, there are provisions within the IDE regulations that allow for compassionate use of the device. If the treating physician believes that the investigational device may be the best option and provide a benefit to the patient, this provision can be used. Compassionate use must be approved by the MCS device developer (study sponsor) and the FDA prior to use. Another important provision of the IDE regulation is the emergency use provision. The emergency use provision can be used for an MCS device in situations where it is necessary to protect the life or physical well-being of a patient in an emergency. Although prior approval for shipment or emergency use of the investigational MCS device is not required prior to implant, the emergency use case is required to be reported post hoc to the FDA, confirming that in fact it was an emergency case and that patient protection measures were not violated. This would involve assuring informed consent, institutional clearance as specified by their policies, concurrence from the institutional review board (IRB) chair, independent assessment from an uninvolved physician, and approval by the IDE study sponsor (MCS device developer).

The required contents of an IDE application and details of both compassionate and emergency use are described in detail in 21 CFR Part 812[28] and in FDA Guidance documents,[26] available online from the FDA's website.

Prior to the submission of an IDE, MCS device developers are able and encouraged to meet with the FDA in a presubmission meeting (pre-IDE meeting). There are many advantages to doing this, and while this is an optional step, it may result in the least burdensome and quickest route to beginning the study. This is a nonbinding interactive meeting where the MCS device developer gains feedback on the proposed study design and other requirements relative to supporting documentation. Once the formal IDE is submitted to the FDA for consideration, they will evaluate the proposed study and supporting documentation to ensure that they meet an appropriate level of scientific rigor and comply with regulatory requirements as previously outlined and that the results from this study will likely provide adequate safety and effectiveness data to support future regulatory approval applications.

If clinical trials are planned in other countries, the MCS device developer should seek local regulatory expertise to ensure all in-country and appropriate regulatory requirements are met. For example, in the EU, if a clinical trial is planned in several EU member states, the MCS device developer should plan to meet with an appropriate accredited Notified Body and plan to gain in-country ministry of health approval, as well as hospital ethics committee (EC) and, in some cases, regional EC approvals before initiating the study. Canada, Australia, and Japan are examples of other countries that all have well-defined regulatory pathways to gain clinical trial approvals for high-risk, life-sustaining devices, including MCS devices.

Many countries such as Japan, France, and Belgium require that local patients be enrolled in the trial to secure reimbursement.[29] Each country has different requirements to gain reimbursement. A positive clinical trial supporting the clinical benefit to a defined population will greatly support in-country reimbursement.

While prospective randomized controlled trials are considered the gold standard design for new MCS devices, other trial designs can and have been used successfully to gain market approvals. Noncontrolled prospective study designs utilizing prespecified Objective Performance Criteria can be used if sufficient prior clinical data exist within a stable patient population. Other nonrandomized study designs can draw upon device registry data as a historical or concurrent control group, resulting in comparable outcomes that can be acceptable to regulatory agencies to support market approvals. The key to use of these alternatives is early collaboration with investigators and the appropriate regulatory bodies in the country where the clinical trial is planned to ensure that risks and benefit tradeoffs are well understood before proceeding. The goal of any prospective clinical trial should be to minimize patient risk, provide measurable benefit, allow evaluation to be completed in the shortest time possible, and produce valid scientific evidence that can be used to determine if the MCS device is safe and effective for its intended use. A well-designed study, executed properly and carefully controlled, can produce the desired results in the least burdensome way.

Another aspect of clinical trial design is planning for cost analysis of the procedure to support the value of the technology to the healthcare system. Data can be collected multiple ways, but the most common are either to collect claim-level data for each implant admission or readmission or to use big data sets, like the Medicare Limited Dataset inpatient data, or the Truven Marketscan data. With LVAD devices, a combination of claims data collected prospectively as part of the clinical trial and payer administrative claims databases was used, and all cost studies have been published.

Premarket Approval

High-risk, life-sustaining medical devices like an MCS device have the highest premarket regulatory approval requirements of any single use medical device. Most premarket regulatory reviews, regardless of country or region, can take a minimum of 6 months of substantive review time. More often, it can take somewhere between 12 and 18 months before a final market approval decision is rendered. In the United States, for an MCS device to gain commercial approval, a PMA Application must be submitted to the FDA. The PMA must contain sufficient valid scientific evidence to demonstrate reasonable assurance of safety and effectiveness when used for its intended use. The application includes information obtained from all prior studies (clinical and nonclinical) such as biocompatibility, device characterization and performance, durability, reliability, sterilization, shelf-life, and if applicable, software, electromagnetic compatibility, and electrical safety. The PMA must also include any other relevant bench or animal data, data from foreign studies, and most importantly, the final comprehensive results from the prospective studies described in the previous section (see "Clinical Testing" section).

In addition to being a time-consuming, thorough, and often interactive process, a PMA review performed by the FDA also requires the device developer to submit a user fee at the time the PMA is submitted. These fees are substantial and cover the cost of the FDA resources necessary to complete rigorous reviews. Once the FDA has completed an initial administrative review of the PMA, it is accepted for substantive review, and it can take several months before the MCS device developer will receive feedback on the progress of the review. Usually, by the third month of review, the FDA will provide the MCS device developer with a list of questions/deficiencies that must be addressed before the substantive review process can continue. Once adequate responses are submitted, the process becomes more interactive as each detail of the submission is carefully evaluated. The PMA process and regulatory requirements are in 21 CFR 814,[30] and refer to the PMA related Guidance documents[31] located on the FDA website.

Another option that may be an appropriate regulatory pathway to commercial use of certain MCS devices that are intended for use in a small and often underserved patient population is a humanitarian device exemption (HDE).[32] To qualify for HDE approval by the FDA, the MCS device developer must first gain a humanitarian use device (HUD) designation. To qualify for the HUD, the MCS device must be intended to benefit patients in the treatment or diagnosis of a disease or condition that affects or is manifested in fewer than 8000 individuals per year in the United States.[33] An HDE application is similar in both form and content to the PMA application previously described. The HDE application must provide the same level of assurance of safety as in a PMA, but the HDE is exempt from the requirements to demonstrate a reasonable assurance of effectiveness; rather, the MCS device sponsor must demonstrate that the probable benefit outweighs the probable risk. Once FDA approves the HDE application, the MCS device developer is authorized to market the HUD in the United States after obtaining IRB approval at each institution for the specific FDA-approved indication.

When FDA has completed its comprehensive review of the MCS device PMA or HDE application, it may decide to seek additional scientific review from expert advisory panels that are composed of independent external experts, familiar with the medical and surgical use of these devices and with knowledge of the disease state and patient populations, to help the FDA with important unanswered questions that must be addressed before the PMA or HDE application can be approved. Often, these expert advisory panels may help the FDA address important aspects such as which patients may benefit from the MCS device and other aspects concerning the use of the device to ensure that it is safe and effective for its intended purpose. Ultimately, the FDA carefully considers the totality of the data contained within the PMA and includes the recommendations/comments from the advisory panel in making a final decision on approvability.

Outside the United States, the regulatory approval process for MCS devices can vary greatly. In Europe, the process is well defined and similar to that in the United States. It requires data from prospective clinical trials conducted within the European community to gain authority commercially. An accredited Notified Body from an EU member state must be involved. The regulatory process involves demonstrating conformity to EU Directives (active implantable devices) and submitting a design dossier to an appointed Notified Body for review. The design dossier is similar in content to the PMA required in the United States. The overall review timeframe mirrors the FDA process and the Notified Body also has an independent scientific review committee that must review and approve the Design Dossier before they can grant the authority to affix the CE Mark to the MCS device. Once this is granted, the MCS device may be marketed within the 28 countries that comprise the EU.

Most of the Tier I countries have a similar process for the premarket evaluation of MCS devices and therefore will not be further delineated within this chapter.

CREATING REIMBURSEMENT FOR LEFT VENTRICULAR ASSIST DEVICES

LVADs used as DT are an example of expansion of an existing technology, but because of the complexity involved with creating reimbursement, the timeframe is more reflective of the most complicated type, or "innovative therapy," described earlier. In 2002, the REMATCH (Randomized Evaluation of Mechanical Assistance for the Treatment of Congestive Heart Failure) trial had been completed, showing efficacy of the device over medical therapy, but there was no payer coverage, no administrative codes, and no payment for devices used for DT.[34] Every reimbursement structure had to be created—from influencing Health Technology Assessments for commercial payer coverage and defining a Medicare National Coverage Decision to clarifying coding in every system. Payment had to be established under the Medicare inpatient diagnosis-related group (DRG) system and, when possible, during clinical trials. Reimbursement for the physician's surgical procedures, replacement of outpatient accessories and supplies required to support discharge of the LVAD patient, and interrogation of the LVAD itself were also necessary. As MCS patient care evolves, new reimbursement structures will need to be analyzed and, when appropriate, created.

So how were these roads to reimbursement created? All reimbursement starts with the concept that the technology is "reasonable and necessary" to warrant payment. All coverage starts with clinical studies that show clinical benefit to the population treated.

Today, ventricular assist device (VAD) therapy is a well-established treatment for end-stage heart failure, with more than 45,000 long-term VAD implants performed in hospitals across the United States since the early 1980s.[35] VADs have been covered by Medicare and most other commercial payers for postcardiotomy use since 1993 and for BTT since 1996. In October 2003, CMS issued a National Coverage Determination (NCD) for VADs used for DT, which was updated in 2007, in 2010, and again in 2013.[36] The initial NCD was based on key studies, which showed significant clinical and quality-of-life benefits to end-stage heart failure patients who were implanted with VADs for DT and the updates provided additional clarifications on center-specific certification.

The 2000s saw a different era in VADs emerge. With a limited number of donor hearts available, VADs were presented as the solution for end-stage heart failure patients who became refractory to medical management. Thoratec Corporation (Pleasanton, CA, now part of Abbott), in conjunction with the National Institutes of Health, conducted a study of VADs for end-stage heart failure patients ineligible for cardiac transplant, either because of age or other complicating factors, referred to as DT. The FDA provided expedited review of the PMA application based on the landmark REMATCH trial results and granted approval in November 2002. Blue Cross Blue Shield conducted its own Technology Evaluation Center report on DT and concluded that the therapy met its criteria for coverage in October 2002.[37]

During 2001, when the REMATCH trial outcomes had been published in the *New England Journal of Medicine*, Thoratec Corporation began working with CMS to open a dialogue around the potential for an NCD for DT before FDA approval. Numerous meetings with CMS officials were held over the next 2 years to establish the clinically appropriate conditions for coverage, with the support of multiple clinical societies. The technology received Medicare Evidence Development and Coverage Advisory Committee (MEDCAC) endorsement in March 2003. This led to Medicare's decision in October 2003 to establish coverage nationally for a narrow population (limiting the definition of DT to the clinical parameters of the REMATCH trial), and Medicare required certification of centers that would perform these surgeries.[38]

In the 1990s, private payers were somewhat familiar with VAD technologies but did not have coverage for DT.

For the first time, a coalition of hospitals, providers, medical societies, and manufacturers came together to advocate for patients to have access to a very innovative technology, which was disruptive to the current standard of care. With that support, commercial payers modified their policies to include DT within 3 months of the CMS NCD.

The body of clinical evidence and how it is used significantly affects CMS coverage determinations. The hierarchy of evidence favors randomized, double-blind, placebo-controlled studies published in a peer-reviewed (preferably US) journal. Less attractive are open-label trials in which both patients and physicians know that the patient is receiving the product or retrospective studies in which charts are reviewed sometime after a group of patients has received a treatment. Case studies are rarely considered in a technology coverage decision. Fig. 21.2 illustrates this hierarchy of clinical evidence and the impact on coverage.

In the case of the VAD, the strength of the published controlled studies supported both CMS and private payers' national DT coverage decisions. With the determination that DT was effective, the question of efficiency or value of the technology in treating end-stage heart failure patients was raised. Determining the cost of a technology is one way of defining value.

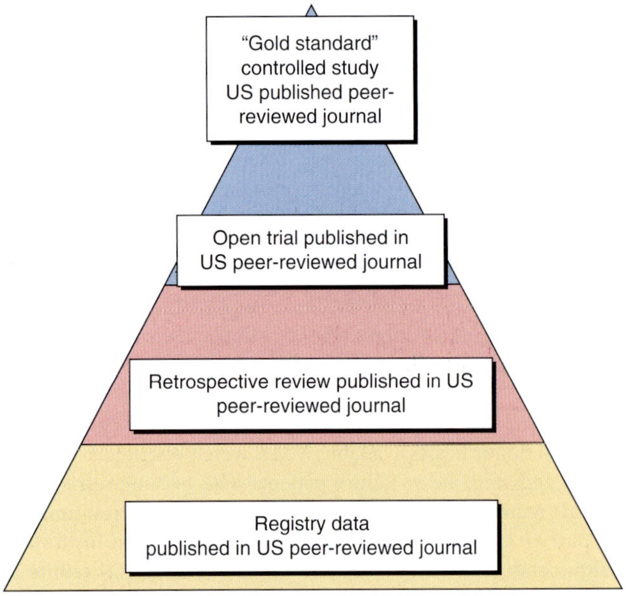

Fig. 21.2 Hierarchy of clinical evidence.

TABLE 21.3 Mechanical Circulatory Support Diagnosis-Related Group Assignment Changes

Fiscal Year	DRG	Description	Approx. Payment
Before 2003	DRG 108	Other cardiothoracic procedures	(>$35,000[a])
2003	DRG 104/105	Cardiac valve and other major cardiothoracic procedures with or without catheterization	($35,000[a])
2004	DRG 525	Heart assist system implants	($54,000[a])
2005	DRG 103	Heart transplant and implanted heart assist + CMS Destination Therapy coverage[b]	($98,000[a])
2008 forward	MS-DRG 1/2	Heart transplant and implanted heart assist with or without complications	($140,000–$300,000[a])

[a]Payment is based on CMS DRG rates and varies by hospital
[b]Inpatient hospital payment increased with CMS destination therapy coverage.
CMS, Centers for Medicare and Medicaid Services; *DRG*, diagnosis-related group.

Pathways to Payment

After obtaining national coverage for DT in 2003, it was important to establish adequate payment to cover the cost of the therapy. Historically, hospitals were reimbursed approximately $35,000 for the VAD implant hospitalization, because there was no specific DRG used to identify the procedure. Table 21.3 shows the DRG assignment and base rate payment over time.

During the coverage process in 2002, 2 years of claims data for DT cases were provided to CMS, reflecting the need to increase the inpatient hospital DRG payment. Implanting hospital champions worked tirelessly with clinical and cost data to educate CMS about the clinical benefits and value of the technology. As a result, payment for DT hospitalizations increased over time, culminating in assignment of VAD procedures to the heart transplant DRG in October 2003. This was a phenomenal achievement, as the typical path to adequate payment for an innovative technology can take 2 to 3 years. In 2018, the current average hospital Medicare payment for DT is approximately $196,000.[39]

Cost-effectiveness

The evolution of VAD therapy for advanced heart failure has been unique when compared to other devices and pharmacological therapy. The change from pulsatile- to continuous-flow VAD technology was relatively rapid as clinicians identified the benefits of the smaller and more durable devices. The "learning curve" associated with the application of the continuous-flow devices was relatively short, and outcomes have improved steadily over the 15 years since their inception. In this same timeframe, the Incremental Cost Effectiveness Ratio (ICER) for pulsatile VADs during the REMATCH trial was $602,361, which then decreased to $187,989 in the posttrial time, and then to $107,569 with the use of the current continuous-flow devices (Fig. 21.3).[40] This progress in cost-effectiveness is compelling, yet controlled unbiased data from clinical trials that guides policy decisions is still needed. Furthermore, because VAD technology is constantly evolving and patient care improves with experience, cost-effectiveness analysis also needs to be continuous and its methods developed.

POSTMARKET STUDIES/SURVEILLANCE

Regardless of country or region of the world where the MCS device was approved, the developer/manufacturer of the MCS device may be required to conduct additional postapproval studies and this is mandated in the United States.[41] The purpose of these studies is to gain additional experience on the safety and performance of the MCS device in a commercial setting. Postapproval studies are beneficial for collecting additional data regarding real-world use, longer-term device reliability, usefulness of training programs, subgroup evaluation within the approved patient population, and evaluation of rare adverse events. Postapproval studies often require 2- to 5-year follow-up on patients implanted with the MCS device and require ongoing clinical summary evaluations to be developed as part of the continuing postapproval reporting to meet the regulatory conditions of approval.

Postmarket surveillance is another tool that can help regulatory bodies gather additional data on the safety and performance in a commercial setting. In the United States, FDA has authority to mandate postmarket surveillance studies under Section 522 of the Food, Drug, and Cosmetic Act[42] and often does so when a Class III medical device such as an MCS device could fail and, if it did so, would be reasonably likely to cause serious injury or have serious adverse health consequences. In May 2016, FDA also released its most recent final guidance document on postmarket surveillance,[43] which can be found on FDA's website. MCS device developers/manufacturers also are subject to Medical Device Reporting regulations.[44] This postmarket surveillance tool requires mandatory reporting requirements for manufacturers, importers, and device user facilities to report certain device-related adverse events and product problems to the FDA.

In Europe, the European Medical Device Directive[45] states that medical device manufacturers are legally required to report adverse incidents to the EU Competent Authorities. Similar rules and regulations exist in many countries throughout the world, but as previously mentioned, no effort has yet been made to harmonize these requirements into a single standard reporting criterion. These postmarket surveillance and vigilance reporting requirements go on for the life of the device. Devices that are investigational and under clinical evaluation are not required to meet these requirements until they are available for commercial use.

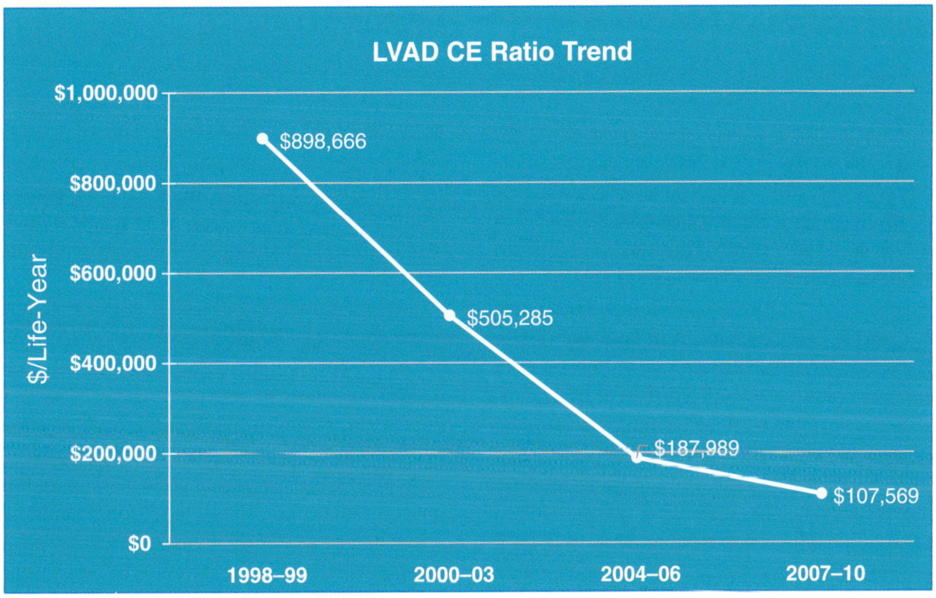

Fig. 21.3 Left ventricular assist device *(LVAD)* cost-effectiveness *(CE)* over time.

DEVICE TRACKING

MCS devices are implantable, high-risk, life-sustaining medical devices and as such are subject to US Federal Medical Device Tracking Regulations.[46] These regulations are intended to ensure that subject medical devices can be tracked from the place they were manufactured to the person in whom the device was implanted (the patient). This regulation also comes with significant requirements for the MCS device developer/manufacturer to maintain very specific patient-related information throughout the use of the device, and these records must be maintained for as long as the device remains implanted in the patient or the MCS device remains in distribution, whichever is longer.

MECHANICAL CIRCULATORY SUPPORT DEVICE REGISTRIES

In October 2003, when CMS created their NCD for VADs, a registry was required as part of the coverage with evidence development. In December 2003, the National Heart, Lung, and Blood Institute (NHLBI) put out a Request for Information, seeking interested parties in the development of an MCS device registry. This led to a collaborative effort between the NHLBI, the FDA, the CMS, and the advanced heart failure/MCS device community to establish the Interagency Registry for Mechanically Assisted Circulatory Support, known as INTERMACS. Data collection in this registry began in June 2006 with 15 participating MCS device implanting centers.[47] Today, it is considered a model for postmarket registries, with more than 26,000 noninvestigational MCS device implants at 180 centers within the United States. Hundreds of publications and presentations have stemmed from this registry, and it has been the genesis for improvements in quality of care not only at the individual participating hospital level but also across the world for patients treated with MCS device therapy. INTERMACS served its purpose, meeting the continual evidence requirement from CMS. INTERMACS was one of the first interagency registries created to report ongoing outcomes of patients supported by an implantable device. This was the first Coverage With Evidence Development program that CMS created, long before they coined the phrase. The 2012 Medicare Evidence Development and Coverage Advisory Committee (MEDCAC) determined that enough data had been collected, which further validated the clinical benefit of LVAD therapy to the Medicare population; therefore, CMS no longer required participation in INTERMACS as they felt the data gathered was sufficient to ensure the safety and effectiveness of LVADs per the 2013 update to the NCD.[27] However, participation in a national, audited registry is still a requirement of the Joint Commission,[38] one of the bodies that certifies centers for DT implantation, and so it remains in widespread use.

The INTERMACS registry has stimulated the development of numerous other MCS device registries worldwide, including European Registry for Patients With Mechanical Circulatory Support (EUROMACS)[48] (a pan-European registry), JMACS[49] (a Japanese registry), Pediatric Interagency Registry for Mechanical Circulatory Support (PEDIMACS)[50] (a US registry to collect data on MCS device use in the pediatric population), and International Registry for Mechanical Circulatory Support (IMACS)[51] (an international registry sponsored by International Society Heart and Lung Transplantation (ISHLT) aimed at consolidating individual registry data on the worldwide use of MCS devices).

The INTERMACS registry can only be described as a revolution in the field of MCS. It has been used as both a historical and concurrent control for prospective MCS device studies and for collecting data to meet the condition of approval mandated postmarket studies. Beginning in January 2018, the oversight and management of this important registry have shifted from the University of Alabama/NHLBI to the Society of Thoracic Surgeons,[52] a change that promises only further continuous improvement that serves as a vital backbone of the advanced heart failure/MCS device community.

MECHANICAL CIRCULATORY SUPPORT DEVICE CORRECTIONS AND REMOVALS (RECALLS)

MCS devices are tested for durability and reliability over the expected life of the product and during actual clinical studies for several years of real-world use before they are finally approved for commercial use. We now know that MCS devices continue to be used to sustain life in advanced heart failure patients for much longer periods than initially anticipated. These patients resume normal activities, which can create wear and tear on the MCS device for support periods exceeding

10 years. Much has been learned since the early 2000s about MCS device use, but as much as is now known, it is very difficult to anticipate every possible use and failure mode that can occur over the expected life of the MCS device.

As the MCS device developer/manufacturer learns more about the use of these devices through the product complaint process, postmarket studies, normal commercial use, and through data collected in registries such as INTERMACS, it periodically may become necessary to provide the patients and user community with additional information about the safe use of the device. Additionally, unanticipated adverse events may occur at any time or component/software-related failures may necessitate the MCS device manufacturer to initiate the device correction and removal process (recall). This can be in the form of additional safety information, a physical modification or software update, or in the worst-case scenario, a physical device removal from the market. Like all other processes within the TPLC, there are formal regulatory procedures that must be followed when such actions are initiated by the MCS device developer/manufacturer. In the United States, it comes in the form of a Code of Federal Regulations 21 CFR Part 806 entitled Medical Device Correction and Removals.[53] These actions are considered a recall and are usually taken voluntarily by the MCS device developer/manufacturer. In rare incidences, if the action is not taken voluntarily, the FDA can mandate a recall to protect public health.[54] Specific information and regulatory requirements associated with a correction and removal activity can be found in Guidance documents on FDA's website.

Similar regulatory processes exist in other countries outside the United States. Usually, when such actions are necessary, it is important to know the correction and removal (recall) regulatory requirements in all countries where the product is marketed to ensure compliance as these actions are most often global in nature and not limited to a specific country or regions of the world.

OBSOLESCENCE

The final phase of the TPLC is obsolescence. Given that MCS devices have a relatively long TPLC, by the time of obsolescence, much has been learned about the use of the device, training, and complication factors. A typical MCS device will have a TPLC of 15+ years accumulating extensive patient years of support experience by this phase of the TPLC. The product experience, both good and bad, is useful in the development of the next-generation device. Also, the risk analysis information for all intended uses can be updated and utilized in the development of next-generation devices. Through this evolutionary process, MCS device developers can improve the patient care experience. While MCS devices have proven to be mechanically very reliable over many years of use, the man-machine interfacing components such as cables, controllers, batteries, and software can and must be improved in iterative generations of MCS devices. Also, several nagging adverse events remain, namely, bleeding, infection, and strokes. Future generations must be designed to eliminate these complications. If MCS device developers can do this successfully, making implant techniques simple and extremely reproducible, MCS will vastly improve the patient's quality of life, and this important therapeutic option will become the standard of care for advanced heart failure and a viable alternative for orthotopic heart transplantation.

Although products may become obsolete, and iterative changes may be made, the health policy that supports its usage for a specific population will continue to evolve based upon the next generation of device. As the clinical trials further expand and define the appropriate population who can most benefit, the health policy must also be modified to reflect these changes.

LESSONS LEARNED

In a perfect world, device regulatory and reimbursement would be more simply laid out. Randomized, double-blinded, placebo-controlled studies would report clear, statistically significant long-term clinical benefits for patients in need and simultaneously demonstrate cost-effectiveness to regulators. An independent patient registry would follow, monitored by a medical group with no connections to the manufacturer, and ongoing peer-reviewed publications would be produced from this registry.

Many companies designing innovative devices are start-ups with one technology. Financial resources are limited. Meetings with investors seem continuous, with reimbursement an important issue in investors' decisions to provide funding. The need to show any clinical benefit early often outweighs the need to construct a comprehensive body of clinical evidence that will satisfy payers' requirements. Despite early positive trials, payers often require additional studies specific to their population or simply additional studies so that substantial evidence demonstrates the benefit of the device. Although such requirements sometimes seem, at best, arbitrary by the payers, identifying the likely payers for a product, and even "partnering" with them in planning studies so the results address their needs, can save years in the reimbursement process.

Reimbursement can translate to financial viability, which can mean life or death to a technology or a field. During product development, attention to clinical, regulatory, sales, and marketing should be coupled with attention to reimbursement. Almost immediately, a company must start defining who will primarily receive the product and who then will pay for it. In addition, other issues such as who will "own" the product (the patient, the payer, the hospital, the physician) and who will do the procedure and in what setting become important in defining a reimbursement plan.

Ideally, reimbursement should be considered before the creation of the first clinical protocol. Attention should be directed to what potential indications are being studied and what effects this product will have on the quality of life for populations such as the Medicare and private payer populations. Once this is determined, meetings with medical directors of the payers who will potentially reimburse for the technology are helpful, if not essential. In preparation for meeting with potential payers, the company should consider how the resulting indications benefit this payer's population.

A positive coverage decision also drives the need for a code to identify the product and/or procedures. These codes help to establish payment by Medicare and private payers. However, confirmation of existing codes that can be used for the product can be determined before FDA approval. Applications for new codes usually require 6 months of FDA postmarket approval volume of at least 300 procedures to demonstrate a need for a new code, and two publications from different authors. Companies must also anticipate costs to the health care system, because it is increasingly necessary to prove a product is not only clinically beneficial but also cost effective and has value to the health care system.

CONCLUSIONS

The regulatory and reimbursement processes for life-sustaining medical devices have evolved significantly and expanded globally during the past 50 years. Despite efforts to harmonize requirements across Tier 1 developed countries, the goal of a single regulatory and reimbursement framework for medical devices remains elusive. A regulatory and reimbursement product plan should be created together during the early phase of development and adjusted throughout the product life cycle with the emphasis on creating ongoing evidence to support the appropriate device use. The goal of these regulatory and reimbursement processes is to deliver a commercially successful product that is both safe and effective (regulatory standard) as well as reasonable and necessary (reimbursement standard). If each is treated separately and implemented linearly rather than collectively, significant market access delays and restrictions can be anticipated.

REFERENCES

1. Act of June 25, 1938 (Federal Food, Drug, and Cosmetic Act), Public Law 75-717, 52 STAT 1040, which prohibited the movement in interstate commerce of adulterated and misbranded food, drugs, devices, and cosmetics.
2. Milestones in medical technology from eyeglasses to the stethoscope to imaging the brain at work, a long list of inventions and innovation have changed medicine. *The New York Times*, October 10, 2012. https://archive.nytimes.com/www.nytimes.com/interactive/2012/10/05/health/digital-doctor.html#/#time15_375. Accessed May 3, 2018.
3. Fair Packaging and Labeling Act. *First enactment*. November 3, 1966. Pub. L. 89-. 755,80 Stat. 1296. Amended: October 22, 1968, Pub. L. 90-. 628,2 82 Stat. 1320. January 2,. 1975, Pub. L. 93-608, 88 Stat. 1972. Current law: l. 15 U.S.C. §§1451-1461.
4. 94th U.S. Congress (December 11, 1975). "H.R.11124: Medical Device Amendments." *U.S. House of Representative Bill Summary & Status*. Library of Congress THOMAS.
5. 101st U.S. Congress (August 2, 1989). "H.R.3095: Safe Medical Devices Act of 1990." *U.S. House of Representative Bill Summary & Status*. Library of Congress THOMAS.
6. 105th U.S. Congress (April 23, 1997). "H.R.1411: Food and Drug Administration Regulatory Modernization Act of 1997." *U.S. House of Representative Bill Summary & Status*. Library of Congress THOMAS.
7. 107th U.S. Congress (October 15, 2002). "H.R. 5651:" Medical Device User Fee and Modernization Act of 2002.
8. 109th U.S. Congress (August 1, 2005) "H.R. 3423 (109th):" Medical Device User Fee Stabilization Act of 2005.
9. 110th U.S. Congress (September 27, 2007) H.R. 3580: Food and Drug Administration Amendments Act of 2007.
10. 112th U.S. Congress (July 9, 2012) S.3187: Food and Drug Administration Safety and Innovation Act of 2012.
11. (Public Law 106-554, December 21, 2000) The Medicare, Medicaid and SCHIP Benefits Improvement and Protection Act of 2000 (BIPA), enacted as part of the appropriations bill for the Departments of Labor and Health and Human Services (Public Law 106-554, 12/21/2000).
12. Medicare Prescription Drug, Improvement, and Modernization Act (MMA) of 2003, Public Law 108–173. https://www.gpo.gov/fdsys/pkg/PLAW-108publ173/pdf/PLAW-108publ173.pdf. Accessed May 3, 2018.
13. Patient Protection and Affordable Care Act, Public Law 111–148—March 23, 2010. https://www.gpo.gov/fdsys/pkg/PLAW-111publ148/pdf/PLAW-111publ148.pdf. Accessed May 3, 2018.
14. 21st Century Cures Act, HB6, passed the House of Representatives 7/10/16. https://www.congress.gov/bill/114th-congress/house-bill/6. Accessed May 3, 2018.
15. Thomasson Melissa. In: Whaples Robert, ed. *Health Insurance in the United States*; April 17, 2003. EH.Net Encyclopedia. Tucson, AZ: Economic History Association. Accessed May 1, 2018.
16. 12002E095; Treaty establishing the European Community (Nice consolidated version) Part Three: Community policies—Title VI: Common rules on competition, taxation and approximation of laws—Chapter 3: Approximation of laws—Article 95—EC Treaty.
17. EU Publications; Guide to the implementation of directives based on new approach and the global approach; Published 2000-05-16; Catalog #: CO-22-99-014-EN-C.
18. Regulation (EU) 2017/745 of the European Parliament and of the Council of 5 April 2017. on medical devices, amending Directive 2001/83/EC, Regulation (EC) No 178/2002 and Regulation (EC) No 1223/2009 and repealing Council Directives 90/385/EEC and 93/42/EEC.
19. Title 21—Food and Drugs Chapter 9—Federal Food, Drug, and Cosmetic Act, Section 802; Listed (Tier 1) Countries; February 20, 2018.
20. Title 21—Food and Drugs Chapter I—Food and Drug Administration; Department of Health and Human Services; Subchapter H—Medical Devices; part 860 Medical Device Classification Procedures CFR—Code of Federal Regulations Title 21. U.S. Food and Drug Administration 15 Oct 2010.
21. AdvaMed, https://www.advamed.org/sites/default/files/resource/advamedreportshortpaper_08v2.pdf. Accessed May 3, 2018.
22. Hausman ED, Altaie SS. Regulatory aspects of total product life cycle. *Diabetes Technol Ther*. 2004;6(6):761–766.
23. ANSI AAMI ISO 14708-5:2010 (R2015) Implants for surgery—active implantable medical devices—part 5: Circulatory support devices.
24. Request for Feedback on Medical Device Submissions; the Pre-Submission Program and Meetings with FDA Staff—final guidance; February 18, 2014.
25. Heatley G, Sood P, Goldstein D, et al. Clinical trial design and rationale of the Multicenter Study of MagLev Technology in Patients undergoing Mechanical Circulatory Support Therapy with HeartMate 3 (MOMENTUM 3) investigational device exemption clinical study protocol. *J Heart Lung Transplant*. 2016;35(4):528–536.
26. U.S. Food and Drug Administration. Medical Devices; Investigation Device Exemption (IDE). *Investigational Approval Process*. December 22, 2017;.
27. CMS Coverage Website at. http://www.cms.gov/Medicare/Coverage/IDE/index.html.
28. Code of Federal Regulations; Title 21, Volume 8, Part 812, Subchapter H - Medical Devices, Investigational Device Exemptions, April 1, 2017.
29. Haute Autorité de Santé, https://www.has-sante.fr/portail/upload/docs/application/pdf/2010-03/guide_dm_gb_050310.pdf. Accessed May 3, 2018.
30. Code of Federal Regulations; Title 21, Volume 8, Part 814, Subchapter H - Medical Devices, Premarket Approval of Medical Devices, April 1, 2017.
31. U.S. Food and Drug Administration. Medical Devices. *Premarket Approval Process (PMA)*. March 27, 2018.
32. U.S. Food and Drug Administration. Medical Devices. *Humanitarian Device Exemption (HDE)*. March 27, 2018.
33. Code of Federal Regulations. *Title 21, Volume 8, Part 814, Subchapter H - Medical Devices, Premarket Approval of Medical Devices, Section 8143 Definitions*. April 1, 2017. Subpart (n) Humanitarian Use Device (HUD).
34. Rose EA, Gelijns AC, Moskowitz AJ, et al. Long-term use of a left ventricular assist device for end-stage heart failure. *N Engl J Med*. 2001;345:1435–1443.
35. INTERMACS, internal Abbott proprietary database, Medtronic Annual Report.
36. CMS Decision Memo for Ventricular Assist Devices as Destination Therapy (CAG-00119R). https://www.cms.gov/medicare-coverage-database/details/nca-decision-memo.aspx?NCAId=243&NcaName=Ventricular+Assist+Devices+as+Destination+Therapy+(2nd+Recon)&fromdb=true. Accessed May 3, 2018.
37. Blue Cross Blue Shield Association Medical Advisory Panel. Special report: Cost effectiveness of left ventricular assist devices as destination therapy for end stage heart failure. *Blue cross Blue Shield Technology Evaluation Center Bulletin*. 2004;19(2):1–29.
38. Joint Commission. http://jointcommission.org/CertificationPrograms/LeftVentricularAssistDevices/. Accessed May 3, 2018.
39. Centers for Medicare and Medicaid Services. The FY 2018 Hospital Inpatient Prospective Payment System Final Rule.
40. Gelijn A, et al. Dynamics of Device Innovation. *INTL J J of Technology Assessment in Health Care*. 2013;29(4).
41. Code of Federal Regulations; Title 21, Volume 8, Part 814, Subchapter H—Medical Devices, Premarket Approval of Medical Devices, Subpart E—Post Approval Requirements, Section 814.82, Post Approval Requirements.
42. United States Food and Drug Administration (2013) 522 Postmarket Surveillance Studies. http://www.accessdata.fda.gov/scripts/cdrh/cfdocs/cfPMA/pss.cfm. Accessed May 3, 2018.
43. U.S. Food and Drug Administration. *Center for Devices and Radiological Health, Office of Surveillance and Biometrics, Division of Epidemiology, Post Market Surveillance Under Section 522 of the Federal Food, Drug and Cosmetic Act, Guidance for industry and FDA Staff*; May 16, 2016.
44. Code of Federal Regulations, Title 21, Subchapter H—Medical Devices, Part 803. *Medical Device Reporting*. February 14, 2014.

45. Council Directive 93/42/EEC of 14 June 1993[1] concerning medical devices, OJ No L 169/1 of 1993-07-12.
46. Code of Federal Regulations, Title 21, Subchapter H—Medical Devices, Part 803. *Medical Device Reporting*. February 14, 2014.
47. Miller MA, Ulisney K, Baldwin JT. INTERMACS (Interagency Registry of Mechanically Assisted Circulatory Support): a new paradigm for translating registry data into clinical practice. *J Am Coll Cardiol*. 2010;56(9):738–740.
48. EUROMACS Registry. https://www.euromacs.org/about. Accessed May 3, 2018.
49. JMACS Registry. https://www.pmda.go.jp/english/safety/surveillance-analysis/0003.html. Accessed May 3, 2018.
50. PEDIMACS Registry. https://www.uab.edu/medicine/intermacs/pedimacs. Accessed May 3, 2018.
51. IMACS Registry. https://ishlt.org/registries/international-registry-for-mechanically-assisted-c. Accessed May 3, 2018.
52. The Society of Thoracic Surgeons, Registries and Research Center, STS National Database. STS INTERMACS Database. https://www.sts.org/registries-research-center/sts-national-database/sts-intermacs-database. Accessed May 3, 2018.
53. Code of Federal Regulations. *Title 21, Subchapter H—Medical Devices, Part 806 Medical Device Reports of Corrections and Removals*; August 14, 2017.
54. FDA Brings Patients Into the Process. Posted September 20, 2013 by FDA Voice. https://blogs.fda.gov/fdavoice/index.php/2013/09/fda-brings-patients-into-the-process/.

22

The Future of Mechanical Circulatory Support

James W. Long, Richard Wampler

KEY POINTS

I. THE TRAIL BLAZED AND THE PATHWAY AHEAD

As the field of Mechanical Circulatory Support (MCS) reaches into its sixth decade beyond first laboratory experimentation, it behooves us to reflect on the historical, pioneering advances on which the future will be leveraged. Such reflection is most valuable when it inspires the thoughtful to blaze new trials.

Much has been accomplished. The field is tantalizingly close to the holy grail of delivering amazing technologies for (1) extending *life* with (2) *quality* and (3) *safety* with (4) *easier-to-use* therapies applied at the (5) optimum *time* in (6) properly selected heart failure *patients* while (7) achieving *cost-effectiveness*.

And, yet, much remains. The good news is that the pace of progress is accelerating. Hopefully, we are in the final decade of pioneering.

Survival with durable MCS devices is finally approaching that of heart transplantation. The vision of suitable *quality of life* is within sight.

However, we are still in the early stages of assuring *safety*, which has been limited by *adverse events* (AEs). This problem continues to compromise patients with *morbidity and mortality*, to burden caretakers with the *rigors of management*, and to strain our healthcare systems with *excessive costs*. All of that inhibits expansion into earlier stages of heart failure.

Despite the marvels of engineering underlying today's blood pumps, their interface and interactions with their hosts remain to be perfected. The single most important opportunity to reduce AEs is through preventing sublethal blood damage. Advances in the science of *hemocompatibility*, as applied to device design and testing, have opened the door for a next generation of devices that will overcome factors that contribute to bleeding, thrombosis, strokes, infection, and inflammation. Other device-host interfaces to be addressed include those that deliver improved durability, enhanced functionality, expanded indications for use, quality of life, and ease of use.

Fortunately, we have learned that it is not only technology, but also management and patient factors, that impacts outcomes in the MCS field. While we continue to await perfected *technology*, the field will continue to see improvements through advances in *management*, of both pumps and patients, and through advances in optimizing *patients* and their selection. That will best be facilitated by *organization* and integration of MCS field-wide efforts.

Indeed, the future is promising. Our mission now is to deliver on the goals so long envisioned.

II. THE FUTURE IS LEVERAGING THE PAST

There is much to be learned by understanding historical roots. In the words of Winston Churchill, "those who fail to learn from history are doomed to repeat it."

Early Goals of Life, and then Life Outside the Hospital

The pioneering, clinical experience with durable, implantable blood pumps began in earnest in the late 1980s. In that early era, it was a remarkable breakthrough to offer *hope of life* to patients declining while awaiting heart transplantation and then, ultimately, offer *hope for quality of life*.

The first device to complete a controlled, clinical trial culminating in US Food and Drug Administration (FDA) approval in 1994 for bridging to transplantation was the HeartMate IP (Thermo CardioSystems, Boston, MA), an implantable, pulsatile left ventricular assist device (LVAD) powered pneumatically by a 90-pound external console. Patients received a survival benefit but remained hospital bound.[1] A portable, 25-pound, pneumatic driver subsequently offered patients greater mobility and early experience with discharge. Electrically powered blood pumps, emerging with the next-generation HeartMate series, the VE and XVE LVADs, were the next to receive FDA approval. This opened the era of outpatient LVAD support and improved quality of life with patients engaging in light recreation and with some returning to their occupations.

That first-generation implantable technology[2] was limited by *durability*, with mechanical bearing and tissue valve failures occurring on average at 1.5 years. *Infections* were problematic, especially with the early, large, rigid percutaneous leads. However, an advantage of that technology that has yet to be reproduced is *freedom from anticoagulation* more than aspirin.

Exploring Long-Term Life with 'Destination Therapy'

A decade later, in the late 1990s, the field began the transition to long-term implantation, introducing the era of so-called *destination therapy* (DT), moving beyond bridging to transplantation. The National Institutes of Health (NIH)-supported Randomized Evaluation of Mechanical Assistance for the Treatment of Congestive Heart Failure (REMATCH) trial became the setting for the first randomized controlled trial of LVAD therapy with the HeartMate XVE compared to optimum medical management over a 2-year period of observation.[3]

Patients receiving an LVAD lived longer, demonstrating a survival benefit greater than any other heart failure therapy previously studied. The hoped-for improvement in quality of life appeared believable. However, mortality (23% survival at 2 years) and morbidity (especially with pump failures and infections) were still considerable, well behind outcomes with heart transplantation. That was not too surprising considering that the population studied had the most advanced level of heart failure ever studied up to that time.

The REMATCH trial served as an early catalyst to the field, opening the door to the long sought-after goal of life-long therapy. Data from that trial were used to secure Medicare approvals for *reimbursement* at levels that permitted cautious growth of the field. And, *clinical teams* began forming, with the important, high-profile entry of heart failure cardiologists joining the efforts of the heart surgeons whose leadership had been instrumental during the early startup stages of the MCS field.

The Pathway to Improvement

The pioneering efforts of the late 1980s through the 1990s were leveraged into an era of progressive improvement throughout the decade of the 2000s.[4,5] Blood pump therapy had to improve substantially to begin approaching heart transplantation, the 'gold-standard' for end-stage heart failure at that time. It would have to follow the precedent observed with heart transplantation in which humble beginnings during the initial pioneering stages gave way to progressively improving outcomes.

Three areas of improvement would be necessary:

1. *Technology*, including a new-generation of blood pumps;
2. *Management*, of both the patients and devices; and
3. *Patient selection*, based on new insight into patient risk factors.

The course to be followed for outcomes improvement, throughout that next era and into the future, is illustrated in Fig. 22.1. The survival outcomes for the pioneering phase of MCS, represented by the 2-year survival curve with LVADs observed during the REMATCH trial, are superimposed on the 17-year survival curve for heart transplantation in the current era. Improving outcomes with MCS would be driven by the three factors most responsible: technology, management, and patient selection.

TECHNOLOGY Breakthroughs

It once was considered dogma that *continuous-flow pumps* with rotors spinning at high speeds would not be suitable for blood, given expectations of unacceptable hemolysis. This myth was dispelled with the

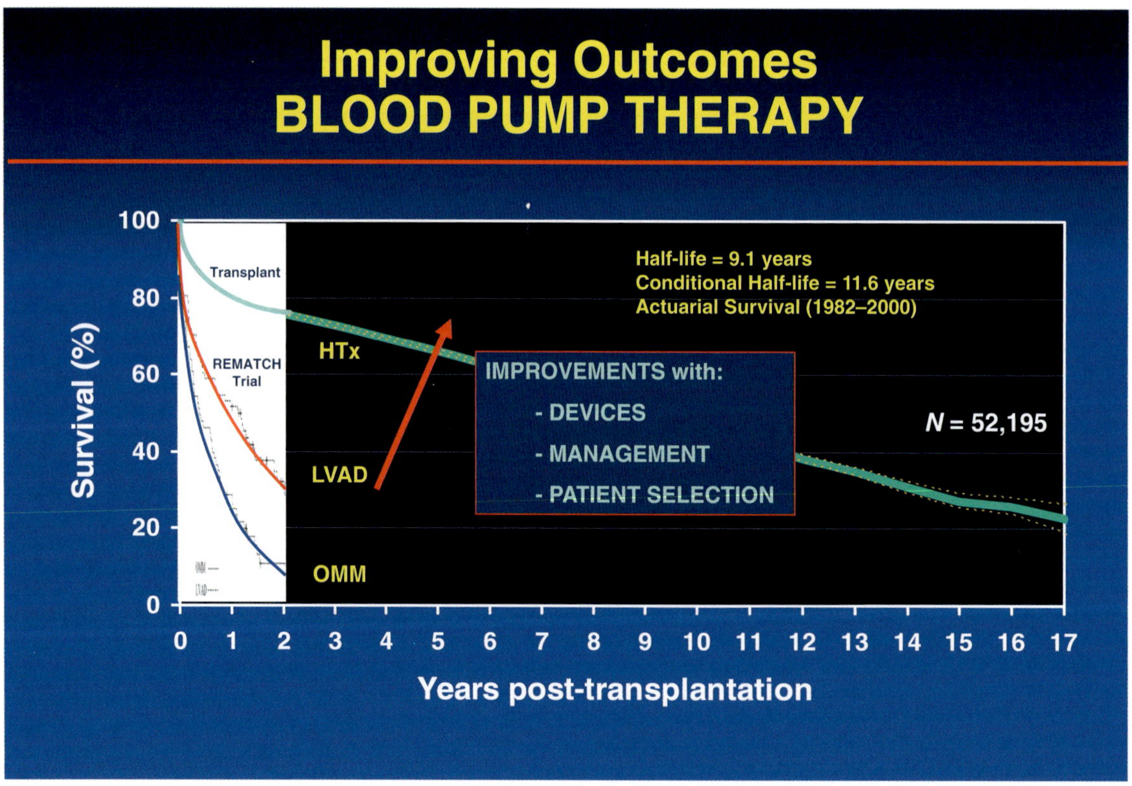

Fig. 22.1 Improving outcomes with blood pump therapy. The 2-year survival curves for LVADs vs. OMM from the pioneering era REMATCH Trial *(in white)* superimposed on the long-term survival curve for heart transplantation. Progress with LVAD outcomes beyond the first trial of long-term destination therapy was enabled by improvements in devices, management and patient selection. *HTx*, Heart transplantation; *LVAD*, left ventricular assist device; *OMM*, optimum medical management; *REMATCH*, Randomized Evaluation of Mechanical Assistance for the Treatment of Congestive Heart Failure.

arrival of the Hemopump,[6,7] after which a whole new generation of implantable blood pumps incorporating rotary blood pump designs, axial or centrifugal, was introduced. These pumps afforded smaller size, elimination of noise and vibration, improved durability, and easier implantation than the previous, pioneering generation of large, pulsing, displacement pumps.

The decade of the 2000s witnessed expanding use of these rotary pumps. Following clinical trials, incorporating randomization against a previous-generation, approved pump, the HeartMate II axial flow LVAD (Thoratec, Pleasanton, CA) received FDA approval in 2008[8] for bridging to transplantation and 2010 for long-term DT.[9] The HeartWare HVAD centrifugal pump (HeartWare, Boston, MA) received FDA approvals for the same indications in 2012[10] and 2017.[11]

MANAGEMENT Improvements and Guidelines

How patients and devices are managed markedly affects outcomes. Good management can offset some technological imperfections. The 2010 decade saw the rise of efforts to establish consensus around management issues, the publication of guidelines,[12–14] and the application of best practices.

PATIENT Selection and Risk Mitigation

Early in the history of the MCS field, patients implanted with devices were extremely high-risk patients, literally on death's door. Moving to earlier-stage patients would be expected to improve outcomes through lower exposure to perioperative risk. If pushed prematurely, however, the benefits of device therapy could be outweighed by the risks associated with good, but less-than-perfect, technology. The search for appropriate 'equipoise' balancing risk versus benefit at a given time with a given technology, has been a subject of considerable discussion.

The US national Interagency Registry for Mechanically Assisted Circulatory Support (INTERMACS) has afforded guidance with patient risk factor characterization and relevant outcomes data. Fig. 22.2 illustrates the breakdown of New York Heart Association (NYHA) class IV patients into six categories from highest severity of illness (IM 1) to lowest (IM 6), followed by NYHA class III (IM 7). The INTERMACS data confirm a lower likelihood of survival in the higher-acuity categories (lower IM levels), indicating the importance of careful patient selection.[16] Preoperative optimization to reduce risk has been recognized as essential.

The Era of Improving Survival

A review of survival with LVADs throughout multiple clinical trials starting with the REMATCH trial demonstrates progressive improvement, now approaching that of heart transplantation, at least within the first 3 to 5 years. This is illustrated in Fig. 22.3, demonstrating progressive improvement in survival from early clinical trials to more recent ones.

Real-world experiences have supported this trend. Individual center and small group experiences have excelled, approaching equivalence to survival with heart transplantation.

III. THE FUTURE IS OPTIMIZING THE PRESENT

How the challenges of preceding decades have been addressed, and what remains to be improved, serves as guidance for future directions in MCS. If remaining challenges represent opportunity, there is plenty of opportunity available.

RECOGNIZING the OPPORTUNITIES

The most important prospect in the near-term to improve the MCS field is to address the ominous challenge of *adverse events* (AEs). Data from the INTERMACS illustrates this and serves as a wake-up call.[17] By 12 months after implantation with current-generation ventricular assist devices (VADs), 70% of patients will have experienced one major AE, whether it be bleeding, stroke, device thrombosis/malfunction, infection, or death.[17] This is illustrated in Fig. 22.4, which graphically displays the sobering magnitude of the AE challenge[18] and summarizes the estimated rates of occurrence of the most troublesome AEs. The cumulative impact of the AEs year after year is considered the most significant impediment to responsible growth of the MCS field, whether that be through limiting the number of patients served or slowing expansion into earlier-stage heart failure.

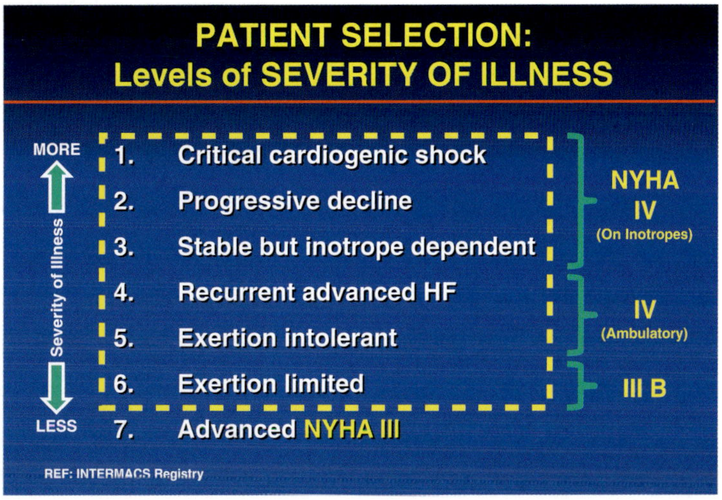

Fig. 22.2 INTERMACS levels of severity of heart failure. Descriptions of INTERMACS levels for IM 1 (greater severity) through IM 7 (less severity), grouped by NYHA class and by inotrope dependence or ambulatory status. *HF*, Heart failure; *INTERMACS*, Interagency Registry for Mechanically Assisted Circulatory Support; *NYHA*, New York Heart Association.

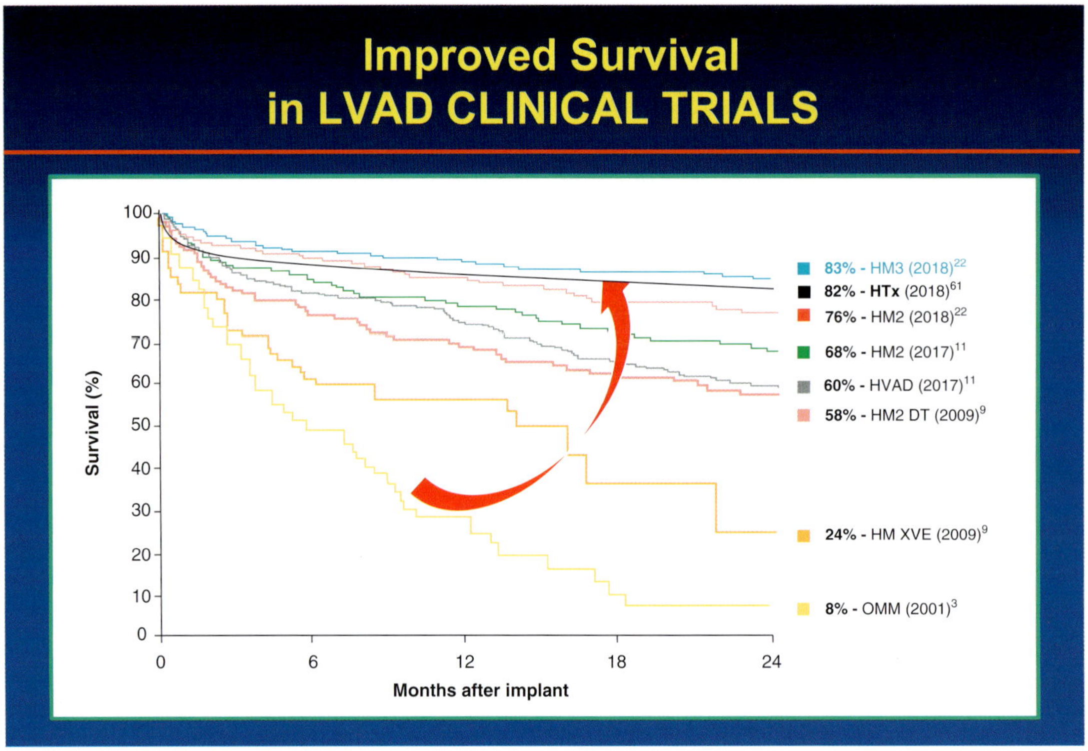

Fig. 22.3 Progressive improvement in LVAD survival. Survival curves from separate, controlled clinical trials of LVADs indicating progressive improvement in outcomes from 2001 onward. A survival curve for heart transplantation is superimposed. Superscript numbers are references. (Based on published data originating from controlled trials involving separate patient populations—presented to illustrate trends with MCS outcomes.) *HM*, HeartMate; *HTx*, heart transplantation; *LVAD*, left ventricular assist device (HM XVE, HM2, HVAD, HM3); *OMM*, optimum medical management (REMATCH trial); *REMATCH*, Randomized Evaluation of Mechanical Assistance for the Treatment of Congestive Heart Failure.

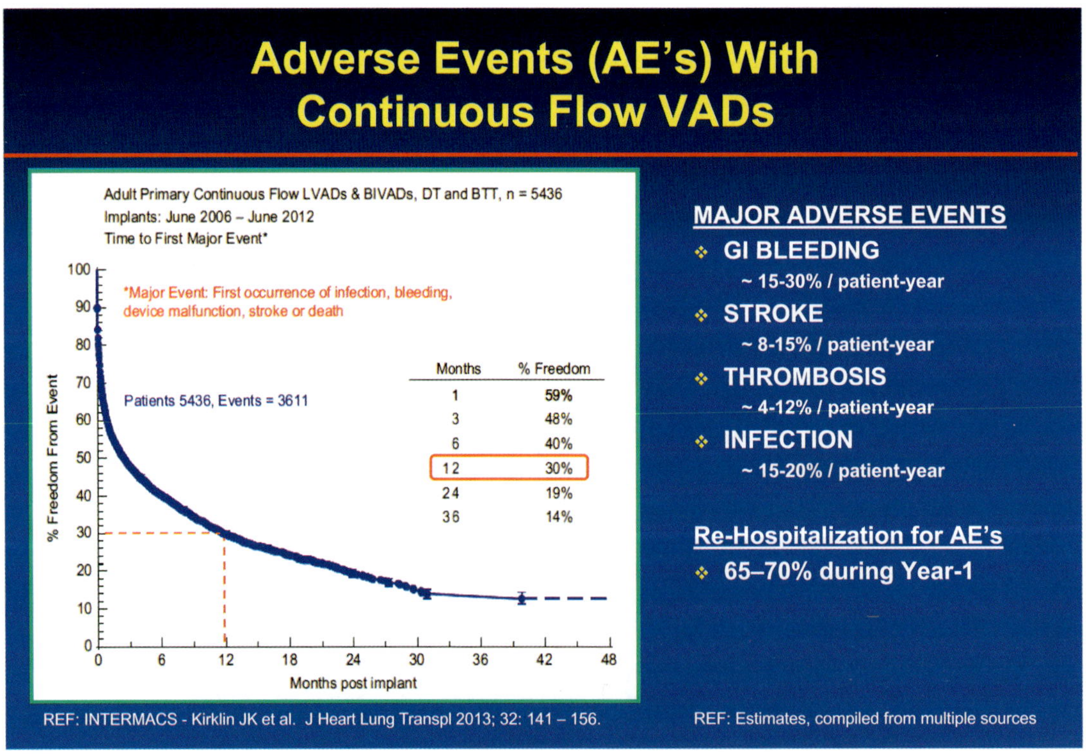

Fig. 22.4 AEs with current LVADs. This INTERMACS analysis indicates a high level of AEs, with only 30% freedom from the first occurrence of a major AE at 1-year post LVAD implantation. Field-wide estimates of the rates of major AEs and impact on re-hospitalizations are provided. *AE*, Adverse event; *INTERMACS*, Interagency Registry for Mechanically Assisted Circulatory Support; *LVAD*, left ventricular assist device (continuous flow).

In addition to the substantial clinical impact of AEs, the *economic challenge* created by the AEs is enormous. Underlying this is the high frequency of re-hospitalizations.[19] The costs of device replacement, rehospitalizations, diagnostic workups, and therapeutic interventions quickly add up. While the initial implantation costs remain high, it is the long-term costs that represent the greatest challenge. While there are encouraging trends with the most recent clinical experience,[20] this opportunity for improving cost-effectiveness through improving AEs cannot be ignored.

MAPPING the Pathway to OPTIMIZATION

As was noted throughout the history of the MCS field, ongoing improvements with technology, management, and patient selection will be fundamental to overcoming the challenges. While requests abound for better technology, it is clear that outcomes can be improved even with existing technology by improving management and patient selection.

Insight into this is garnered from observations of large differences in outcomes, varying from center to center even with the same devices. For example, wide differences in rates of pump thrombosis have been noted even with the same LVAD. Stroke rates have varied considerably between centers and across eras even with the same device.

Evidence exists to support the idea that improvements in thrombosis with HeartMate II LVADs can be achieved as a result of minimizing variation in management by standardization around best practices, either evidence based or through consensus.[15] Improvements in stroke rates with HVAD LVADs have been noted with better management of blood pressure.[21] Certainly, patient factors contribute varying degrees of risk for the occurrence of AEs—either through a state of compromise and deterioration induced by progressive heart failure—or through inherent biologic or genetically induced conditions that may predispose a particular patient to specific risks.

OPTIMIZING TECHNOLOGY

A wish list of technological improvements is presented in Fig. 22.5. These improvements are broadly categorized into those for safety, for performance, and for utility. Safety is the highest priority given that the greatest challenge in MCS is the AE issue.

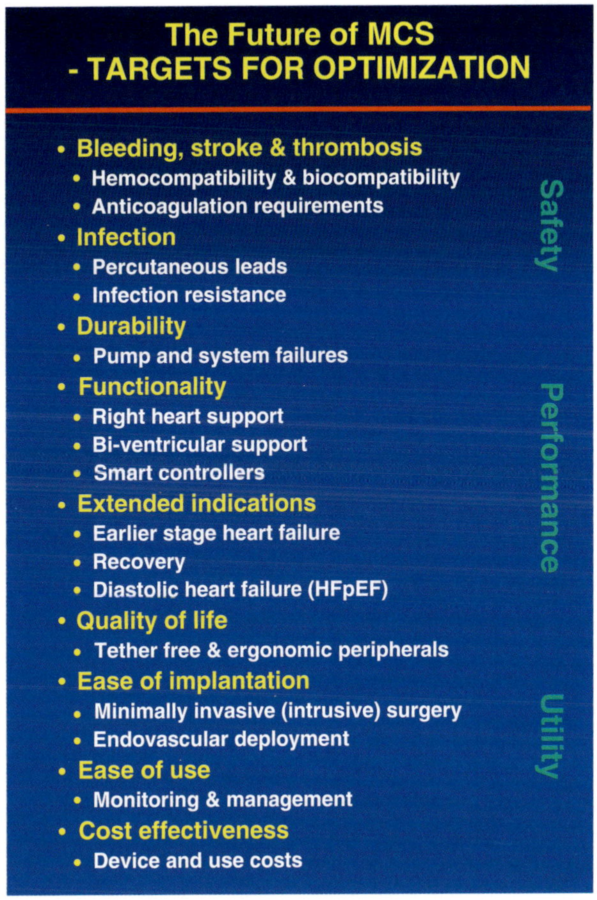

Fig. 22.5 Targets for optimization of mechanical circulatory support *(MCS)* technology. Opportunities for improving MCS technology, broadly categorized in relationship to safety, performance, and utility, with safety being the highest priority.

Improving HEMOCOMPATIBILITY

Hemocompatibility, a subset of biocompatibility, is the term used to describe the avoidance of damage to blood elements. The device-associated AEs of bleeding, thrombosis, and stroke are largely related to hemocompatibility.

Early goals for achieving hemocompatibility were focused on preventing major hemolysis due to shear-mediated damage to red blood cells. Given the relative freedom from significant hemolysis in current pumps, attention has turned to other blood elements, including the von Willebrand factor (vWF), platelets, and white blood cells (WBCs). Damage to the vWF has been associated with clinical bleeding, notably mucosal bleeding, particularly gastrointestinal (GI). Platelet damage and activation have been associated with thrombosis. Damage to WBCs can trigger inflammatory responses and impact defenses against infection.

The recent arrival of a blood pump designed intentionally to improve hemocompatibility has been met with enthusiasm, as evidenced by robust participation in the largest randomized trial ever in the MCS space.[22] The HeartMate 3 LVAD (Abbott, Lake Bluff, IL, USA) is a centrifugal pump employing (a) magnetics to levitate its rotor instead of two other preceding designs: (b) miniature mechanical bearings lubricated by blood or (c) hydrodynamic bearings using inclined planes fabricated into the rotor edges to lift the rotor away from the pump body, suspending it on a thin, blood fluid film created when the rotor turns above a minimum speed, analogous to hydroplaning or skiing across the surface of water. By employing magnetics to continuously suspend the rotor, even when stopped, the gaps between the rotor and housing can be wider, resulting in lower shear forces between the rotor and housing.[23] The HeartMate 3 also employs intermittent, intrinsic speed oscillation to avoid areas of stagnation. In theory, these device improvements could lead to lower rates of bleeding, thrombosis, and stroke.

An overall improvement in hemocompatibility-related AEs with the HeartMate 3 in comparison to the HeartMate II has been reported.[24] Pump thrombosis has been markedly improved, now occurring rarely. However, stroke rates are still higher than ideal, although there are early indications of the potential for improvement. And bleeding remains a frequent, vexing problem. Further improvements in outcomes will depend upon device engineering advances supplemented by changes in clinical management.

The emerging science of hemocompatibility applied to device design. Fortunately, additional improvement with the hemocompatibility of pumps, especially regarding bleeding, appears plausible. This ray of optimism is rooted in the evolving science of hemocompatibility as outlined in Fig. 22.6.[25]

Fundamental to this endeavor has been the characterization of biomarkers that signal the mal-effects of MCS pumps on an array of blood components, including vWF, platelets, and WBCs, resulting in their

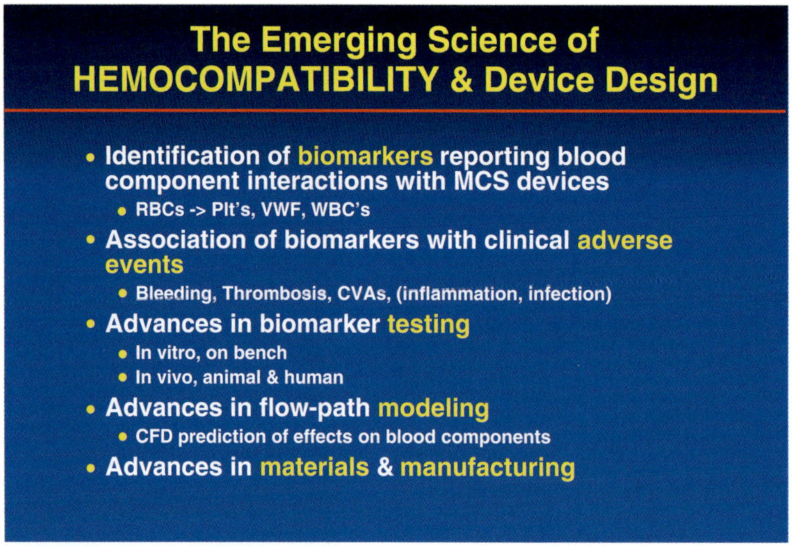

Fig. 22.6 The emerging science of hemocompatibility and device design. Advances in the science of hemocompatibility as applied to the design of blood pumps may contribute to (1) improving pump-related blood trauma, (2) enhancing preclinical testing and its predictability, and (3) reducing clinical adverse events. *CFD*, Computation fluid dynamics; *CVA*, cerebrovascular accident; *MCS*, mechanical circulatory support; *Plt*, platelets; *RBC*, red blood cell; *VWF*, von Willebrand factor; *WBC*, white blood cell.

damage and/or activation. These biomarkers signal alterations that have associations with clinical AEs, including bleeding, thrombosis, and strokes, as well as inflammation and infection.

Advances in biomarker testing have enabled in vitro side-by-side comparisons of one device configuration against another in the laboratory.[26–28] In vivo testing in animals allows for preclinical evaluation and clinical testing in patients will continue to refine our understanding of the relationships between the preclinical testing and clinical outcomes.

Research into how these biomarkers are affected under various pump operating conditions will enable further evolution of computation fluid dynamic modeling predictive of blood element damage. The influence of (1) shear forces, (2) flow perturbations, and (3) time of exposure to those conditions on damage to the different components of blood will be better understood. Such tools will enable optimizing pumps for hemocompatibility during the earliest phases of design.

Advances in material science will be increasingly important for identifying metallics, polymers, and ceramics, as well as surface textures, most compatible with blood. Enhanced manufacturing methodologies aid in assuring hemocompatibility, especially important as blood pumps are miniaturized further.

As this field of endeavor matures, it will enable the emergence of devices designed to improve hemocompatibility. The timeframe in which a device can move from concept to clinical reality can hopefully be shortened. And, this new wave of advanced, preclinical testing should have predictive value, raising the level of confidence about how a device will perform in humans even before reaching clinical experience.[29]

Improving BIOCOMPATIBILITY

Biocompatibility involves the degree to which a foreign device is viewed as unobtrusive, relatively inert, and compatible with its host. Achieving biocompatibility is fundamental to avoiding Adverse Events resulting from disturbances originating at the interfaces of an implanted, synthetic device with adjacent tissues.

Especially important is the pump inlet cannula as it interfaces with the surrounding tissues, that being the left ventricle in the case of an LVAD. There is good reason to believe that this interface is a source for thrombus formation contributing to pump thrombosis, strokes, and thromboembolic events either by ingestion or by embolization through the pump or embolization directly out of the left ventricle.

Further understanding of this phenomenon is important as efforts are made to prevent this problem. Solutions may include better cannula designs with more biocompatible surfaces promoting a better interface of the device with surrounding tissue, perhaps with full incorporation within the surrounding tissue.

Blood flow dynamics through the LV to a pump inlet at the LV apex may predispose the region to stasis and thrombosis.[30,31] Here, too, better cannula designs may be helpful. So might pump operating conditions designed to promote intermittent washout of the regions at risk.

Synthetic vascular grafts and conduits may contribute to thrombosis and thromboembolism. The redesign of these conduits may be part of a future strategy with pump designs, including their elimination with endovascular pumps that reside fully contained within the walls of the cardiovascular pathways.

Eliminating the need for ANTICOAGULATION

The goal of operating a blood pump with little to no anticoagulation has only ever been achieved with one implantable blood pump design, the first-generation HeartMate LVAD IP/VE/XVE series. Aspirin was the only anticoagulation required. This was enabled by the use of non-mechanical tissue valves, carefully engineered blood flow pathways, and notably, textured surfaces promoting a biocompatible, neointimal lining on the blood contacting surfaces and at the myocardial tissue interface.

Whether blood pumps will traverse a journey 'back to the future' and revisit this standard has yet to be determined. It should, however, be maintained as a goal, to be pursued through advances with the science of hemocompatibility as applied to device design.

Reducing INFECTION

MCS device infections remain problematic, involving percutaneous lead exit sites, deep infections of the percutaneous leads, or the pumps themselves. They are a leading cause of readmission and are an unfortunate cause of long-term death. New approaches are needed.

The MCS field has been looking forward to *transcutaneous energy transmission* systems, or TETS, as a long-awaited solution to *percutaneous lead infections*.[32] Early clinical experience with an LVAD that incorporated TETS (LionHeart, Arrow International)[33] exposed the field to tantalizing images of tether-free life without percutaneous leads. However, those limited experiences faded with the exodus of those systems from clinical use.

Enthusiasm for MCS devices employing TETS in lieu of percutaneous leads has been rekindled. Developers of the two VADs most in clinical use today (HeartMate 3 and HVAD) will be incorporating TETS into their own systems. Independent developers are working on TET systems with potential universal applicability and adaptation for use with different devices.

Progress is needed to overcome barriers to the development and adoption of TETS. Some of the challenges are (1) technical with engineering design and development; (2) clinical with the additional complexities of implantation and the bulk of implanted components, along with infection risk of additional implanted hardware and component replacement, including periodic reoperations to replace batteries; (3) related to human factors and ergonomics; (4) business development related; and (5) financial, given development costs and expected increases in system pricing.

A less elegant, but yet worthy, approach to reducing the burden of percutaneous lead infections has been in practice with the Jarvik technology.[34] The internal cable for that LVAD is exteriorized at a connector configured with a *skull-mounted pedestal* that serves as the interface to a flexible, small-diameter external cable attached to the controller and batteries. Two enabling features are a well-incorporated skin-subcutaneous interface and stabilization to reduce traction-related trauma at the exit site. In the future, alternative locations for such *skin-button connector* approaches should improve implantability, ease of access, and cosmesis. With an implanted battery and controller electronics, it would be possible to enjoy periods of uncoupled, tether-free mobility, adding quality of life while reducing infections.

Like all implanted foreign bodies, MCS devices have an inherent vulnerability to *surface infections* at the interface of the synthetic materials with surrounding host tissues. In the future, MCS devices may be able to incorporate features to reduce external infections, perhaps (1) with surfaces promoting tissue ingrowth, (2) by using materials with greater infection resistance or (3) the capacity to release antimicrobial materials, and (4) by adopting surface topologies to reduce dead-space pockets in which wound seromas accumulate, serving as culture medium for infections.

A unique vulnerability of MCS devices to infections is related to hemocompatibility, given that blood trauma to white blood cells (WBCs) could alter *immune defenses to infections*. Far less attention has been given to this aspect of hemocompatibility than to bleeding, thrombosis, and strokes. Much has yet to be learned about shear and flow-related effects on WBCs. Minimizing shear-induced damage and/or activation of white cells should be considered as a goal for next-generation devices.

Extending Device DURABILITY

The incidence of primary *mechanical failure* with current blood pumps has improved markedly since first-generation technology that was compromised by 50% pump failure rates at only 1.5 years. The elimination of mechanical bearings and reduction of the many moving parts to a single, rotating rotor has helped. Other causes of *pump system failure*, however, remain problematic[35] and must be improved to allow freedom from pump replacement to extend beyond 5 to 7 years or more.

Percutaneous lead failures occur too frequently, generally the result of use-related trauma. Improved lead designs would make them more durable—perhaps achieved by more flexible, smaller-diameter leads and improved resistance to bend- or cut-related damage.

No matter how well designed, as long as there are percutaneous leads, there will be failures necessitating replacement. Lead failures in exteriorized sections can be managed by splicing in new lead segments externally. However, at the present time, lead failures within internal, implanted sections require pump replacement along with the lead.

Complete lead replacement without replacing the pump, as is currently required, should be made available by incorporating *implantable connectors* on a pump at the site where the lead is attached to the pump, or in near proximity. This approach awaits further development and adoption, having only ever been achieved with one LVAD (WorldHeart's Levacor), which is no longer available.

Electronic controller and *peripheral component* (e.g., batteries, chargers etc.) failures remain troublesome and expensive even though less impactful than pump or lead failures. As many as one-third of the electronic controllers fail each year.[35] More robust designs will be needed anticipating the rigors of routine use, and even abuse. Improved preclinical testing methods should be sought that will better simulate the real-world "torture-testing" by patients to better predict readiness of the devices to meet such challenges.

Expanding FUNCTIONALITY

The implantable MCS field today is dominated by LVAD's providing full-flow, univentricular LV support in patients with late-stage, mostly NYHA class IV, systolic heart failure. As safer technologies with lower adverse event profiles emerge, the freedom to move to earlier-stage patients will gain traction. Likewise, attention will be turned to enhanced performance afforded by *expanded functionalities*.

Right Heart Support. Obviously missing from the MCS armamentarium is dedicated right heart support. This is despite an increasingly recognized need to address the morbidity and mortality invoked by RV failure post-LVAD and by late RV dysfunction. Without dedicated implantable RV assist device (RVADs), the MCS field has explored off-label and off-specification use of implantable LVADs deployed as RVADs.

Right heart support is needed post-LVAD implantation more often than is indicated by the current use of RVADs. The single greatest cause of perioperative mortality following LVAD implantation is multiorgan failure (MOF) resulting from organ and tissue hypoperfusion. MOF is really a surrogate for RV failure, given that the only reason that a full-flow LVAD (normally capable of delivering 7–8+ liters per minute) cannot maintain adequate organ perfusion is because there is not enough blood pumped through the right heart to maintain adequate filling of the LVAD.

The perioperative burden of RV dysfunction is underappreciated. Patients with RV dysfunction require prolonged inotrope use and have a greater likelihood of experiencing bleeding, sustained inflammatory responses, prolonged intubation, and long lengths of stay in expensive intensive care units (ICUs).

Acute RV support technology is available but limited by having to reoperate to remove surgically placed devices or by restricted patient mobility due to femoral cannulation with percutaneous technology (Abiomed Impella RP). A dual-lumen cannula (Protek Duo, Tandem Heart/LivaNova) placed in the right internal jugular vein is available for use with an external pump drawing blood from the right atrium and returning it to the pulmonary artery. It allows for ambulatory mobilization and percutaneous removal, but patients must remain hospitalized.

It should be considered a high priority for developers to deliver RVADs designed for both early mobilization and percutaneous removal, offering intermediate duration right heart support for up to a 30-day use, knowing that the greatest need will be for the first 1–2 weeks postoperatively. Besides improved clinical outcomes, cost-effectiveness should be possible given expected reductions in hospital costs due to reductions in costly ICU care and long hospital lengths of stay.

Bi-ventricular Support. The MCS field awaits chronic, long-term biventricular support devices on par with advanced LVAD technology. While the pneumatic total artificial heart (TAH; Syncardia) still serves a useful role with patients, it is based on decades-old technology, with significant limitations of utility and quality of life.

Fortunately, newer technology is reaching early clinical use with a pulsatile, electric TAH (Carmat, Paris). Continuous-flow technology, designed for biventricular support as a TAH-equivalent, is also in development (e.g., Bivacor). For those patients who start with an LVAD but develop late RV failure, durable RVADs are needed that are integrated with LVAD systems providing combination LVAD + RVAD support without requiring two controllers and separate leads.

Smart Controllers. Today's continuous-flow LVADs are the culmination of highly intelligent pump engineering. On the other hand, with regard to physiologic engineering, they fall short, essentially devoid of intelligence. This has ramifications for safety, for performance, and for quality of life.

These pumps function at a single set speed as essentially 'dumb devices' with no active auto-regulation capability. That one speed setting is established by clinical studies ramping speed up and down while imaging the LV with echocardiography to find a condition at which the risk of LV collapse with LVAD flow interruption will be minimized in balance with the need to avoid LV overload and distention.[36] Only a limited margin of error is allowed—and, if exceeded, patients will be exposed to undue risks should they become dehydrated or volume overloaded or develop extremes of hypo- or hypertension.

Today's continuous-flow rotary pumps operating at fixed speeds[37] have an extremely limited capacity to increase output in response to increasing preload pressure, as occurs with the increased hemodynamic demands of exercise.[38] Any increase in pump output is solely an innate, passive response related to the behavioral properties of continuously flowing pumps in which pump flow at a given speed is affected by preload pressure and afterload pressure. Flow through these pumps increases modestly in response to increasing preload, mimicking a very muted Starling-curve-like physiologic response. However, that physiologic-like response can be countered, or even defeated, by high afterload pressures which impede flows through these pumps.

To achieve autoregulation, future generations of continuous-flow pump systems will have to incorporate *sensors* to provide physiologic and hemodynamic information, preload pressure, for example, by which smart controllers will modulate pump speed and other settings.

Alternatively, the field could 'return to the future' redeploying modernized versions of the original MCS pulsatile pumps using volume displacement pumping mechanisms.[39] Such pumps are able to electronically detect, or sense, varying filling conditions as preload and respond with appropriate speed changes.

In the meantime, until pumps behave more physiologically, smarter controllers will have to leverage whatever pump performance information is available electronically.[40] Advanced analyses of the data available in *pump system logs* are gaining traction for identifying patterns that can be correlated to clinical events. It is hoped that such information may guide preemptive intervention to prevent AEs or to improve pump performance.

Pulsatility. Interest is recurring in reexploring the utility of physiologically meaningful pulsatility. To achieve that, either a new generation of volume displacement pumps or adding the ability to ramp up, then ramp down, the speed of continuous-flow pumps to produce pulsatile output is required. The degree and character of pulsatility that is physiologically useful have yet to be determined.

Advocates for pulsatility suggest that it may be important for preserving the microscopic architecture of blood vessels and vascular endothelial cell linings. Others believe its absence plays some role in mucosal bleeding. However, given generally favorable outcomes observed clinically with long-term exposure to diminished pulsation and with some of the challenging tradeoffs that are obligatory to generating pulsatility, more analysis will be necessary before justifying pulsatility as a standard for next-generation devices.

Extending INDICATIONS

The greatest usage of MCS devices has been in patients with systolic heart failure (heart failure with reduced ejection fraction [HFrEF]), nearing end-stage, mostly in NYHA class IV, primarily in one of two groups, bridge to transplantation (BTT) or long-term DT. Given increasingly blurred lines of distinction between BTT and DT, these endpoint categories are changing in favor of duration of support, either short-term (<6 months) or long-term (>6 months).

In the future, there will be a shift in the systolic heart failure population from near-end-stage patients to those with earlier-stage heart failure, extending into NYHA class III/IIIB—as it becomes justified to do so based on improving MCS outcomes. Two other populations are expected to receive increasing attention in the future: candidates for *cardiac recovery* and patients with *diastolic heart failure* (heart failure with preserved ejection fraction [HFpEF]).

Recovery. The phenomenon of ventricular reverse remodeling in patients with chronic heart failure has been met with considerable enthusiasm but has yet to be established as a meaningful and predictable target for therapeutic intervention. Important examples have illustrated the potential for cardiac recovery—sometimes spontaneously as with acute myocarditis, sometimes facilitated by drugs or cardiac resynchronization pacing.

Numerous approaches have been proposed to augment cardiac recovery, but none have been as hopeful as the use of VADs to provide chronic mechanical unloading. The amazing experience described by the Harefield group[41] reporting 60%–70% recovery rates with either a pulsatile or continuous-flow LVAD supplemented with clenbuterol stimulated the field to pursue this. Such encouraging rates of recovery have been difficult to reproduce—at least until the recent multicenter study, the RESTAGE-HF, reporting findings of a 50% rate of recovery to LVAD explantation.[42]

LVADs as tools to augment recovery may be at the early stage of a new era with new opportunities.[43] The beauty of mechanical unloading is that it stabilizes a patient with decompensated heart failure and creates a durable and sustainable myocardial recovery test-bed in which many different interventions facilitating recovery may be explored—whether pharmacologic, biologic, cellular, genetic, or bioengineered.

The door should be wide open for the development of MCS devices tailored to support cardiac recovery. Well-engineered devices with sensing capabilities will be able to provide diagnostic information about the stage of recovery and the hemodynamic/physiologic conditions for supporting recovery. Next-generation pumps with smart controllers will enable optimum unloading during an initial period of ventricular shape restoration, followed by controlled loading for enhanced retraining while avoiding degenerative apoptosis. Greater success with LVAD-supported recovery will set the stage for even further advances as the science of reverse remodeling matures at the cellular, extracellular, metabolic and genomic levels.[44]

Heart failure with preserved ejection fraction. The large, and growing, population of patients with HFpEF (alternatively referred to as diastolic heart failure) experiences a burden of heart failure as great as those with HFrEF (systolic heart failure). Unfortunately, there are no proven, effective treatment options.

Traditional LVADs with LV apical cannulation have seen only limited use in the HFpEF population. LV cannulation with hypertrophic hearts, as seen with HFpEF, is challenging and generally avoided, given the small LV cavity size and associated risk of obstruction to inflow.

On the other hand, HFpEF patients consistently have enlarged left atria (LA). Thus, a pump designed for HFpEF patients would preferentially employ LA uptake, based on anatomic considerations alone.

Besides the anatomic advantages, there are physiologic benefits of LA to aortic pumping in HFpEF. During exercise, patients with HFpEF markedly increase LA pressures. When the LA pressures become extreme (three to four times normal), patients can no longer exercise. With active pumping from the LA to the aorta, the LA pressure can be decompressed to a level low enough to accommodate exercise while the pump contributes net forward blood flow from the heart to the body. Plus, the LV can still function to support exercise when LA pressures are maintained high enough to allow effective LV filling and ejection from the stiff, poorly compliant LV (as is the case with HFpEF)—but at LA pressures low enough to permit exercise.

Thus a partial-flow pump with output in the 2–4 liter per minute range should be sufficient given that it is working in parallel to supplement a functional LV with preserved systolic ejection capacity. This has been demonstrated by modeling encouraged by clinical experience with the Circulite device,[45] a miniaturized pump with an uptake in the LA and arterial return to the subclavian artery. With expectations of improved pump safety along with less invasive implantation, possibly even with percutaneous delivery, use in earlier-stage heart failure may be warranted. Advanced controller features will be needed to accommodate the unique HFpEF (patho)physiology.[46]

Enhancing QUALITY OF LIFE

The phrase 'forgettable technology' has been used to describe an ideal state for the coexistence of patients with their MCS devices. Today, it is a dream beyond foreseeable reach—but the vision of "forgettable technology" should not be forgotten.

Every effort must be made to reduce the burden of MCS therapy for patients. It is one type of achievement to make implantation 'less invasive'; it is a different accomplishment to make the daily experience 'less intrusive'. Smaller incisions may sound attractive at the time of implantation—but that attraction soon disappears when patients are obliged to carry an unwieldy bulk of peripherals, every day, for the rest of their lives.

Hardware components to be targeted for improving quality of life include: (1) percutaneous lead elimination or alternatives for periodic untethering; (2) controller size, ergonomics, and user interface, including visuals and alarms; (3) battery size and duration; and (4) external cables and connectors with consideration for wireless interconnectivity, for example, Bluetooth.

Functional features to be addressed for improving quality of life include autoresponsive controllers enabling greater exercise tolerance.[47]

Facilitating IMPLANTATION

Adoption and responsible dissemination of a new therapy are wholly dependent on standardization, reproducibility, and ease of use. Being able to move beyond the pioneering experimental phase and assure successful transfer into the 'real world' depends on that.

For MCS implantation, that means making the surgical process less burdensome, reducing complexity, and reducing risk. Much of the responsibility for that is left in the hands of surgeons who develop, adapt, and optimize surgical techniques.

Device developers can take it a step further by providing well-designed *surgical tools* to simplify implantation. That could include tools designed to support 'keyhole' surgery through small incisions. Tools that could make it possible to decrease or eliminate cardiopulmonary bypass could include devices that allow for *bloodless insertion* of uptake cannulas or for connecting outflow grafts to blood vessels with *auto-anastamotic devices* and readily accessible *imaging tools* to help with selecting best anatomic locations to avoid risks related to blind insertion, such as dislodging thrombi or calcified plaques.

Enthusiasm is developing for *percutaneous, endovascular deployment* of chronic, implantable MCS devices. This approach will have to be reserved for patient populations in which miniaturized, partial-flow devices will be effective. The development of such devices for long-term implantation will necessitate overcoming the engineering challenges of down-scaling while still maintaining manufacturability, performance, durability, and hemocompatibility. Further, the challenges of percutaneous delivery, internal stabilization, endovascular connections, lead exteriorization, etc., will require new, creative developmental effort.

Easing Device USE

Remote Monitoring and Management. The burden for caretakers of managing an increasing number of MCS outpatients at home is substantial and will become onerous with escalating growth of the field. *Remote monitoring* of pump systems has been demonstrated (e.g., Reliant Heart) and may serve to ease the burden of care. Data security and patient confidentiality must be assured. Adapting existing remote monitoring platforms already in widespread use today such as those for pacemakers and diabetic therapy may be helpful (e.g., Abbott's Merlin.net and Medtronic's CareLink networks).

Remote management of pump systems could further ease the burden of care. However, extensive effort will be necessary given the challenges of engineering, information transfer, and regulatory requirements. Automated algorithms for closed-loop responses should reduce the manual burden but will face extensive development and regulatory challenges.

While such capabilities will enable remote care and make it less burdensome, it will not eliminate the need for readily available and responsive *clinical teams* to engage and intervene as necessary. Efficiency will be important, enabled by high-reliability information and technology.

OPTIMIZING MANAGEMENT

Ongoing advances with management are extremely important to the future of MCS. As essential as improvements in technology are, the future depends on making best use of whatever technology is available at any point in time. Furthermore, innovative management will even circumvent limitations with technology, until further perfected, as has been demonstrated repeatedly since the inception of the MCS field. Clinical teams and care providers will have numerous opportunities to optimize management, whether it be surgical, medical, or lifelong.

Optimizing SURGICAL Management

Enthusiasm for *less invasive surgery* to implant MCS devices is expected to increase. This trend follows what has been happening with conventional cardiovascular surgery. The less invasive surgical approach most often involves a left thoracotomy for LVAD implantation combined with an upper hemi-sternotomy (or right paramedian approach) for aortic graft anastomosis.[48–50]

The nonsternotomy approach is sometimes required when the risks associated with a reoperative sternotomy are considered prohibitive. Avoiding a median sternotomy is believed by some as useful with the BTT indication, sparing the median sternotomy for the subsequent transplantation procedure. Other proposed advantages of the non-sternotomy approach may include less bleeding, faster recovery, and better preservation of right heart function. On the other hand, a sternotomy approach is sometimes necessary, for example, when concurrent cardiac surgical procedures such as valve repair or replacement are indicated.

Further advances with minimally invasive *implantation tools* will be beneficial for less invasive approaches. Until the techniques are well refined and readily reproducible, enabled by expertise and easier-to-use hardware, it seems prudent to exercise caution with widespread dissemination of procedures that can quickly become extraordinarily complicated.

Another approach to the "less is more" concept is what might be referred to as *less intrusive surgery*. The reduction or elimination of cardiopulmonary bypass time may offer advantages avoiding the potential mal-effects of inflammation and bleeding. This too will be enabled by the development of surgical tools to minimize blood loss and facilitate control.

The presumed advantages of less invasive or less intrusive approaches should be validated by more extensive clinical studies allowing for carefully controlled comparison to traditional, conventional approaches. Among the outcome variables for consideration would be surgical complications, impact on right heart function, impact of loss of access for concomitant surgical procedures, recovery time, pain, impact of surgeon experience and enabling technology, etc.

Another area for optimizing surgical management is to intensify efforts to improve *surgical outcomes*. This is well exemplified by a wide-open opportunity for surgeons to play a major role in reducing the incidence of strokes that are seen at implantation or in the weeks to early months thereafter.

The neurologic outcomes within the MOMENTUM (Multicenter Study of MagLev Technology in Patients Undergoing Mechanical Circulatory Support Therapy With HeartMate 3) Trial of the HeartMate 3 include an amazingly low stroke rate beyond 6 months of 0.04 per patient-year.[51] Assuming such outcomes can be carried into real-world practice, it would be considered a remarkable advance for LVAD therapy. The greatest opportunity for further improvement in neurologic outcomes occurs within the first 6 months after implantation, wherein the stroke rate is 0.15 per patient-year, with 50% of those occurring in the immediate perioperative period, within the first 30 days after the operation.

So, how can surgical management make meaningful contributions to reducing stroke rates? The answer may lie with implementing intensive efforts to mitigate risks for perioperative strokes while encouraging field-wide adoption of surgical best practices incorporating *neuroprotective guidelines*. Fig. 22.7 provides a list of risk factors that may exist during the implantation of an LVAD.

To avoid stokes, consideration must be given to factors contributing to thrombo-emboli developing near the site of insertion of the LVAD uptake cannula, including the location of the cannula avoiding impingement on the septum, cannula angulation to avoid tissue contact with the tip of the cannula, removal of LV thrombus, avoiding apical calcification, and resecting thick portions of myocardial tissue that could leave myocardium overhanging the cannula.

With the outflow graft, factors to consider include proper length, route, and position to avoid kinking, twisting, or pulling the inflow

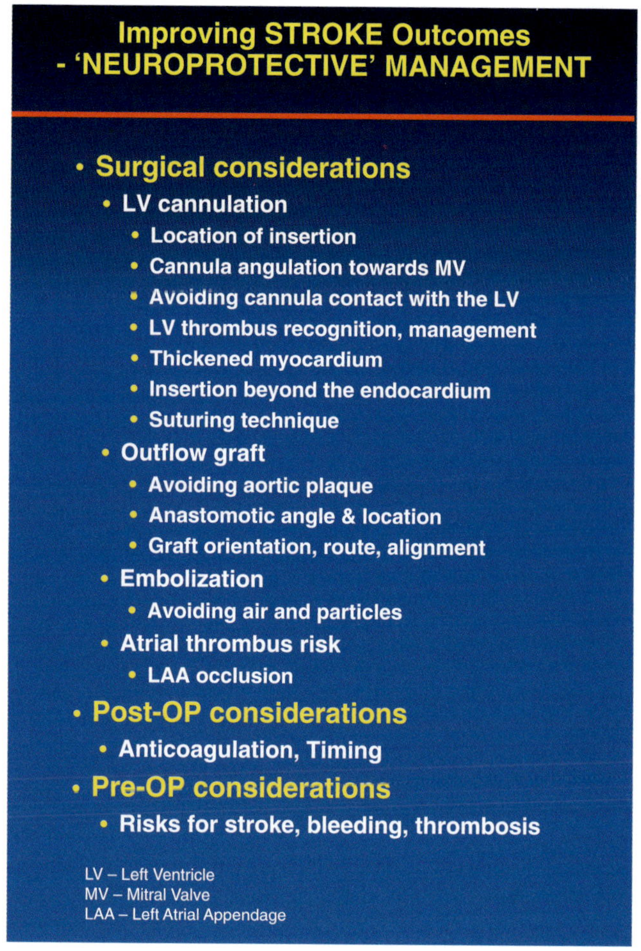

Fig. 22.7 Improving stroke outcomes with neuroprotective management. Perioperative management factors to be considered for mitigating the risk of strokes with left ventricular assist devices. These deserve a high level of attention given that the greatest opportunity for reducing strokes occurs at the time of implantation and for the 30 days following.

cannula out of correct orientation, as well as the location and angulation of the aortic anastomosis with the graft and avoiding aortic plaque and calcification that could be dislodged during clamping.

For those at risk for thrombo-emboli from the LA appendage, including patients with atrial fibrillation, oversewing or clipping the appendage should be considered. Care must be exercised to avoid air or particle embolization.

Preoperatively, care should be exercised with patients at known risk for perioperative strokes. Postoperatively, anticoagulation should be balanced to avoid thrombo-embolic events while avoiding bleeding.

Optimizing MEDICAL Management

Bleeding, especially GI and mucosal bleeding, remains challenging despite near-elimination of pump thrombosis. It is anticipated that with the next generation of pumps, hemocompatibility improvements will address blood damage–related factors that contribute to such bleeding. Until that occurs, however, the best hope for improvement rests with exploring *opportunities to lower anticoagulation requirements*, doing so cautiously to avoid reintroducing thrombosis.

Anecdotal experience with lowering anticoagulation indicates that this can be achieved without thrombotic complications in some LVAD patients who have been removed from anticoagulation due to prohibitive bleeding. There have been suggestions that aspirin can be eliminated safely,[52] although more study is needed. Early experience with lowering warfarin intentionally in HeartMate 3 LVAD patients is starting to emerge. One pilot study suggests that lowering anticoagulation to an international normalized ratio target of 1.5–1.9 (versus the traditional goal of 2.0–2.5) is achievable and safe with the HeartMate 3, at least in the short-term out to 6 months postimplantation.[53] A large-scale trial is warranted.

Alternative anticoagulants, other than current approaches using aspirin, warfarin, and bridging heparin, have received little attention in the MCS field. This is in stark contrast to the world of coronary artery interventions and stenting, wherein anticoagulation regimens have become highly sophisticated.

Other approaches in the future to reduce GI bleeding might involve therapies directed at correcting factors that are deranged, either directly or indirectly, as a result of blood trauma and pump flow characteristics. Further research into the mechanisms of GI bleeding with MCS patients is needed to identify suitable targets and effective therapies that may modulate the effects of vWF, angiopoietin II, or others.[54–56]

Optimizing LIFE-LONG Management

The *lifelong management* of MCS patients is challenging and represents an opportunity for improvement. Preventative maintenance and routine management of both technology and patients need to be less burdensome. The need to intervene for device problems or for patients experiencing AEs must decrease. Progress toward those goals may be facilitated by distributing management activities across integrated networks of care with good information exchange, enabled by remote monitoring and advances in medical informatics.

Until improvements arrive with technology or therapies for overcoming the remaining deficiencies with current devices, however, the MCS field will need to gear up to handle these issues. Additional resources will be required. Growth in the number of patients cannot be allowed to outstrip the capacity to care for them.

OPTIMIZING PATIENTS

Addressing *patient factors* affecting outcomes is important, just as is optimizing technology and management. Selecting the *right patients* and/or *preparing them to be the right patients* within a given set of risk-benefit tradeoffs is essential. In a future era of enhanced, personalized medicine, precision around this process may be refined with greater understanding of individually distinct, patient-specific factors.

Movement to EARLIER-STAGE PATIENTS

As noted in the INTERMACS registry, implanting patients with a lower risk profile can result in improved outcomes.[16] How far that can be taken depends on the benefits versus risks of the therapy at any point in time.

Any movement of the MCS field toward earlier-stage patients should take into consideration a combination of (1) existing *justification* based on evidence derived from historical experience and (2) the realistic *expectations* that new improvements will occur in the proximate future. The importance of reliable *data* is obvious, having guided evidence-based practice for years in situations where seeking standardization and validating incremental change are the primary goals. The value of *belief* in a better future may have less scientific merit but is essential in a dynamically evolving world of pioneering unchartered territory within which there is little or no experience. *Expectations* for the future exceed mere *hope* when they are based on consistent, near-real-time trends of delivering progressive improvement.

Because of its complexities, the MCS field has been in a prolonged phase of extended pioneering and innovation. It has been a dynamic field throughout its history, delivering continuous, ongoing improvements over three decades, despite occasional oscillations in that trajectory.

Finding the right equipoise for any clinical trial of earlier-stage patients therefore must account for both where we are today and where we will be in the near term even before the trial is completed. Adaptive trial designs may be helpful with that—lessening the burden of getting predications perfect ahead of the trial.

The MCS field has toyed with trials intended to study LVADs in earlier-stage patients. The REVIVE-IT (Randomized Evaluation of VAD InterVEntion before Inotropic Therapy) trial, sponsored by the NIH, was abandoned in 2015 because the field felt at that time that equipoise could not be achieved with either HVADs or HeartMate II's implanted in NYHA class III heart failure patients because of concerns about the AE profile of these devices, namely, stroke or thrombosis.[57]

Following that was the ROADMAP (Risk Assessment and Comparative Effectiveness of Left Ventricular Assist Device and Medical Management in Ambulatory Heart Failure Patients) trial trial looking at HeartMate II experience in class IIIB/IV non-inotrope dependent patients (INTERMACS level 4-6 as in Fig. 22.2)[58,59]. While trends favoring the LVAD were apparent, the overall impact was not motivating enough to move the field substantially toward earlier-stage patients. There are still a lot of higher acuity INTERMACS level 1–3 patients being implanted - 87% as recorded in the INTERMACS registry - and that has not changed much over the last decade.[17]

Data from the recent report of the MedaMACS (Medical Arm of Mechanically Assisted Circulatory Support) US national registry tracking the natural history of ambulatory heart failure patients provide some additional guidance.[60] Patients with INTERMACS (IM) profiles 4 through 7 receiving medical therapy were compared to a comparable cohort of LVAD recipients (mostly HeartMate II and HVAD LVADs) from the INTERMACS. With ambulatory heart failure patients IM 4 and IM 5, survival favored LVAD over medical management. Further, it was recommended that all patients in IM 4 through 7 be referred to LVAD and heart transplantation centers for consideration of life-saving treatment options.

Is the MCS field ready for another look at a clinical trial involving earlier-stage patients? Findings from the MOMENTUM randomized controlled trial of the HeartMate 3 LVAD[22] provide recent evidence that the risk profile with LVAD therapy has been improved since the 2015 analysis for the REVIVE-IT trial that concluded the HeartMate II was not ready for NYHA class III heart failure patients. Assuming that the posttrial, real-world experience with the HeartMate 3 will reflect this clinical trial experience, significant improvements in outcomes will have been achieved: 2-year survival reaching 83% (comparing favorably with 82% for heart transplantation)[61]; a stroke rate at 2 years of 0.08 per patient-year and 0.04 per patient-year beyond the first 6 months; pump thrombosis occurrence of 1.1% at 2 years; and need for pump replacement at 1.6% at 2 years.

Counterbalancing these advancements is the persistence of some AEs, notably GI bleeding and infections. In addition, quality of life perceptions, increasingly important to earlier stage patents, are affected by factors yet to be improved, such as activity limitations associated with tethering to external controllers and batteries via percutaneous leads.

The new improved outcome benchmarks, coupled with trends and expectations for continuing improvement, serve as the underpinning by which the field could consider that the threshold for equipoise has been moved far enough in favor of MCS to justify a trial of earlier-stage patients. In the meantime, anecdotal experience will accrue as it can be expected that a drift toward LVAD use in earlier-stage patients will occur, driven by those who have been encouraged by this recent favorable trend with outcomes.

Addressing PATIENT-SPECIFIC Characteristics

No two patients are alike, given genetic and biologic variation. The recognition that individual patients may respond differently to the same treatment is the basis for individualizing therapies around *patient-specific characteristics*. Tailoring therapy to individual patient characteristics is rooted in the concept of *personalized medicine*, now attracting considerable attention in health care. How can that approach be adapted to the field of MCS?

In patients receiving current MCS devices, GI bleeding occurs in some patients, sometimes repeatedly, while not occurring in others at all, even though exposed to the exact same technology and same management. As greater understanding emerges about the etiologic factors that play into individual patient-specific characteristics related to mucosal bleeding, it may be possible to design therapies targeting those specific factors and to modulate those therapies around unique patient-specificities.

Addressing patient-specific *responsiveness to anticoagulants* used with MCS may have benefit. Patient-specific variations in response to anticoagulation therapies are well known.

Variation in responsiveness to *aspirin* as an antiplatelet agent serves to illustrate the point. How do we know that 80 mg or 325 mg of aspirin is the right daily dose for a given patient with a given MCS device when the effects on platelet activity vary from one device to another and from patient to patient? This may be an opportunity for further analysis and intervention.

Genetic variation in *warfarin* responsiveness has been identified, and testing is available for determining the related genotypes. The risks for thrombosis or bleeding during the initiation of warfarin vary between genotypes. Warfarin genotype testing may help identify genetic susceptibilities to these AEs in MCS patients and lead to safer use of anticoagulation.[62] Expanded studies to evaluate the benefits and cost-effectiveness of genotyping to guide warfarin therapy are warranted.

Hemocompatibility varies from one blood pump to another. The degree to which an individual patient may experience blood damage with a specific device may vary from patient to patient. The ability to test a patient's blood in a laboratory with a microfluidic facsimile capable of simulating a specific VAD's shear-mediated blood damage risk-profile has been proposed.[63] The use of this approach to optimize outcomes by *matching a specific VAD to a specific patient* may represent a new, innovative direction in the future of personalized medicine with MCS devices.

IV. THE FUTURE REQUIRES ORGANIZATION

The future of MCS looks promising given the myriad of opportunities to improve technology, to optimize management, and to address patient factors. To achieve the penultimate results, *organization* is paramount. So much more can be accomplished by integrating efforts in a spirit of cooperation and mutual commitment.

Heart Failure Networks

Coordinated efforts to support responsible growth and development of the MCS field should be most effective when exercised within a framework of organized heart failure management at large. Best practices for MCS will be enabled by best practices for heart failure within *integrated care delivery networks*.

Heart failure is a complex, chronic disease. It encompasses a spectrum of severities, a spectrum of therapies, and a spectrum of care providers. *Heart failure teams* are needed to integrate the efforts of all those who are involved in the care of heart failure patients wherever they are.

Heart failure therapy is filled with options that require diverse skills and understanding for best use of medications, cardiology interventions, surgery, devices, and novel therapies. Optimum patient care requires careful integration of effort between care providers to enable (1) best decisions, for (2) management that is optimum, timely, efficient, and cost-effective, and for (3) triaging patients between care providers.

Consider the following framework for these networks. Operating at the center, or hub, of the integrated care delivery network is the *expert heart failure team* composed of all disciplines engaged in advanced heart failure care. That team is usually based at a quaternary care center where a full spectrum of advanced heart failure therapies, including MCS, are available. Emanating from the hub are spokes connected to peripheral, satellite care providers, usually community-based, comprising the *extended-care team*.

Spanning across the networks are all the care providers, including the following:

1. the patient and family caring for themselves at home;
2. home and community health providers;
3. primary care clinicians;
4. general cardiologists; and
5. advanced cardiac care specialists.

Within this framework, it should be possible to (1) *track* a patient with heart failure from the time of first diagnosis throughout life, wherever they are, (2) to *assess* severity and need for intervention, (3) offer *guidance* for treatment and prevention, (4) facilitate seamless referral and *transition* of care, (5) ease the burden of *documentation*, (6) assure *compliance*, (7) demonstrate *quality*, and (8) optimize *cost-effectiveness* and reimbursement.

Presently, the process of maintaining such a network requires extensive manual effort. In the future, *electronic information management* based around electronic health records will provide the necessary (1) *data* repositories, or warehouses, (2) *analytics* to identify the status of patients and call attention to abnormalities, and (3) *guidance* tools for enabling best practices for care and best recommendations for triage of care.

Field-wide Collaboration

Advances across the MCS field at-large will benefit from field-wide collaboration. Stakeholders providing leadership include clinicians, engineers, scientists, developers, and payers. The MCS field is best served when these resources are working together on behalf of advancing field-wide initiatives. No matter how well organized all processes are, it takes a *culture* that is harmoniously integrated to deliver success with complex processes and lofty goals.

We tend to operate in silos with myopic presumptions of narrowly focused responsibility. Allowing for some exaggeration, *clinicians* expect the developers to deliver perfected technology, *developers* expect the clinicians to obtain perfected outcomes with their technology, and both clinicians and developers expect *patients* to deliver perfected results with the therapy.

The world of marketplace competition among device developers is too often skewed toward merely redistributing existing market share rather than growing the market at large. It is not totally irrational to believe that if developers joined together to support the clinical community in efforts to improve outcomes, the field would break through the barriers to market growth faster. Expanding the field would expand the market, which would enhance competitive opportunity in a healthy way that should stimulate field-wide improvements.

Is it too farfetched to speculate about a unified, field-wide clinical study in which consensus around best clinical practices with any MCS device would be applied in anticipation of reducing AEs? Standardization of care would result in improved quality and cost-effectiveness. And, head-to-head comparisons of different therapies and devices for given indications in different patient populations would enable best use of *all* devices. There is precedent in the medical device field, at large, for field-wide cooperation, joining efforts to improve field-wide practices on behalf of responsible growth and dissemination. Why not with MCS?

V. THE FUTURE IS NOW

Once the future has been envisioned and the pathway mapped out, the timeline to the future is set beginning with the here and now. Mother Teresa put it this way, "Yesterday is gone. Tomorrow has not yet come. We only have today. Let us begin."

Overcoming the remaining challenges is clearly within our grasp—but nothing can be taken for granted. In fact, there are looming threats—time and costs—both of which will undermine decades of incremental progress, if not addressed with intensity.

Overall *costs* of MCS remain high.[64] MCS therapy is at risk of being categorized as a heroic intervention impacting a limited population. Some will consider it an unaffordable luxury given growing concerns about health care costs in general and the persistent challenges of delivering even the most basic, fundamental health care for all. These societal perspectives cannot be disregarded, nor should they be.

The MCS field must do more with less. In general, the field has been blessed with sustainable reimbursement levels. Current payments accommodate the present state of financial affairs, allowing individual MCS programs to maintain solvency. As reimbursement levels decline, as should be anticipated, financials will become prohibitive unless matched by concomitant cost reductions.

The overall *price of MCS devices* should be lowered as the market expands and economies of scale prevail. More importantly, the *costs of long-term care* for recurrent hospitalizations, AE complications, and device exchanges must continue to improve, even beyond what could be expected with recent, encouraging trends.

Addressing the overall *costs of care of heart failure* in general is essential. That is achievable with cost-effective integrated care delivery networks, as proposed. Heart failure is one of the most expensive of the expensive chronic diseases. When addressed effectively, cost savings across the entire spectrum of heart failure should support appropriate use of advanced therapies, including MCS.

Finally, *time* is of the essence. It has been a long journey toward the goals of delivering amazing technologies for (1) extending *life* with (2) *quality* and (3) *safety* with (4) *easier-to-use* therapies applied at the (5) optimum *time* in (6) properly selected heart failure *patients* while (7) achieving *cost-effectiveness*.

The potential for the future of MCS is invigorating. It is time to deliver on the promises long awaited.

REFERENCES

1. Frazier OH, Rose EA, McCarthy P, et al. Improved mortality and rehabilitation of transplant candidates treated with a long-term implantable left ventricular assist system. *Ann Surg*. 1995;222:327–336. discussion 336-8.
2. Long JW. Advanced mechanical circulatory support with the HeartMate left ventricular assist device in the year 2000. *Ann Thorac Surg*. 2001;71:S176–S182. discussion S183-4.
3. Rose EA, Gelijns AC, Moskowitz AJ, et al. Long-term use of a left ventricular assist device for end-stage heart failure. *N Engl J Med*. 2001;345:1435–1443.
4. Long JW, Kfoury AG, Slaughter MS, et al. Long-term destination therapy with the HeartMate XVE left ventricular assist device: improved outcomes since the REMATCH study. *Congest Heart Fail*. 2005;11:133–138.
5. Long JW, Healy AH, Rasmusson BY, et al. Improving outcomes with long-term destination therapy using left ventricular assist devices. *J Thorac Cardiovasc Surg*. 2008;135:1353–1360. discussion 1360-1.
6. Frazier OH, Wampler RK, Duncan JM, et al. First human use of the Hemopump, a catheter-mounted ventricular assist device. *Ann Thorac Surg*. 1990;49:299–304.
7. Wampler R, Frazier OH. The Hemopump, The first intravascular ventricular assist device. *ASAIO J*. 2019;65:297–300.
8. Frazier OH, Delgado 3rd RM, Kar B, Patel V, Gregoric ID, Myers TJ. First clinical use of the redesigned HeartMate II left ventricular assist system in the United States: a case report. *Tex Heart Inst J*. 2004;31:157–159.
9. Slaughter MS, Rogers JG, Milano CA, et al. Advanced heart failure treated with continuous-flow left ventricular assist device. *N Engl J Med*. 2009;361:2241–2251.
10. Slaughter MS, Pagani FD, McGee EC, et al. HeartWare ventricular assist system for bridge to transplant: combined results of the bridge to transplant and continued access protocol trial. *J Heart Lung Transplant*. 2013;32:675–683.
11. Rogers JG, Pagani FD, Tatooles AJ, et al. Intrapericardial left ventricular assist device for advanced heart failure. *N Engl J Med*. 2017;376:451–460.
12. Slaughter MS, Pagani FD, Rogers JG, et al. Clinical management of continuous-flow left ventricular assist devices in advanced heart failure. *J Heart Lung Transplant*. 2010;29:S1–39.
13. Feldman D, Pamboukian SV, Teuteberg JJ, et al. The 2013 International Society for Heart and Lung Transplantation guidelines for mechanical circulatory support: executive summary. *J Heart Lung Transplant*. 2013;32:157–187.
14. Goldstein DJ, John R, Salerno C, et al. Algorithm for the diagnosis and management of suspected pump thrombus. *J Heart Lung Transplant*. 2013;32:667–670.
15. Maltais S, Kilic A, Nathan S, et al. PREVENtion of HeartMate Ii pump thrombosis through clinical management: The PREVENT multi-center study. *J Heart Lung Transplant*. 2017;36:1–12.
16. Kormos RL, Cowger J, Pagani FD, et al. The Society of Thoracic Surgeons Intermacs database annual report: evolving indications, outcomes, and scientific partnerships. *J Heart Lung Transplant*. 2019;38:114–126.
17. Kirklin JK, Pagani FD, Kormos RL, et al. Eighth annual INTERMACS report: special focus on framing the impact of adverse events. *J Heart Lung Transplant*. 2017;36:1080–1086.
18. Kirklin JK, Naftel DC, Kormos RL, et al. Fifth INTERMACS annual report: risk factor analysis from more than 6,000 mechanical circulatory support patients. *J Heart Lung Transplant*. 2013;32:141–156.
19. Akhter SA, Badami A, Murray M, et al. Hospital readmissions after continuous-flow left ventricular assist device implantation: incidence, causes, and cost analysis. *Ann Thorac Surg*. 2015;100:884–889.
20. Mehra MR, Salerno C, Cleveland JC, et al. Healthcare resource use and cost implications in the MOMENTUM 3 long-term outcome study. *Circulation*. 2018;138:1923–1934.

21. Milano CA, Rogers JG, Tatooles AJ, et al. HVAD: the ENDURANCE supplemental trial. *JACC Heart Fail.* 2018;6:792–802.
22. Mehra MR, Goldstein DJ, Uriel N, et al. Two-year outcomes with a magnetically levitated cardiac pump in heart failure. *N Engl J Med.* 2018;378:1386–1395.
23. Bourque K, Cotter C, Dague C, et al. Design rationale and preclinical evaluation of the HeartMate 3 left ventricular assist system for hemocompatibility. *ASAIO J.* 2016;62:375–383.
24. Uriel N, Colombo PC, Cleveland JC, et al. Hemocompatibility-related outcomes in the MOMENTUM 3 trial at 6 months: a randomized controlled study of a fully magnetically levitated pump in advanced heart failure. *Circulation.* 2017;135:2003–2012.
25. Long JW, Snyder T, Stanfield JR. Emerging science of hemocompatibility as applied to VAD design and pre-clinical evaluation. *J Heart Lung Transplant.* 2017;36:S60.
26. Coghill PA, Kanchi S, Azartash-Namin ZJ, Long JW, Snyder TA. Benchtop von Willebrand factor testing: comparison of commercially available ventricular assist devices and evaluation of variables for a standardized test method. *ASAIO J.* 2018.
27. Chan CH, Pieper IL, Hambly R, et al. The CentriMag centrifugal blood pump as a benchmark for in vitro testing of hemocompatibility in implantable ventricular assist devices. *Artif Organs.* 2015;39:93–101.
28. Bartoli CR, Kang J, Zhang D, et al. Left ventricular assist device design reduces von Willebrand factor degradation: a comparative study between the HeartMate II and the EVAHEART left ventricular assist system. *Ann Thorac Surg.* 2017;103:1239–1244.
29. Snyder TA, Watach MJ, Litwak KN, Wagner WR. Platelet activation, aggregation, and life span in calves implanted with axial flow ventricular assist devices. *Ann Thorac Surg.* 2002;73:1933–1938.
30. Wong K, Samaroo G, Ling I, et al. Intraventricular flow patterns and stasis in the LVAD-assisted heart. *J Biomech.* 2014;47:1485–1494.
31. May-Newman K, Vu V, Herold B. Modeling the link between left ventricular flow and thromboembolic risk using Lagrangian coherent structures. *Fluids.* 2016;1:38.
32. Pae WE, Connell JM, Adelowo A, et al. Does total implantability reduce infection with the use of a left ventricular assist device? The LionHeart experience in Europe. *J Heart Lung Transplant.* 2007;26:219–229.
33. Mehta SM, Pae Jr. WE, Rosenberg G, et al. The LionHeart LVD-2000: a completely implanted left ventricular assist device for chronic circulatory support. *Ann Thorac Surg.* 2001;71:S156–S161. discussion S183-4.
34. Westaby S, Jarvik R, Freeland A, et al. Postauricular percutaneous power delivery for permanent mechanical circulatory support. *J Thorac Cardiovasc Surg.* 2002;123:977–983.
35. Kormos RL, McCall M, Althouse A, et al. Left ventricular assist device malfunctions: it is more than just the pump. *Circulation.* 2017;136:1714–1725.
36. Uriel N, Levin AP, Sayer GT, et al. Left ventricular decompression during speed optimization ramps in patients supported by continuous-flow left ventricular assist devices: device-specific performance characteristics and impact on diagnostic algorithms. *J Card Fail.* 2015;21:785–791.
37. Moazami N, Fukamachi K, Kobayashi M, et al. Axial and centrifugal continuous-flow rotary pumps: a translation from pump mechanics to clinical practice. *J Heart Lung Transplant.* 2013;32:1–11.
38. Gross C, Marko C, Mikl J, et al. LVAD pump flow does not adequately increase with exercise. *Artif Organs.* 2018.
39. Wappenschmidt J, Autschbach R, Steinseifer U, et al. Rotary piston blood pumps: past developments and future potential of a unique pump type. *Expert Rev Med Devices.* 2016;13:759–771.
40. Clifford R, Robson D, Gross C, et al. Beat-to-beat detection of aortic valve opening in HeartWare left ventricular assist device patients. *Artif Organs.* 2018.
41. Birks EJ, Tansley PD, Hardy J, et al. Left ventricular assist device and drug therapy for the reversal of heart failure. *N Engl J Med.* 2006;355:1873–1884.
42. Birks EJ, Drakos SG, Lowes BD, et al. Outcome and primary endpoint results from a prospective multi-center study of myocardial recovery using LVADs: Remission from Stage D Heart Failure (RESTAGE-HF). *J Heart Lung Transplant.* 2018;37:S142.
43. Drakos SG, Pagani FD, Lundberg MS, Baldwin TJ. Advancing the science of myocardial recovery with mechanical circulatory support: a working group of the National, Heart, Lung, and Blood Institute. *J Thorac Cardiovasc Surg.* 2017;154:165–170.
44. Uriel N, Kim G, Burkhoff D. Myocardial recovery after LVAD implantation: a vision or simply an illusion? *J Am Coll Cardiol.* 2017;70:355–357.
45. Meyns BP, Simon A, Klotz S, et al. Clinical benefits of partial circulatory support in New York Heart Association Class IIIB and Early Class IV patients. *Eur J Cardiothorac Surg.* 2011;39:693–698.
46. Burkhoff D, Maurer MS, Joseph SM, et al. Left atrial decompression pump for severe heart failure with preserved ejection fraction: theoretical and clinical considerations. *JACC Heart Fail.* 2015;3:275–282.
47. Fresiello L, Buys R, Jacobs S, et al. Exercise capacity in left ventricular assist device patients with full and partial support. *Eur J Prev Cardiol.* 2017;24:168–177.
48. Maltais S, Anwer LA, Tchantchaleishvili V, et al. Left lateral thoracotomy for centrifugal continuous-flow left ventricular assist device Placement: An Analysis from the Mechanical Circulatory Support Research Network. *Asaio j.* 2018;64:715–720.
49. Schmitto JD, Krabatsch T, Damme L, Netuka I. Less invasive HeartMate 3 left ventricular assist device implantation. *J Thorac Dis.* 2018;10:S1692–s1695.
50. Strueber M, Cheung A, Mokadam NA, et al. Impact of the thoracotomy implant approach on average length of stay and rehospitalizations in the HVAD LATERAL trial. *J Heart Lung Transplant.* 2018;37:S83–S84.
51. Colombo PC, Mehra MR, Goldstein DJ, et al. Comprehensive analysis of stroke in the long-term cohort of the MOMENTUM 3 study. *Circulation.* 2019;139:155–168.
52. Netuka I, Litzler PY, Berchtold-Herz M, et al. Outcomes in HeartMate II patients with no antiplatelet therapy: 2-year results from the European TRACE study. *Ann Thorac Surg.* 2017;103:1262–1268.
53. Netuka I, Ivak P, Tucanova Z, et al. Evaluation of low-intensity anti-coagulation with a fully magnetically levitated centrifugal-flow circulatory pump-the MAGENTUM 1 study. *J Heart Lung Transplant.* 2018;37:579–586.
54. Houston BA, Schneider AL, Vaishnav J, et al. Angiotensin II antagonism is associated with reduced risk for gastrointestinal bleeding caused by arteriovenous malformations in patients with left ventricular assist devices. *J Heart Lung Transplant.* 2017;36:380–385.
55. Proudfoot AG, Davidson SJ, Strueber M. von Willebrand factor disruption and continuous-flow circulatory devices. *J Heart Lung Transplant.* 2017;36:1155–1163.
56. Tabit CE, Chen P, Kim GH, et al. Elevated angiopoietin-2 level in patients with continuous-flow left ventricular assist devices leads to altered angiogenesis and is associated with higher nonsurgical bleeding. *Circulation.* 2016;134:141–152.
57. Pagani FD, Aaronson KD, Kormos R, et al. The NHLBI REVIVE-IT study: understanding its discontinuation in the context of current left ventricular assist device therapy. *J Heart Lung Transplant.* 2016;35:1277–1283.
58. Shah KB, Starling RC, Rogers JG, et al. Left ventricular assist devices versus medical management in ambulatory heart failure patients: an analysis of INTERMACS Profiles 4 and 5 to 7 from the ROADMAP study. *J Heart Lung Transplant.* 2018;37:706–714.
59. Starling RC, Estep JD, Horstmanshof DA, et al. Risk assessment and comparative effectiveness of left ventricular assist device and medical management in ambulatory heart failure patients: the ROADMAP study 2-year results. *JACC Heart Fail.* 2017;5:518–527.
60. Ambardekar AV, Kittleson MM, Palardy M, et al. Outcomes with ambulatory advanced heart failure from the Medical Arm of Mechanically Assisted Circulatory Support (MedaMACS) Registry. *J Heart Lung Transplant.* 2018. Article Online.

61. Khush KK, Cherikh WS, Chambers DC, et al. The International Thoracic Organ Transplant Registry of the International Society for Heart and Lung Transplantation: Thirty-fifth adult heart transplantation report—2018; focus theme: multiorgan transplantation. *J Heart Lung Transplant.* 2018;37:1155–1168.
62. Topkara VK, Knotts RJ, Jennings DL, et al. Effect of CYP2C9 and VKORC1 gene variants on warfarin response in patients with continuous-flow left ventricular assist devices. *ASAIO J.* 2016;62:558–564.
63. Slepian M, Rasponi, M., Bluestein, D., Redaelli A. HyperShear in a Channel: A Microfluidic Facsimile of Ventricular Assist Devices to Reduce Thrombotic Risk and Enhance Patient Safety. Tech Launch Arizona.
64. Patel N, Kalra R, Doshi R, Bajaj NS, Arora G, Arora P. Trends and cost of heart transplantation and left ventricular assist devices: impact of proposed Federal cuts. JACC Heart Fail. 2018;6:424–432.

INDEX

Note: Page numbers followed by *f* indicate figures, *t* indicate tables, and *b* indicate boxes.

D

M

Q

R